Perinatal Depression: Detection and Treatment

Perinatal Depression: Detection and Treatment

Edited by Larry Stone

hayle medical
New York

Hayle Medical,
750 Third Avenue, 9th Floor,
New York, NY 10017, USA

Visit us on the World Wide Web at:
www.haylemedical.com

ISBN: 978-1-63241-462-5

Printed in China.

Cataloging-in-Publication Data

Perinatal depression : detection and treatment / edited by Larry Stone.
p. cm.
Includes bibliographical references and index.
ISBN 978-1-63241-462-5
1. Depression, Mental. 2. Postpartum depression. 3. Postpartum depression--Diagnosis.
4. Postpartum depression--Treatment. I. Stone, Larry.
RC537 .P47 2017
616.852 7--dc23

Table of Contents

Preface

This book was inspired by the evolution of our times; to answer the curiosity of inquisitive minds. Many developments have occurred across the globe in the recent past which has transformed the progress in the field.

Perinatal depression is defined as depression caused by stress and strain experienced during childbirth. It also studies mood disorders occurring before as well after pregnancy. It combines the diagnosis and treatment of perinatal and postpartum depression. The two most common methods of treatment for perinatal depression are psychotherapy and medication. This book presents the complex subject of perinatal depression in the most comprehensible and easy to understand language. From theories to research to practical applications, case studies related to all contemporary topics of relevance have been included in this book. This book will prove to be helpful for both students and researchers in the field of neurological disorders, gynaecology and psychotherapy.

This book was developed from a mere concept to drafts to chapters and finally compiled together as a complete text to benefit the readers across all nations. To ensure the quality of the content we instilled two significant steps in our procedure. The first was to appoint an editorial team that would verify the data and statistics provided in the book and also select the most appropriate and valuable contributions from the plentiful contributions we received from authors worldwide. The next step was to appoint an expert of the topic as the Editor-in-Chief, who would head the project and finally make the necessary amendments and modifications to make the text reader-friendly. I was then commissioned to examine all the material to present the topics in the most comprehensible and productive format.

I would like to take this opportunity to thank all the contributing authors who were supportive enough to contribute their time and knowledge to this project. I also wish to convey my regards to my family who have been extremely supportive during the entire project.

Editor

The Effect of Short-Term Aerobic Exercise on Depression and Body Image in Iranian Women

Sareh Zarshenas, Parsa Houshvar, and Ali Tahmasebi

Department of Occupational Therapy, School of Rehabilitation Sciences, Isfahan University of Medical Sciences, Isfahan, Iran

Correspondence should be addressed to Sareh Zarshenas; zarshenas.otr@gmail.com

Academic Editor: Charles B. Nemeroff

The purpose of this study was to determine the effect of short-term aerobic exercise on depression symptoms and body image attitudes among Iranian women. In this quasiexperimental study, 82 females were assigned to experimental group (aerobic exercise group, $n = 41$) or control group (waiting list, $n = 41$) and evaluated by Beck Depression Inventory-second edition (BDI-II) and Multidimensional Body Self-Relation Questionnaire (MBSRQ), respectively. The experimental group received four-week aerobic exercise program, and control group had been asked to wait for the next four weeks. Results of this study confirmed the significant decrease in depression symptoms at the experimental group compared to control group ($P < 0.5$). For the body image dependent variables, significant improvement was also found in appearance evaluation, appearance orientation, health orientation, and illness orientation in aerobic exercise group ($P < 0.5$).

1. Introduction

Negative body image and body-image dissatisfaction are two cognitive symptoms in depression which can also be the cause of depression [1–4]. Body image refers to the accuracy of an individual's perception about body size and thoughts and feelings associated with his or her body [5]. It has profound implications for various psychological disorders and disturbances such as low self-esteem, depression, social anxiety, sexual dysfunction, anorexia nervosa, and body-dysmorphic disorder [2, 6].

Over the last decades, increasing sociocultural emphasis on physical attractiveness and fitness by most of the mass media has raised very deep concern among psychologists and sociologists which may contributed to the increasing rate of body-image dissatisfaction among women [2, 7–9].

Traditional treatment of these disorders is based on pharmacology and psychotherapy, which can be very expensive and time consuming [10]. The symptoms of depression do not however respond to antidepressant drugs until they have been administered for 10 to 20 days which also suggests that a similar period of exercise is needed for adaptations in neural regulation. Thus, approximately four-week adherence to aerobic exercise may be needed to observe changes in mood state and depression. In aerobic exercise sessions that were conducted in gymnasium settings, motivation to get exercise is provided, respectively. However, it remains to be seen how effective short-term exercise could be. In addition, recent research has not considered the effect of short-term exercise on body image and depression with most published studies being conducted in western countries and Asian societies [11]. This study investigated the effect of short-term aerobic exercise on body image and depression among Iranian women. It was hypothesized that aerobic exercise would significantly improve body image attitudes and decrease depression symptoms in comparison with a control group.

2. Methods

2.1. Participants. Eighty-two participants volunteered to participate in this study. All of them were matched in age, education, and marital status before being assigned to an aerobic exercise group ($n = 41$) or control group ($n = 41$). The subjects were registered in order to begin their program at gymnasiums. The first 41 registrants were selected as exercise group, and the next 41 volunteers were asked to wait for the next four weeks. The study was approved by the Ethics Committee for Human Experiments, University of Welfare and Rehabilitation Sciences, Tehran, Iran, and informed consent was obtained from participants before assignment. Their age ranged from 18 to 45 years, with a mean of 26 years of age (SD = 6.9) in the exercise group and 27 years of age (SD = 6.5) in the control group. Inclusion criteria for participants were as follows:

(a) aged between 18 and 45 years;

(b) BDI-II score of 14 or above, [12].

Exclusion criteria were receiving any treatment for depression during the last six months prior to volunteering to participate in the study, participating in any exercise program during the previous three months prior to commencement of the study, and diagnosis of physical and other neurological psychotic disorders.

2.2. Measures. Descriptive information of age, education, and marital status were obtained from all participants. Body image was measured by using MBSRQ.

The Multidimensional Body Self-Relation Questionnaire is a self-report inventory for the assessment of self-attitudinal aspects of the body-image construct, which includes The Body Self-Relation Questionnaire (54 items), The Body Areas Satisfaction Scale (BASS) (nine items), The Overweight Preoccupation Scale (four items), and The Self-Classified Weight Scale (two items). The Body Self-Relation Questionnaire consists of three somatic domains: physical appearance, fitness, and health-illness. Within each of these domains, items address either evaluation or orientation to the domain. Participants were asked to indicate their agreement or disagreement with each statement in the survey using a five-point Likert scale. Tests on internal consistency of each subscale yielded a coefficient alpha ranging from 0.73 to 0.95 [13]. Yuen and Hanson (2002) demonstrated that the Multidimensional Body Self-Relation Questionnaire has adequate construct validity [14]. Internal consistency for all subscales in the present sample was acceptable (Cronbach's α: 70% to 87%).

BDI-II includes 21-item self-reporting inventory so as to assess the severity of clinical depression and change in depression symptoms across time. This inventory has demonstrated good internal consistency [12] and has been widely used to assess changes in depressive symptoms across time. Cut-off points for scoring the inventory are <14 (minimal), 14 to 19 (mild), 20 to 28 (moderate), and 29 to 63 (severe) depression. The validity and reliability of the Persian version of the Beck Depression Inventory (second edition) have been confirmed [15].

2.3. Study Protocol

2.3.1. Exercise Group. The exercise sessions were designed by the exercise instructors and followed the same format with specific intensity and frequency across all sessions. All participants completed both measurements before and after allotted time. Exercise group was then informed about the frame of the sessions and exercise by occupational therapist so that each subject was competent in measuring their wrist pulse.

Resting heart rate was measured several times to ensure subjects had the ability to obtain consistent heart rate values at rest. The resting heart rate measurement was repeated in the next exercise session to further ensure. It was no undue variation in the first and second exercise session measures. Maximum heart rate was estimated from the subject's age as follows:

Maximum heart rate = 220 − age (in years).

The overall target of heart rate for the exercise sessions was 70% of maximal heart rate. All participants in the exercise group were required to accomplish their aerobic exercise in front of mirrors to be oriented on details of their movements completely; in addition, the exercise sessions included appropriate music which was adjusted to the intensity of movements which made it possible for all subjects to become well practiced at about 70% of maximal heart rate.

Each exercise session included the following sequence of steps.

(1) Before starting the exercise, resting heart rate was measured by the participants from the wrist pulse. Aerobic exercise commenced with a "warm up," followed by dynamic stretching, concentrating on breathing and then continued with slow jogging (10 minutes).

(2) In the next phase of the exercise which took 30 to 35 minutes, the movements were performed with higher intensity in the range of 60% to 80% of maximal heart rate. This step included faster unilateral and bilateral hands and feet movements. Some exercise equipments such as bench, box, ball, wooden stick, and weight were used by participants in this regard. Heart rate was measured and recorded after this step (Active heart rate).

(3) In the third step, the intensity of movements was decreased, and movements were carried out on mat which included static stretching and muscle relaxation. Immediately after this step, heart rate was measured (15 to 20 minutes).

2.3.2. Control Group. Control group did not participate in any exercises in this duration as waiting list and received the papers which researchers indicated that they would be provided the same exercise protocol in the next four weeks if the results confirmed the exercise effectiveness. It should be noted that all of these participants were newly registered members of gym and had not participate in any other type of exercise.

2.4. Analysis. In this study, SPSS was used to analyse the data. Independent t-test was used to compare the effect of aerobic exercise between the exercise group and the control group. Paired t-test also was used to compare the heart rate response to aerobic exercise before and after performing each step.

Table 1: Heart rates of aerobic exercise.

Aerobic exercise scale	Minimum rate	Maximum rate	Mean	SD
MHR	175	202	193.951	6.884
THR (Session 1)	105	121.20	116.370	4.130
THR (Session 2)	148.75	171.70	164.858	5.851
AHR (Session 1)	120	140	118.829	18.33
AHR (Session 2)	120	150	135.365	6.744
RHR (Session 1)	60	90	78.658	8.196
RHR (Session 2)	63	90	79.414	8.285

HR: heart rate; M: maximum; T: target; A: active; R: rest.

Table 2: Pretest and posttest, mean and standard deviations of body-image variables.

Multidimensional Body Self-Relation Questionnaire Subscales	Exercise group		Control group	
	Pretest Mean ± SD	Posttest Mean ± SD	Pretest Mean ± SD	Posttest Mean ± SD
AE	3.10 ± 0.28	3.53 ± 0.29	3.13 ± 0.46	3.10 ± 0.45
AO	3.41 ± 0.30	3.60 ± 0.26	3.37 ± 0.38	3.33 ± 0.41
FE	3.24 ± 0.50	3.30 ± 0.40	3.13 ± 0.50	3.58 ± 0.58
FO	3.21 ± 0.30	3.30 ± 0.18	3.24 ± 0.33	3.30 ± 0.47
HE	3.18 ± 3.39	3.19 ± 3.35	3.08 ± 0.26	3.19 ± 0.35
HO	3.46 ± 0.46	3.73 ± 0.27	3.45 ± 0.61	3.41 ± 0.60
IO	3.15 ± 0.48	3.54 ± 0.24	3.04 ± 0.42	3.02 ± 0.50
BS	3.34 ± 0.73	3.57 ± 0.66	3.46 ± 0.76	3.48 ± 0.74
OWP	3.06 ± 1.007	2.70 ± 1.78	2.95 ± 1.22	2.99 ± 1.09
SCW	3.42 ± 0.95	2.92 ± 0.96	3.21 ± 0.77	3.20 ± 0.70

AE: appearance evaluation; AO: appearance orientation; FE: fitness evaluation; FO: fitness orientation; HE: health evaluation; HO: health orientation; IO: illness orientation; BS: body areas satisfaction; OWP: overweight preoccupation; SCW: self-classified weight.

Chi-square was conducted to examine the matches of age, education, and marital status among both groups.

3. Results

According to a Chi-square test, all participants had the same range of education in both groups. Most of them had an undergraduate bachelor degree ($P = 0.139$) (53.3%) and were mostly single ($P = 0.114$) (67.1%), with a mean value of 26.5 SD = 6.9 years in the exercise group and mean value of 26.85, SD = 6.9 years in the control group ($P = 0.285$).

Maximum target and active heart rate showed that exercise was within the prescribed exercise protocol (see Table 1). Table 2 depicts the pretest and posttest, mean and standard deviations for each body-image variable (see Table 2). Pretest independent t-test confirmed no significant differences between both groups before aerobic exercise in body image subscales while the result of the posttest showed significant differences in appearance evaluation or orientation and health and illness orientation subscales between two groups after undertaking a short-term aerobic exercise program (see Table 3).

Paired t-test conducted on posttest body-image variables revealed significant differences before and after exercise training in the exercise group (see Table 4). Table 5 depicts the pretest and posttest mean and standard deviations for each body-image variable. Posttest independent t test revealed a significant interaction between decreasing depression and exercise training in the exercise group compared with the control group (see Table 5). Paired t test conducted on posttest depression variables revealed significant differences between before and after the exercise training program undertaken by the exercise group (see Table 6).

4. Discussion

The exercise group showed a significant decrease in levels of depression coupled with an improved body image in comparison with the control group. The measures of depression in the exercise group had decreased after four-week short-term exercise training program. Symptoms of depression diminished from a moderate level to a mild level in the exercise group.

Overall, the ability of aerobic exercise to reduce symptoms of depression in this study is consistent with previous published research [16]. Exercise produces changes in the concentration of several biologically active molecules such as Adrenocorticotrophic hormone, Cortisol, Catecholamines, Opioid peptides, and cytokines [17, 18]. Moreover, some evidence suggests that exercise can modify the concentration of retroactive substances in central nervous system [17, 19]. However, such factors as motivation, expectancy, self-esteem,

Table 3: The result of t-test among exercise and control group in body-image subscales.

*P value	AE	AO	FE	FO	HE	HO	IO	BS	OWP	SCW
Before exercise	0.715	0.634	0.311	0.688	0.882	0.114	0.289	0.464	0.677	0.285
After exercise	0 < 0.05	0.001	0.141	0.888	0.072	0.003	0.002	0.089	0.167	0.156

*($P < 0.05$); AE: appearance evaluation; AO: appearance orientation; FE: fitness evaluation; FO: fitness orientation; HE: health evaluation; HO: health orientation; IO: illness orientation; BS: body areas satisfaction; OWP: overweight preoccupation; SCW: self-classified weight.

Table 4: The result of paired t-test in exercise group in body-image subscales.

*P value	AE	AO	FE	FO	HE	HO	IO	BS	OWP	SCW
Exercise group	0 < 0.05	0 < 0.05	0 < 0.05	0.046	0.040	0 < 0.05	0 < 0.05	0 < 0.05	0 < 0.05	0 < 0.05

*($P < 0.05$) AE: appearance evaluation; AO: appearance orientation; FE: fitness evaluation; FO: fitness orientation; HE: health evaluation; HO: health orientation; IO: illness orientation; BS: body areas satisfaction; OWP: overweight preoccupation; SCW: self-classified weight.

Table 5: Pretest and posttest mean and standard deviations of depression.

	Exercise group		Control group	
	Pretest	Posttest	Pretest	Posttest
	Mean ± SD	Mean ± SD	Mean ± SD	Mean ± SD
Depression	20.58 ± 7.40	5.42 ± 22.04	15.92 ± 5.12	19.95 ± 4.31

Table 6: The result of t-test among exercise and control group in depression.

*P value	Depression
Before exercise	0.304
After exercise	0.005

*($P < 0.05$).

and human contact may also have influence on the mood of the participants [20–22]. These factors are known to have a direct correlation with the exercise in a social setting [23–25].

It should be noted that some studies do not support the results of the present study regarding reduced depression symptoms with exercise training. Chalder et al. (2012) in a randomized controlled trial concluded that the addition of a facilitated physical activity intervention to usual care does not improve depression outcome or reduce use of antidepressants compared with usual care alone. However, the TREAD (treatment of depression with physical activity) is designed to improve long-term adherence to physical activity [26]. Evidence of a long-term beneficial effect of exercise in patients with clinical depression is limited [27].

Group activity provided an opportunity for participants to develop more interpersonal relationships with each other and also to reinforce and motivate each other to continue exercise, gain self-efficacy, and improve their mood [21, 28, 29]. All sessions were accompanied by music in order to decrease depression [29]. Another factor that could affect the depression score was the intensity of aerobic exercise [30]. Legrand and Heuze (2007) in their research also confirmed that intense and moderate aerobic exercises appear to have a greater impact on decreasing depression compared with exercise undertaken at a mild intensity [30].

After four weeks, exercise training resulted in significant positive impact on appearance evaluation and orientation and health and illness orientation in comparison with the control group. Improvements in appearance orientation indicated that after exercise training they invested more time on their appearance. Thus, participants in the exercise training program reduced their symptoms of depression and felt well about themselves when they spent more time making sure their appearance was presentable. In addition, higher scores in appearance evaluation after the exercise training program means they had positive feelings about their physical attractiveness. This result revealed that the exercise group became more health conscious and opted to seek medical attention. Several factors can explain this improvement in body-image variables.

Body esteem is one of the factors that can affect improvement of the body image. The construct of body-esteem places emphasis on person's affective evaluation of their body and is associated with their particular body image [31]. All exercise sessions were undertaken in a gym where mirrors were positioned on the walls and ceiling. Past research has demonstrated that mirror exposure can reduce stress and body dissatisfaction through exercise [32, 33]. Like the depression measures, an exercise program in the form of group activity can also affect the bodyimage, because participants experience more interpersonal relationships and verbal encouragement and persuasion from others [11, 21, 22].

However, scores of other subscales such as fitness orientation or evaluation, health evaluation, and BASS scale did not show any significant differences in the exercise group compared with the control group. Some possible reasons that may explain these results are as follows.

One factor is the multidimensional nature of physical fitness [2]. The evaluation of physical fitness is characterized by measures of strength, endurance, speed, power output, and flexibility which are governed by a range of body systems including cardiac and respiratory systems. However, the present study emphasized on the heart-rate response and worked on skills and different dimensions of coordination in physical fitness.

A further factor that may influence the results of the present study was the type of exercise undertaken (aerobic exercise) while previous research included resistance exercise for increasing strength and shape of muscles [34]. The duration of exercise is another challenging factor that can affect the result. It seems that for making change in BASS and fitness attitudes, more than four-week exercise is required. It should be noted that this study did not use any weight watcher to avoid interruptions that could affect attitudes of participants especially about BASS scale; furthermore, some studies confirmed that weight perception is more related to depressive symptoms than actual weight [1].

The present research study is limited by a relatively low number of participating subjects, a short exercise training intervention, and the use of a nonclinical participants and nonrandom assignment which may represent a bias. Replication of this study in a larger sample size with random assignment and third group to evaluate regular treatment would be beneficial. Nevertheless, such studies provide a comprehensive insight to the potential value of a short duration exercise program as a treatment strategy. We consider that the present study could be a catalyst to the conduct of larger clinical trials designed to investigate the efficacy of regular moderate exercise in the treatment of depression.

5. Conclusion

According to the results of this study, four-week aerobic exercise can effectively reduce depression symptoms and improve some aspects of body-image attitudes in women. Short-term aerobic exercise can be used as an effective method of treatment for these disorders.

References

[1] M. L. Frisco, J. N. Houle, and M. A. Martin, "The image in the mirror and the number on the scale: weight, weight perceptions, and adolescent depressive symptoms," *Journal of Health and Social Behavior*, vol. 51, no. 2, pp. 215–228, 2010.

[2] S. H. Hessenly, *The effect of aerobic on state and trait body-image and physical fitness among college women [Ph.D. thesis]*, Old Dominion University, 1995.

[3] M. Santos, C. Steven Richards, and M. Kathryn Bleckley, "Comorbidity between depression and disordered eating in adolescents," *Eating Behaviors*, vol. 8, no. 4, pp. 440–449, 2007.

[4] B. Xie, J. B. Unger, P. Gallaher, C. A. Johnson, Q. Wu, and C.-P. Chou, "Overweight, body image, and depression in asian and hispanic adolescents," *American Journal of Health Behavior*, vol. 34, no. 4, pp. 476–488, 2010.

[5] T. F. Cash, "Body-image attitudes: evaluation, investment, and affect," *Perceptual and Motor Skills*, vol. 78, no. 3, pp. 1168–1170, 1994.

[6] K. A. Phillips, "Quality of life for patients with body dysmorphic disorder," *Journal of Nervous and Mental Disease*, vol. 188, no. 3, pp. 170–175, 2000.

[7] T. F. Cash and T. Pruzinsky, *Body-Image: A Handbook of Theory, Research, and Clinical Practice*, Guilford Press, New York, NY, USA, 2002.

[8] S. Grabe, L. M. Ward, and J. S. Hyde, "The role of the media in body image concerns among women: a meta-analysis of experimental and correlational studies," *Psychological Bulletin*, vol. 134, no. 3, pp. 460–476, 2008.

[9] S. S. O'Riordan and B. L. Zamboanga, "Aspects of the media and their relevance to bulimic attitudes and tendencies among female college students," *Eating Behaviors*, vol. 9, no. 2, pp. 247–250, 2008.

[10] T. F. Cash and M. D. Strachan, "Cognetive-behavioral approaches to changing body-image," in *Body-Image: A Handbook of Theory, Research, and Clinical Practice*, pp. 478–486, Guilford Press, New York, NY, USA, 2004.

[11] G. Chen, S. M. Gully, and D. Eden, "General self-efficacy and self-esteem: toward theoretical and empirical distinction between correlated self-evaluations," *Journal of Organizational Behavior*, vol. 25, no. 3, pp. 375–395, 2004.

[12] A. T. Beck, C. H. Ward, M. Mendelsohn, J. Mock, and J. Erbaugh, "An inventory for measuring depression," *Archives of general psychiatry*, vol. 4, pp. 561–571, 1961.

[13] T. F. Cash, *User's Manual for the Multidimensional Body-Self Relations Questionnaire*, Old Dominion University, Norfolk, UK, 2000.

[14] H. K. Yuen and C. Hanson, "Body image and exercise in people with and without acquired mobility disability," *Disability and Rehabilitation*, vol. 24, no. 6, pp. 289–296, 2002.

[15] H. Ghassemzadeh, R. Mojtabai, N. Karamghadiri, and N. Ebrahimkhani, "Psychometric properties of a Persian-language version of the Beck Depression Inventory-second edition: BDI-II-Persian," *Depression and Anxiety*, vol. 21, no. 4, pp. 185–192, 2005.

[16] S. A. Paluska and T. L. Schwenk, "Physical activity and mental health: current concepts," *Sports Medicine*, vol. 29, no. 3, pp. 167–180, 2000.

[17] P. Callaghan, "Exercise: a neglected intervention in mental health care?" *Journal of Psychiatric and Mental Health Nursing*, vol. 11, no. 4, pp. 476–483, 2004.

[18] F. Dimeo, M. Bauer, I. Varahram, G. Proest, and U. Halter, "Benefits from aerobic exercise in patients with major depression: a pilot study," *British Journal of Sports Medicine*, vol. 35, no. 2, pp. 114–117, 2001.

[19] G. Stathopoulou, M. B. Powers, A. C. Berry, J. A. J. Smits, and M. W. Otto, "Exercise interventions for mental health: a quantitative and qualitative review," *Clinical Psychology*, vol. 13, no. 2, pp. 179–193, 2006.

[20] D. D. Luxton and R. M. Wenzlaff, "Self-esteem uncertainty and depression vulnerability," *Cognition and Emotion*, vol. 19, no. 4, pp. 611–622, 2005.

[21] F. Pajares, "Current directions in self-efficacy research," *Advances in Motivation and Achievement*, vol. 10, no. 149, 1997.

[22] P. Strelan, S. J. Mehaffey, and M. Tiggemann, "Self-objectification and esteem in young women: the mediating role of reasons for exercise," *Sex Roles*, vol. 48, no. 1-2, pp. 89–95, 2003.

[23] L. L. Craft, "Exercise and clinical depression: examining two psychological mechanisms," *Psychology of Sport and Exercise*, vol. 6, no. 2, pp. 151–171, 2005.

[24] R. W. Motl, J. F. Konopack, E. McAuley, S. Elavsky, G. J. Jerome, and D. X. Marquez, "Depressive symptoms among older adults: long-term reduction after a physical activity intervention," *Journal of Behavioral Medicine*, vol. 28, no. 4, pp. 385–394, 2005.

[25] S. Vocks, T. Hechler, S. Rohrig, and T. Legenbauer, "Effects of a physical exercise session on state body image: the influence of pre-experimental body dissatisfaction and concerns about weight and shape," *Psychology and Health*, vol. 24, no. 6, pp. 713–728, 2009.

[26] M. Chalder, N. J. Wiles, J. Campbell et al., "Facilitated physical activity as a treatment for depressed adults: randomised controlled trial," *British Medical Journal*, vol. 344344, Article ID e2758, 2012.

[27] J. Krogh, M. Nordentoft, J. A. C. Sterne, and D. A. Lawlor, "The effect of exercise in clinically depressed adults: Systematic review and meta-analysis of randomized controlled trials," *Journal of Clinical Psychiatry*, vol. 72, no. 4, pp. 529–538, 2011.

[28] P. Dijkstra and D. P. H. Barelds, "Women's meta-perceptions of attractiveness and their relations to body image," *Body Image*, vol. 8, no. 1, pp. 74–77, 2011.

[29] T. MacDonald, *The relative effectiveness of aerobic exercise and yoga in reducing depression symptoms among female clinical sample [M.S. thesis]*, Clinical psychology, Acadia University, 2006.

[30] F. Legrand and J. P. Heuze, "Antidepressant effects associated with different exercise conditions in participants with depression: a pilot study," *Journal of Sport and Exercise Psychology*, vol. 29, no. 3, pp. 348–364, 2007.

[31] S. S. Banfield and M. P. McCabe, "An evaluation of the construct of body image," *Adolescence*, vol. 37, no. 146, pp. 372–393, 2002.

[32] S. S. Delinsky and G. T. Wilson, "Mirror exposure for the treatment of body image disturbance," *International Journal of Eating Disorders*, vol. 39, no. 2, pp. 108–116, 2006.

[33] A. Jansen, D. Bollen, B. Tuschen-Caffier, A. Roefs, A. Tanghe, and C. Braet, "Mirror exposure reduces body dissatisfaction and anxiety in obese adolescents: a pilot study," *Appetite*, vol. 51, no. 1, pp. 214–217, 2008.

[34] A. Sarsan, F. Ardiç, M. Özgen, O. Topuz, and Y. Sermez, "The effects of aerobic and resistance exercises in obese women," *Clinical Rehabilitation*, vol. 20, no. 9, pp. 773–782, 2006.

2

Short-Term Psychodynamic Psychotherapy in Patients with "Male Depression" Syndrome, Hopelessness, and Suicide Risk

Gloria Angeletti,[1] Maurizio Pompili,[2] Marco Innamorati,[2] Chiara Santucci,[1] Valeria Savoja,[1] Mark Goldblatt,[3,4] and Paolo Girardi[1,2,5]

[1] *Department of Neurosciences, Mental Health and Sensory Functions and Department of Psychiatry, Sant'Andrea Hospital, Sapienza University of Rome, 00189 Rome, Italy*
[2] *Department of Neurosciences, Mental Health and Sensory Functions and Department of Psychiatry, Suicide Prevention Center, Sant'Andrea Hospital, Sapienza University of Rome, 1035 Via di Grottarossa, 00189 Rome, Italy*
[3] *McLean Hospital, Belmont, MA, USA*
[4] *Department of Psychiatry, Harvard Medical School, Cambridge, MA 02138, USA*
[5] *Villa Rosa Medical Research Centre, Viterbo, Italy*

Correspondence should be addressed to Maurizio Pompili; maurizio.pompili@uniroma1.it

Academic Editor: H. Grunze

Objectives and Methods. This was an observational study of the efficacy of short-term psychodynamic psychotherapy (STPP) in a sample of 35 (30 women and 5 men) patients with moderate-to-severe "male depression" (Gotland Scale for Male Depression (GSMD) ≥ 13) comorbid with unipolar mood disorder (dysthymia and major depression) or anxiety disorder. Outcome measures were GSMD and BHS (Beck Hopelessness Scale) score changes from baseline. *Results.* Patients had a strong response to STPP on the GSMD (estimated mean score change ($\pm$SE) = -9.08 ± 2.74; $P < 0.01$; partial eta squared = 0.50), but not on the BHS (estimated mean score change ($\pm$SE) = -0.92 ± 1.55; $P = 0.57$; partial eta squared = 0.03). BHS score changes were significantly associated with GSMD score changes (Pearson's $r = 0.56$; $P < 0.001$), even when controlling for the severity of hopelessness at the baseline (partial $r = 0.62$; $P < 0.001$). *Conclusions.* STPP proved to be effective in patients suffering from "male depression" although hopelessness was only marginally reduced by this treatment which points to the need to better understand how STPP can be involved in the reduction of suicide risk.

1. Introduction

The term "depression" encompasses a wide range of conditions that may occur along a continuum, ranging from milder forms of discomfort to more severe and persistent form, as in the case of major depression. Depression is the leading cause of disability and the 4th leading contributor to the global burden of disease [1, 2] and by the year 2020, it is projected to become the 2nd leading contributor to the global burden of disease in all ages and both sexes [1].

Major depression is the most frequent mental illness in the world [3–6]. For example, in the US, the Epidemiological Catchment Area (ECA) Study indicated a one-month prevalence between 1.7% and 3.4% [7], and more recently, the National Comorbidity Survey Replication (NCS-R) estimated a 12-month prevalence of 6.6% [8]. Nevertheless, prevalence of moderate-to-severe depressive symptoms could be much higher [9–11].

In 2010, the British National Institute for Health and Clinical Excellence (NICE) commissioned the development of an updated version of the guideline on the treatment and management of depression in adults [12]. The NICE guideline pointed out that people who suffer from depression usually prefer psychological treatments to medication

[13] and value outcomes beyond symptom reduction [14]. The NICE guideline indicated that it was not possible to demonstrate a consistent picture of any clinically important benefit for short-term psychodynamic psychotherapy (STPP) in depression. While cognitive-behavioral therapy and interpersonal therapy continue to have the most evidence for efficacy [15], however, some randomized trials and meta-analyses indicated that STPP could be effective in reducing symptoms and in improving functional ability of patients with mild or moderate depression [16–20].

Based on the experiences of the Gotland Study, Wålinder and Rutz [21] identified a male depressive syndrome including low stress tolerance, acting-out behavior, poor impulse control, substance abuse and family history of depression, alcoholism, and suicidality. The authors also devised an instrument to measure such syndrome, the Gotland Scale for Male Depression [22]. Despite its name, male depression is common in women; for example, female students showed a greater risk of male depression than their male counterparts in one study [23]. Male depression was found to be equally severe in men and women who had made a nonviolent suicide attempt [24]. Both men and women with substance abuse have a higher probability of having male depression and higher suicide risk than those without substance abuse [25].

To date, no psychological therapies have been assessed for their efficacy in the treatment of male depression. Thus, the aim of this study was to assess the efficacy of STPP in reducing "male depression" symptoms comorbid with mood disorders or anxiety disorders in an outpatient setting. Our hypothesis is that STPP can be effective in reducing male depression. Furthermore, we hypothesize that the reduction in male depression will be significantly associated with a reduction of hopelessness, a proxy of suicide risk.

2. Materials and Methods

2.1. Participants. This was an observational study of the efficacy of STPP in a sample of 35 consecutive (30 women and 5 men) outpatients with moderate to severe "male depression" (*Gotland Scale for Male Depression* (GSMD) $\geq$ 13) comorbid with an unipolar mood disorder (dysthymia and major depression) or an anxiety disorder. Patients were admitted between January and June 2009 at the Department of Psychiatry of the Sant'Andrea Hospital, Rome, Italy. Inclusion criteria were the presence of moderate-to-severe "male depression" syndrome as assessed by the GSMD, ages between 18 and 64 years old, and a diagnosis of a mood disorder or anxiety disorder. Exclusion criteria were the presence of lifetime diagnosis of delirium, dementia, amnesic or other cognitive disorders, schizophrenia or other psychotic disorders, anorexia nervosa and bulimia nervosa, comorbid cluster B personality disorder, current presence of severe suicide intent, a score on the *Hamilton Depression Rating Scale* [26] of 28 or higher, and the inability to complete the assessment for illiteracy or the denial of informed consent.

As concomitant psychotropic medication, only benzodiazepines at a maximum of 3 mg lorazepam equivalent per day were allowed.

All the patients participated voluntarily in the study and gave their informed consent. The study was approved by the local IRB.

2.2. Measures. At intake the participants were assessed for psychopathology by expert clinical psychologists through a clinical interview based on the DSM-IV-TR [27]. The patients were also administered the GSMD and the Beck Hopelessness Scale (BHS: [28]).

The GSMD [21, 22, 29] is a screening instrument for male depression, consisting of 13 items which are rated on a 4-point Likert scale from 0 (not present) to 3 (present to a high degree). A score of 12 or lower indicates no depression, scores in the 13–26 range indicate moderate depression, and scores >26 indicate severe depression [22]. The GMDS has good validity [30–32].

The BHS is a 20-item scale for measuring the cognitive component of the syndrome of depression. This scale assesses three major aspects of hopelessness: feelings about the future, loss of motivation, and expectations. Responding to the 20 true or false items on the Beck Hopelessness Scale, individuals have to either endorse a pessimistic statement or deny an optimistic statement. Research consistently supports a positive relationship between BHS scores and measures of depression, suicidal intent, and current suicidal ideation. In addition, Beck et al. [33] carried out a prospective study of 1,958 outpatients and found that BHS scores were related significantly to eventual completed suicide. A cutoff score of 9 or above identified 16 (94%) of the 17 patients who eventually committed suicide. The high-risk group identified by this cutoff score was 11 times more likely to commit suicide than the rest of the outpatients. The BHS may, therefore, be used as an indicator of suicide potential. An Italian version of the BHS has validated by the authors of the present study [34, 35].

2.3. Interventions. Our intervention was derived from Malan's focused short-term technique [36, 37].

The treatment was administered in individual 45-minute sessions per week for no longer than 40 sessions. STPP explores those aspects of self not fully known, especially as they are manifested and potentially influenced in the therapy relationship [38]. It requires the psychological work to be organized around a focus (i.e., a specific, strategic conflictual area to reach an understanding of the psychopathological picture manifesting as a crisis), and that the therapist takes an active role working through the central conflictual area in the psychic life of the patient.

The psychotherapists were psychologists or psychiatrists certified as psychotherapists from the Italian Board with a previous training in STPP. Group supervision sessions were carried out weekly allowing psychotherapists to discuss their cases with senior psychotherapists/supervisor.

2.4. Analysis. The primary outcome measure was the mean GSMD score changes from baseline.The secondary outcome

TABLE 1: Outcomes.

Variables		Estimated differences ($M \pm$ SE)	$P <$	Effect size (partial eta squared)
Men—%	14.3			
Women—%	85.7			
Age—$M \pm$ SD	40.00 ± 12.57			
Therapy duration—months	7.21 ± 2.03			
Baseline BHS—$M \pm$ SD	10.53 ± 4.90	−0.92 ± 1.55	0.57	0.03
Follow-up BHS—$M \pm$ SD	9.03 ± 5.17			
Baseline GMDS—$M \pm$ SD	23.57 ± 6.06	−9.08 ± 2.74	0.01	0.50
Follow-up GMDS—$M \pm$ SD	15.54 ± 8.89			

Multivariate test of within subject effect: Wilks' $\lambda = 0.49$; $F_{2;10} = 5.11$; $P < 0.05$; $\eta_p^2 = 0.51$.
GMDS ≤ 13: no depression; GMDS between 13 and 26: moderate depression; GMDS > 26: severe depression. BHS ≤ 3: no hopelessness; BHS between 4 and 8: mild hopelessness; BHS ≥ 9 moderate-to-severe hopelessness.

was mean score changes from baseline on the BHS. Response to treatment was assessed with a general linear model for repeated measures. Differences between baseline and followup are calculated on the estimated marginal means (M_e). Partial eta squared (η_p^2) are reported as measures of effect size. Associations between response on the GSMD and on the BHS were assessed through Pearson's r and partial indices of correlations. All the analyses were performed with the statistical package for social sciences SPSS for Windows 19.0.

3. Results

The mean age of the patients was 40.0 years (SD = 12.6; Min./Max.: 20/62), 40.3 ± 19.6 years for men and 40.0 ± 12.1 years for women. Sixty percent of the patients had a diagnosis of anxiety disorders (mostly, generalized anxiety, panic attack disorder, and anxiety disorder not otherwise specified), 26% were diagnosed with dysthymia, and 14% were diagnosed with a major depressive disorder.

Psychotherapy sessions were carried out for a mean of 7.2 months (SD = 2.0; range, 5–10) (see Table 1). At baseline, mean GSMD scores were 23.6 (SD = 6.1; range, 14–37). Sixty-three percent of patients scored 9 or more on the BHS at baseline (10.5 ± 4.9).

Patients had a significant strong response to the psychodynamic psychotherapy on the GSMD ($M_e \pm$ SE $= -9.08 \pm 2.74$; $P < 0.01$; $\eta_p^2 = 0.50$), but not on the BHS ($M_e \pm$ SE $= -0.92 \pm 1.55$; $P = 0.57$; $\eta_p^2 = 0.03$). Mean changes on outcome measures were neither associated with the length of the treatments (Pearson's r from −0.06 to 0.16), nor with the baseline severity of male depression (Pearson's r between 0.05 and 0.07), or hopelessness (Pearson's $r = 0.05$). Only mean BHS score change was moderately associated with baseline severity of hopelessness ($r = 0.50$; $P < 0.01$).

Furthermore, mean GSMD score change was significantly associated with BHS score change (Pearson's $r = 0.56$; $P < 0.001$), even when controlling for the severity of hopelessness at the baseline (partial $r = 0.62$; $P < 0.001$).

4. Discussion

The results of this pilot study of short-term psychodynamic psychotherapy for "male depression" are mixed. We found that self-ratings of depressive symptoms were significantly improved, suggesting that this therapy is effective for depressive symptoms in these patients.

Self-ratings associated with increased suicide risk were not significantly affected over the course of treatment. Even those patients who reported a significant response on the MINI-based suicidal risk after treatment showed no improvement on the BHS. This result is consistent with other studies, such as that of Linehan et al. [39], which showed a reduction in the risk of suicide after a psychotherapeutic intervention, but no significant changes between baseline and posttreatment in BHS scores. However, cognitive behavioural therapy proved to be superior in the reduction of hopelessness (a proxy of suicide risk) compared to other therapeutic interventions [40].

Although suicide risk has most often been studied in the context of depressive symptoms, it remains unclear what distinguishes those depressions with lethal outcome from those in which the patients do not attack themselves.

It should also be noted that these treatments took place in a public psychiatric setting where their sessions are part of the government supported public health system, and patients paid a small additional fee. While there are differences between sessions taking place in a therapist's office and those in the rooms of an outpatient clinic (due to changes in the setting from time to time, hospital furniture, white coats around, etc.), every effort was made to maintain standard procedures and provide a good test of STPP. Nevertheless, we must admit that discussion over the delivery of such psychotherapy in public environment was often raised nationwide, pointing to caution in the generalization of our results.

Such important considerations may explain deficits in outcomes as compared with modalities in which STPP is currently practiced.

It should also be noted that our original model was derived from Malan's technique; our approach shared principles with Davanloo's method [41, 42]. Although it is generally acknowledged that Malan espoused the methods of Davanloo, seeing in them a radical fulfilment of his own work, recent eminent evidence also support a valid role for Malan's approach. Malan's proposals, both in direct or modified forms, have been thoroughly tested in efficacy studies [43]. Moreover, common principles among short-term psychotherapies can be identified, which points to the fact that Malan and Davanloo's approaches have similarities that are nowadays acknowledged among experts [44].

This study has noteworthy limitations, including moderate sample size and treatment duration, mix of diagnoses, nonrandomized and largely uncontrolled treatment regimens, including use of benzodiazepine—all of which may limit generalization of findings. However, all subjects were selected for having specific features of depression and suicide risk so that the sample was overall homogeneous. Despite the fact that all psychotherapists involved in this study were trained under the principles of the brief psychodynamic psychotherapy [45], treatment bias might have been appeared, even though all the therapists were routinely supervised by senior psychotherapists. Although all psychotherapists took careful notes and reported detailed description of each session, there was no videotape or audiotape. No doubt, this constitutes a limitation, however, concordant with the limited facilities provided by the public service.

5. Conclusions

This study of the use of short-term psychodynamic therapy for "male depression" with features of suicidality reveals how difficult it is to clearly address the suicide risk factors in such patients. Although depressive symptoms appear to improve relatively soon after initiating therapy, suicidality lingers for a much longer time. Further research is needed to clarify the positive effects of such therapy and the interaction between depression and suicidality. Further studies are also needed to distinguish what kinds of therapies are useful in rapidly addressing suicide risk.

Authors' Contribution

All authors have made substantial contributions to conception and design or acquisition of data or analysis and interpretation of data, have been involved in drafting the paper or revising it critically for important intellectual content, and have given final approval of the version to be published.

Conflict of Interests

The authors declare that they have no conflict of interests for this research.

References

[1] World Health Organisation, *Depression. What is depression?*, World Health Organisation, Geneva, Switzerland, 2011, http://www.who.int /mental_health/management/depression/depression/definition/en/.

[2] T. B. Üstün, J. L. Ayuso-Mateos, S. Chatterji, C. Mathers, and C. J. L. Murray, "Global burden of depressive disorders in the year 2000," *The British Journal of Psychiatry*, vol. 184, pp. 386–392, 2004.

[3] D. S. Hasin, R. D. Goodwin, F. S. Stinson, and B. F. Grant, "Epidemiology of major depressive disorder: results from the National Epidemiologic Survey on Alcoholism and Related Conditions," *Archives of General Psychiatry*, vol. 62, no. 10, pp. 1097–1106, 2005.

[4] C. Blanco, M. Okuda, J. C. Markowitz, S. M. Liu, B. F. Grant, and D. S. Hasin, "The epidemiology of chronic major depressive disorder and dysthymic disorder: results from the National Epidemiologic Survey on Alcohol and Related Conditions," *The Journal of Clinical Psychiatry*, vol. 71, no. 12, pp. 1645–1656, 2010.

[5] V. Lehtinen and M. Joukamaa, "Epidemiology of depression: prevalence, risk factors and treatment situation," *Acta Psychiatrica Scandinavica*, vol. 377, pp. 7–10, 1994.

[6] M. M. Ohayon, "Epidemiology of depression and its treatment in the general population," *Journal of Psychiatric Research*, vol. 41, no. 3-4, pp. 207–213, 2007.

[7] D. A. Regier, J. H. Boyd, J. D. Burke Jr. et al., "One-month prevalence of mental disorders in the United States, based on five epidemiologic catchment area sites," *Archives of General Psychiatry*, vol. 45, no. 11, pp. 977–986, 1988.

[8] R. C. Kessler, P. Berglund, O. Demler et al., "The epidemiology of major depressive disorder: results from the National Comorbidity Survey Replication (NCS-R)," *The Journal of the American Medical Association*, vol. 289, no. 23, pp. 3095–3105, 2003.

[9] J. L. Rushton, M. Forcier, and R. M. Schectman, "Epidemiology of depressive symptoms in the National Longitudinal Study of Adolescent Health," *Journal of the American Academy of Child and Adolescent Psychiatry*, vol. 41, no. 2, pp. 199–205, 2002.

[10] D. Blazer, D. C. Hughes, and L. K. George, "The epidemiology of depression in an elderly community population," *The Gerontologist*, vol. 27, no. 3, pp. 281–287, 1987.

[11] S. Win, K. Parakh, C. M. Eze-Nliam, J. S. Gottdiener, W. J. Kop, and R. C. Ziegelstein, "Depressive symptoms, physical inactivity and risk of cardiovascular mortality in older adults: the Cardiovascular Health Study," *Heart*, vol. 97, no. 6, pp. 500–505, 2011.

[12] National Collaborating Centre for Mental Health, *Depression. The NICE Guideline on the Treatment and Management of Depression in Adults*, The British Psychological Society & The Royal College of Psychiatrists, London, UK, 2010.

[13] M. A. Prins, P. F. M. Verhaak, J. M. Bensing, and K. van der Meer, "Health beliefs and perceived need for mental health care of anxiety and depression—the patients' perspective explored," *Clinical Psychology Review*, vol. 28, no. 6, pp. 1038–1058, 2008.

[14] M. Zimmerman, I. Chelminski, J. B. McGlinchey, and D. Young, "Diagnosing major depressive disorder X: can the utility of the DSM-IV symptom criteria be improved?" *The Journal of Nervous and Mental Disease*, vol. 194, no. 12, pp. 893–897, 2006.

[15] S. V. Parikh, Z. V. Segal, S. Grigoriadis et al., "Canadian Network for Mood and Anxiety Treatments (CANMAT) clinical guidelines for the management of major depressive disorder in adults. II. Psychotherapy alone or in combination with antidepressant medication," *Journal of Affective Disorders*, vol. 117, supplement 1, pp. S15–S25, 2009.

[16] J. K. Salminen, H. Karlsson, J. Hietala et al., "Short-term psychodynamic psychotherapy and fluoxetine in major depressive

disorder: a randomized comparative study," *Psychotherapy and Psychosomatics*, vol. 77, no. 6, pp. 351–357, 2008.

[17] E. Driessen, P. Cuijpers, S. C. M. de Maat, A. A. Abbass, F. de Jonghe, and J. J. M. Dekker, "The efficacy of short-term psychodynamic psychotherapy for depression: a meta-analysis," *Clinical Psychology Review*, vol. 30, no. 1, pp. 25–36, 2010.

[18] A. A. Abbass, "Intensive short-term dynamic psychotherapy of treatment-resistant depression: a pilot study," *Depression and Anxiety*, vol. 23, no. 7, pp. 449–452, 2006.

[19] C. Bressi, M. Porcellana, P. M. Marinaccio, E. P. Nocito, and L. Magri, "Short-term psychodynamic psychotherapy versus treatment as usual for depressive and anxiety disorders: a randomized clinical trial of efficacy," *The Journal of Nervous and Mental Disease*, vol. 198, no. 9, pp. 647–652, 2010.

[20] M. J. Hilsenroth, S. J. Ackerman, M. D. Blagys, M. R. Baity, and M. A. Mooney, "Short-term psychodynamic psychotherapy for depression: an examination of statistical, clinically significant, and technique-specific change," *The Journal of Nervous and Mental Disease*, vol. 191, no. 6, pp. 349–357, 2003.

[21] J. Wålinder and W. Rutz, "Male depression and suicide," *International Clinical Psychopharmacology*, vol. 16, supplement 2, pp. S21–S24, 2001.

[22] W. Rutz, "Improvement of care for people suffering from depression: the need for comprehensive education," *International Clinical Psychopharmacology*, vol. 14, supplement 3, pp. S27–S33, 1999.

[23] A. M. Moller-Leimkuhler and M. Yucel, "Male depression in females?" *Journal of Affective Disorders*, vol. 121, no. 1, pp. 22–29, 2010.

[24] A. Rihmer, S. Szilagyi, S. Rozsa et al., "The role of childhood abuse in adult suicidal behaviour," *Neuropsychopharmacologia Hungarica*, vol. 11, no. 4, pp. 237–246, 2009.

[25] M. Pompili, M. Innamorati, D. Lester et al., "Substance abuse, temperament and suicide risk: evidence from a case-control study," *Journal of Addictive Diseases*, vol. 28, no. 1, pp. 13–20, 2009.

[26] M. Hamilton, "A rating scale for depression," *Journal of Neurology, Neurosurgery, and Psychiatry*, vol. 23, pp. 56–62, 1960.

[27] D. V. Sheehan, Y. Lecrubier, K. H. Sheehan et al., "The Mini-International Neuropsychiatric Interview (M.I.N.I.): the development and validation of a structured diagnostic psychiatric interview for DSM-IV and ICD-10," *The Journal of Clinical Psychiatry*, vol. 59, supplement 20, pp. 22–33, 1998.

[28] A. T. Beck, A. Weissman, D. Lester, and L. Trexler, "The measurement of pessimism: the hopelessness scale," *Journal of Consulting and Clinical Psychology*, vol. 42, no. 6, pp. 861–865, 1974.

[29] W. Rutz, L. von Knorring, H. Pihlgren, Z. Rihmer, and J. Walinder, "Prevention of male suicides: lessons from Gotland study," *The Lancet*, vol. 345, no. 8948, p. 524, 1995.

[30] R. Strmberg, L. G. Backlund, and M. Lfvander, "A comparison between the Beck's Depression Inventory and the Gotland Male Depression Scale in detecting depression among men visiting a drop-in clinic in primary care," *Nordic Journal of Psychiatry*, vol. 64, no. 4, pp. 258–264, 2010.

[31] F. Zierau, A. Bille, W. Rutz, and P. Bech, "The Gotland Male Depression Scale: a validity study in patients with alcohol use disorder," *Nordic Journal of Psychiatry*, vol. 56, no. 4, pp. 265–271, 2002.

[32] M. Innamorati, Z. Rihmer, M. Amore et al., "Psychometric properties of the Gotland Scale for Depression in Italian psychiatric inpatients and its utility in the prediction of suicide risk," *Journal of Affective Disorders*, vol. 132, no. 1-2, pp. 99–103, 2011.

[33] A. T. Beck, G. Brown, R. J. Berchick, B. L. Stewart, and R. A. Steer, "Relationship between hopelessness and ultimate suicide: a replication with psychiatric outpatients," *American Journal of Psychiatry*, vol. 147, no. 2, pp. 190–195, 1990.

[34] M. Pompili, P. Iliceto, D. Lester et al., *BHS Beck Hopelessness Scale: Manuale*, Giunti O.S. Organizzazioni Speciali, Firenze, Italy, 2009.

[35] M. Pompili, R. Tatarelli, J. R. Rogers, and D. Lester, "The Hopelessness Scale: a factor analysis," *Psychological Reports*, vol. 100, no. 2, pp. 375–378, 2007.

[36] D. H. Malan, *Toward the Validation of Dynamic Psychotherapy: A Replication*, Plenum Medical Book Co., New York, NY, USA, 1976.

[37] D. H. Malan and F. Osimo, *Psychodynamics, Training, and Outcome in Brief Psychotherapy*, Butterworth-Heinemann, Boston, Mass, USA, 1992.

[38] J. Shedler, "The efficacy of psychodynamic psychotherapy," *The American Psychologist*, vol. 65, no. 2, pp. 98–109, 2010.

[39] M. M. Linehan, H. L. Heard, and H. E. Armstrong, "Naturalistic follow-up of a behavioral treatment for chronically parasuicidal borderline patients," *Archives of General Psychiatry*, vol. 50, no. 12, pp. 971–974, 1993.

[40] A. T. Beck and R. A. Steer, *Beck Hopelessness Scale—Manual*, Harcourt Brace Javanovich, San Antonio, Tex, USA, 1988.

[41] H. D. Davanloo, *Basic Principles and Techiniques in the Short-Term Dynamic Psychotherapy*, Spectrum, New York, NY, USA, 1978.

[42] H. D. Davanloo, *Selcted Papers*, Wiley, New York, NY, USA, 1990.

[43] F. Leichsenring, S. Rabung, and E. Leibing, "The efficacy of short-term psychodynamic psychotherapy in specific psychiatric disorders: a meta-analysis," *Archives of General Psychiatry*, vol. 61, no. 12, pp. 1208–1216, 2004.

[44] M. Trujillo, "Intensive dynamic psychotherapy of anxiety and depression," *Primary Psychiatry*, vol. 13, no. 5, pp. 77–86, 2006.

[45] P. Crits-Christoph, "The efficacy of brief dynamic psychotherapy: a meta-analysis," *The American Journal of Psychiatry*, vol. 149, no. 2, pp. 151–158, 1992.

3

Prospective Associations between Religiousness/Spirituality and Depression and Mediating Effects of Forgiveness in a Nationally Representative Sample of United States Adults

Loren L. Toussaint,[1] Justin C. Marschall,[1] and David R. Williams[2,3,4]

[1] *Department of Psychology, Luther College, 700 College Dr., Decorah, IA 52101, USA*
[2] *Department of Society, Human Development, and Health, Harvard University, Boston, MA 02115, USA*
[3] *Department of African and African American Studies, Harvard University, Cambridge, MA 02138, USA*
[4] *Department of Sociology, Harvard University, Cambridge, MA 02138, USA*

Correspondence should be addressed to Loren L. Toussaint, touslo01@luther.edu

Academic Editor: Harold G. Koenig

The present investigation examines the prospective associations of religiousness/spirituality with depression and the extent to which various dimensions of forgiveness act as mediating mechanisms of these associations. Data are from a nationally representative sample of United States adults who were first interviewed in 1998 and reinterviewed six months later. Measures of religiousness/spirituality, forgiveness, and various sociodemographics were collected. Depression was assessed using the Composite International Diagnostic Interview administered by trained interviewers. Results showed that religiousness/spirituality, forgiveness of oneself and others, and feeling forgiven by God were associated, both cross-sectionally and longitudinally, with depressive status. After controlling for initial depressive status, only forgiveness of oneself and others remained statistically significant predictors of depression. Path analyses revealed that religiousness/spirituality conveyed protective effects, prospectively, on depression by way of an indirect path through forgiveness of others but not forgiveness of oneself. Hence, forgiveness of others acts as a mechanism of the salutary effect of religiousness/spirituality, but forgiveness of oneself is an independent predictor. Conclusions regarding the continued development of this type of research and for the treatment of clients with depression are offered.

1. Introduction

The present study examines the associations of religiousness/spirituality with depression in a nationally representative sample of United States adults. A parallel aim is to investigate the extent to which various dimensions of forgiveness may act as mechanisms of the connection between religiousness/spirituality and depression. Though research on religiousness/spirituality and its connections to depression and broader mental health has proliferated for several decades, only a small fraction of this research has utilized longitudinal designs and population-based samples. The present study aims to address this void in the literature and contribute to our understanding in this area.

In the *Handbook of Religion and Health*, Koenig et al. [1] define religion as "an organized system of beliefs, practices, rituals, and symbols" (page 18) intended to encourage a close relationship with God or higher power/truth/reality and to help individuals understand their connection to others living in a community. Spirituality is defined as the search for understanding and meaning in life that may or may not be related to religious rituals and community [1]. Koenig et al. devote an entire chapter in this handbook to the review of published research on religiousness/spirituality and depression. These authors provide an overall synopsis of this literature and suggest that generally religious and spiritual individuals experience less depression, as compared to non-religious/spiritual individuals. Over 100 studies are indexed that on the whole support this conclusion. The size of this correlation is modest, but not trivial, and meta-analytic reviews have estimated the overall effect size to be in the neighborhood of $r \approx .20$ [2]. In about a decade since the publication of this comprehensive review, more than 60 studies have been added to this literature that again support the conclusion that religiousness/spirituality shows salutary associations with mental health [3]. As one example, recent longitudinal work showed that church attendance was associated with reduced development of subsequent depressed mood over the course of eight years in older Australian adults [4]. Despite sustained interest in the potentially beneficial effects of religiousness/spirituality on mental health, few studies have examined the question using similar longitudinal designs or population-based samples. Hence, there remains a gap in the literature that cannot be filled by cross-sectional analyses of convenience samples. Prospective designs are needed to discern the temporal ordering of the association between religiousness/spirituality and depression. Evaluating the generalizability of any such effect will require representative, population-based samples. The present study offers both of these advantages.

In addition to testing the prospective relationship between religiousness/spirituality and depression, the present study offers the opportunity to examine several dimensions of forgiveness as potential mechanisms of this association. A number of psychosocial, health, and health-behavior mechanisms have been invoked to explain the salutary associations of religiousness/spirituality and depression; yet the question of what accounts for these effects has yet to be entirely answered [5]. Perhaps forgiveness is a viable mechanism.

Forgiveness is a multidimensional phenomenon that involves the voluntary letting go of negative thoughts, feelings, and behaviors and potentially even replacing these with positive thoughts, feelings, and behaviors [6]. Often the focus of forgiveness is toward another individual, but the focus of forgiveness can also involve oneself [7], God/higher power [8], and sometimes involves the process of seeking the forgiveness of others [9]. Forgiveness has been shown to be related to religious and spiritual variables, but often it is not related at the levels of magnitude that one might expect [10, 11]. Further, investigations of the connections between religiousness/spirituality and forgiveness almost exclusively regard forgiveness of others, and do not consider other dimensions of forgiveness. Nonetheless, there is a modest but reliable association between religiousness/spirituality and forgiveness of others and it may likely extend to other dimensions of forgiveness as well, especially feeling forgiven by God and seeking others' forgiveness.

Given its association with religiousness/spirituality, forgiveness might be considered a viable mechanism of the salutary associations of religiousness/spirituality with depression if it too were associated with depression or other related mental health conditions. Indeed, associations between forgiveness and a variety of mental health outcomes have been documented [12]. A vast majority of these studies have examined cross-sectional associations in convenience samples or highly specific patient populations. A few exceptions do exist in which, for instance, forgiveness has been linked to diagnosable depression in a nationally representative sample of United States adults [13] or in a prospective fashion demonstrating that forgiveness predicts subsequent mental distress [14]. These recent findings suggest that forgiveness may have meaningful prospective associations with mental health outcomes.

Given the research findings reviewed above, we believe that a prospective study of religiousness/spirituality, forgiveness, and depression will offer useful insights and add to what we estimate is only a handful of studies of this type. Based on our review, we have built a model to examine four hypotheses. First, we hypothesize that religiousness/spirituality will show a prospective, protective (inverse) association with depression. Second, we hypothesize that religiousness/spirituality will be positively associated with multiple dimensions of forgiveness. Third, we hypothesize that forgiveness will show a prospective, protective (inverse) association with depression. Fourth, we hypothesize that the protective (inverse) association of religiousness/spirituality with depression will operate via the mechanism of forgiveness. Put another way, we expect that religious and spiritual individuals will experience a greater proclivity toward multiple forms of forgiveness, and this tendency will in turn yield benefits for depression risk.

2. Method

2.1. Sample. Participants responded to the Survey of Consumers, a telephone survey of adults age 18, and older conducted by the University of Michigan's Institute for Social Research. The sample was nationally representative and was randomly selected using the two-stage random-digit-dialing (RDD) procedure described by Waksberg [15]. The survey employs a rotating panel design to gather data from approximately 500 respondents on a monthly basis. Each monthly sample consists of about 300 new respondents and 200 respondents being re-interviewed six months after their initial interview. The initial sample for this study consisted of the new national sample selected each month for five months for a total of 1,423 respondents. The reinterview target sample consisted of approximately three-fourths of the original respondents who were randomly selected for a total of 1,055 respondents. Both the initial and reinterview samples are nationally representative. The response rate for the survey ranged from .69 to .71. After listwise deletion of missing data, the final sample consisted of 966 respondents who participated at both times 1 and 2.

2.2. Measures

2.2.1. Depression. The measurement of major depressive episode was based on the definitions and criteria specified in the revised edition of the American Psychiatric Association's Diagnostic and Statistical Manual of Mental Disorders (DSM-III-R). Major depressive episode was assessed using a brief, screening version [16, 17] of the depression module of the World Health Organization's (WHO) Composite International Diagnostic Interview, Version 1.0 (CIDI) [18, 19]. The CIDI is a structured interview schedule designed to be used by trained interviewers who are nonclinicians to assess the prevalence of specific psychiatric disorders [20]. WHO field trials and other methodological studies have

Table 1: Forgiveness scales, items, and alphas.

Scale (alpha)
Forgiveness of self (α = .67)
I often feel that no matter what I do now I will never make up for the mistakes I have made in the past.[a]
I find it hard to forgive myself for some of the things I have done wrong.[a]
Forgiven by God (α = .64)
Knowing that I am forgiven for my sins gives me the strength to face my faults and be a better person.[a]
I know that God forgives me.[a]
Forgiveness of others (α = .72)
When someone hurts you, how often do you hold resentment or keep it inside?[b]
When someone hurts you, how often do you try to get even in some way?[b]
When someone hurts you, how often do you try to forgive the other person?[b]
I have grudges that I have held on for months or years.[a]
I have forgiven those who have hurt me.[a]
Seeking forgiveness (α = .64)
How often do you ask God's forgiveness when the respondent had hurt someone?[b]
How often do you ask the other person's forgiveness when the respondent had hurt someone?[b]
How often do you pray for someone who had hurt the respondent?[b]

[a]Response scale: strongly agree, agree, disagree, or strongly disagree.
[b]Response scale: never, hardly ever, not too often, fairly often, and very often.

shown good test-retest reliability and clinical validity of these CIDI diagnoses [21, 22].

2.2.2. Forgiveness. Four dimensions of forgiveness were assessed, and, as with all following scales, all scoring was done so that higher scores represented higher levels of the construct. All reported alpha values for forgiveness and all following scales are based on the present study's data. Forgiveness measures used in the present investigation were adapted from those originally used by Watson et al. [23, 24], Mauger et al. [25], Idler et al. [26], and Gorsuch and Hao [27]. For a complete list of the items utilized to measure forgiveness, see Table 1.

2.2.3. Religiousness/Spirituality. 4 religiousness/spirituality factors were assessed as follows: *service attendance* was measured by asking respondents how often they went to religious services. Response categories ranged from (1) never to (6) more than once a week. Frequency of *prayer* was measured by asking how often they prayed in places other than church and synagogue. Responses ranged from (1) never to (6) more than once a day. Respondents were also asked to rate how *religious* and how *spiritual* they were on a ten-point scale.

The four religiousness/spirituality items were combined to form a single index of religiousness/spirituality. This decision was made for five reasons. First, the items had virtually identical patterns and magnitudes of association with depression. Second, when factor analyzed (maximum likelihood extraction) the items loaded on a single latent factor (loadings = attend (.67), pray (.71), how religious (.92), and how spiritual (.80)). Third, using a single religiousness/spirituality composite offered parsimony in testing more complex religiousness/spirituality → forgiveness → depression mediation models. Fourth, multiitem composites contain less measurement error than single items. Finally, Koenig et al. caution researchers about multicollinearity in the use of multiple religiousness/spirituality indices in regression models. The average correlation between religious/spiritual variables in this study was r = .55, similar to the magnitude of the associations used to illustrate multicollinearity problems in Koenig et al.'s [1] discussion. Using a composite instead of individual measures of religiousness/spirituality eliminates potential multi-collinearity issues in our regression models. The religiousness/spirituality composite index had an internal consistency of .85.

2.2.4. Control Variables. Covariates assessed included: gender (male = reference category), age (in years), race (white = reference category), marital status (0 = not married; 1 = married), education (years completed), and income (13-point continuum ranged from under $10,000 to $100,000 or more). Exploratory analyses revealed that there were no noticeable differences between this coding scheme and other schemes that included dummy variables for separated and divorced, never married, and widowed respondents.

2.3. Statistical Analyses. Data were weighted for age, gender, and race to take into account differential probabilities of selection and to adjust the demographics of the sample to that of the United States population using the Current Population Survey. Analyses proceeded in three phases. First, we computed and examined descriptive statistics (means/counts and standard deviations/ranges) and bivariate correlations. Second, we used a hierarchical logistic regression model to examine the prospective relations of religiousness/spirituality and forgiveness with depressive diagnosis six months later. This model was structured so that on step one depressive diagnosis at time one was entered. On step two, sociodemographic control variables were entered. On step three, the religiousness/spirituality index was entered. On step four, the four forgiveness variables were entered. In this way, religiousness/spirituality was tested for its longitudinal association with depressive status, and initial evaluations of the mediating effects of forgiveness were also considered.

The third phase of analysis involved a more thorough and sophisticated examination of the mediating mechanisms that might explain the prospective relationship of religiousness/spirituality with six-month depressive diagnosis. Although the design of the hierarchical logistic regression model allows one to examine the extent to which the religiousness/spirituality coefficient is accounted for by forgiveness variables entered on the subsequent step, it does not allow for a specific test of the indirect effect of religiousness/spirituality through forgiveness to six-month depressive status.

Traditionally, a hierarchical model of this type might have been seen as sufficient for establishing that forgiveness acts as a mediating mechanism, but thanks to recent work [28], it has become clear that the traditional mediation approach is limited in two important ways. First, the traditional mediation approach requires a statistically significant total effect between religiousness and depressive diagnosis to be present. Second, it does not guarantee an explicit test of the indirect effect. A better manner in which to proceed is to simply test the indirect effects of interest [28]. However, when the outcome variable is dichotomous, calculating an indirect effect requires that any logistic regression coefficients in the estimated mediation model be standardized. There are at least six different methods for standardizing logistic regression coefficients, but an efficient and effective method requires simply that the predictors be standardized before entry into the logistic model [29]. Following this requirement, our mediation models are constructed so that coefficients representing the associations between religiousness/spirituality and forgiveness are *unstandardized* ordinary least squares regression coefficients. Coefficients representing associations between forgiveness variables and depressive diagnosis are *standardized* logistic regression coefficients. The indirect effect is computed by multiplying the unstandardized coefficient for religiousness/spirituality predicting forgiveness with the standardized coefficient for forgiveness predicting depressive diagnosis. The indirect effect can then be tested for statistical significance using the Sobel method [30].

3. Results

Table 2 gives the means and proportions, standard deviations and ranges, and bivariate associations for all study variables. Looking at columns one and two shows the associations between all predictors and depression both cross-sectionally and six months lagged. Lagged associations showed that the strongest predictor of depression at time two was prior depression at time one. Religiousness/spirituality showed a modest protective association, as did feeling forgiven by God. Protection against depression offered by forgiveness of oneself and others was noticeably larger. Bivariate associations for religiousness/spirituality and forgiveness variables with depression were similar for cross-sectional and lagged analyses.

Intercorrelations between religiousness/spirituality and forgiveness are contained in the lower right-hand portion of Table 2. Religiousness/spirituality was positively correlated at moderate levels with forgiveness of others and feeling forgiven by God. Religiousness/spirituality showed its highest positive correlation with seeking forgiveness and its lowest positive correlation with forgiveness of oneself. Forgiveness of others was moderately, positively correlated with forgiveness of oneself, feeling forgiven by God, and seeking forgiveness. Forgiveness of oneself was modestly, positively correlated with feeling forgiven by God and not correlated with seeking forgiveness. Feeling forgiven by God and seeking forgiveness were moderately, positively correlated.

Also evident in the table are small cross-sectional associations of sex and age with depression. Women showed slightly greater risk of depression at time one, and older participants showed slightly less risk. Age and income also showed a small protective, prospective association with depressive diagnosis. Hispanics were at increased risk, prospectively, of developing a depressive diagnosis.

Table 3 summarizes the results of the hierarchical logistic regression analysis. Unlike the bivariate associations reported above, the logistic model allows for an examination of the unique, prospective predictors of depressive diagnosis at time two, controlling the effects of initial depressive diagnosis. Model one examined the association of time one depression with time two depression. The odds ratio indicated that individuals with likely depressive diagnosis at time one showed over 12 times increased odds of depression at time 2. Regarding sociodemographic predictors of depression at time two, Hispanic respondents showed 3.6 times increased odds of depression, whereas higher-income respondents showed .08 times reduced odds of depression. The most theoretically meaningful results of the logistic regression model were those showing effects for religiousness/spirituality and forgiveness. Religiousness/spirituality showed no influence on the odds of depression at time two, but forgiveness of oneself and others showed .28 and .32 reduced odds of depression, respectively.

Based on the results of our bivariate and logistic analyses, we constructed a path model examining the indirect effects of religiousness/spirituality through forgiveness of oneself and others on depressive diagnosis at time two (see Figure 1). We did not include feeling forgiven by God or seeking forgiveness because neither variable had an independent direct effect on depression—a requirement for a mediating variable. The mediation model controlled the effects of depressive diagnosis at time one and all socio-demographic variables. The results of the model showed that religiousness/spirituality was significantly, positively associated with both forgiveness of oneself and others. Forgiveness of oneself and others were also significantly, negatively associated with depressive diagnosis at time two. The indirect effect of religiousness/spirituality through forgiveness of oneself on depressive diagnosis at time two was not statistically significant ($B = .02$, $Z = -1.63$, $P = .10$). The indirect effect of religiousness/spirituality through forgiveness of others on depressive diagnosis at time two was statistically significant ($B = .03$, $Z = -1.98$, $P < .05$). Hence, religiousness/spirituality shows a prospective, protective association with depression through forgiveness of others but not forgiveness of oneself.

4. Discussion

This study set out to examine the prospective association of religiousness/spirituality with depression and the extent to which this association might be mediated through various dimensions of forgiveness. Our findings both confirm and disconfirm our expectations. As is typical in this type of

TABLE 2: Means/proportions, standard deviations/ranges, and bivariate correlations for all study variables.

(a)

	Dep T2	Dep T1	Fem	Age	Blk	Hsp	Ed	Inc
Depression time 1	.41***	1.00						
Sex (female = 1)	.05	.09**	1.00					
Age	−.08*	−.10**	.04	1.00				
Black (other = 0)	.02	−.03	−.03	−.10**	1.00			
Hispanic (other = 0)	.10**	.00	.09**	−.14***	−.07	1.00		
Years of education	−.03	−.01	−.06	−.11**	−.09**	−.07*	1.00	
Income	−.12***	−.07	−.16***	−.11**	−.14***	−.10**	.46***	1.00
Separated/divorced (other = 0)	.04	.02	−.05	.06	.05	.01	−.09**	−.14***
Widowed (other = 0)	−.01	−.04	.16***	.37***	.01	−.05	−.22***	−.28***
Never married (other = 0)	.05	.01	−.07*	−.41***	.21***	−.02	.03	−.12***
Religiousness/spirituality	−.09*	−.12***	.14***	.17***	.01	−.05	.01	−.04
Forgiven oneself	−.25***	−.28***	.05	.00	−.12***	.02	.22***	.23***
Forgiven others	−.25***	−.30***	.10**	.13***	−.08*	−.04	.04	.03
Forgiven by God	−.09**	−.08*	.14***	.07*	.06	−.02	−.11**	−.06
Seek forgiveness	−.04	−.04	.27***	−.02	.15***	−.02	−.09**	−.16***
Mean/proportion	.11	.12	.55	45.90	.10	.06	14.03	8.02
SD/range	0-1	0-1	0-1	16.11	0-1	0-1	2.49	3.60

(b)

	Sep/Div	Wid	Nvr Mar	Rel/Sp	FS	FO	FG	SF
Separated/divorced (other = 0)	1.00							
Widowed (other = 0)	−.11**	1.00						
Never married (other = 0)	−.20***	−.14***	1.00					
Religiousness/spirituality	−.01	.09*	−.14***	1.00				
Forgiven oneself	−.07*	−.07*	−.08*	.07*	1.00			
Forgiven others	−.02	.08*	−.13***	.32***	.39***	1.00		
Forgiven by God	.06	.07*	−.14***	.39***	.10**	.26***	1.00	
Seek forgiveness	.02	.02	−.03	.57***	.02	.32***	.38***	1.00
Mean/proportion	.15	.07	.19	5.28	4.03	4.03	4.70	3.87
SD/range	0-1	0-1	0-1	1.76	1.15	.74	.66	.99

$^*P < .05$, $^{**}P < .01$, $^{***}P < .001$. Listwise $N = 966$. Dep = depression, Fem = female, Blk = black, Hsp = Hispanic, Ed = years of education, Inc = household income, Sep/Div = separated/divorced, Wid = widowed, Nvr Mar = never married, FS = forgiven self, FO = forgiven others, FG = forgiven by God, and SF = seek forgiveness. Values in the "mean/proportion" row represent means for continuous variables and proportions for dichotomous variables; likewise, values in the "SD/Range" row represent standard deviations for continuous variables and range of possible values for dichotomous variables.

Table 3: Unstandardized logistic regression coefficients, standard errors, and odds ratios for the association of time 1 depression, sociodemographics, religiousness/spirituality, and Forgiveness Predicting Time 2 Depression.

	Model 1				Model 2				Model 3				Model 4			
	B	S.E.	OR		B	S.E.	OR		B	S.E.	OR		B	S.E.	OR	
Depression time 1																
Depressed	2.52	.26	12.46	***	2.54	.28	12.70	***	2.50	.28	12.21	***	2.07	.30	7.91	***
Not depressed (referent)	—	—	—		—	—	—		—	—	—		—	—	—	
Sex																
Female					−.01	.28	.99		.02	.28	1.02		.22	.30	1.24	
Male (referent)					—	—	—		—	—	—		—	—	—	
Age					−.01	.01	.99		−.01	.01	.99		−.01	.01	.99	
Race ethnicity																
Black					.25	.41	1.28		.26	.42	1.29		.17	.42	1.19	
Hispanic					1.28	.54	3.61	*	1.26	.54	3.54	*	1.36	.55	3.90	**
White (referent)					—	—	—		—	—	—		—	—	—	
Years of education					.05	.06	1.05		.05	.06	1.05		.09	.07	1.10	
Income					−.09	.04	.92	*	−.09	.04	.92	*	−.06	.05	.94	
Marital status																
Separated/divorced					.39	.37	1.48		.37	.37	1.45		.39	.39	1.48	
Widowed					.28	.59	1.32		.28	.59	1.32		.35	.62	1.42	
Married (referent)					—	—	—		—	—	—		—	—	—	
Never married					.24	.37	1.27		.18	.38	1.20		.16	.39	1.17	
Religiousness/spirituality									−.06	.08	.94		−.01	.10	.99	
Forgiveness of oneself													−.32	.12	.72	**
Forgiveness of others													−.39	.20	.68	*
Forgiveness by God													−.21	.20	.81	
Seeking forgiveness													.09	.20	1.09	

$^{*}P < .05$, $^{**}P < .01$, $^{***}P < .001$; listwise $N = 966$; model 1 pseudo $R^2 = .22$, model 2 pseudo $R^2 = .26$, model 3 pseudo $R^2 = .26$, model 4 pseudo $R^2 = .31$.

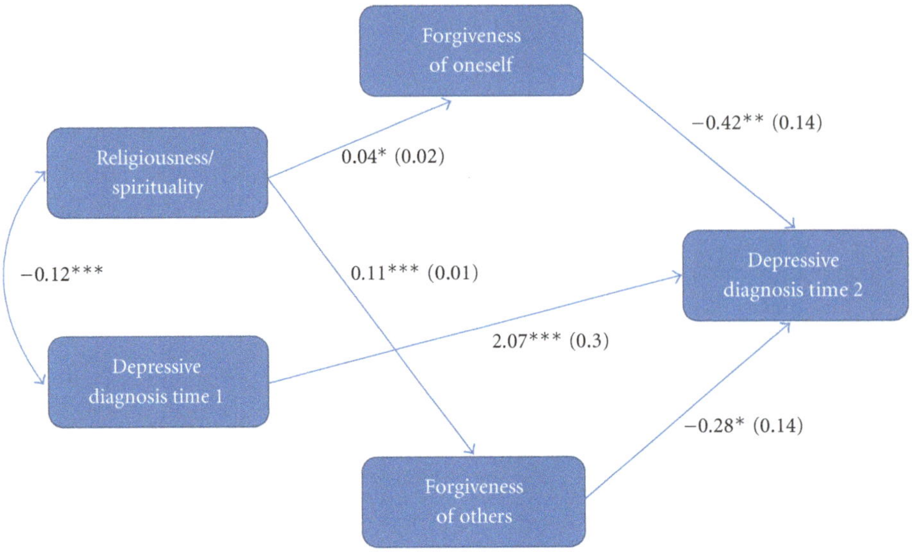

FIGURE 1: Path analysis of the prospective effects of religiousness/spirituality and prospective mediating effects of forgiveness on depression. Paths from religiousness/spirituality to forgiveness of oneself and others are unstandardized ordinary least-squares regression coefficients (standard errors). Paths from forgiveness of oneself and others to depression are standardized logistic regression coefficients (standard errors). All coefficients are net of the effects of gender, age, race, education, income, and marital status. $R^2 = .32$ for depression at time 2. Listwise $N = 966$.

design, the strongest predictor of depression at time 2 was depression at time 1. More importantly, bivariate analyses confirmed that religiousness/spirituality and forgiveness of oneself, forgiveness of others, and feeling forgiven by God were inversely associated with depression, and this was true both cross-sectionally and longitudinally. Unexpectedly, religiousness/spirituality did not show prospective associations with depression after controlling for initial depressive status in logistic models. As expected, forgiveness of oneself and others remained statistically significant, prospective predictors of depression, even after controlling for initial depressive status.

4.1. No Prospective Effect of Religiousness/Spirituality on Depression. Although unadjusted associations between religiousness/spirituality and depression do exist in the present study, religiousness/spirituality does not predict depression prospectively after adjusting for initial depressive status and other controls. The lack of a prospective association flies in the face of existing, sound empirical work suggesting the opposite [1–3, 5]. Furthermore, the results of the present study run contrary to those of dozens of studies showing that religiousness/spirituality offers protective advantages in multiple mental health domains [3]. As noted earlier, hundreds of other studies show salutary effects of religiousness/spirituality for physical health outcomes [1]. Given this outcome, there is good reason to consider what this might mean.

Although there are probably several reasons for the results observed in the present study, a couple of issues deserve discussion. First, as noted above, Koenig et al. [1] identified over 100 studies of religiousness/spirituality and depression that were conducted prior to 2001, and Toussaint et al. [3] identified an additional 66 that were conducted between 2001 and 2009. The majority of these studies reported at least one result suggestive of a protective connection between religiousness/spirituality and depression [3]. However, these studies have been overwhelmingly cross-sectional in nature, and most have relied on convenience samples. Koenig et al. [1] in their exhaustive review identified only 22 prospective cohort studies, and Toussaint et al. [3] identified little more than a handful of additional prospective studies in recent years. Of the 22 prospective cohort studies identified by Koenig et al. [1], only four utilized population-based samples, and in two of the four studies the beneficial effects of religiousness/spirituality were confined to a particular group (e.g., blacks, men). As such, the overreliance on cross-sectional methods to inform us about the relationships between religiousness/spirituality and depression seems a risky enterprise. Longitudinal research continues to be badly needed. The present study offers exactly that, a prospective examination of associations between religiousness/spirituality and depression in a representative sample of United States adults. Given how much faith we have placed in cross-sectional studies and how few and nuanced the prospective relations are, perhaps the current findings are not all that surprising. Rather, the present study might offer an initial point of reference for future prospective, population-based work.

A second issue in the present study regards the measurement of religiousness/spirituality. There has been great debate regarding what is the core essence of religiousness/spirituality and how it should be measured. Nevertheless, three key constructs have emerged [1, 31]. These include organizational religiousness, private religious practices, and religious importance. Indicators of each of these constructs were included in the present study; however, we chose to combine each of the items into an overall religiousness/spirituality index. Some may question the utility of this approach arguing that these are different constructs worthy of individual investigation. We would agree. However, as we indicated in the methods, there are several reasons for this decision. First, the direction and magnitude of the effects were all highly similar for each of the individual items. Second, all items factored onto a single factor that resulted in an index with good internal consistency. Third, examining single-item indicators has an untoward effect on predictive efficiency due to increased measurement error, and including multiple variables in regression models increases the likelihood of multicollinearity problems. Fourth, although we captured multiple dimensions of religiousness/spirituality, we used single-item indicators of each construct and did not comprehensively capture all relevant dimensions of religion/spirituality. As a result, the decision was made to combine the items into a single index. This allowed for a more sensitive test of the association between religiousness/spirituality and depression and allowed us to focus on the important mediating effects of forgiveness without requiring 8 to 16 paths from initial religiousness/spirituality variables to mediating forgiveness variables. The end result of creating a religiousness/spirituality composite was a sensitive yet parsimonious model of the prospective relations between religiousness/spirituality, forgiveness, and depression.

4.2. Indirect Effects of Religiousness/Spirituality on Depression Operate through Forgiveness of Others but Not Oneself. The absence of a prospective relationship between religiousness/spirituality and depression offered the opportunity to refocus on an important and vexing question. That question is why might religiousness/spirituality have salutary effects? Though numerous psychological, social, and health mechanisms have been proposed and examined [1, 5, 32], the answer to why religiousness/spirituality has mental health benefits has not been entirely answered. Based on the present findings, we believe that forgiveness is an important piece of the puzzle.

Our data show that religiousness/spirituality promotes forgiveness of others, which in turn has a moderate protective relationship with depression, and our path model bears out that this indirect effect is statistically significant. This is not so for forgiveness of oneself. In this case, the connection between religiousness/spirituality and forgiveness of oneself is not sufficiently large, even though it is statistically significant, to result in a significant indirect effect. It is clear that the indirect effect breaks down in this connection and not elsewhere, because the connection between forgiveness of self and depression is almost twice the size of the connection between forgiveness of others and depression. Furthermore, the prospective direct effect of forgiveness of oneself on depression is over twice the size of the typical effect of religiousness/spirituality on depression ($r \approx .20$) [2]. Clearly, there is a meaningful benefit of forgiveness of oneself in terms of depression. But interestingly, this type of forgiveness is not strongly driven by religiousness/spirituality.

To summarize, the results of our path model suggest that religious and spiritual persons secure mental health benefits through their increased likelihood to forgive others but not because they forgive themselves. This may reflect the emphasis on forgiveness of others that is present in organized religion [11, 33, 34] and the relative lack of religious teaching on forgiveness of oneself [35]. It appears there is a stark delineation between the forgiving mechanisms that convey benefit of religiousness/spirituality to depression. That said, forgiveness of oneself remains the most powerful prospective predictor of depression, outside of preexisting depression. Clearly, this dimension of forgiveness deserves more attention.

Forgiving oneself has clearly been "The Stepchild of Forgiveness Research" [7]. That said, recent conceptual and empirical work has outlined some of the key correlates/predictors of self-forgiveness and its likely outcomes. Hall and Fincham [7] provide what might be considered the most comprehensive review of self-forgiveness and discuss several constructs which are likely to be causal antecedents of self-forgiveness. These include causal attributions, offense severity, shame/guilt, empathy, perceived forgiveness from victim/higher power, and conciliatory behavior. Nowhere is there mention of religiousness/spirituality in this conceptual model. This is a striking irony, because the general notion of forgiveness is infused with such religious and spiritual overtones that for years its study was thought not to be appropriate within science [11]. Moreover, Barry [35] indicates that the Bible offers no instance in which self-forgiveness is discussed. Given this context, perhaps it is not surprising that forgiveness of oneself emerged as an independent prospective predictor of depression and did not act as a mediating mechanism of the influence of religiousness/spirituality.

Recent empirical work confirms the importance of self-forgiveness for mental health. Macaskill [36] examined self-forgiveness in two studies involving over 500 participants. In her path analyses, self-forgiveness consistently showed robust associations with mental health. Importantly, in one of her path models where both self- and other forgiveness were modeled simultaneously, self-forgiveness showed statistically significant and moderate associations with both mental illness symptoms and life dissatisfaction while other forgiveness did not show significant associations with either variable. While these were cross-sectional studies and causal effects cannot be inferred, they do provide confirming evidence of the particular importance of self-forgiveness in our path models predicting depression.

4.3. Limitations. As with studies of this type, there are some limitations to this work. First, the number of religious/spiritual and forgiveness items could have been greater. This would have allowed for broader assessment coverage of these constructs and would have helped to reduce measurement error. Nonetheless, even after a decade of enthusiastic forgiveness research, we are hard pressed to find measures that provide equally efficient and broad coverage of these four different forgiveness dimensions. Second, the elapsed time span between initial data collection and followup was six months. Though this provides ample time for changes to occur in mental health status, diagnosable depression likely changes less in this period of time. A longer follow-up would allow for even greater change, more variability, and potentially more predictive power. Third, given the paucity of longitudinal studies utilizing population-based samples, we feel that the findings from the present study provide a useful contribution to the existing literature. Nevertheless, we would encourage future investigators to consider collecting data from three or more waves so that growth modeling and latent trajectories could be established. Our two time-point data are useful in establishing prospective effects but do not allow for this type of more sophisticated understanding of change, variability in change, and latent trajectory analysis. Fourth, religiousness/spirituality and forgiveness are both measured at time one, and as such it is not possible to infer causal direction. Though religiousness/spirituality are often thought to be causally antecedent to forgiveness [11], it is also possible that being a more forgiving person might influence one's tendencies toward a religious/spiritual life. Future work utilizing three panels of data collection would be advisable and would improve on mediation models of the present type. Fifth, it is important to consider that respondents reporting on religiousness, spirituality, and forgiveness can be influenced by social desirability. Finally, in looking at depression as the main outcome in this study, it would have been useful to have controlled for other co-morbid disorders.

5. Conclusions

The present study provides a prospective, population-based analysis of relationships between religiousness/spirituality and depression. To our knowledge, approximately five other studies have investigated this question using prospective designs and representative, population-based samples. As a result of the scantiness of this literature, our understanding of the influence of religiousness/spirituality on depression is limited. Continued development of this literature will inform us about the extent to which religiousness/spirituality can truly be considered a causal factor that impacts the risk of depression or whether it is merely a side effect of psychiatric disturbance.

Prospective relationships between multiple dimensions of forgiveness and depression were tested in our analyses. Forgiveness of oneself and others proved to be important predictors of depression. Forgiveness of self is an independent predictor not connected to religiousness/spirituality as a mediating mechanism. Forgiveness of others, however, was found to convey the beneficial effects of religiousness/spirituality to depression. This is most likely the first demonstration, of which we are aware, of the prospective relations between forgiveness of oneself and others and diagnosable depression risk.

Continued attention to the connections between religiousness/spirituality, forgiveness, and depression will undoubtedly shed light on the causal linkages between these constructs. To the extent that religious and spiritual persons reap benefit from forgiveness of others but not of oneself, there may be potential for tailored patient-centered forgiveness therapy; that is, religious and spiritual clients may be helped more by addressing issues regarding forgiveness of others, whereas self-forgiveness may be more important for less religious/spiritual clients or nonreligious. Future work might do well to examine the interaction effects of religiousness/spirituality and forgiveness. If synergistic effects were observed, this might suggest the importance of client-centered forgiveness interventions. With continued attention, the importance of religiousness/spirituality and forgiveness for depression care and treatment will be better understood, and we will gain improved resolution on the implications of religiousness/spirituality and forgiveness in the treatment of depression and related mental illnesses.

Acknowledgments

This study was supported in part by the Fetzer Institute as part of the John Templeton Foundation's campaign for forgiveness research, by Grant T32-MH16806 from the National Institute of Mental Health, and by a Faculty Research Grant from the Office of the Vice President for Research at the University of Michigan.

References

[1] H. G. Koenig, M. E. McCullough, and D. B. Larson, *Handbook of Religion and Health*, Oxford University Press, 2001.

[2] M. E. McCullough and D. B. Larson, "Religion and depression: a review of the literature," *Twin Research*, vol. 2, no. 2, pp. 126–136, 1999.

[3] L. Toussaint, J. Webb, and W. Keltner, "Religion, spirituality, and mental health," in *The Psychology of Religion and Spirituality for Clinicians: Using Research in Your Practice*, J. D. Aten, K. A. O'Grady, and E. L. Worthington Jr., Eds., pp. 331–356, Routledge, New York, NY, USA , 2012.

[4] R. W. Law and D. A. Sbarra, "The effects of church attendance and marital status on the longitudinal trajectories of depressed mood among older adults," *Journal of Aging and Health*, vol. 21, no. 6, pp. 803–823, 2009.

[5] D. R. Williams, "Scientific research on the study of religion/spirituality and mental health: lessons, positive affirmations, and disquieting questions," in *A Christian Worldview and Mental Health: A Seventh-Day Adventist Perspective*, C. Fayard, B. C. Hernandez, B. Anderson, and G.T. HardingIV, Eds., pp. 185–208, Andrews University Press, Berrien Springs, Mich, USA, 2011.

[6] E. L. Worthington, "More questions about forgiveness: research agenda for 2005–2015," in *Handbook of Forgiveness*, E. L. Worthington, Ed., pp. 557–573, Brunner-Routledge, New York, NY, USA, 2005.

[7] J. H. Hall and F. D. Fincham, "Self-forgiveness: the stepchild of forgiveness research," *Journal of Social and Clinical Psychology*, vol. 24, no. 5, pp. 621–637, 2005.

[8] J. J. Exline and A. Martin, "Anger toward God: a new frontier in forgiveness research," in *Handbook of Forgiveness*, E. L. Worthington, Ed., pp. 73–88, Brunner-Routledge, New York, NY, USA, 2005.

[9] S. J. Sandage, E. L. Worthington, T. L. Hight, and J. W. Berry, "Seeking forgiveness: theoretical context and an initial

empirical study," *Journal of Psychology & Theology*, vol. 28, no. 1, pp. 21–35, 2000.

[10] M. E. McCullough and E. L. Worthington, "Religion and the Forgiving Personality," *Journal of Personality*, vol. 67, no. 6, pp. 1140–1164, 1999.

[11] M. E. McCullough, G. Bono, and L. M. Root, "Religion and forgiveness," in *Handbook of the Psychology of Religion and Spirituality*, R. F. Paloutzian, C. L. Park, R. F. Paloutzian, and C. L. Park, Eds., pp. 394–411, Guilford Press, New York, NY, USA, 2005.

[12] L. Toussaint and J. Webb, "Theoretical and empirical connections between forgiveness, mental health, and well-being," in *Handbook of Forgiveness*, E. L. Worthington, Ed., pp. 349–362, Brunner-Routledge, New York, NY, USA, 2005.

[13] L. Toussaint and A. C. D. Cheadle, "Unforgiveness and lifetime prevalence of psychopathology: findings from an epidemiological study of United States adults," in *Religion and Psychology*, M. T. Evans and E. D. Walker, Eds., p. 2009, Nova Publishers, New York, NY, USA.

[14] H. K. Orcutt, "The prospective relationship of interpersonal forgiveness and psychological distress symptoms among college women," *Journal of Counseling Psychology*, vol. 53, no. 3, pp. 350–361, 2006.

[15] J. Waksberg, "Sampling methods for random digit dialing," *Journal of the American Statistical Association*, vol. 73, pp. 40–46, 1978.

[16] R. C. Kessler, H. U. Wittchen, J. M. Abelson et al., "Methodological studies of the composite international diagnostic interview (CIDI) in the US national comorbidity survey (NCS)," *International Journal of Methods in Psychiatric Research*, vol. 7, no. 1, pp. 33–55, 1998.

[17] R. C. Kessler, H.-U. Wittchen, J. Abelson, and S. Zhao, "Methodological issues in assessing psychiatric disorder with self-reports," in *The Science of Self-Report: Implications for Research and Practice*, A. A. Stone, J. S. Turrkan, C. A. Bachrach, J. B. Jobe, H. S. Kurtzman, and V.S. Cain, Eds., pp. 229–255, Lawrence Erlbaum Associates, Mahwah, NJ, USA, 2000.

[18] World Health Organization, *CIDI, Version 1.0.*, World Health Organization, Geneva, Switzerland, 1990.

[19] R. C. Kessler, K. D. Mickelson, and D. R. Williams, "The prevalence, distribution, and mental health correlates of perceived discrimination in the United States," *Journal of Health and Social Behavior*, vol. 40, no. 3, pp. 208–230, 1999.

[20] L. N. Robins, J. Wing, H. U. Wittchen et al., "The Composite International Diagnostic Interview: an epidemiologic instrument suitable for use in conjunction with different diagnostic systems and in different cultures," *Archives of General Psychiatry*, vol. 45, no. 12, pp. 1069–1077, 1988.

[21] H. U. Wittchen, "Reliability and validity studies of the WHO-Composite international diagnostic interview (CIDI): a critical review," *Journal of Psychiatric Research*, vol. 28, no. 1, pp. 57–84, 1994.

[22] D. G. Blazer, R. C. Kessler, K. A. McGonagle, and M. S. Swartz, "The prevalence and distribution of major depression in a national community sample: The National Comorbidity Survey," *American Journal of Psychiatry*, vol. 151, no. 7, pp. 979–986, 1994.

[23] P. Watson, R. Hood, R. Morris, and J. Hall, "Religiosity, sin, and self-esteem," *Journal of Psychology and Theology*, vol. 13, pp. 116–128, 1985.

[24] P. Watson, R. Morris, and R. Hood, "Antireligious humanistic values, guilt, and self-esteem," *Journal for the Scientific Study of Religion*, vol. 26, pp. 535–546, 1987.

[25] P. Mauger, J. Perry, T. Freeman, D. Grove, A. McBride, and K. McKinney, "The measurement of forgiveness: preliminary research," *Journal of Psychology and Christianity*, pp. 170–180, 1992.

[26] E. L. Idler, M. A. Musick, C. G. Ellison et al., "Measuring multiple dimensions of religion and spirituality for health research: conceptual background and findings from the 1998 general social survey," *Research on Aging*, vol. 25, no. 4, pp. 327–365, 2003.

[27] R. Gorsuch and J. Hao, "Forgiveness: an explanatory factor analysis and its relationships to religious variables," *Review of Religious Research*, vol. 34, pp. 333–347, 1993.

[28] A. F. Hayes, "Beyond Baron and Kenny: statistical mediation analysis in the new millennium," *Communication Monographs*, vol. 76, no. 4, pp. 408–420, 2009.

[29] S. Menard, "Six approaches to calculating standardized logistic regression coefficients," *American Statistician*, vol. 58, no. 3, pp. 218–223, 2004.

[30] D. P. MacKinnon and J. H. Dwyer, "Estimating mediated effects in prevention studies," *Evaluation Review*, vol. 17, no. 2, pp. 144–158, 1993.

[31] D. R. Williams, "The measurement of religion in epidemiologic studies: problems and prospects," in *Religion in Aging and Health: Theoretical Foundations and Methodological Frontiers*, J. S. Levin, Ed., pp. 125–148, Sage, Thousand Oaks, Calif, USA, 1994.

[32] J. S. Levin, L. M. Chatters, and H. G. Koenig, "Research on religion and mental health: an overview of empirical findings and theoretical issues," in *Handbook of Religion and Mental Health*, pp. 33–50, Academic Press, San Diego, Calif, USA, 1998.

[33] M. Rye, K. Pargament, and A. Ali, "Religious perspectives on forgiveness," in *Forgiveness: Theory, Research, and Practice*, M. E. McCullough, K. I. Pargament, and C. E. Thoresen, Eds., pp. 17–40, Guilford, New York, NY, USA, 2000.

[34] L. Toussaint and D. Williams, "National survey results for Protestant, Catholic, and nonreligious experiences of seeking forgiveness and of forgiveness of self, of others, and by God," *Journal of Psychology and Christianity*, vol. 27, pp. 120–130, 2008.

[35] M. Barry, *The Forgiveness Project: The Startling Discovery of How to Overcome Cancer, Find Health, and Achieve Peace*, Kregel, Grand Rapids, Mich, USA, 2011.

[36] A. Macaskill, "Differentiating dispositional self-forgiveness from other-forgiveness: associations with mental health and life satisfaction," *Journal of Social and Clinical Psychology*, vol. 31, pp. 28–50, 2012.

4

Prevalence and Impact of Anxiety and Depression on Type 2 Diabetes in Tunisian Patients over Sixty Years Old

Jawaher Masmoudi,[1] Rahma Damak,[1] Hela Zouari,[2] Uta Ouali,[1] Anouar Mechri,[3] Nouri Zouari,[2] and Abdelaziz Jaoua[1]

[1] *Department of Psychiatry A, University Medical Center Hédi Chaker, 3000 Sfax, Tunisia*
[2] *Department of Functional Exploration and Metabolic Diseases, University Medical Center Habib Bourguiba, 3000 Sfax, Tunisia*
[3] *Department of Psychiatry, University Medical Center Fattouma Bourguiba, 5000 Monastir, Tunisia*

Correspondence should be addressed to Rahma Damak; d_rahma@live.com

Academic Editor: H. Grunze

Objectives. To estimate the prevalence of anxiety and depression using the Hospital Anxiety and Depression Scale (HADS) in a population aged over sixty years with type 2 diabetes and to study the impact of anxiety and depression on glycemic balance and disease outcome. *Results.* The prevalence of anxiety and depression in the 62 subjects included in the study was, respectively, 40.3% and 22.6%. We found a relationship between these disorders and complicated diabetes. The subjects having an imperfectly balanced diabetes had a higher average anxiety score than those having a good glycemic control (9.1 ± 4.2 versus 6.5 ± 3.1; $P = 0.017$). No relationship was found between diabetes balance and depression. *Conclusion.* Association between anxiety and depressive disorders and diabetes is frequent and worsens patients' outcome, in terms of diabetes imbalance as well as in terms of diabetic complications. Our study shows that there is need for physicians to detect, confirm, and treat anxiety and depressive disorders in elderly diabetic patients.

1. Introduction

In Tunisia, the proportion of individuals over 60 years is increasing, and it reached 9% in 2004 [1].

Diabetes is a major public health problem in Tunisia. Its prevalence has increased steadily and is currently about 9.9% [2]. Prevalence increases with age (11.9% for 60 years or older) [3, 4]. In addition, depression and anxiety, at the top of mental disorders list, mainly remain undiagnosed [5, 6], in particular in the elderly [7, 8] and consequently untreated [9]. Studying the link between diabetes and depressive as well as anxiety disorders in elderly subjects is useful for several reasons. First, diabetes as well as depression constitutes a major source of functional incapacity, and thus of loss of autonomy, in the elderly population [10]. Second, the association of these two pathologies in the same person worsens total health outcome [11] and quality of life [6, 12]. Finally, this association increases health care expenditures [11] and mortality [13]. The aim of this study is to estimate the prevalence of anxiety and depression in a population of elderly subjects aged over sixty suffering from type 2 diabetes and to study the impact of anxiety and depression on glycemic control and the evolution of the disease.

2. Methods

We undertook a descriptive and analytical cross-sectional study on 62 patients who have consulted during September and October 2010 at the Department of Functional Explorations and Metabolic Diseases of Habib Bourguba University Hospital, Sfax, Tunisia. Recruitment was carried out on an ad hoc basis.

The patients included were those who had agreed to take part in the investigation and who were 60 years old or over. We used this age limit because under Tunisian law, 60 is the retirement age.

Exclusion criteria were the incapacity to answer the questions because of cognitive deterioration and refusal to take part in the study.

TABLE 1: Sociodemographic characteristics of the sample.

Sociodemographic characteristics	Number (%)
Sex	
Male	16 (25.8)
Female	46 (74.2)
Marital status	
Single	0 (0)
Married	40 (64.5)
Divorced	1 (1.6)
Widowed	21 (33.9)
Socioeconomic level	
Low	26 (42)
Medium	25 (40.3)
High	11 (17.7)
Resides	
With family	42 (88.7)
Alone	20 (11.3)
Profession	
No professional qualifications	45 (72.6)
Retired	15 (24.2)
Active	2 (3.2)

TABLE 2: Clinical and therapeutic characteristics of the sample.

Clinical and therapeutic characteristics	Number (%)
Somatic comorbidity	
Hypertension	45 (72.6)
Dyslipidemia	31 (50)
Heart disease	15 (24.2)
Obesity	13 (21)
Dysthyroidism	8 (12.9)
Balanced diabetes	
Yes	42 (67.7)
No	20 (32.3)
Diabetes complications	
Macro angiopathy	25 (40.3)
Peripheral neuropathy	24 (38.7)
Retinopathy	22 (35.5)
Nephropathy	8 (12.9)
Erectile dysfunction	3 (18.7)
Treatment compliance	
Yes	57 (91.1)
No	5 (8.9)
Follow a balanced diet	
Yes	37 (59.7)
No	25 (41.3)
Practice of physical activity	
Yes	19 (30.6)
No	45 (69.4)
Consultation mode	
Regular	60 (96.8)
Irregular	2 (3.2)

We used a semistructured questionnaire composed of sociodemographic and professional characteristics which was administered by the same investigator. We collected the clinical data relating to diabetes (duration, personal medical history: dyslipidemia, cardiac and vascular disorders, obesity, and diabetic complications such as macroangiopathy, nephropathy, peripheral neuropathy, and erectile dysfunction) and therapeutic data (physical exercise, diet, regular followup, treatment compliance). The balance of diabetes was assessed by the last rate of glycated hemoglobin (HbA1) and/or fasting glycaemia. Diabetes was considered as balanced if HbA1 <7% and/or fasting glycaemia ≤6 mmol/L.

To evaluate the mood and anxiety state of subjects, we used the Hospital Anxiety and Depression Scale (HADS), a self-assessment scale that has been developed and found to be a reliable instrument for detecting states of depression and anxiety in the setting of a hospital medical outpatient clinic. The anxiety and depressive subscales are also valid measures of severity of the emotional disorder. It is suggested that the introduction of HADS into general hospital practice would facilitate the large task of detection and management of emotional disorder in patients under investigation and treatment in medical and surgical departments. The thresholds for pathological anxiety and depression were 10 on each of the two subscales (A for anxiety and D for depression) of HADS [14]. We used a validated Arabic version of this questionnaire [15]. The subjects having an elevated score (≥10) were referred to the psychiatric outpatient clinic for specialized evaluation and treatment.

Data analysis was made using the software SPSS for Windows version 11. For the quantitative variables, we calculated averages and standard deviations. We then compared the sub groups: anxious: $A \geq 10$ to nonanxious: $A < 10$ and depressed: $D \geq 10$ to not depressed by chi-square test of Pearson or the Fisher exact test as well as Student's "t" test of. Statistical significance was designated as P less than 0.05.

3. Results

3.1. Sociodemographic Characteristics. Sociodemographic characteristics are summarized in Table 1. In our sample, a female predominance was observed. The average age of included subjects was 66.8 years (standard deviation = 4.8) with patients aged 60 years minimum/80 years maximum. More than two-thirds of the subjects were married. The socioeconomic level was qualified as average in more than 40% of the participants. A little less than three quarters of the subjects had no professional qualifications.

3.2. Clinical and Therapeutic Characteristics. The various clinical and therapeutic characteristics are presented in Table 2. The average age of diabetes onset was 54.5 years (standard deviation = 9.4), ranging from 25 to 74 years. The average duration of the diabetes was 12.4 years (standard deviation = 8.1), ranging from 0 to 36 years. The near total of included subjects (90.3%) had a somatic comorbidity associated with the diabetes. Hypertension was the most

TABLE 3: Distribution of prevalence and average scores of anxiety and depression.

	Average score (%)
$A \geq 10$	12.4 ± 2.4 (40.3)
$A < 10$	5.5 ± 2.1 (59.7)
$D \geq 10$	12.2 ± 3.6 (22.6)
$D < 10$	4.4 ± 2.7 (77.4)

$A \geq 10$: anxious; $A < 10$: not anxious; $D \geq 10$: depressed; $D < 10$: not depressed.

frequent comorbidity. More than two-thirds of the sample had poor glycemic control. The average fasting glycaemia was 9.4 mmol/L (standard deviation = 4.4 mmol/L) and average HbA1 was 9% (standard deviation = 2.1%). Fifty-seven subjects affirmed having a good compliance with treatment.

3.3. Prevalence of Anxiety and Depression. The prevalence of anxiety and depression was, respectively, 40.3% and 22.6%. The average score of anxiety was 8.3 ± 4.4. The average score of depression was 6.1 ± 4.3 (Table 3).

3.4. Relationship between Anxiety and Depression and Sociodemographic Characteristics. According to the HADS scale, women were significantly more anxious than men. The subjects with no professional qualifications scored higher on the anxiety subscale than did subjects with a profession. In our study, we did not find a link between depression and the different sociodemographic variables (Table 4).

3.5. Relationship between Anxiety and Depression and Diabetes Clinical Characteristics. In our study, we did not note a statistically significant correlation between duration of diabetes and anxiety and depression (13.1 ± 7.1 years in anxious subjects versus 11.9 ± 8.7 years in nonanxious subjects; P = 0.59 and 13.7 ± 8.3 years in depressed subjects versus 12 ± 8 years in nondepressed subjects, P = 0.48). When we studied the link between anxiety/depression and diabetes somatic comorbidities, we found that the average anxiety score of the subjects having a somatic comorbidity was higher, except for subjects having obesity as a comorbidity. However, this correlation was statistically significant only for hypertension. A similar correlation was not found when we studied the relationship between depression and somatic comorbidity. As to glycaemic control, average anxiety score was significantly higher amongst patients whose diabetes was badly managed. Nevertheless, there was no relationship between depression and diabetes balance in our sample. We noted that patients with complicated diabetes had a significantly higher average anxiety score (9.4 ± 3.9 versus 6.3 ± 3.7; P = 0.004). Indeed, anxious subjects had more diabetes complications, especially nephropathy and retinopathy. Subjects suffering from peripheral neuropathy, and retinopathy had a higher depression average score (Table 5).

Logistic regression analysis showed that anxiety was principally related to female gender (P = 0.008) and to the presence of nephropathy (P = 0.032). On the other hand, depression was correlated with the two variables: peripheral neuropathy (P = 0.004) and retinopathy (P = 0.05)

3.6. Relationship between Anxiety, Depression, and Diabetes Treatment Characteristics. In our study, we did not find a correlation between diabetes treatment characteristics, anxiety, and depression.

4. Discussion

The prevalence of anxiety and depression, according to HADS scores, was, respectively, 40.3% and 22.6% in our sample of elderly diabetic subjects.

In the literature, the prevalence of depression in elderly type 2 diabetics varies from 4.5% [11] to 17% [10]. Contrary to depression, there are few studies [16–18] examining anxiety in type 2 diabetics, particularly in older subjects. A study on a sample of 1,066 elderly type 2 diabetics aged 69 to 74 years [17], showed an average anxiety score of 5.7 ± 3.9 on the HADS scale and an average depression score of 3.9 ± 2.9. The anxiety and depression scores of the patients in our sample were higher. This difference could be explained by our sample being derived from subjects consulting at a hospital. Indeed, diabetic subjects who consulted at the hospital were generally referred there due to difficulties during treatment in first line structures. Consequently, they might have had a higher risk to present anxiety and depression. That is why it seems to be important to detect and treat these disorders as early as possible.

The relationship between mood disorders and diabetes is bidirectional [10, 13, 19]. Several explanations are proposed that are inevitably interconnected; mood disorders are associated with an unhealthy lifestyle (tobacco abuse, little or no exercise, and excessive caloric intake) [20]. Depression is also related to obesity, which in turn is responsible for intolerance to glucose. Furthermore, depression is associated with physiological abnormalities, including the activation of the hypothalamus-pituitary-adrenal axis, the sympathetic nervous system, and the proinflammatory cytokines [18, 20], which can induce a resistance to insulin, and thus increase the risk of diabetes. Diabetes might increase the risk of depression and anxiety because of feelings of threat and loss related to the announcement of the diagnosis and the need to make lifestyle changes [11]. Finally, the association between mood disorders and diabetes can be partly explained by the existence of comorbidities [3, 18].

In our study, patients having a poorly controlled diabetes presented a significantly higher average anxiety score (P = 0.017). Indeed, these patients might be worried about complications related to their poor glycemic control. In addition, anxiety could deteriorate glycemic balance via adrenergic hyperactivity [21, 22]. We did not find a relationship between depression and diabetes balance; this has also been the case in several other studies on the subject [13, 23, 24].

In our study, subjects having high scores of anxiety and depression had significantly more complications of nephropathy, peripheral neuropathy and retinopathy. Indeed, depressed and anxious subjects are less likely to conform to

TABLE 4: Relationship between sociodemographic characteristics, anxiety, and depression.

	$A \geq 10/A < 10$	P	$D \geq 10/D < 10$	P
Sexe M/F	2/23; 14/23	**0.008**	5/9; 11/37	0.36
Marital status				
Married	14/26		7/33	
Divorced	0/1	0.29	1/0	0.10
Widowed	11/10		6/15	
Profession				
Active	1/1		0/2	
Retired	1/14	**0.009**	1/14	0.15
No professional qualifications	23/22		13/32	
Resides				
Alone	5/2	0.07	1/6	0.57
With family	20/37		13/42	
Socioeconomic level				
Low	13/14		6/20	
Medium	8/17	0.40	7/18	0.45
High	4/7		1/10	

N: number of patients; M/F: male/female; $A \geq 10$: anxious; $A < 10$: not anxious; $D \geq 10$: depressed; $D < 10$: not depressed.

TABLE 5: Clinical and therapeutic characteristics of diabetes according to depression and anxiety average scores.

Clinical and therapeutic characteristics	AAS (SD)	P	DAS (SD)	P
Balanced diabetes				
Yes	6.5 (3.1)	**0.017**	5 (3.1)	0.14
No	9.1 (4.2)		6.7 (4.7)	
Comorbidity type				
Dyslipidemia				
Yes	9.1 (4)	0.14	6.5 (4.6)	0.47
No	7.5 (4)		5.7 (4.1)	
Heart disease				
Yes	9 (4.6)	0.47	7.6 (4.8)	0.15
No	8.1 (3.9)		5.7 (4.1)	
HTA				
Yes	9 (4.1)	**0.03**	6.5 (4.6)	0.24
No	6.5 (3.6)		5.1 (3.4)	
Obesity				
Yes	7.5 (4)	0.43	6.9 (5.3)	0.49
No	8.5 (4)		5.9 (4.1)	
Dysthyroidism				
Yes	8.2 (3.7)	0.94	5.1 (2.8)	0.47
No	8.3 (4)		6.3 (4.5)	
Complication type				
Macroangiopathy				
Yes	8.9 (3.8)	0.33	6.9 (4.5)	0.27
No	7.9 (4.3)		5.6 (4.2)	
Nephropathy				
Yes	**11.3** (3.2)	**0.024**	8.1 (4.7)	0.18
No	7.8 (4)		5.8 (4.3)	
Retinopathy				
Yes	**10.3** (4.1)	**0.004**	7.9 (4.6)	**0.017**
No	7.2 (3.7)		5.2 (3.9)	
Peripheral neuropathy				
Yes	9.4 (3.9)	0.10	8.1 (5.4)	**0.005**
No	7.6 (4.1)		4.9 (3)	
Erectile dysfunction				
Yes	7.3 (3.5)	0.67	7.3 (2.3)	0.64
No	8.3 (4.1)		6.1 (4.4)	

AAS: anxiety average score; DAS: depression average score; (SD): standard deviation.

recommendations concerning their diabetes that could affect glycemic control and consequently might impact the outcome of the disease [11, 13, 16]. Moreover, subjects suffering from diabetes are exposed to continuous stress generated by these complications, which may worsen or precipitate depression [11, 13, 18, 19]. Lastly, depression might constitute an etiopathologic factor responsible for the development of micro and macroangiopathy via pathophysiological modifications induced by deterioration of cellular immunity (diminished proliferative response of lymphocytes and reduction of NK activity) [11].

5. Limits of the Study

Although diabetes has a high prevalence in elderly subjects, our sample size was small. The reasons for this are varied. Our exclusion criteria left out a large proportion of patients, specifically those who were illiterate, those with cognitive impairments, and those who refused to join the study. Furthermore, the majority of diabetic patients in Tunisia are treated in first line health care facilities (private and public general practitioners). Thus, the hospital population represents only a part of the patients, most often those who had a diabetes which was difficult to manage.

Our study has a cross-sectional design; therefore, a causal relationship between clinical variables related to diabetes and symptoms of anxiety and depression cannot be established.

We used a psychometric scale, rather than a structured interview, to evaluate anxiety and depression. However, this instrument is frequently used as a screening tool in units for somatic diseases in order to detect psychiatric disorders and refer patients to a more specialized consultation. The interest of the HADS scale lies in the fact that it does not take into account the physical dimension of psychiatric symptoms, which could be a source of confusion. Indeed, symptoms which could be attributed to physical diseases such as insomnia, tiredness, headaches, and disturbances of appetite were omitted to avoid false positive findings amongst people with somatic diseases.

Another limit to the study is the nature of the studied population. As was mentioned above, patients consulting at a hospital might have a higher prevalence of anxiety and depression than the patients consulting in first line facilities.

6. Conclusion

Diabetes, anxiety, and depression, are frequent pathologies, and each constitutes a public health problem in Tunisia. These pathologies are known to be more frequent in elderly people. Whereas diabetes is easy to detect and diagnose, this is not always the case with anxiety and mood disorders. According to recent estimates, more than three quarters of these psychiatric pathologies might not be detected. Several factors might explain this: the frequent expression of depression through somatic symptoms in the elderly, the tendency to attribute psychical suffering in the elderly to physical symptoms only the fear of being stigmatized as a psychiatric patient. Our results, in major part, are comparable to those of the literature and confirm the high prevalence of anxiety and depression in elderly subjects suffering from diabetes. The causal link between these two conditions seems to be bidirectional. In any case and according to our results, the association of these two types of pathologies impairs global outcome in terms of a greater diabetes imbalance and more frequent complications. Thus the need to detect, confirm, and treat anxiety and depressive disorders in elderly diabetic subjects. This will only be possible through close collaboration between geriatrists, diabetologists, nutritionists, and psychiatrists.

References

[1] M. Ben Ferjani and A. Ben Brahim, "Demographic developments in Tunisia and its impact on the labor market and human resources policies," Mediterranean Federation of Human Resources, 2012, http://www.fmrh.org/ .

[2] Evaluation of the Nutritional Status of the Tunisian Population, "National survey 1996/1997," National Report, Ministry of Public Health, Tunisia.

[3] C. Maraldi, S. Volpato, B. W. Penninx et al., "Diabetes mellitus, glycemic control, and incident depressive symptoms among 70- to 79-year-old persons: the health, aging, and body composition study," *Archives of Internal Medicine*, vol. 167, no. 11, pp. 1137–1144, 2007.

[4] J. Dirmaier, B. Watzke, U. Koch et al., "Diabetes in primary care: prospective associations between depression, nonadherence and glycemic control," *Psychotherapy and Psychosomatics*, vol. 79, no. 3, pp. 172–178, 2010.

[5] A. S. Rigaud, C. Bayle, F. Latour et al., "Psychiatry of the elderly," *EMC: Psychiatrie*, vol. 2, no. 4, pp. 259–281, 2005.

[6] C. Lloyd, "The impact of diabetes on depression and depression on diabetes," *Diabetesvoice*, vol. 53, no. 1, pp. 23–26, 2008.

[7] S. Baudic, L. Traykov, A. S. Rigaud, and P. Césaro, "Place and role of neuropsychological exam in elderly depression," *Revue de Medecine Interne*, vol. 26, no. 8, pp. 637–642, 2005.

[8] R. Trouillet and M. C. Gély-Nargeot, "Depression of elderly persons and defence mechanisms in nursing homes," *Annales Medico-Psychologiques*, vol. 167, no. 2, pp. 119–126, 2009.

[9] J. Y. Guo, C. C. Han, and Y. M. Liu, "A contemporary treatment approach to both diabetes and depression by cordyceps sinensis, Rich in Vanadium," *Evidence-Based Complementary and Alternative Medicine*, vol. 7, no. 3, pp. 387–389, 2010.

[10] M. D. Pawaskar, R. T. Anderson, and R. Balkrishnan, "Self-reported predictors of depressive symptomatology in an elderly population with type 2 diabetes mellitus: a prospective cohort study," *Health and Quality of Life Outcomes*, vol. 5, article 50, 2007.

[11] D. G. Bruce, W. A. Davis, S. E. Starkstein, and T. M. E. Davis, "A prospective study of depression and mortality in patients with type 2 diabetes: the fremantle diabetes study," *Diabetologia*, vol. 48, no. 12, pp. 2532–2539, 2005.

[12] S. Hardy, M. Scanlan, and R. Gray, "Identifying and managing anxiety and depression in diabetes: a need for training," *Journal of Diabetes Nursing*, vol. 14, no. 5, pp. 190–195, 2010.

[13] E. H. B. Lin, C. M. Rutter, W. Katon et al., "Depression and advanced complications of diabetes: a prospective cohort study," *Diabetes Care*, vol. 33, no. 2, pp. 264–269, 2010.

[14] J. P. Lépine, M. Godchau, P. Brun, and T. Lemperiere, "Assessment of anxiety and depression in patients hospitalized in a department of internal medicine," *Annales Medico-Psychologiques*, vol. 143, no. 2, pp. 175–189, 1985.

[15] T. H. Malasi, I. A. Mirza, and M. F. El-Islam, "Validation of the hospital anxiety and depression scale in arab patients," *Acta Psychiatrica Scandinavica*, vol. 84, no. 4, pp. 323–326, 1991.

[16] M. M. Collins, P. Corcoran, and I. J. Perry, "Anxiety and depression symptoms in patients with diabetes," *Diabetic Medicine*, vol. 26, no. 2, pp. 153–161, 2009.

[17] D. G. Bruce, W. A. Davis, S. E. Starkstein, and T. M. E. Davis, "A prospective study of depression and mortality in patients with type 2 diabetes: the Fremantle Diabetes Study," *Diabetologia*, vol. 48, no. 12, pp. 2532–2539, 2005.

[18] A. Engum, "The role of depression and anxiety in onset of diabetes in a large population-based study," *Journal of Psychosomatic Research*, vol. 62, no. 1, pp. 31–38, 2007.

[19] L. C. Brown, S. R. Majumdar, S. C. Newman, and J. A. Johnson, "Type 2 diabetes does not increase risk of depression," *Canadian Medical Association Journal*, vol. 175, no. 1, pp. 42–46, 2006.

[20] T. W. Strine, A. H. Mokdad, S. R. Dube et al., "The association of depression and anxiety with obesity and unhealthy behaviors among community-dwelling US adults," *General Hospital Psychiatry*, vol. 30, no. 2, pp. 127–137, 2008.

[21] S. H. Golden, "A review of the evidence for a neuroendocrine link between stress, depression and diabetes mellitus," *Current Diabetes Reviews*, vol. 3, no. 4, pp. 252–259, 2007.

[22] U. Ehlert, J. Gaab, and M. Heinrichs, "Psychoneuroendocrinological contributions to the etiology of depression, posttraumatic stress disorder, and stress-related bodily disorders: the role of the hypothalamus-pituitary-adrenal axis," *Biological Psychology*, vol. 57, no. 1–3, pp. 141–152, 2001.

[23] S. R. Heckbert, C. M. Rutter, M. Oliver et al., "Depression in relation to long-term control of glycemia, blood pressure, and lipids in patients with diabetes," *Journal of General Internal Medicine*, vol. 25, no. 6, pp. 524–529, 2010.

[24] L. E. Egede and C. Ellis, "The effects of depression on metabolic control and quality of life in indigent patients with type 2 diabetes," *Diabetes Technology and Therapeutics*, vol. 12, no. 4, pp. 257–262, 2010.

5

Prevalence of Depression among University Students

Diana Sarokhani,[1,2] Ali Delpisheh,[3,4] Yousef Veisani,[1,4] Mohamad Taher Sarokhani,[1,5] Rohollah Esmaeli Manesh,[6] and Kourosh Sayehmiri[4,7]

[1] *Student Research Committee, Ilam University of Medical Science, P.O. Box 69311-57793, Ilam, Iran*
[2] *Department of Computer, Faculty of Engineering, Malayer University, P.O. Box 95863-65719, Hamadan, Iran*
[3] *Department of Clinical Epidemiology, Ilam University of Medical Sciences, P.O. Box 69315-138, Ilam, Iran*
[4] *Psychosocial Injuries Research Center, Ilam University of Medical Science, P.O. Box 69315-138, Ilam, Iran*
[5] *Science and Research Branch, Islamic Azad University, Kermanshah, Iran*
[6] *Eslamabad Payame Noor University, Kermanshah, Iran*
[7] *Social Medicine Department, Medicine Faculty, Ilam University of Medical Sciences, P.O. Box 69315-138, Ilam, Iran*

Correspondence should be addressed to Mohamad Taher Sarokhani; m_taher_sarokhani@yahoo.com

Academic Editor: Verinder Sharma

Introduction. Depression is one of the four major diseases in the world and is the most common cause of disability from diseases. The aim of this study is to estimate the prevalence of depression among Iranian university students using meta-analysis method. *Materials and Methods.* Keyword depression was searched in electronic databases such as PubMed, Scopus, MAGIran, Medlib, and SID. Data was analyzed using meta-analysis (random-effects model). Heterogeneity of studies was assessed using the I^2 index. Data was analyzed using STATA software Ver.10. *Results.* In 35 studies conducted in Iran from 1995 to 2012 with sample size of 9743, prevalence of depression in the university students was estimated to be 33% (95% CI: 32–34). The prevalence of depression among boys was estimated to be 28% (95% CI: 26–30), among girls 23% (95% CI: 22–24), single students 39% (95% CI: 37–41), and married students 20% (95% CI: 17–24). Metaregression model showed that the trend of depression among Iranian students was flat. *Conclusions.* On the whole, depression is common in university students with no preponderance between males and females and in single students is higher than married ones.

1. Introduction

Depression among university students is extremely prevalent and widespread problem across the country [1–3]. University students are a special group of people that are enduring a critical transitory period in which they are going from adolescence to adulthood and can be one of the most stressful times in a person's life. Trying to fit in, maintain good grades, plan for the future, and be away from home often causes anxiety for a lot of students [4]. As a reaction to this stress, some students get depressed. They find that they cannot get themselves together. They may cry all of the time, skip classes, or isolate themselves without realizing they are depressed. Previous studies reported that depression in university students is noted around the world [5–7] and the prevalence seems to be increasing [8].

The average age of onset is also on the decline, making depression a particularly salient problem area for university student populations [8]. Over two-thirds of young people do not talk about or seek help for mental health problems [9].

In Iran, preliminary studies on emotional distress have emerged in recent years including depression in Iranian university. Within the abovementioned background, the aim of this study is to estimate the prevalence of depression among university students using meta-analysis method.

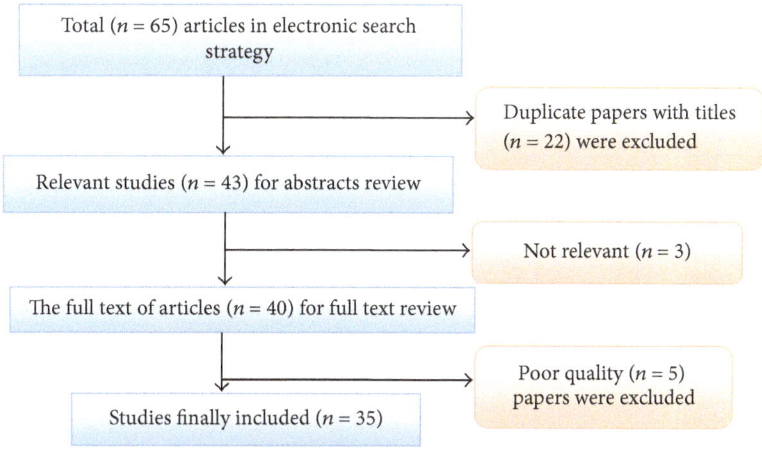

FIGURE 1: Results of the systematic literature search.

2. Methods and Materials

2.1. Literature Search. Our search strategy, selection of publications, and the reporting of results for the review will be conducted in accordance with the PRISMA guidelines [10]. Literatures on the depression among student were acquired through searching Scientific Information Databases (SID), Global Medical Article Limberly (Medlib), Iranian Biomedical Journal (Iran Medex), Iranian Journal Database (Magiran), and international databases including PubMed/Medline, Scopus and ISI Web of Knowledge. The search strategy was limited to the Persian and/or English language and articles published up until February 2012 were considered. All publications with medical subject headings (MeSh) and keywords in title, abstract, and text for words including student depression were investigated. Iranian scientific databases were searched only using the keyword "student depression," as these databases do not distinguish synonyms from each other and do not allow sensitive search operation using linking terms such as "AND," "OR" or "NOT." Consequently, this single keyword search was the most practical option.

2.2. Selection and Quality Assessment of Articles. All identified papers were critically appraised independently by two reviewers. Disagreements between reviewers were resolved by consensus. Appraisal was guided by a checklist assessing clarity of aims and research questions. The inclusion criteria were as follows: (1) studies in the mentioned databases with full text, despite the language of original text; (2) having a standardized assessment of depression (either self-report or observer-rated). Exclusion criteria were (1) studies upon student overlapping time intervals of sample collection from the same origin; (2) low-quality design (STROBE checklist score's below 7.75 [11]); (3) inadequate reporting of results.

2.3. Data Extraction. Data were extracted using a standardized and prepiloted data extraction form. Data extraction will be undertaken by the first reviewer, and checked by a second reviewer although the process will be discussed and piloted by both reviewers. All identified papers will be critically appraised independently by both reviewers. Disagreements were resolved through discussion. Appraisal will be guided by a checklist assessing clarity of aims and research questions. Information was extracted from each included study (including author, title, year and setting of study, methods of sample selection, sample size, study type, age, STROBE score, and prevalence). These data abstraction forms were reviewed and eligible papers were entered into the meta-analysis.

2.4. Statistical Analysis. The random effects model was used for combining results of studies in meta-analysis. Variance for each study was calculated using the binomial distribution formula. The presence of heterogeneity was determined by the DerSimonian-Laird (DL) approach [12]. Significance level was <0.1 and I^2 statistic for estimates of inconsistency between studies. The I^2 statistic estimates the percent of observed between-study variability due to heterogeneity rather than to chance and ranges from 0 to 100 percent (values of 25%, 50% and 75% were considered representing low, medium and high heterogeneity, resp.). A value of 0% indicates no observed heterogeneity whilst 100% indicates significant heterogeneity. For this review, we determined that I^2 values above 75 percent were indicative of significant heterogeneity warranting analysis with a random effects model as opposed to the fixed effects model to adjust for the observed variability [13]. This heterogeneity was further explored through subgroup analyses and metaregression. Univariate and multivariate approach were employed to assess the causes of heterogeneity among the selected studies. Egger test was conducted to examine potential publication bias. Data manipulation and statistical analyses were done using STATA software, version 10. P values < 0.05 were considered as statistically significant.

3. Results

According to the literature search strategies, 65 studies were identified, but 30 studies were excluded as they did not meet the inclusion criteria. Finally, 35 studies were published between 1995 and 2012 and included in meta-analysis (Table 1 and Figure 1).

Table 1: Feature and characteristic studies included in study.

Study number/author(s)/no. of reference	Place	Publication year	No. of population	Prevalence (%)	Instrument assessment	Cut point
(1) Bahrami Dashtaki [14]	Tehran	2005	100	—	BDI	15
(2) Mohammadian [15]	Tehran	2010	302	—	BDI	16
(3) Alavi [16]	Mashhad	2011	20	—	BDI	16
(4) Hosseini [17]	Kermanshah	2002	162	23.5	BDI	15
(5) Bahadori Khosroshahi [18]	Zahedan	2010	200	—	BDI	16
(6) Biani [19]	Tabriz	2008	571	—	BDI	16
(7) Mohammad-Bigi et al. [20]	Arak	2009	304	52.3	BDI	15
(8) Amani et al. [21]	Ardabil	2004	324	54.7	BDI	16
(9) Dadkhah [22]	Ardabil	2009	409	50.8	BDI	16
(10) Pahlavan-Zadeh et al. [23]	Isfahan	2010	50	38	GHQ 28	22
(11) Ranjbar-Kohan and Sajjadi Nejad [24]	Isfahan	2010	40	—	BDI	16
(12) Makvandi et al. [25]	Ahvaz	2012	185	—	BDI	17
(13) Makvandi [26]	Ahvaz	2010	215	—	BDI	16
(14) Ahmadi [27]	Ahvaz	1995	200	45	BDI	16
(15) Hasan Zadeh Taheri et al. [28]	Birjand	2011	231	12.1	BDI	14
(16) Moghareb et al. [29]	Birjand	2009	400	45	BDI	16
(17) Frotani [3]	Lar	2005	134	42.5	BDI	16
(18) Najafipour and Yektatalab [30]	Jahrom	2008	150	45.4	BDI	15
(19) Ildar Abadi et al. [1]	Zabol	2002	175	64.3	BDI	16
(20) Ahmadi-Tehrani et al. [31]	Qom	2009	250	62.8	BDI	14
(21) Partoi-Nejad [32]	Qom	2011	600	33.3	GHQ 28	22
(22) Karami [33]	Kashan	2009	208	48	GHQ 28	22
(23) Sooky et al. [34]	Kashan	2010	307	35.8	BDI	16
(24) Raenai et al. [35]	Kordestan	2010	400	37.5	BDI	17
(25) Eslami et al. [36]	Gorgan	2002	202	15.5	BDI	16
(26) Abdollahi et al. [37]	Golestan	2011	132	—	BDI	16
(27) Tavakoli et al. [38]	Gonabad	2001	291	13.4	BDI	15
(28) Ghasemi et al. [39]	Mashhad	2009	780	28.6	BDI	15
(29) Mohtashami-Poor et al. [40]	Mashhad	2001	264	45.3	BDI	16
(30) Abedini et al. [2]	Bandaradas	2007	190	30.2	BDI	16
(31) Hashemi et al. [41]	Yasuj	2003	421	69.2	BDI	16
(32) Hashemi et al. [42]	Hormozgan	2004	452	62	BDI	14
(33) Hashemi and Kamkar [43]	Yasuj	2001	464	35.6	BDI	17
(34) Baghiani Moghadam and Ehrampoosh [44]	Yazd	2006	125	42.4	BDI	16
(35) Baghiani Moghadam et al. [45]	Yazd	2011	185	30	BDI	15

The overall prevalence of depression among university students was 33% (CI 95%: 32–34) (Figure 2). Prevalence of depression among subgroup including male and female students and single and married students was 28% (CI 95%: 26–30), 23% (CI 95%: 22–24), 39% (95%: 37–41), and 20% (CI 95%: 17–24) respectively (Figure 3).

The meta regression of the prevalence of student depression again sample size of studies showed no statistically significant relationship ($P = 0.66$) (Figure 4). Scatter plot year of study and the prevalence of student depression meta regression showed a negative and no statistically significant relationship ($P = 0.70$). Since 1995, the student depression showed a stable trend (Figure 5).

4. Discussion

In this systematic review, we have fully described our search strategy, study selection, data summary, and analysis to allow sensitivity analysis of any aspect of our approach. We have included every study that to our knowledge satisfies our inclusion criteria and employed techniques of estimation that allow integration of studies with high heterogeneity. In situations with high between-study heterogeneity (93.3%), the use of random-effects models is recommended as it produces study weights that primarily reflect the between-study variation and thus provides close-to-equal weighting [13].

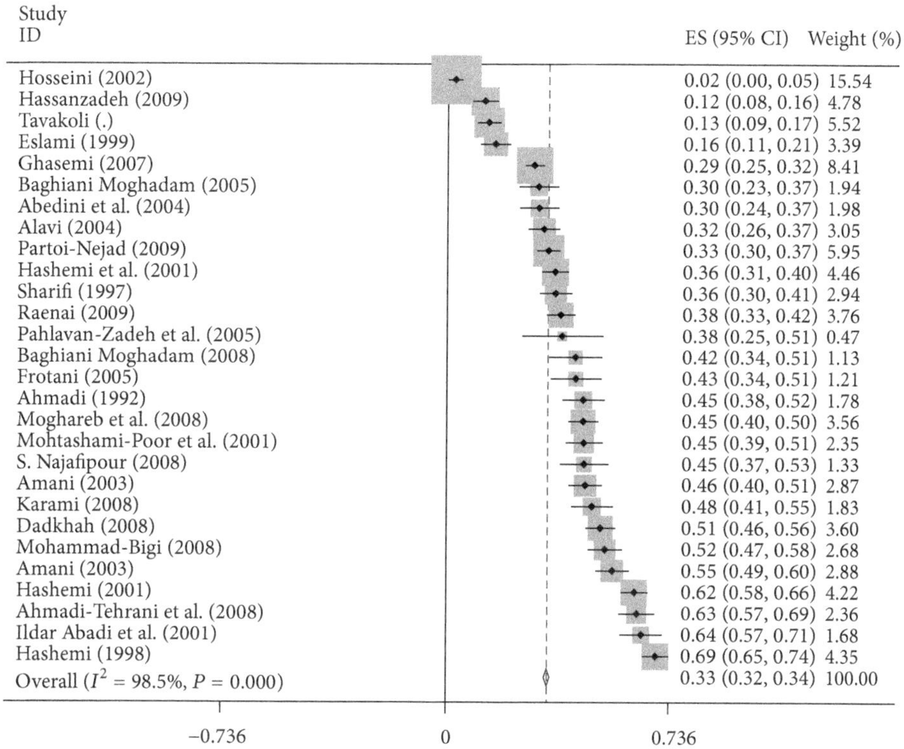

FIGURE 2: Forest plots of student depression for random effects meta-analyses. (Squares represent effect estimates of individual studies with their 95% confidence intervals of depression with size of squares proportional to the weight assigned to the study in the meta-analysis. The diamond represents the overall result and 95% confidence interval of the random-effects meta-analysis.)

In the current study, the Beck depression inventory (BDI) has been utilized to detect the prevalence of depression among university students. Although it is not designed for diagnostic purposes, its epidemiologic utility has been evaluated in several studies, which concluded that it is a reliable and valid instrument for detecting depressive disorders in nonclinical populations. Several studies support the BDI's usefulness in measuring and predicting depression in adolescent samples [46, 47].

The study showed that the prevalence of depression among university student was 33% (CI 95%: 32–34). Steptoe et al. showed that Asian countries had the highest level depressive symptoms [48], which was consistent with our result. The incidence of depression in our study was higher than in other studies, and as Bayram and Bilgel reported that depression were found in 27.1% of Turkish university students [49], Bostanci reported that out of all university students in Denizli, 26.2% had a BDI score of 17 or higher [50]. This variation has been explained to be due to cultural differences, different measurement tools, different methods, and different appraisal standards. University is an important transient life stage, with special academic, financial, and interpersonal pressures. Undergoing these transitions may lead to an increased risk of depression. However, the prevalence of depressive symptoms in the present study is a high incidence rate, more than that seen in average people. Most students who join university in Iran are leaving their homes for the first time. This might subject them to loss of the traditional social support and supervision, in addition to residing with other students and peer relationships. Moreover, there is a change in the style of learning from what the students are used to in school. These changes may act as risk factors to depression in university students in Iran.

We found no differences in depression between genders in our study. Similar to our results, some previous studies [49–51] showed that no differences in depression were observed among male and female students. This might originate from the fact that Iranian female university students have equal experience of the same pressure. However, some studies findings are contrary to our results and found higher levels of depression among female students [50–52].

We found that single students were susceptible to depression compared with married students. This may be because the single students face more stressful events than the married students, such as employment, economic, graduation, and marriage pressures. Contrary to our study, some studies showed that married students reported higher levels of depression [49].

One of the limitations of this study is that the difference in assessment tools and researchers varies in their choice of cut point according to the study location. Secondly, the more studies were observational and patients were not randomly chosen in addition our ability to assess study quality was limited by the fact that many studies failed to offer detailed information on selected subjects or valid data on important factors. Therefore selection bias and confounding

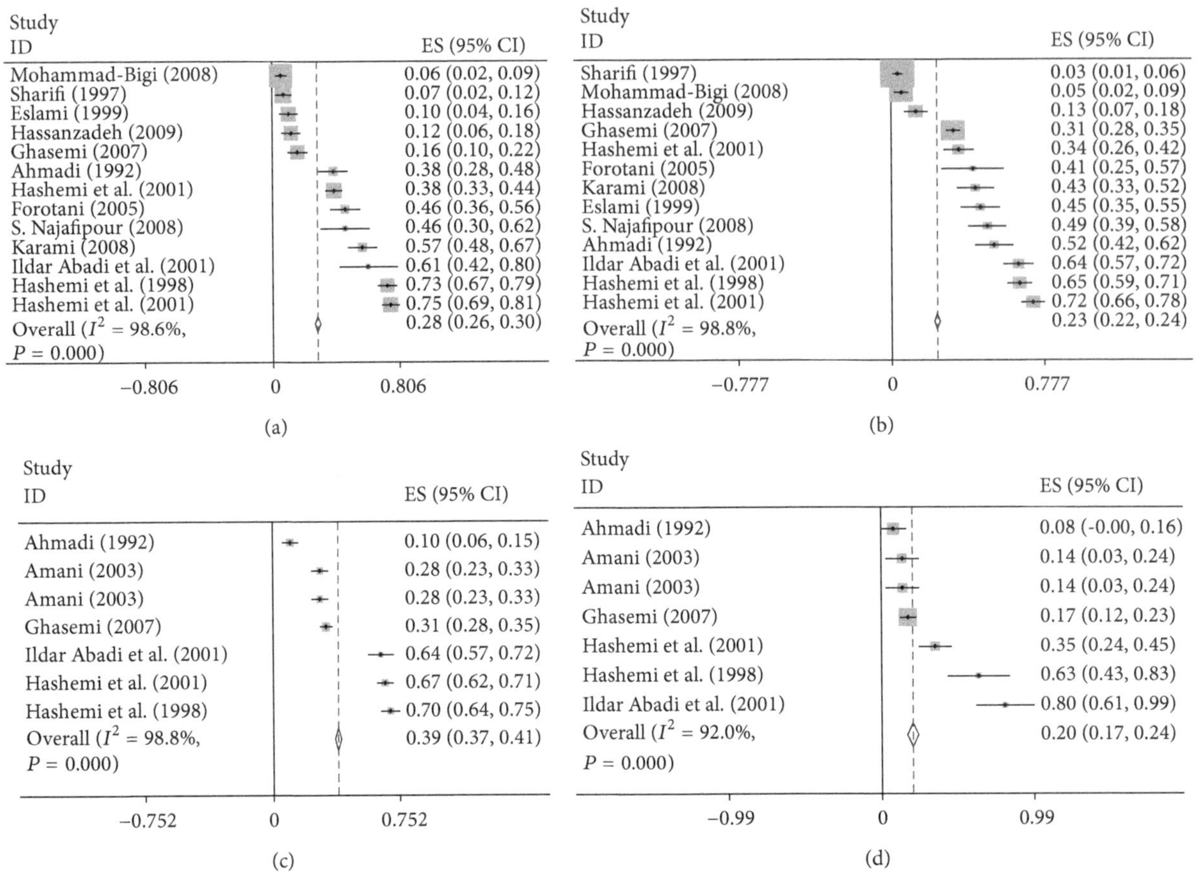

FIGURE 3: Forest plots of student depression for subgroups analysis (forest plot (a) depression among male students, (b) among female students, (c) among single students, and (d) among married students).

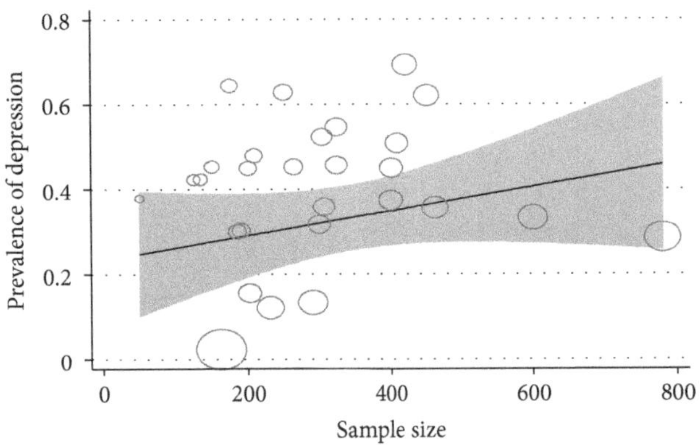

FIGURE 4: Meta-regression plots of change in depression according to changes in continuous study moderator's sample size.

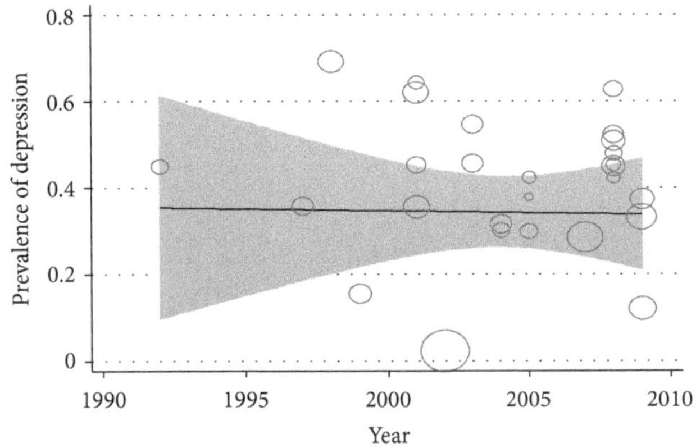

FIGURE 5: Meta-regression plots of change in depression according to changes in continuous study moderator's year.

seem inevitable. Thirdly, many of our data were extracted from the internal databases in Iran.

5. Conclusion

In summary, we found that depression is common in university students with no preponderance between males and females and in single students is higher than married ones. Our findings point to importance of screening of this vulnerable population and taking appropriate interventional measures to prevent the complications of depression. Further research studying sociodemographic factors and the effect of depression on the academic performance is needed.

Conflict of Interests

The authors declare no conflict of interests.

Acknowledgment

This study was supported financially by Ilam University of Medical Sciences, Ilam, Iran.

References

[1] E. Ildar Abadi, M. Firouz Kouhi, S. Mazloum, and A. Navidian, "Prevalence of depression among students of Zabol Medical School, 2002," *Journal of Shahrekord University of Medical Sciences*, vol. 6, no. 2, pp. 15–21, 2004.

[2] S. Abedini, A. Davachi, F. Sohbaee, M. Mahmoodi, and O. Safa, "Prevalence of depression in nursing students in Hormozgan University of Medical Sciences," *Hormozgan Medical Journal*, vol. 11, 42, no. 2, pp. 139–145, 2007.

[3] M. Frotani, "Depression in students of higher education centers," *Iranian Journal of Nursing Research*, vol. 18, no. 41-42, pp. 13–27, 2005.

[4] J. L. Buchanan, "Prevention of depression in the college student population: a review of the literature," *Archives of Psychiatric Nursing*, vol. 26, no. 1, pp. 21–42, 2012.

[5] T. Eller, A. Aluoja, V. Vasar, and M. Veldi, "Symptoms of anxiety and depression in Estonian medical students with sleep problems," *Depression and Anxiety*, vol. 23, no. 4, pp. 250–256, 2006.

[6] A. K. Ibrahim, S. J. Kelly, and C. Glazebrook, "Reliability of a shortened version of the Zagazig Depression Scale and prevalence of depression in an Egyptian university student sample," *Comprehensive Psychiatry*, vol. 53, no. 5, pp. 638–647, 2012.

[7] J. S. R. Mahmoud, R. T. Staten, L. A. Hall, and T. A. Lennie, "The relationship among young adult college students' depression, anxiety, stress, demographics, life satisfaction, and coping styles," *Issues in Mental Health Nursing*, vol. 33, no. 3, pp. 149–156, 2012.

[8] N. Reavley and A. F. Jorm, "Prevention and early intervention to improve mental health in higher education students: a review," *Early Intervention in Psychiatry*, vol. 4, no. 2, pp. 132–142, 2010.

[9] J. M. Castaldelli-Maia, S. S. Martins, D. Bhugra et al., "Does ragging play a role in medical student depression—cause or effect?" *Journal of Affective Disorders*, vol. 139, no. 3, pp. 291–297, 2012.

[10] P. Grossman, L. Niemann, S. Schmidt, and H. Walach, "Mindfulness-based stress reduction and health benefits: a meta-analysis," *Journal of Psychosomatic Research*, vol. 57, no. 1, pp. 35–43, 2004.

[11] E. von Elm, D. G. Altman, M. Egger, S. J. Pocock, P. C. Gøtzsche, and J. P. Vandenbroucke, "The Strengthening the Reporting of Observational Studies in Epidemiology (STROBE) statement: guidelines for reporting observational studies," *The Lancet*, vol. 370, no. 9596, pp. 1453–1457, 2007.

[12] R. Der Simonian and N. Laird, "Meta-analysis in clinical trials," *Controlled Clinical Trials*, vol. 7, no. 3, pp. 177–188, 1986.

[13] A. E. Ades, G. Lu, and J. P. T. Higgins, "The interpretation of random-effects meta-analysis in decision models," *Medical Decision Making*, vol. 25, no. 6, pp. 646–654, 2005.

[14] H. Bahrami Dashtaki, "Spirituality as a way of teaching effectiveness in reducing depression in students," *Counseling Research & Developments*, vol. 5, no. 19, pp. 47–73, 2005.

[15] Y. Mohammadian, "Evaluating the use of poetry to reduce signs of depression in students," *Journal of Ilam University of Medical Sciences*, vol. 18, no. 2, pp. 9–16, 2010.

[16] K. Alavi, "Effectiveness of dialectical behavior therapy group practices (with emphasis on the fundamental components of pervasive awareness, distress tolerance, and emotional regulation), on depressive symptoms in students," *The Journal of Fundamentals of Mental Health*, vol. 13, no. 50, pp. 35–47, 2011.

[17] A. Hosseini, "Introduction of changes in medical students' attitudes and Depression—using group education," *The Journal of Fundamentals of Mental Health*, vol. 4, no. 13-14, pp. 13–23, 2002.

[18] J. Bahadori Khosroshahi, "Relationship between stressful life events and sense of humor with depression in students," *Zahedan Journal of Research in Medical Sciences*, vol. 9, no. 51, pp. 27–53, 2010.

[19] A. Biani, "The relationship between religious orientation and depression and anxiety in students," *The Journal of Fundamentals of Mental Health*, vol. 10, no. 39, pp. 191–199, 2008.

[20] A. Mohammad-Bigi, N. Mohammad-Salehi, F. Ghamari, and B. Salehi, "Prevalence of depressive symptoms, general health status and risk factors in students of Arak University dormitory 2008," *Arak Medical University Journal*, vol. 12, 48, no. 3, pp. 116–124, 2009.

[21] F. Amani, B. Sohrabi, S. Sadeghieh, and M. Mash'oufi, "Prevalence of depression in students of medical sciences 2003," *Journal of Ardabil University of Medical Sciences*, vol. 4, no. 11, pp. 7–9, 2004.

[22] B. Dadkhah, "Prayer association with depression in medical students," *Teb va Tazkiyeh*, vol. 18, no. 3-4, pp. 23–29, 2009.

[23] S. Pahlavan-Zadeh, M. Kiassat Poor, and M. Nassiri, "Depression in athletes and non-athlete students of Isfahan University of Medical Sciences," *Journal of Research in Behavioural Sciences*, vol. 4, 8, no. 1-2, pp. 26–32, 2006.

[24] Z. Ranjbar-Kohan and M. Sajjadi Nejad, "Effect of assertiveness training on self-esteem and depression in university students," *Birjand University of Medical Sciences*, vol. 17, 45, no. 4, pp. 308–316, 2010.

[25] B. Makvandi, A. Heidari, M. Shahany, B. Najarian, and P. Askari, "The relationship between alexithymia and anxiety and depression in female students of Islamic Azad University of Ahvaz," *Knowledge & Research in Applied Psychology*, vol. 13, 47, no. 1, pp. 83–92, 2012.

[26] B. Makvandi, "The relationship between alexithymia and anxiety and depression in female students of Islamic Azad University of Ahvaz," *Journal of Women in Culture Arts*, vol. 2, no. 6, pp. 83–92, 2010.

[27] J. Ahmadi, "Rate of depression among medical students (Ahwaz 1992)," *Thought and Behavior in Clinical Psychology*, vol. 1, no. 4, pp. 13–21, 1995.

[28] M. Hasan Zadeh Taheri, M. Moghareb, E. Ekhbari, M. Raissun, and M. Hassanzadeh Taheri, "Prevalence of depression among new students of Birjand University of Medical Sciences in the year 2009-2010," *Birjand University of Medical Sciences*, vol. 18, 47, no. 2, pp. 109–117, 2011.

[29] M. Moghareb, M. Qnadkafy, and N. Rezaei, "The relationship between prayer and depressive in Birjand University of Medical Sciences," *Journal of Nursing and Midwifery, Birjand University of Medical Sciences*, vol. 6, 24, no. 1–4, pp. 54–60, 2009.

[30] S. Najafipour and S. Yektatalab, "The prevalence of depression in University of Medical Sciences of Jahrom," *Journal of Jahrom Uiversity of Medical Sciences*, vol. 6, no. 6, pp. 27–38, 2008.

[31] H. Ahmadi-Tehrani, A. Haidari, A. Kachuei, M. Moghiseh, and M. Irani, "The association between depression and religious

attitude towards Qom University of Medical Sciences, 2008," *Qom University of Medical Sciences Journal*, vol. 3, 11, no. 3, pp. 51–56, 2009.

[32] Partoi-Nejad, "Comparison of depression in medical college students and scholars of Qom Seminary, 2008," *Qom University of Medical Sciences Journal*, vol. 5, no. 3, pp. 49–52, 2011.

[33] M. Karami, "Depression in college of paramedical kashan university of medical sciences, 2008," *Journal of Urmia Nursing and Midwifery Faculty*, vol. 7, no. 3, pp. 166–172, 2009.

[34] Z. Sooky, K. Sharifi, Z. Tagharrobi, H. Akbari, and E. Mesdaghinia, "Depression prevalence and its correlation with the psychosocial need satisfaction among Kashan high-school female students," *Feyz Journal of Kashan University of Medical Sciences*, vol. 14, no. 3, serial 55, pp. 257–263, 2010.

[35] F. Raenai, F. Ardalan, and F. Zaheri, "Attitude and practice of prayer and its relationship with depression in students of Kurdistan University of Medical Sciences in 2009," *Teb va Tazkiyeh*, vol. 19, no. 4, pp. 75–85, 2010.

[36] A.-A. Eslami, M.-A. Vakili, and J. Faraji, "Depression among medical students of Gorgan and its relation to spend leisure time," *Journal of Gorgan University of Medical Sciences*, vol. 4, no. 9, pp. 52–60, 2002.

[37] A. Abdollahi, H. Asaiesh, Y. Jafari, and M. Rezaeian, "University of Medical Sciences Students' Mental Health: arrival in university and after one year," *Journal of Gorgan Bouyeh Faculty of Nursing & Midwifery*, vol. 8, 19, no. 1, pp. 52–59, 2011.

[38] J. Tavakoli, M. Ghahramani, F. Haddizadeh Talasaz, and H. Chamanzari, "Mental health status of in young smokers and non smokers Gonabad city," *Horizon of Medical Sciences*, vol. 9, no. 1, pp. 1–9, 2001.

[39] M. Ghasemi, F. Rajbnia, V. Seadtian, and M. Meshkat, "Depression and its influencing factors in medical and paramedical students of Islamic Azad University of Mashhad, 2008-2009," *Journal of Medival Science*, vol. 4, 15, no. 3, pp. 173–180, 2009.

[40] E. Mohtashami-Poor, M. Mohtashami-Poor, F. Shadlou Mashhadi, A. Emadzadeh, and H. Hassan Abadi, "Prayer relationship with depression in college students Mashhad University of Medical Sciences," *Horizon of Medical Sciences*, vol. 9, no. 1, pp. 61–69, 2001.

[41] N. Hashemi, M. Baghri, and H.-R. Ghafarian, "Factors associated with depression in university students Yasuj—2001," *Journal of Medical Research*, vol. 2, 5, no. 1, pp. 19–28, 2003.

[42] N. Hashemi, Z. Hoseini, and M.-A. Shahami, "Epidemiological studies of depression among university students Yasouj," *Teb va Tazkiyeh*, vol. 13, no. 2, p. 128, 2004.

[43] N. Hashemi and A. Kamkar, "Prevalence of depression in students of medical sciences," *Armaghan Danesh, Biomonthly Yasuj University of Medical Research Sciences Journal*, vol. 6, no. 21, pp. 14–21, 2001.

[44] M.-H. Baghiani Moghadam and M.-H. Ehrampoosh, "Depression in of medical sciences students of Yazd and its relationship to academic factors," *Tolooe Behdasht*, vol. 5, no. 1-2, p. 92, 2006.

[45] M.-H. Baghiani Moghadam, M.-H. Ehrampoosh, B. Rahimi, A.-H. Aminian, and M. Aram, "Assessment of depression among college students in health and nursing Yazd University of Medical Sciences in 2008," *Journal of Medical Education Development Center*, vol. 6, no. 1, pp. 17–24, 2011.

[46] S. K. Ganesh, J. Animesh, and H. Supriya, "Prevalence of depression and its associated factors using Beck Depression Inventory among students of a medical college in Karnataka," *Indian Journal of Psychiatry*, vol. 54, no. 3, pp. 223–226, 2012.

[47] L. Teri, "The use of the Beck Depression Inventory with adolescents," *Journal of Abnormal Child Psychology*, vol. 10, no. 2, pp. 277–284, 1982.

[48] A. Steptoe, A. Tsuda, Y. Tanaka, and J. Wardle, "Depressive symptoms, socio-economic background, sense of control, and cultural factors in university students from 23 countries," *International Journal of Behavioral Medicine*, vol. 14, no. 2, pp. 97–107, 2007.

[49] N. Bayram and N. Bilgel, "The prevalence and socio-demographic correlations of depression, anxiety and stress among a group of university students," *Social Psychiatry and Psychiatric Epidemiology*, vol. 43, no. 8, pp. 667–672, 2008.

[50] M. Bostanci, O. Ozdel, N. K. Oguzhanoglu et al., "Depressive symptomatology among university students in Denizli, Turkey: prevalence and sociodemographic correlates," *Croatian Medical Journal*, vol. 46, no. 1, pp. 96–100, 2005.

[51] K. Grant, P. Marsh, G. Syniar et al., "Gender differences in rates of depression among undergraduates: measurement matters," *Journal of Adolescence*, vol. 25, no. 6, pp. 613–617, 2002.

[52] T. J. Wade, J. Cairney, and D. J. Pevalin, "Emergence of gender differences in depression during adolescence: national panel results from three countries," *Journal of the American Academy of Child & Adolescent Psychiatry*, vol. 41, no. 2, pp. 190–198, 2002.

6

Predicting Depression with Psychopathology and Temperament Traits: The Northern Finland 1966 Birth Cohort

Jouko Miettunen,[1,2] Matti Isohanni,[1,2] Tiina Paunio,[3] Nelson Freimer,[4] Anja Taanila,[5,6] Jesper Ekelund,[7] Marjo-Riitta Järvelin,[5,8] Matti Joukamaa,[9,10] Dirk Lichtermann,[11] Heli Koivumaa-Honkanen,[12,13,14,15,16,17] and Juha Veijola[1,2]

[1] *Department of Psychiatry, Institute of Clinical Medicine, University of Oulu, P.O. Box 5000, 90014 Oulu, Finland*
[2] *Clinic of Psychiatry, Oulu University Hospital, Oulu, Finland*
[3] *Department of Chronic Disease Prevention, National Institute for Health and Welfare, Haartmaninkatu 8, 00251 Helsinki, Finland*
[4] *UCLA Center for Neurobehavioral Genetics, Semel Institute for Neuroscience and Human Behavior, Gonda Building, Room 3506, 695 Charles E. Young Drive South, Los Angeles, CA 90095, USA*
[5] *Institute of Health Sciences, University of Oulu, P.O. Box 5000, 90014 Oulu, Finland*
[6] *Unit of General Practice, Oulu University Hospital, 90029 Oulu, Finland*
[7] *Department of Mental Health and Substance Use Services, National Institute for Health and Welfare, P.O. Box 30, 00271 Helsinki, Finland*
[8] *Department of Epidemiology and Biostatistics, Imperial College London, London SW7 2AZ, UK*
[9] *Social Psychiatry Unit, School of Health Sciences, University of Tampere, 33014 Tampere, Finland*
[10] *Department of Psychiatry, Tampere University Hospital, Tampere, Finland*
[11] *Methadone Maintenance Clinic "Café Ersatz", Münsterstraße 18, 53111 Bonn, Germany*
[12] *Department of Psychiatry, University of Eastern Finland and Kuopio University Hospital, P.O. Box 1777, 70211 Kuopio, Finland*
[13] *Department of Psychiatry, South-Savonia Hospital District, Mikkeli, Finland*
[14] *Department of Psychiatry, North Karelia Central Hospital, Joensuu, Finland*
[15] *Department of Psychiatry, SOSTERI, Savonlinna, Finland*
[16] *Department of Psychiatry, SOTE, Iisalmi, Finland*
[17] *Department of Psychiatry, Lapland Hospital District, Rovaniemi, Finland*

Correspondence should be addressed to Jouko Miettunen, jouko.miettunen@oulu.fi

Academic Editor: Toshinori Kitamura

We studied the concurrent, predictive, and discriminate validity of psychopathology scales (e.g., schizotypal and depressive) and temperament traits for hospitalisations due to major depression. Temperament, perceptual aberration, physical and social anhedonia, Depression Subscale of Symptom Checklist (SCL-D), Hypomanic Personality Scale, Schizoidia Scale, and Bipolar II Scale were completed as part of the 31-year follow-up survey of the prospective Northern Finland 1966 Birth Cohort ($n = 4941$; 2214 males). Several of the scales were related to depression. Concurrent depression was especially related to higher perceptual aberration (effect size when compared to controls, $d = 1.29$), subsequent depression to high scores in SCL-D ($d = 0.48$). Physical anhedonia was lower in subjects with subsequent depression than those with other psychiatric disorders ($d = -0.33$, nonsignificant). Participants with concurrent ($d = 0.70$) and subsequent ($d = 0.54$) depression had high harm avoidance compared to controls, while differences compared to other psychiatric patients were small. Subjects with depression differed from healthy controls in most of the scales. Many of the scales were useful predictors for future hospital treatments, but were not diagnosis-specific. High harm avoidance is a potential indicator for subsequent depression.

1. Introduction

Several studies have attempted to predict psychiatric symptoms or disorders using various psychological and psychiatric instruments [1, 2]. These scales have clinical importance, for example, when identifying high-risk individuals. They may also help to detect intermediate phenotypes for psychiatric disorders [3]. Potential psychopathological intermediate phenotypes of depression include, for example, depressed mood and anhedonia [4]. The objectiveness of these scales adds to their usefulness in etiological research of psychiatric disorders [5].

Numerous instruments have been used to evaluate depressive symptoms in the general population. For instance, the Symptom Checklist was developed to screen for depression and anxiety in the general population [6]. Personality traits, such as those measured with Cloninger's [7] temperament dimensions, have been associated with several psychiatric disorders [8]. Particularly high harm avoidance has been associated with depression [8]. The previous longitudinal studies in relation to depression are very few and have included relatively short follow-up period [9, 10]. These studies indicate that harm avoidance may be a phenotypic indicator for risk of depressive episodes [10]. Schizotypal traits, such as anhedonia, are key features both in schizophrenia and depression. In patients with schizophrenia, anhedonia has been strongly associated with the depressive syndrome [11].

The aim of the present study was to evaluate the concurrent, predictive, and discriminate validity of several psychological scales for depression, using a large representative population based sample of adults, with adequate followup. Our hypothesis was that subjects with either concurrent or subsequent depression would score differently in schizotypal and depressive symptom scales and temperament dimensions, when compared to subjects with other psychiatric disorders or healthy controls.

2. Material and Methods

2.1. Participants. The Northern Finland 1966 Birth Cohort (NFBC 1966) is an unselected, general population-based birth cohort ascertained during mid-pregnancy. It comprised of 12,058 live-born children in the Finnish provinces of Lapland and Oulu [12]. We required that all subjects had been living in Finland at the age of 16 (n = 10,933; 5,589 males and 5,344 females), as we have previously validated psychiatric diagnoses from the Finnish Hospital Discharge Register in this subsample [13, 14]. Permission to gather data was obtained from the Ministry of Social and Health Affairs and the study design has been approved by, and is under review of, the Ethical Committee of The Northern Ostrobothnia Hospital District. After complete description of the study, written informed consent was obtained from study participants.

In 1997, the questionnaires used for the 31-year followup of the cohort included a large collection of psychopathology scales and four temperament dimensions that were given to all cohort members who participated in a clinical examination [15]. Participants completed these scales at home and returned them in the envelopes provided. The 12-item version of the Infrequency Scale [16] was used to assess careless responding. It contains items that are very unlikely to be true and identifies random response styles. Participants who endorsed three or more items (n = 105) on this scale were excluded from further analyses. The Symptom Checklist-25 [6, 17, 18] was sent, by post, in a different set of questions, together with several sociodemographic questions and an invitation letter for the clinical examination. In total, 4,941 participants (2,214 males and 2,727 females) adequately completed at least one of these scales.

The Finnish Hospital Discharge Register (FHDR) covers all mental and general hospitals as well as beds in local health centres, prison and military hospitals and private hospitals nationwide. All cohort members, over 16 years old, appearing on the FHDR until the end of 1997 for any mental disorder were identified and their diagnoses were rechecked twice by psychiatrists using DSM-III-R criteria [19]. The reliability of this procedure was moderate for depression κ = 0.57). A more detailed description of the validation process is presented elsewhere [13, 14].

Data was also collected from postal questionnaires sent to all subjects in 1977 and outpatient treatments with self-re- ported diagnoses. Subjects were asked whether they had any of the following: depression, psychosis, alcohol use disorder, other substance use disorder, or any other psychiatric disorder diagnosed by a medical doctor. Three groups were formed: "depressive disorder" (n = 204; 68 males, 33%), "other psychiatric disorders" (n = 150; 77 males, 51%), and "no psychiatric disorders" (n = 4587; 2069 males, 45%). The "depressive disorder" group included subjects with validated hospital care diagnoses of psychotic depression (DSM-III-R codes: 296.24 and 296.34; n = 2) or nonpsychotic depression (296.22, 296.23, 296.31, 296.33, and 311.00; n = 20), or self-reported depressions (n = 182). "Other psychiatric disorders" included subjects with other psychiatric diagnoses based on either hospital (n = 70) or self-reported data (n = 80). In the followup, the same groups were used, but only with nonvalidated data from the FHDR from 1998 to 2010, classified as described above. The distribution of the diagnoses for major depressive disorders (ICD-10 diagnoses: F32-F33 and F341) are presented in Section 3.

When comparing the final sample at the 31-year followup to subjects alive at the age of 16 years, females participated more commonly than males (51.4% versus 40.4%; χ^2 134.81, $P < 0.001$) and those with tertiary (more than 12 years) and secondary level (10–12 years) education more commonly than those with basic level (9 or less years) education (49.5% and 49.7% versus 25.1%; χ^2 343.73, degrees of freedom = 2, $P < 0.001$). The attrition analyses for the 31-year follow-up study have previously been described in detail. For individuals with psychiatric hospital diagnoses until 1997, the participation rate was 42% among those with mood disorders and 54% among controls [15].

2.2. Instruments. The questionnaire given to subjects consisted of mental health related true/false questions, which were collected from several psychopathology (e.g., schizotypal) scales and four temperament subscales. All these items, and the 12 items from the Infrequency Scale, were randomly rearranged into a 354-item questionnaire, called "Survey of Opinions and Experiences." We used the temperament subscales (novelty seeking, harm avoidance, reward dependence, and persistence) from the Temperament and Character Inventory (TCI). The schizotypal scales were the following: Physical Anhedonia Scale (PAS), Social Anhedonia Scale (SAS), Perceptual Aberration Scale (PER), Hypomanic Personality Scale (HPS), Bipolar II Scale (BIP2), and Schizoidia Scale (SCHD). From a separate survey, we included the depression subscale (15 items) of Symptom Checklist (SCL-D) in order to also assess depressive symptoms. The answers to SCL are scored on a scale from 1 (not bothered) to 4 (extremely bothered) [6]. The references and short descriptions for the scales are presented in Table 1. Firstly, we studied these scales in respect to previous hospitalization or current self-reported psychiatric diagnosis in 1997. Secondly, among those without previous psychiatric diagnosis in 1997, these scales were studied in respect to subsequent hospitalizations due to psychiatric causes between 1998 and 2010.

The original English versions of the scales, except SCL-25, were translated into Finnish by one investigator and then back-translated blindly to the original English scale by a professional English translator. The original version and the back-translation were compared, and corrections were made accordingly. The translation was tested in a sample of 50 laboratory workers, and the results indicated that no questions required revision. We used an earlier Finnish translation of the SCL in the current study. We have previously presented validity results in this sample for the SCL-25 [18], temperament [26], and schizotypal scales [27].

2.3. Statistical Methods. We present means, standard deviations (SD), and Student's t-tests for continuous variables. Mean scores between different groups were compared using effect sizes (Cohen's d) and two-way analysis of variance, where diagnostic group and gender were used as grouping variables and scale scores as dependent variables. Gender was used as a covariate, as previous meta-analyses have found gender differences in these scales [28, 29]. Cohen [30] interpreted d values of 0.2 to 0.5 as small, 0.5 to 0.8 as medium, and 0.8 or over as large effects. We studied associations of all the scales both to depressions and to other psychiatric disorders in order to estimate the specificity of the scales. As substance use disorder is a common diagnosis in other psychiatric diagnoses and a common comorbid diagnosis in depression, we performed additional analysis with substance abuse as a covariate in analysis of variance. All tests are two-tailed. The data was analyzed using the IBM SPSS v. 20.

3. Results

Table 2 shows mean (SD) values for the different scales in categories of concurrent depression, other psychiatric disorders, and no psychiatric disorders. In 1997, those with depression scored statistically significantly ($P < 0.05$) higher than those without previous psychiatric disorders in all studied psychopathology scales, except PAS. The difference was highest in SCL-D (means 1.78 versus 1.33, $d = 1.29$) followed by perceptual aberration scale (means 5.09 versus 2.24, $d = 0.90$). In temperament dimensions, this difference was statistically significant only in TCI-HA, with higher scores among those with depression ($d = 0.70$). Almost all the scales were related to depression. However, it was only in SCL-D that those with depression differed statistically significantly from those with other psychiatric disorders with a small effect size ($d = 0.20$). No significant differences between these two groups were found in temperament dimensions (Table 2).

Among those with no psychiatric disorders until 1997, 51 (26 males, 51%) new cases with depression requiring hospitalizations emerged during the subsequent followup of thirteen years. This group included subjects with psychotic depression (F323, F333), $n = 9$ and nonpsychotic depression (F32-F33, not F323, F33; F341), $n = 42$. In this followup, 57 (36 males, 63%) individuals were hospitalized for other psychiatric disorders. This group included various psychiatric diagnoses. The most common diagnoses were substance use disorder ($n = 30$), nonaffective psychosis ($n = 14$), and anxiety disorders ($n = 12$).

Of the psychopathology scales, the bipolar II scale ($d = 0.52$), SCL-D ($d = 0.48$), SCHD ($d = 0.46$), and SAS ($d = 0.45$) were the strongest predictors for new cases of depression requiring hospitalization. However, the scales were not diagnosis-specific. The greatest difference between depression and other psychiatric disorders requiring hospitalization ($d = -0.33$; NS) was found in PAS.

In temperament dimensions, new cases of depression requiring hospitalization scored high in the harm avoidance when compared to those with no hospitalization due to psychiatric causes (16.96 versus 13.77; $P < 0.001$, $d = 0.54$). No significant differences were found between the two psychiatric groups. Novelty seeking had the highest effect size (ns, $d = -0.32$), with lower scores among those with hospitalization due to depression. In additional analyses, between those with depression and other psychiatric disorders we controlled for substance use disorders. The difference between these two groups was statistically significant in harm avoidance in concurrent analyses ($F = 7.12$, $P = 0.008$) with higher scores among those with hospitalization due to depression. Differences in other temperament traits or in predictive analyses were nonsignificant (Table 3).

4. Discussion

We studied the concurrent, predictive, and discriminate validity of several psychopathology scales and temperamental dimensions in relation to depression. Many of them were related to depression but also to other psychiatric disorders.

Table 1: Psychological scales used in the 31-year followup of the Northern Finland 1966 Birth Cohort.

Instrument (abbreviation)	Number of items	Description of high scorers	Reference(s)
Revised Physical Anhedonia Scale (PAS)	61	Lowered ability to experience physical and sensory pleasures	Chapman et al., [20]
Revised Social Anhedonia Scale (SAS)	40	Schizoid lack of interest in social interaction	Chapman et al., [20]; Eckbladet al., [21]
Perceptual Aberration Scale (PER)	35	Have distorted perception of own body and other objects	Chapman et al., [22]
Hypomanic Personality Scale (HPS)	48	Energetic, upbeat, gregarious people, often able to work long hours	Eckblad and Chapman, [23]
Bipolar II Scale (BIP2)	31	Designed to predict bipolar II disorder among unipolar subjects	Akiskal et al., [24]
Schizoidia Scale (SCHD)	7	Minnesota Multiphasic Personality Inventory (MMPI) items that as pooled best detect schizophrenia	Golden and Meehl, [25]
Symptom Check-List, Depression subscale (SCL-D)	13	Used as a screen for depression in normal population	Derogatis et al., [6]; Fink et al., [17]
Temperament and Character Inventory (TCI) subscales:			
(i) novelty seeking (TCI-NS)	40	Respond with intense excitement to novel stimuli	Cloninger et al., [7]
(ii) harm avoidance (TCI-HA)	35	Subjects with tendency to respond intensively to signals of aversive stimuli, thereby inhibiting/stopping behaviour	Cloninger et al., [7]
(iii) reward dependence (TCI-RD)	24	Respond intensely to signals of reward	Cloninger et al., [7]
(iv) persistence (TCI-P)	8	Subjects with tendency to persevere in behaviours associated with reward	Cloninger et al., [7]

Harm avoidance ($d = 0.54$) as a temperament dimension and the bipolar II scale ($d = 0.52$) best predicted depression, and also the depression subscale of the SCL associated with depression, especially concurrently ($d = 1.29$). These findings reflect the relatively high predictive value of the scales and confirm their utility as clinical tools for the identification of individuals at risk for psychiatric disorders. None of the scales discriminated well subjects with depression from subjects with other psychiatric disorders. However, when we took into account substance use disorders as a covariate in concurrent analyses, individuals with depression scored statistically significantly higher in harm avoidance than those with other psychiatric disorders.

4.1. Schizotypal Scales. We found that many of the psychopathology scales related to both concurrent and subsequent depression. However, these scales were not diagnosis-specific as these traits were also common in other psychiatric disorders. In the schizotypal (PAS, SAS, and PER) scales, there have been some previous case-control studies in depression, with small sample sizes. These studies have found large effect sizes between psychiatric cases and healthy controls (e.g., students), with cases scoring higher in all of them. In physical anhedonia, effect sizes have varied between 0.92 [31] and 1.79 [32], and in social anhedonia between 0.86 [33] and 1.19 [34]. In perceptual aberration, Katsanis et al. [33] found depressive patients scored higher than healthy controls, with an effect size of 0.57. Loas et al. [35] note that physical anhedonia in depressed patients seems to relate to the severity of the depression and does not appear to identify quantitatively distinct subgroup.

We have previously studied these schizotypal scales in schizophrenia [36]. Individuals with concurrent depression ($n = 202$) scored lower than those with schizophrenia ($n = 29$) in all schizotypal scales, for example, in physical anhedonia, mean score in schizophrenia was 18.38 and in depression 14.68. When predicting these disorders, differences in scores were smaller; however, those with subsequent schizophrenia scored substantially higher in perceptual aberration (means 4.30 versus 2.96) and hypomanic personality (17.10 versus 12.37) than those with subsequent depression. Interestingly, our results contradict some previous studies such as Blanchard et al. [34], who found that depressive patients had higher scores for social anhedonia than schizophrenia patients (means 18 versus 15). They concluded that schizophrenia patients seem to have stable high scores in social anhedonia whereas, in depressive patients, it correlates with the clinical state. These differences may relate to our sample being based on lifetime diagnoses in population, including also individuals without current treatment or symptoms.

Table 2: Mean and standard deviation (SD) of psychological scales in the 31-year followup (in 1997) for those with self-report or previous hospitalisation due to depression, other psychiatric disorders, and for those without psychiatric disorders.

	(A) Depression until 1997			(B) Other psychiatric disorders until 1997			(C) No psychiatric disorders until 1997			Effect sizes (Cohen's *d*)		
	N	Mean	SD	*N*	Mean	SD	*N*	Mean	SD	(A) versus (B) *F* (*d*)	(A) versus (C) *F* (*d*)	(B) versus (C) *F* (*d*)
Psychopathology scales:												
Physical Anhedonia Scale (PAS)	202	14.68	8.19	149	16.34	7.86	4572	15.02	6.97	0.74 (−0.21)	0.49 (−0.05)	5.24* (0.19)
Social Anhedonia Scale (SAS)	200	11.60	6.78	146	11.99	6.75	4569	9.33	5.43	0.00 (−0.06)	48.43*** (0.41)	31.54*** (0.49)
Perceptual Aberration Scale (PER)	202	5.09	5.64	147	4.29	5.85	4568	2.24	3.04	3.86 (0.14)	149.00*** (0.90)	34.05*** (0.65)
Hypomanic Personality Scale (HPS)	201	15.11	7.44	147	15.07	8.78	4571	11.07	6.92	0.26 (0.01)	60.89*** (0.58)	29.44*** (0.57)
Bipolar II Scale (BIP2)	202	12.99	4.46	148	12.91	4.39	4577	10.47	3.73	0.57 (0.02)	88.75*** (0.67)	42.63*** (0.65)
Schizoidia Scale (SCHD)	202	3.51	1.61	147	3.31	1.56	4578	2.51	1.39	1.21 (0.13)	89.90*** (0.72)	39.89*** (0.57)
SCL-Depression (SCL-D)	202	1.78	0.58	144	1.66	0.56	4571	1.33	0.33	4.54* (0.20)	310.90*** (1.29)	92.19*** (0.97)
Temperament dimensions:												
novelty seeking (TCI-NS)	200	21.29	5.82	145	21.84	6.13	4534	20.34	5.86	0.83 (−0.09)	3.62 (0.16)	6.91** (0.26)
harm avoidance (TCI-HA)	200	18.09	7.36	145	17.21	6.64	4534	13.82	6.00	0.94 (0.12)	86.49*** (0.70)	42.03*** (0.56)
reward dependence (TCI-RD)	200	14.95	3.95	145	14.30	3.89	4534	14.74	3.78	0.23 (0.16)	0.31 (0.05)	1.40 (−0.12)
persistence (TCI-P)	200	4.28	1.86	145	4.09	1.89	4534	4.31	1.74	0.66 (0.10)	0.02 (−0.02)	2.76 (−0.12)

TCI: Temperament and Character Inventory. Mean values in categories are compared using two-way analysis of variance (ANOVA), with diagnostic group and gender as independent variables. Statistical significant effect sizes are marked with asterisks as follows: $^{*}P < 0.05$, $^{**}P < 0.01$, and $^{***}P < 0.001$.

Table 3: Mean and standard deviation (SD) of psychological scales in the 31-year followup (in 1997) for those with hospitalisation of depression or other psychiatric disorders and for those without hospitalization due to psychiatric disorders in 1998–2010.

	(A) Depression in 1998–2010			(B) Other psychiatric disorders in 1998–2010			(C) No psychiatric disorders until 2010			Effect sizes (Cohen's *d*)		
										(A) versus (B)	(A) versus (C)	(B) versus (C)
	N	Mean	SD	*N*	Mean	SD	*N*	Mean	SD	*F* (*d*)	*F* (*d*)	*F* (*d*)
Psychopathology scales:												
Physical Anhedonia Scale (PAS)	51	15.88	6.08	57	18.07	7.24	4464	14.97	6.97	1.77 (−0.33)	0.43 (0.13)	6.16* (0.44)
Social Anhedonia Scale (SAS)	51	11.69	5.82	57	11.98	6.78	4461	9.27	5.39	0.00 (−0.05)	9.37** (0.45)	9.75** (0.50)
Perceptual Aberration Scale (PER)	51	2.96	2.75	57	2.95	3.45	4460	2.22	3.04	0.04 (0.00)	3.30 (0.24)	4.12* (0.24)
Hypomanic Personality Scale (HPS)	51	12.37	6.65	57	12.32	8.19	4463	11.04	6.91	0.00 (0.01)	2.10 (0.19)	2.62 (0.18)
Bipolar II Scale (BIP2)	51	12.37	3.56	57	11.68	4.50	4469	10.44	3.71	0.81 (0.17)	13.49*** (0.52)	5.75* (0.33)
Schizoidia Scale (SCHD)	51	3.14	1.66	57	2.65	1.62	4470	2.50	1.38	1.97 (0.30)	12.09*** (0.46)	1.77 (0.11)
SCL-Depression (SCL-D)	51	1.49	0.46	55	1.45	0.41	4465	1.33	0.33	2.38 (0.09)	12.46*** (0.48)	9.22** (0.36)
Temperament dimensions:												
novelty seeking (TCI-NS)	51	19.78	6.20	57	21.68	5.75	4426	20.33	5.86	3.30 (−0.32)	0.33 (−0.09)	4.08* (0.23)
harm avoidance (TCI-HA)	51	16.96	6.28	57	15.02	7.68	4426	13.77	5.96	1.44 (0.28)	16.11*** (0.54)	4.29* (0.21)
reward dependence (TCI-RD)	51	14.24	3.99	57	13.68	3.51	4426	14.76	3.78	0.22 (0.15)	0.52 (−0.14)	1.46 (−0.29)
persistence (TCI-P)	51	4.53	1.76	57	4.07	1.93	4426	4.31	1.73	1.86 (0.25)	0.65 (0.13)	1.91 (−0.14)

TCI: Temperament and Character Inventory. Mean values in categories are compared to using two-way analysis of variance (ANOVA), with diagnostic group and gender as independent variables. Statistical significant effect sizes are marked with asterisks as follows: *$P < 0.05$, **$P < 0.01$, and ***$P < 0.001$.

4.2. Depressive Symptoms. Sandanger et al. [37] previously conducted a cross-sectional study of the specificity of SCL-25 for depression. They found that a cutoff of 1.75 points in average was a powerful predictor for depression (crude odds ratio, OR 14.0). However, the scale was also significantly associated with different anxiety disorders (ORs 2.2 to 4.4) and with any disorder (OR 3.9). In a previous study of the NFBC 1966, Veijola et al. [18] compared the SCL-25 with Structured Clinical Interview for DSM-III-R (SCID) diagnoses in a subsample of the cohort. They concluded that SCL-25 might be useful for screening purposes in primary health care and epidemiological surveys. They noted that cases with psychiatric comorbid disorders were screened successfully using the instrument. According to the present study, the depression subscale of the SCL was a quite good ($d = 0.48$) predictor of new cases of depression requiring hospitalization, when compared to those with no new psychiatric disorders requiring hospitalization during the followup. However, specificity was poor ($d = 0.09$), indicating that depressive symptoms also relate to other subsequent psychiatric disorders (Table 3).

4.3. Temperament Dimensions. We found a strong association between depression and harm avoidance, as has also been noted in a recent meta-analysis comparing different psychiatric disorders [8]. This meta-analysis also found a small negative effect size ($d = -0.20$) of lower novelty seeking in major depression, whereas the effect in harm avoidance was very large ($d = 1.64$) when compared to controls. High harm avoidance in depression has been shown to remain, after controlling for age, gender, diagnosis, and depressive state effects [38]. Harm avoidance has also been shown to decrease after treatment response [39]. Interestingly, never-depressed siblings of the probands with major depression are reported as having higher harm avoidance compared to never-depressed siblings of never-depressed controls. Thus, the authors suggested that harm avoidance might be a trait-like characteristic related to a familial vulnerability to depression [40].

In our sample, individuals with concurrent or previous depression had very similar temperament when compared to individuals with other psychiatric disorders, with all the effect sizes being below 0.20. In the extensive meta-analysis by Miettunen and Raevuori [8], depression (23 studies) had higher P, RD, and HA than schizophrenia, but quite similar temperament when compared to alcohol use disorders. It is worth mentioning that, in the present study, about half of the patients with subsequent other psychiatric disorder had a substance use diagnosis (as their only diagnosis or in addition to some other diagnosis). Because of this, we performed additional analyses substance use disorder as additional covariate. We found that in concurrent, but not in predictive analyses, individuals with depression scored significantly higher than those with other psychiatric disorders in harm avoidance.

When we compared current results to our previous schizophrenia study with the NFBC 1966 [36], in those who have already received a diagnosis, harm avoidance was lower ($d = -0.50$) and novelty seeking higher ($d = 0.48$) in depression than in schizophrenia. Those with subsequent depression substantially had higher scores, especially in reward dependency, than those with subsequent schizophrenia (mean scores 14.2 versus 11.8; $d = 0.65$).

4.4. Strengths and Limitations. The sample was relatively large and population-based. Unlike many of the previous studies, we also included a comparison group with other psychiatric disorders. The extensive set of scales used is also an advantage. A limitation of the sample is that, although it was large, a low number of cases during the followup also meant that it was not possible to predict diagnoses more specifically. Due to cohort design, it only consists of one age group. As we used the nationwide hospital register to find new cases of depression, our outcome only indicates a very severe form of depression. We cannot avoid the possibility that, at the end of followup, high scorers without psychiatric diagnosis may have a depression diagnosis not requiring hospitalization, as most of the subjects with depressive episode are not treated in psychiatric hospital facilities [41]. It should also be noted that quite a large proportion of eligible subjects did not participate or gave inadequate answers [15].

5. Conclusions

In most of the scales, subjects with depression differed from healthy controls. Many of the scales were useful predictors for subsequent new hospitalisations due to depression. With lack of diagnosis specificity, these scales also predicted other psychiatric diagnoses. Thus, these scales are useful both in clinical work and in etiological research of psychiatric disorders.

Conflict of Interests

The authors declare that they have no conflict of interests.

Acknowledgments

This study has been supported by the Academy of Finland, the European Commission (EURO-BLCS, Framework 5 award QLG1-CT-2000-01643), NARSAD: Brain and Behavior Research Fund (Dr. Mortimer D. Sackler Developmental Psychobiology Research Program), the Sigrid Jusélius Foundation, DAAD (German Academic Exchange Service), and US National Institutes of Health (NIMH) (5R01MH63706:02).

References

[1] M. E. Maruish, Ed., *The Use of Psychological Testing for Treatment Planning and Outcomes Assessment*, Lawrence Erlbaum Associates, Mahwah NJ, USA, 1999.

[2] American Psychiatric Association, *Handbook of Psychiatric Measures*, American Psychiatric Association, Washington, DC, USA, 2000.

[3] I. I. Gottesman and T. D. Gould, "The endophenotype concept in psychiatry: etymology and strategic intentions," *American Journal of Psychiatry*, vol. 160, no. 4, pp. 636–645, 2003.

[4] G. Hasler, W. C. Drevets, H. K. Manji, and D. S. Charney, "Discovering endophenotypes for major depression," *Neuropsychopharmacology*, vol. 29, no. 10, pp. 1765–1781, 2004.

[5] C. E. Bearden and N. B. Freimer, "Endophenotypes for psychiatric disorders: ready for primetime?" *Trends in Genetics*, vol. 22, no. 6, pp. 306–313, 2006.

[6] L. R. Derogatis, R. S. Lipman, and L. Covi, "SCL-90: an outpatient psychiatric rating scale—preliminary report," *Psychopharmacology Bulletin*, vol. 9, no. 1, pp. 13–28, 1973.

[7] C. R. Cloninger, D. M. Svrakic, and T. R. Przybeck, "A psychobiological model of temperament and character," *Archives of General Psychiatry*, vol. 50, no. 12, pp. 975–990, 1993.

[8] J. Miettunen and A. Raevuori, "A meta-analysis of temperament in axis I psychiatric disorders," *Comprehensive Psychiatry*, vol. 53, pp. 152–166, 2011.

[9] C. R. Cloninger, D. M. Svrakic, and T. R. Przybeck, "Can personality assessment predict future depression? A twelve-month follow-up of 631 subjects," *Journal of Affective Disorders*, vol. 92, no. 1, pp. 35–44, 2006.

[10] R. F. Farmer and J. R. Seeley, "Temperament and character predictors of depressed mood over a 4-year interval," *Depression and Anxiety*, vol. 26, no. 4, pp. 371–381, 2009.

[11] G. Loas, P. Boyer, and A. Legrand, "Anhedonia in the deficit syndrome of schizophrenia," *Psychopathology*, vol. 32, no. 4, pp. 207–219, 1999.

[12] P. Rantakallio, "Groups at risk in low birth weight infants and perinatal mortality," *Acta Paediatrica Scandinavica*, vol. 193, pp. 1–71, 1969.

[13] M. Isohanni, T. Mäkikyrö, J. Moring et al., "A comparison of clinical and research DSM-III-R diagnoses of schizophrenia in a Finnish national birth cohort. Clinical and research diagnoses of schizophrenia," *Social Psychiatry and Psychiatric Epidemiology*, vol. 32, no. 5, pp. 303–308, 1997.

[14] K. Moilanen, J. Veijola, K. Läksy et al., "Reasons for the diagnostic discordance between clinicians and researchers in schizophrenia in Northern Finland 1966 Birth Cohort," *Social Psychiatry and Psychiatric Epidemiology*, vol. 38, no. 6, pp. 305–310, 2003.

[15] M. Haapea, J. Miettunen, E. Läärä et al., "Non-participation in a field survey with respect to psychiatric disorders," *Scandinavian Journal of Public Health*, vol. 36, no. 7, pp. 728–736, 2008.

[16] L. J. Chapman and J. P. Chapman, *Infrequency Scale for Personality Measures*, TR Kwapil Department of Psychology, University of North Carolina, Greensboro, NC, USA, 1986.

[17] P. Fink, J. Jensen, L. Borgquist et al., "Psychiatric morbidity in primary public health care: a Nordic multicentre investigation Part I: method and prevalence of psychiatric morbidity," *Acta Psychiatrica Scandinavica*, vol. 92, no. 6, pp. 409–418, 1995.

[18] J. Veijola, J. Jokelainen, K. Läksy et al., "The Hopkins Symptom Checklist-25 in screening DSM-III-R axis-I disorders," *Nordic Journal of Psychiatry*, vol. 57, no. 2, pp. 119–123, 2003.

[19] American Psychiatric Association, *DSM-III-R: Diagnostic and Statistical Manual of Mental Disorders*, American Psychiatric Association, Washington, DC, USA, 3rd edition, 1987.

[20] L. J. Chapman, J. P. Chapman, and M. L. Raulin, "Scales for physical and social anhedonia," *Journal of Abnormal Psychology*, vol. 85, no. 4, pp. 374–382, 1976.

[21] M. Eckblad, L. J. Chapman, J. P. Chapman, and M. Mishlove, *The Revised Social Anhedonia Scale*, University of Wisconsin, Madison, Wis, USA, 1982.

[22] L. J. Chapman, J. P. Chapman, and M. L. Raulin, "Body-image aberration in schizophrenia," *Journal of Abnormal Psychology*, vol. 87, no. 4, pp. 399–407, 1978.

[23] M. Eckblad and L. J. Chapman, "Development and validation of a scale for hypomanic personality," *Journal of Abnormal Psychology*, vol. 95, no. 3, pp. 214–222, 1986.

[24] H. S. Akiskal, J. D. Maser, P. J. Zeller et al., "Switching from "unipolar" to bipolar II: an 11-year prospective study of clinical and temperamental predictors in 559 patients," *Archives of General Psychiatry*, vol. 52, no. 2, pp. 114–123, 1995.

[25] R. R. Golden and P. E. Meehl, "Detection of the schizoid taxon with MMPI indicators," *Journal of Abnormal Psychology*, vol. 88, no. 3, pp. 217–233, 1979.

[26] J. Miettunen, L. Kantojärvi, J. Ekelund et al., "A large population cohort provides normative data for investigation of temperament," *Acta Psychiatrica Scandinavica*, vol. 110, no. 2, pp. 150–157, 2004.

[27] J. Miettunen, J. Veijola, N. Freimer et al., "Data on schizotypy and affective scales are gender and education dependent—study in the Northern Finland 1966 Birth Cohort," *Psychiatry Research*, vol. 178, no. 2, pp. 408–413, 2010.

[28] J. Miettunen, J. Veijola, E. Lauronen, L. Kantojärvi, and M. Joukamaa, "Sex differences in Cloninger's temperament dimensions-a meta-analysis," *Comprehensive Psychiatry*, vol. 48, no. 2, pp. 161–169, 2007.

[29] J. Miettunen and E. Jääskeläinen, "Sex differences in wisconsin schizotypy scales-a meta-analysis," *Schizophrenia Bulletin*, vol. 36, no. 2, pp. 347–358, 2010.

[30] J. Cohen, "A power primer," *Psychological Bulletin*, vol. 112, no. 1, pp. 155–159, 1992.

[31] G. Loas, "Anhedonia in major depressive disorders. A comparative study between 55 major depressives (RDC) and 54 healthy subjects," *Encephale*, vol. 21, no. 5, pp. 559–562, 1995.

[32] I. Berlin, L. Givry-Steiner, Y. Lecrubier, and A. J. Puech, "Measures of anhedonia and hedonic responses to sucrose in depressive and schizophrenic patients in comparison with healthy subjects," *European Psychiatry*, vol. 13, no. 6, pp. 303–309, 1998.

[33] J. Katsanis, W. G. Iacono, and M. Beiser, "Anhedonia and perceptual aberration in first-episode psychotic patients and their relatives," *Journal of Abnormal Psychology*, vol. 99, no. 2, pp. 202–206, 1990.

[34] J. J. Blanchard, W. P. Horan, and S. A. Brown, "Diagnostic differences in social anhedonia: a longitudinal study of schizophrenia and major depressive disorder," *Journal of Abnormal Psychology*, vol. 110, no. 3, pp. 363–371, 2001.

[35] G. Loas, E. Salinas, J. D. Guelfi, and B. Samuel-Lajeunesse, "Physical anhedonia in major depressive disorder," *Journal of Affective Disorders*, vol. 25, no. 2, pp. 139–146, 1992.

[36] J. Miettunen, J. Veijola, M. Isohanni et al., "Identifying schizophrenia and other psychoses with psychological scales in the generasl population," *Journal of Nervous and Mental Disease*, vol. 199, no. 4, pp. 230–238, 2011.

[37] I. Sandanger, T. Moum, G. Ingebrigtsen, O. S. Dalgard, T. Sørensen, and D. Bruusgaard, "Concordance between symptom screening and diagnostic procedure: the Hopkins Symptom Checklist-25 and the Composite International Diagnostic Interview I," *Social Psychiatry and Psychiatric Epidemiology*, vol. 33, no. 7, pp. 345–354, 1998.

[38] K. Y. Abrams, S. K. Yune, S. J. Kim et al., "Trait and state aspects of harm avoidance and its implication for treatment in major depressive disorder, dysthymic disorder, and depressive personality disorder," *Psychiatry and Clinical Neurosciences*, vol. 58, no. 3, pp. 240–248, 2004.

[39] O. Kampman and O. Poutanen, "Can onset and recovery in depression be predicted by temperament? A systematic review

and meta-analysis," *Journal of Affective Disorders*, vol. 135, pp. 20–27, 2011.

[40] R. F. P. de Winter, R. Wolterbeek, P. Spinhoven, F. G. Zitman, and J. G. Goekoop, "Character and temperament in major depressive disorder and a highly anxious-retarded subtype derived from melancholia," *Comprehensive Psychiatry*, vol. 48, no. 5, pp. 426–435, 2007.

[41] V. Lehtinen and M. Joukamaa, "Epidemiology of depression: prevalence, risk factors and treatment situation," *Acta Psychiatrica Scandinavica, Supplement*, vol. 89, no. 377, pp. 7–10, 1994.

7

Religious versus Conventional Psychotherapy for Major Depression in Patients with Chronic Medical Illness: Rationale, Methods, and Preliminary Results

Harold G. Koenig[1, 2]

[1] *Departments of Psychiatry and Medicine, Duke University Medical Center, Box 3400 Medical Center, Durham, NC 27705, USA*
[2] *Department of Medicine, King Abdulaziz University, Jeddah 21413, Saudi Arabia*

Correspondence should be addressed to Harold G. Koenig, Harold.Koenig@dm.duke.edu

Academic Editor: Rachel E. Dew

This paper (1) reviews the physical and religious barriers to CBT that disabled medically ill-depressed patients face, (2) discusses research on the relationship between religion and depression-induced physiological changes, (3) describes an ongoing randomized clinical trial of religious versus secular CBT in chronically ill patients with mild-to-moderate major depression designed to (a) overcome physical and religious barriers to CBT and (b) compare the efficacy of religious versus secular CBT in relieving depression and improving immune and endocrine functions, and (4) presents preliminary results that illustrate the technical difficulties that have been encountered in implementing this trial. CBT is being delivered remotely via instant messaging, telephone, or Skype, and Christian, Jewish, Muslim, Buddhist, and Hindu versions of religious CBT are being developed. The preliminary results described here are particular to the technologies employed in this study and are not results from the CBT clinical trial whose findings will be published in the future after the study ends and data are analyzed. The ultimate goal is to determine if a psychotherapy delivered remotely that integrates patients' religious resources improves depression more quickly than a therapy that ignores them, and whether religious CBT is more effective than conventional CBT in reversing depression-induced physiological changes.

1. Introduction

Depression is a major public health problem. Based on a joint study conducted by the Harvard School of Public Health and the World Health Organization, depression was the leading cause of disability in the world (measured by years of life lived with disability) in 1990 [1] and, in 2020, is expected to be the world's second leading cause of disability, surpassed only by cardiovascular disease [2]. The lifetime prevalence of depression in the USA is 20% in women and 10% in men [3].

Depression is widespread in patients with chronic disabling medical illness. While the point prevalence of major depression among the general population in the United States is 7% [4], this figure increases to 10% to 45% among patients with medical illness depending on setting [5–8]. Not surprising, the use of antidepressants by primary care physicians has increased dramatically in recent years [9]. Treating with antidepressants, while lifesaving for many, comes with it the risk of side effects in medically frail patients and increases the risk of drug interactions with medications prescribed for nonpsychiatric illness [10]. This is especially true since major depression is already a potent risk factor for disease morbidity, with depressed medical patients having double the mortality of those without depression [11, 12]. Furthermore, medications are expensive, and managing side effects or drug interactions increases the cost further.

Psychotherapy has also been shown to benefit depressed medical patients. The kinds of depression seen in primary care medicine are often situation-specific and due to life changes brought on by physical illness, including day-to-day problems with functioning at home and work. Thus, psychotherapeutic approaches focused on helping patients adjust to difficult real life circumstances are useful in depressed patients seen in primary care settings. Not surprising, psychological approaches such as cognitive-behavioral therapy (CBT) have been particularly effective in treating depression in medical patients, often done by addressing the maladaptive beliefs and thoughts related to medical illness that initiate and maintain depression [13–16].

The aims of this paper are to (1) review the physical and religious barriers to psychotherapy that disabled medically ill-depressed patients face, (2) discuss research on the relationship between religious involvement and depression, and their relationships to physiological changes influencing the course of medical illness, (3) describe an ongoing randomized clinical trial designed to overcome physical and religious barriers to psychotherapy in the medically ill by utilizing remote delivery methods for CBT that integrate religious resources into psychotherapy, and (4) present preliminary results that illustrate the technical difficulties that we have encountered in implementing this trial.

2. Barriers to Psychotherapy

While psychological treatments for depression are known to be effective, there are numerous barriers to referral, compliance, and follow-up of persons with depressive disorders. These include physical, cultural, and religious barriers. Physical barriers to psychotherapy for medically ill-disabled patients are formidable. Medical patients with mobility problems or those who are home bound may have trouble accessing psychotherapy (i.e., traveling to therapists' offices, sitting in waiting rooms, etc.). To address this barrier, online and telephone approaches to delivering CBT have been developed, and are effective in and acceptable to medical patients with depression [17, 18].

2.1. Online Communications. Online communications are now widespread in the United States and around the world. Of 6.8 billion people, 25% (1.7 billion) use the Internet [19]. Of the 341 million people in North America, nearly 75% (252 million) use the Internet. In 2005, close to 75 million Americans used e-mail and search engines on an average day (including 29% of those over age 50) [20, 21]. That number has increased considerably since then, not to mention the millions who now have a MySpace or Facebook account (74% of all Americans ages 18 to 34, and 25% of those ages 55 or older), or the estimated 15 million who use Twitter [22]. One of the fastest growing groups of Internet users is older adults; 77% of all persons over age 55 use the Internet to search for healthcare information [23].

2.2. Online CBT. Individual cognitive-behavior therapy (CBT) can be offered online by a therapist using instant messaging, during which client and therapist communicate in real time with typewritten responses. Benefits of this approach include flexibility and optimal use of patient and therapist time, outreach to patients for whom travel to treatment centers is difficult for reasons of geography or disability, and access to foreign language therapists. Furthermore, this approach is acceptable to depressed patients, and therapy without face-to-face contact may encourage greater disclosure [24].

The Lancet published the first report of a randomized controlled trial (RCT) of therapist-delivered online CBT for moderately severe depression in primary care patients in 2009 [25]. The study found that CBT by this method was significantly more beneficial than usual care provided by primary care physicians. Those benefits were maintained over at least 8 months. This means that a relatively small number of therapists can cover a wide geographical area and be available to patients at a range of times. The way that patients express their feelings may also impact treatment effectiveness. Online CBT takes advantage of the fact that writing about traumatic experiences improves outcomes [26, 27]. This appears especially true when writing about events from a religious viewpoint [28, 29].

2.3. Telephone CBT. An issue with online CBT, particularly when delivered alone on the Internet without therapist guidance, has been "*dropouts*" during treatment [30]. Even with therapist-delivered online CBT, this remains a problem (dropout rate was 28% in the *Lancet* study). To minimize dropouts and boost effects, it has been recommended that a telephone component be added [31] since telephone therapy is known to increase compliance [32]. Furthermore, structured CBT delivered by telephone has been shown to be both clinically effective and cost effective in treating medical patients with depression [33].

3. Religion and Depression

Besides physical barriers that depressed disabled medically ill patients encounter when seeking psychotherapy, there are also religious barriers. When religious patients become depressed, their beliefs may interfere with their acceptance of and compliance with conventional treatments, especially psychotherapy. Many such patients shy away from secular psychotherapy because they perceive it as unsympathetic to their religious beliefs [34]. Religious patients may also feel that seeking therapy means abandoning their faith in favor of secular treatments. Finally, religious persons may feel guilty or ashamed about being depressed and thus fail to address it with their clergy and avoid seeking support within their faith community.

Clergy have traditionally served as front-line mental health providers in communities across the USA, providing nearly as many hours of counseling as does the entire membership of the American Psychological Association [35]. Consider that clergy spend on average 15% of their time in counseling activities, providing over 140 million hours of mental health services each year, not including the activities of nearly 100,000 full-time nuns or chaplains. Furthermore, they do not charge for their services, and there is no stigma associated with this type of counseling. Thus, depressed religious persons often receive their first treatment by clergy or other counselors within their faith community.

Treatment within the faith community, however, is not always effective, especially for more severe depression, requiring referral to mental health professionals for additional treatment. The problem is that the relationship between clergy and mental health professionals has not always been good. In fact, there is a long history of conflict between religious and mental health professionals, beginning with

Freud's description of religion as "the universal obsessional neurosis." [36] There is often open resistance to consideration of religious beliefs in conventional mental health care, resistance that is clear from a recent discussion among British psychiatrists (see e-letters in response to two recent articles in *The Psychiatrist*) [37, 38]. Negative attitudes toward religion by mental health professionals are not limited to Great Britain. A systematic review of the religious content of DSM-III-R found that nearly one-quarter of all cases of mental illness included religious descriptions [39]. More recent publications by mental health professionals continue to emphasize a lack of concern for patients' religious beliefs, [40, 41] and a recent national survey of USA psychiatrists found that 56% never, rarely, or only sometimes inquire about religious/spiritual issues in patients with depression or anxiety [42].

Based on this generally neglectful (and at times disparaging) view held by some mental health professionals toward religion, religious professionals are often reluctant to refer members of their congregation to mental health professionals, especially for psychotherapy that seeks to alter beliefs and attitudes. Failure of clergy to refer may prevent many patients from receiving the treatment they need. Furthermore, if patients are members of a faith community and that community does not reinforce (or perhaps even counteracts) the gains made in psychotherapy, then those gains may not last.

4. Depression, Religion, and Physiological Changes

Whether religion is a resource (as clergy claim) or a liability (as mental health specialists like Freud claim) to depressed medical patients needs to be established before bringing down the barrier that stands between mental health care and religion. Like it or not, religious involvement is important to the vast majority people in the USA and around the world [43]. According to a January 2009 Gallup Poll, 65% of Americans indicated that religion is an important part of their daily life, a figure that increases to over 75% in the southeastern USA [44]. Likewise, according to the Pew Foundation's national survey of 35,000 Americans, 56% indicated that religion was "very important" in their lives, a figure that increases to 69% in the southeastern USA This is especially true for medical patients, who often turn to religious beliefs to cope with illness [45].

Literally hundreds of qualitative and quantitative studies document high rates of religious coping behaviors in those trying to cope with medical illness [46, 47]. In some areas of the USA, nearly 90% of hospitalized patients with medical problems use religion to cope, and of those who do, nearly half (45%) report that religion is the *most important* factor that keeps them going [48]. Furthermore, greater religiosity predicts a faster resolution of depressive symptoms in medical patients over time, increasing the speed of remission by 50 to 70 percent overall, but especially in those with persistent physical disability, in whom it predicts a more than 100 percent increase in speed of remission [49–52].

Religious involvement has also been associated with positive emotions such as optimism and purpose in life [53], as well as gratefulness, generosity, and altruism [54–56]. These characteristics may enhance well-being and counteract maladaptive cognitions and behaviors that maintain depression [57]. Religious people, however, are not exempt from depression, especially when serious health problems strike. In a study at Duke Hospital, 64% of medical inpatients over age 50 with major depression (diagnosed using the Structured Clinical Interview for Depression (SCID)) indicated they were both spiritual and religious and 76% prayed at least once daily [58].

5. Consideration of Religious Beliefs in Therapy

Depression not only destroys quality of life but may also affect the physical body by interfering with immune and endocrine functioning. Religious beliefs and behaviors that facilitate coping with life stress may help to normalize those changes.

5.1. Physiological Effects of Depression. There is evidence that the alterations in immune and endocrine function associated with depression increase medical morbidity by increasing the risk of infection [59], inflammatory disorders [60], and possibly malignancy [61–63]. This relationship, however, is a complex one that is likely bidirectional in nature [64]. Furthermore, depression is known to stimulate some components of the immune system and suppress others. Stimulation of proinflammatory cytokines can lead to sickness behaviors that resemble depression, which has led to consideration of how immune and endocrine functions influence the pathophysiology of depression, especially when depression develops in a setting of chronic stress [65].

Regardless of direction of effect, major depression is associated with a host of immune [66], endocrine [67], and proinflammatory functions [68] that could adversely affect physical health and response to medical treatments. Depression is associated with an altered balance in the Th1/Th2 ratio, that is, higher pro-inflammatory Th1 cytokines (IL-1, IL-12, INF-γ), higher pro-inflammatory monocytic cytokines (IL-6, TNF-α) [69–71], and lower anti-inflammatory Th2 cytokines (IL-4, IL-10) [72]. Depressed patients also have reduced natural killer (NK) cell cytotoxicity [73–75] and diminished lymphocyte responses to phytohemagglutinin and concanavalin A [76, 77].

Impaired immune functions associated with depression also appear to normalize in response to treatment with electroconvulsive therapy (serum TNFα) [78], antidepressant drug therapy (serum TNFα and CRP) [79], and psychological interventions [80] (due in part to a return of the pro-/anti-inflammatory cytokine balance). A number of randomized clinical trials involving psychological interventions that relieve depression or boost positive emotions have reported improvement in immune and/or endocrine functions. For example, Antoni et al. conducted a 10-week CBT stress-management program in human-immunodeficiency-virus- (HIV-) infected men [81]. The intervention significantly increased naïve CD4+ T cells in blood over a 12-month follow-up among those in the CBT group (n = 16) compared to controls (n = 9). This effect was mediated by a reduction in depressive symptoms and a decrease in urinary cortisol levels. A more recent study by Antoni et al. examined the effects of a 10-week cognitive behavioral stress management program in 128 women with breast cancer, finding that the intervention significantly lowered serum cortisol, increased Th_1 pro-inflammatory cytokines (IL-2 and INF-γ), and increased IL-2 : IL-4 ratio [82].

In another clinical trial, Van Middendorp et al. conducted an emotional disclosure intervention (4 weekly sessions) in 68 nondepressed patients with rheumatoid arthritis, finding a reduction in urinary cortisol, a reduction of serum INF-γ, and a trend towards a reduction in IL-6 (P = 0.07) [83]. Also, a recent intervention by Lee Berk et al. to increase positive emotions (via mirthful laughter) in 20 high-risk diabetics with hypertension and hyperlipidemia found that the intervention lowered serum epinephrine, norepinephrine, INF-γ, CRP, TNF-α, and IL-6 [84]. Finally, Roberts et al. found that the hypocortisolism in 41 subjects with chronic fatigue syndrome (a depression-like syndrome) was improved following 15 sessions with CBT [85]; thus, whether cortisol is pathologically high or low, psychological therapies may help normalize levels.

In summary, psychotherapeutic treatments that increase positive emotions (particularly CBT) appear to increase naïve CD4+ cells, increase NK cell cytotoxicity, reduce IL-6, reduce TNF-α, reduce CRP, reduce INF-γ (sometimes increasing in nondepressed female patients), decrease catecholamines, and normalize (decreasing or increasing) cortisol.

5.2. Physiological Effects of Religion. As noted previously, religious involvement has been associated with better mental health. However, it is also associated with better physical health and greater longevity [86, 87]. The mechanisms that explain the association with physical health are unclear but likely involve behavioral and psychosocial factors operating at least partly through immune/endocrine pathways related to stress [88–90]. There is some evidence that religious involvement is associated with better immune and endocrine functions, although no studies have yet examined the effects of a religious psychotherapy on these functions.

For example, Sephton et al. examined the relationship between religious involvement and immune function in 112 women with metastatic breast cancer [91]. Religious expression was positively related to the total number of circulating T cells (r = 0.24, P = 0.01) and helper T cells (r = 0.23, P = 0.01), and controlling for social network size, disease, and medical treatment variables had little effect on these relationships. Investigators also found positive associations between religious expression and cytotoxic T cells (r = 0.18, $P < 0.05$) and a trend towards greater NK cell numbers (r = 0.14, P = 0.07).

Studying a vulnerable population, Ironson et al. examined the effects of changes in spirituality/religiousness (S/R) following the diagnosis of HIV on CD4 counts (T cells) and viral load during 4 years of follow-up [92]. Hierarchical linear modeling was used to examine the effects of changes in S/R over time with the outcome being slopes of change in CD4 cells and viral load during follow-up. Patients who reported an increase in S/R after diagnosis experienced significantly less decrease in CD4 counts and less increase in viral load during the 4-year follow-up. Results were independent of church attendance and initial disease status, medication use, age, gender, race, education, health behaviors, depression, hopelessness, optimism coping, and social support. In fact, among all significant predictors of CD4 cell count and viral load, change in S/R was the most powerful predictor. A number of other studies have found similar connections between religious involvement and other immune functions (T cells, in particular) [93–95], pro-inflammatory indicators (IL-6) [96–98], and endocrine measures (specifically cortisol) [99–103].

In contrast to the numerous observational studies cited perviously, there have been far fewer intervention studies. One that examined nondepressed HIV+ patients reported that a stress management intervention designed to increase spiritual growth led to an increase in lymphocyte proliferation and a 3-fold increase of INF-γ [104]. Likewise, Eastern spiritual meditation has been shown to increase antibody response to influenza vaccine [105], alter the ratio of pro-/anti-inflammatory cytokines [106, 107], increase NK cell activity [107], reduce cortisol [107–110], and decrease catecholamine [111, 112] levels (and in one study, there was a trend toward superiority over conventional CBT [113]).

Thus, psychotherapy for depression that utilizes patients' religious resources in therapy may help to normalize endocrine and immune dysfunctions, perhaps even more so than conventional treatments [114]. Whether or not this is true, however, is completely unknown. The study described below is the first randomized clinical trial to address this gap in the literature and to examine whether religious CBT is equally effective, more effective, or less effective than conventional CBT in depressed patients with chronic medical illness. The effectiveness of religious CBT is suggested both (1) by an earlier study showing that religious CBT was more effective than conventional CBT in religious patients [115] and (2) by a study showing that patients receiving conventional CBT responded more quickly to the therapy if they indicated that religion was important to them [116].

6. Ongoing Randomized Clinical Trial

Psychotherapy that takes into account patients' religious beliefs as potential resources in therapy may not only help to overcome religious barriers to therapy but may also be more effective in resolving depressive symptoms and reversing depression-induced physiological changes. The efficacy of religious psychotherapy, that is, taking into account the religious beliefs and practices of patients and utilizing them in therapy, however, has yet to be examined in medical settings. Religious CBT has been shown to increase the speed of remission in depressed healthy religious patients and do so beyond that achieved by conventional CBT [117–119]. Likewise, a number of studies that utilized patients' religious beliefs in therapy have reported results superior to secular treatments or usual care, especially in religious patients [120–124].

Finally, there is plenty of evidence that many patients in the United States prefer to have their religious beliefs integrated into therapy. For example, one recent study found that 77% to 83% of adults aged 55 or older with depression and comorbid chronic medical illness wished to include religion in their therapy [125]. Likewise, in a survey of a more general population of 74 individuals receiving counseling, Rose et al. found that only 18% of patients said they did not want to discuss religion or spirituality in psychotherapy and only 8% said they wanted to discuss spiritual but not religious issues [126]. Likewise, Kelly found in a national survey that only 19% of respondents did not want to integrate religious/spiritual beliefs and values into therapy [127]. Thus, from the patient's perspective, there appears to be little resistance to utilizing their religious beliefs in therapy.

Benefits resulting from addressing religious beliefs in therapy may stem partly from redirecting attention away from a focus on loss and preoccupation with self and instead centering one's thoughts on positive processes such as gratitude, altruism, and generosity. Such positive cognitions have been shown to predict lower depressive symptoms [128–131]. Furthermore, religious cognitions that promote purpose and meaning in life and a hopeful and optimistic attitude toward circumstances may help to counter the negative cognitions and behaviors associated with depression. Indeed, dozens of studies have reported a link between positive emotions such as optimism and purpose in life, religious involvement, and fewer depressive symptoms [132]. Having a common worldview and explanatory model that gives meaning and purpose to negative life events may also strengthen the therapeutic alliance between patient and therapist, which could contribute to treatment efficacy [133]. This may be particularly true for minority populations who often suffer from disparities in psychiatric care and yet tend to be very religious.

7. The Interventions

We are now in the first phase of a randomized clinical trail being conducted at two sites, Duke University Health Systems in the Triangle region of North Carolina and Glendale Adventist Medical Center in Los Angeles County. During Phase I (Rounsaville 1a) [134], we are developing and further refining a manual to guide the delivery of religious CBT and are conducting an open trial to assess subject recruitment and to allow therapists to gain experience with the treatment and method of delivery. In this preliminary phase, religious and conventional CBT are being delivered online by instant messaging, over the telephone, or by Skype to determine which method of delivery is most acceptable, preferred, and likely to be complied with by patients during the randomized clinical trial in Phase II.

In Phase II (Rounsaville 1b), we will conduct a randomized proof of concept comparison of conventional CBT versus religious CBT that will (1) further demonstrate feasibility of recruitment and subject compliance, (2) confirm the expected clinically meaningful difference (effect size) in the therapies, and (3) show differential effects in reversing depression-induced immune and endocrine functions. In this head-to-head trial, 70 persons who are at least somewhat religious/spiritual and ages 18–85 with an episode of major depression (diagnosed by the Mini International Neuropsychiatric Inventory using DSM-IV criteria), moderate severity of depression based on Beck Depression Inventory (BDI) scores, and at least one chronic medical illness will be randomized to either conventional CBT or religious CBT. Excluded will be patients with significant cognitive impairment, those currently receiving psychotherapy, those that meet criteria on the MINI for psychotic disorder, alcohol or substance abuse, or PTSD, those with a history of bipolar disorder, active suicidal thoughts (passive suicidal thoughts will not exclude), diagnosis of HIV/AIDS, autoimmune diseases, or endocrine disorders likely to affect stress hormone levels, or taking immunosuppressant drugs (due to proposed immune and endocrine analyses).

The trial will consist of ten 50 min sessions, administered by licensed master's level therapists and delivered over 12 weeks. The primary endpoint will be depressive symptoms on the BDI (clinician-rated scales like the Hamilton or MADRS are not being used because nonclinicians blind to study group will be administering outcome assessments). Subjects will be assessed on the BDI at baseline, 4 weeks, 8 weeks, 12 weeks, and 24 weeks. Immune (pro-inflammatory and anti-inflammatory cytokines) and endocrine (urinary cortisol, epinephrine, and norepinephrine) measures will be assessed at baseline, immediately at the end of therapy (12 weeks), and at 24 weeks from baseline.

8. Preliminary Results

Both interventions are taking a CBT approach documented in treatment manuals. Depressed persons with chronic medical illness have often allowed their health problems and disability (i.e., circumstances) to shape the way they think and view their world. Depression is often maintained by a negative worldview that sees the person's situation as hopeless and without meaning or purpose. Both conventional and religious CBT seek to alter these dysfunctional, maladaptive beliefs, replacing them with positive, realistic beliefs and behaviors that generate positive emotions.

8.1. Conventional CBT. CCBT helps depressed patients understand the links between thoughts, emotions, and behavior. It uses guided discovery, Socratic questioning, and challenge of automatic negative thoughts to help patients identify and appraise their cognitions and determine problematic behaviors. Interventions include activity scheduling, along with practice assignments, in which clients test out ideas and behaviors discussed during sessions. In this arm, therapists will be asked to avoid reference to the participant's faith or religious belief. If religious issues come up, therapists will gently redirect the patient to more secular ways of approaching the issue and, if necessary, will address religious issues in the broadest conventional way possible, relating them to other cognitions/behaviors usually addressed in conventional CBT. We felt justified in doing this because most CBT today does not utilize and integrate the religious beliefs of patients into psychotherapy.

8.2. Religious CBT. Religious CBT follows the same process described for CCBT, except that religious beliefs and motivations will be utilized to stimulate changes in thought and behavior. For example, participants may have obsessive guilt about sin or punishment, report religious doubt, or want to discuss the cognitive and emotional elements of their faith. In RCBT all those issues will be considered fully acceptable as part of therapy, including an emphasis on religious resources. In other words, RCBT uses religious rationales (based on the subject's faith tradition) and religious arguments to counter irrational thoughts and utilizes religious behaviors (involvement in the religious community) to increase supportive relationships. RCBT teaches patients to use their own religious teachings, doctrines, and behaviors to help change maladaptive beliefs, values, and behaviors so as to transform their worldview into one that is meaningful, hopeful, and optimistic, one that is incompatible with depression. RCBT seeks to bolster powerful religious beliefs that promote behaviors such as forgiveness, gratitude, generosity, and altruism (focusing on others and on God) that generate meaning and purpose, optimism, and hope, which neutralize depression.

The RCBT manual is initially being developed within a Christian framework and will then be adapted to the subject's faith tradition (i.e., versions of the manual for Jewish, Hindu, Buddhist, and Muslim patients). These versions of the manual will be prepared by experienced psychotherapists well versed each of these faith traditions, who will work under the direction of Ken Pargament, a psychotherapist widely renowned for his writings on integrating spirituality into psychotherapy [135]. The therapists who develop the different religious versions will help supervise study therapists while they are treating patients in these faith traditions.

9. Conclusions

Preliminary results from Phase I indicate that of the first 82 patients screened for inclusion (from North Carolina and Los Angeles County), 78% had a computer at home, 77% had access to the Internet at home, 75% could type easily and quickly on the computer, 68% had a landline telephone, 95% had a cell phone, but only 30% had Skype (or equivalent program) and a webcam. Most (>80%) preferred therapy by telephone, 9% preferred online therapy, and 9% preferred therapy via Skype. Patients were also asked what method of therapy they were not willing to try; 70% said they were unwilling to try online therapy and 78% were unwilling to try Skype.

Of the 82 subjects, 18 met inclusion criteria and were randomized to treatment arm (one to online, two to Skype, and 15 to telephone, based on what subjects were willing to do). Technical issues encountered during therapy have been the biggest problem. The telephone route has had the fewest issues; 84% of telephone sessions (delivered by two-person conference call) had no technical difficulties; 8% had a problem with conference call ending or dropping; 5% had difficulty with sound; and one patient's cell phone battery died. Overall, only 0.6% of telephone therapy session time was wasted dealing with technical issues (during the course of 57 therapy sessions). For the single subject who was willing to try the online method thus far, difficulty connecting to the online platform (PsychologyOnline) was a problem for all sessions; overall, 35% of session therapy time was wasted on dealing with this issue. With regard to Skype, only 30% of 20 sessions proceeded without technical difficulties; 30% had difficulty with sound, 25% had difficulty connecting with Skype over the computer; and 5% had trouble with delay in picture, video call dropped, or session could not be recorded. Overall, 7% of therapy session time for Skype was spent dealing with technical issues. These preliminary findings suggest that the most preferred method of delivering the therapy and the one with the least technical difficulties is therapy by telephone, although we need more experience with the online and Skype methods.

10. Conclusions

Major depression is a common psychiatric illness, especially prevalent among persons with chronic medical illness, that can adversely affect physical health and medical outcomes by altering immune and endocrine functions. Religion is widespread and often used to cope with medical illness and problems with physical functioning. In this study, we are testing whether a psychological therapy that takes advantage of patients' religious resources improves depression more or less quickly than conventional therapy and reverses the adverse physiological changes associated with depression.

The results from this study will be important because they are relevant to therapists other than those who explicitly practice pastoral counseling, extending to secular therapists as well. If 65% of Americans indicate that religion is an important part of daily life and 80% of depressed patients wish to include it in therapy, then all therapists (whether they have explicit training in pastoral counseling or not) are likely to encounter patients among their clientele who will prefer this approach. Interestingly, Propst et al. in their study of religious versus conventional CBT found that delivery of religious CBT by secular therapists was at least as effective (if not more so) than religious CBT delivered by religious therapists [136].

In their 2009 review of religion in psychotherapy, Post and Wade make two points relevant to this issue [137]. First, although therapists in general are less overtly religious than patients, many therapists have spiritual beliefs that should assist them in appreciating the role that patients' religious beliefs play as a resource in their mental health. Second, while it is helpful for therapists to be well versed in the basic tenets of their patients' religious beliefs, it is not necessary for them to be experts in religion: "instead, approaching religious/spiritual clients with an openness and willingness to engage the religious/spiritual conversation will help clients to feel comfortable expressing their needs." These authors concluded that religious interventions in psychotherapy can be effectively delivered by therapists with a wide range of religious/spiritual beliefs, not only pastoral counselors.

Conflict of Interests

The author have no conflict of interests.

Acknowledgments

This work was funded by the John Templeton Foundation. This paper is supported by a grant from the John Templeton Foundation and by support from the Center for Spirituality, Theology and Health.

References

[1] A. D. Lopez and C. C. J. L. Murray, "The global burden of disease, 1990–2020," *Nature Medicine*, vol. 4, no. 11, pp. 1241–1243, 1998.

[2] C. Murray and A. Lopez, *The Global Burden of Disease*, Harvard University Press, Cambridge, Mass, USA, 1996.

[3] D. C. Steffens, I. Skoog, M. C. Norton et al., "Prevalence of depression and its treatment in an elderly population: the Cache County study," *Archives of General Psychiatry*, vol. 57, no. 6, pp. 601–607, 2000.

[4] R. C. Kessler, P. Berglund, O. Demler et al., "The epidemiology of major depressive disorder: results from the National Comorbidity Survey Replication (NCS-R)," *JAMA*, vol. 289, no. 23, pp. 3095–3105, 2003.

[5] M. A. Kitchell, R. F. Barnes, and R. C. Veith, "Screening for depression in hospitalized geriatric medical patients," *Journal of the American Geriatrics Society*, vol. 30, no. 3, pp. 174–177, 1982.

[6] H. G. Koenig, K. G. Meador, H. J. Cohen, and D. G. Blazer, "Depression in elderly hospitalized patients with medical illness," *Archives of Internal Medicine*, vol. 148, no. 9, pp. 1929–1936, 1988.

[7] H. G. Koenig, L. K. George, B. L. Peterson, and C. F. Pieper, "Depression in medically ill hospitalized older adults: prevalence, characteristics, and course of symptoms according to six diagnostic schemes," *American Journal of Psychiatry*, vol. 154, no. 10, pp. 1376–1383, 1997.

[8] T. Rosemann, M. Backenstrass, K. Joest, A. Rosemann, J. Szecsenyi, and G. Laux, "Predictors of depression in a sample of 1,021 primary care patients with osteoarthritis," *Arthritis Care and Research*, vol. 57, no. 3, pp. 415–422, 2007.

[9] M. Olfson and S. C. Marcus, "National patterns in antidepressant medication treatment," *Archives of General Psychiatry*, vol. 66, no. 8, pp. 848–856, 2009.

[10] E. Spina, V. Santoro, and C. D'Arrigo, "Clinically relevant pharmacokinetic drug interactions with second-generation antidepressants: an update," *Clinical Therapeutics*, vol. 30, no. 7, pp. 1206–1227, 2008.

[11] L. R. Wulsin, G. E. Vaillant, and V. E. Wells, "A systematic review of the mortality of depression," *Psychosomatic Medicine*, vol. 61, no. 1, pp. 6–17, 1999.

[12] H. G. Koenig, F. Shelp, V. Goli, H. J. Cohen, and D. G. Blazer, "Survival and health care utilization in elderly medical inpatients with major depression," *Journal of the American Geriatrics Society*, vol. 37, no. 7, pp. 599–606, 1989.

[13] E. Ward, M. King, M. Lloyd et al., "Randomised controlled trial of non-directive counselling, cognitive-behaviour therapy, and usual general practitioner care for patients with depression. I: clinical effectiveness," *British Medical Journal*, vol. 321, no. 7273, pp. 1383–1388, 2000.

[14] P. Bower, S. Byford, B. Sibbald et al., "Randomised controlled trial of non-directive counselling, cognitive-behaviour therapy, and usual general practitioner care for patients with depression. II: cost effectiveness," *British Medical Journal*, vol. 321, no. 7273, pp. 1389–1392, 2000.

[15] M. King, B. Sibbald, E. Ward et al., "Randomised controlled trial of non-directive counselling, cognitive-behaviour therapy and usual general practitioner care in the management of depression as well as mixed anxiety and depression in primary care," *Health Technology Assessment*, vol. 4, no. 19, pp. 1–73, 2000.

[16] M. A. Serfaty, D. Haworth, M. Blanchard, M. Buszewicz, S. Murad, and M. King, "Clinical effectiveness of individual cognitive behavioral therapy for depressed older people in primary care: a randomized controlled trial," *Archives of General Psychiatry*, vol. 66, no. 12, pp. 1332–1340, 2009.

[17] D. Kessler, G. Lewis, S. Kaur et al., "Therapist-delivered internet psychotherapy for depression in primary care: a randomised controlled trial," *The Lancet*, vol. 374, no. 9690, pp. 628–634, 2009.

[18] G. E. Simon, E. J. Ludman, and C. M. Rutter, "Incremental benefit and cost of telephone care management and telephone psychotherapy for depression in primary care," *Archives of General Psychiatry*, vol. 66, no. 10, pp. 1081–1089, 2009.

[19] Internet World Stats: Usage and Population Statistics, 2009, http://www.internetworldstats.com/stats.htm.

[20] Pew Internet and American Life Project, 2005, http://www.flickr.com/photos/cambodia4kidsorg/755159352/.

[21] Harris Poll, Almost three-quarters of all U.S. adults—an estimated 163 million, *Harris Interactive*, 2005, http://www.harrisinteractive.com/Insights/HarrisVault.aspx?PID=569.

[22] D. Weir, One in twenty Americans use Twitter, 2009.

[23] Anonymous, Older adults using Internet more, traditional media less. MarketingVOX: the voice of online marketing, 2006, http://www.marketingvox.com/older_adults_using_internet_more_traditional_media_less-020721/.

[24] A. Beattie, A. Shaw, S. Kaur, and D. Kessler, "Primary-care patients' expectations and experiences of online cognitive behavioural therapy for depression: a qualitative study," *Health Expectations*, vol. 12, no. 1, pp. 45–59, 2009.

[25] D. Kessler, G. Lewis, S. Kaur et al., "Therapist-delivered internet psychotherapy for depression in primary care: a randomised controlled trial," *The Lancet*, vol. 374, no. 9690, pp. 628–634, 2009.

[26] J. W. Pennebaker and J. D. Seagal, "Forming a story: the health benefits of narrative," *Journal of Clinical Psychology*, vol. 55, pp. 1243–1254, 1999.

[27] P. G. Frisina, J. C. Borod, and S. J. Lepore, "A meta-analysis of the effects of written emotional disclosure on the health outcomes of clinical populations," *Journal of Nervous and Mental Disease*, vol. 192, no. 9, pp. 629–634, 2004.

[28] Y. Y. Chen, "Written emotional expression and religion: effects on PTSD symptoms," *International Journal of Psychiatry in Medicine*, vol. 35, no. 3, pp. 273–286, 2005.

[29] P. R. Bennett, Prayers about traumatic experiences as self-disclosure to God: implications for health and well-being [Ph.D. dissertation], University of Nevada, Reno, Nev, USA, 2006.

[30] H. Christensen, K. M. Griffiths, A. J. Mackinnon, and K. Brittliffe, "Online randomized controlled trial of brief and

full cognitive behaviour therapy for depression," *Psychological Medicine*, vol. 36, no. 12, pp. 1737–1746, 2006.
[31] G. Andersson and P. Cuijpers, "Pros and cons of online cognitive-behavioural therapy," *British Journal of Psychiatry*, vol. 193, no. 4, pp. 270–271, 2008.
[32] G. E. Simon, E. J. Ludman, S. Tutty, B. Operskalski, and M. Von Korff, "Telephone psychotherapy and telephone care management for primary care patients starting antidepressant treatment: a randomized controlled trial," *JAMA*, vol. 292, no. 8, pp. 935–942, 2004.
[33] G. E. Simon, E. J. Ludman, and C. M. Rutter, "Incremental benefit and cost of telephone care management and telephone psychotherapy for depression in primary care," *Archives of General Psychiatry*, vol. 66, no. 10, pp. 1081–1089, 2009.
[34] H. G. Koenig, "History of mental health care," in *Faith & Mental Health*, H. G. Koenig, Ed., pp. 17–39, Templeton Foundation Press, Philadelphia, PA, USA, 2005.
[35] A. J. Weaver, "Has there been a failure to prepare and support parish-based clergy in their role as frontline community mental health workers: a review," *Journal of Pastoral Care*, vol. 49, no. 2, pp. 129–147, 1995.
[36] S. Freud, "Future of an illusion," in *Standard Edition of the Complete Psychological Works of Sigmund Freud*, J. Strachey, Ed., p. 43, Hogarth Press, London, UK, 1962.
[37] H. G. Koenig, "Religion and mental health: what are psychiatrists doing and should do?" *Psychiatric Bulletin*, vol. 32, no. 6, pp. 201–203, 2008.
[38] S. Dein, C. C. H. Cook, A. Powell, and S. Eagger, "Religion, spirituality and mental health," *Psychiatrist*, vol. 34, no. 2, pp. 63–64, 2010.
[39] D. B. Larson, S. B. Thielman, M. A. Greenwold et al., "Religious content in the DSM-III-R Glossary of Technical Terms," *American Journal of Psychiatry*, vol. 150, no. 12, pp. 1884–1885, 1993.
[40] W. Watters, *Deadly Doctrine: Health, Illness, and Christian God-Talk*, Prometheus Books, Buffalo, NY, USA, 1992.
[41] H. E. Jones, *Religion: The Etiology of Mental Illness*, Mental Health Education Press, 2007.
[42] F. A. Curlin, R. E. Lawrence, S. Odell et al., "Religion, spirituality, and medicine: psychiatrists' and other physicians' differing observations, interpretations, and clinical approaches," *American Journal of Psychiatry*, vol. 164, no. 12, pp. 1825–1831, 2007.
[43] Pew Forum, U.S. religious landscape survey, 2007, http://religions.pewforum.org/.
[44] The Gallup Poll, State of the States: Importance of Religion, http://www.gallup.com/poll/114022/state-states-importance-religion.aspx.
[45] H. G. Koenig, D. B. Larson, and S. S. Larson, "Religion and coping with serious medical illness," *Annals of Pharmacotherapy*, vol. 35, no. 3, pp. 352–359, 2001.
[46] H. G. Koenig, D. E. King, and V. B. Carson, *Handbook of Religion and Health*, Oxford University Press, New York, NY, USA, 2011.
[47] K. Pargament, *The Psychology of Religion and Coping*, Guilford Press, New York, NY, USA, 1997.
[48] H. G. Koenig, "Religious beliefs and practices of hospitalized medically ill older adults," *International Journal of Geriatric Psychiatry*, vol. 13, pp. 213–224, 1998.
[49] P. Pressman, J. S. Lyons, D. B. Larson, and J. J. Strain, "Religious belief, depression, and ambulation status in elderly women with broken hips," *American Journal of Psychiatry*, vol. 147, no. 6, pp. 758–760, 1990.
[50] H. G. Koenig, H. J. Cohen, D. G. Blazer et al., "Religious coping and depression among elderly, hospitalized medically ill men," *American Journal of Psychiatry*, vol. 149, no. 12, pp. 1693–1700, 1992.
[51] H. G. Koenig, "Religion and remission of depression in medical inpatients with heart failure/pulmonary disease," *Journal of Nervous and Mental Disease*, vol. 195, no. 5, pp. 389–395, 2007.
[52] H. G. Koenig, L. K. George, and B. L. Peterson, "Religiosity and remission of depression in medically ill oder patients," *American Journal of Psychiatry*, vol. 155, no. 4, pp. 536–542, 1998.
[53] H. G. Koenig, D. E. King, and V. B. Carson, *Handbook of Religion and Health*, Oxford University Press, New York, NY, USA, 2nd edition, 2012.
[54] M. E. McCullough, R. A. Emmons, and J. A. Tsang, "The grateful disposition: a conceptual and empirical topography," *Journal of Personality and Social Psychology*, vol. 82, no. 1, pp. 112–127, 2002.
[55] R. A. Emmons and T. T. Kneezel, "Giving thanks: spiritual and religious correlates of gratitude," *Journal of Psychology and Christianity*, vol. 24, no. 2, pp. 140–148, 2005.
[56] A. F. Shariff and A. Norenzayan, "God is watching you: priming God concepts increases prosocial behavior in an anonymous economic game," *Psychological Science*, vol. 18, no. 9, pp. 803–809, 2007.
[57] N. Krause, "Religious involvement, gratitude, and change in depressive symptoms over time," *International Journal for the Psychology of Religion*, vol. 19, no. 3, pp. 155–172, 2009.
[58] H. G. Koenig, "Religion and depression in older medical inpatients," *American Journal of Geriatric Psychiatry*, vol. 15, no. 4, pp. 282–291, 2007.
[59] D. L. Evans, T. R. Ten Have, S. D. Douglas et al., "Association of depression with viral load, CD8 T lymphocytes, and natural killer cells in women with HIV infection," *American Journal of Psychiatry*, vol. 159, no. 10, pp. 1752–1759, 2002.
[60] A. J. Zautra, D. C. Yocum, I. Villanueva et al., "Immune activation and depression in women with rheumatoid arthritis," *Journal of Rheumatology*, vol. 31, no. 3, pp. 457–463, 2004.
[61] P. H. Thaker, S. K. Lutgendorf, and A. K. Sood, "The neuroendocrine impact of chronic stress on cancer," *Cell Cycle*, vol. 6, no. 4, pp. 430–433, 2007.
[62] S. K. Lutgendorf, D. M. Lamkin, K. DeGeest et al., "Depressed and anxious mood and T-cell cytokine expressing populations in ovarian cancer patients," *Brain, Behavior, and Immunity*, vol. 22, no. 6, pp. 890–900, 2008.
[63] S. K. Lutgendorf, K. DeGeest, C. Y. Sung et al., "Depression, social support, and beta-adrenergic transcription control in human ovarian cancer," *Brain, Behavior, and Immunity*, vol. 23, no. 2, pp. 176–183, 2009.
[64] M. R. Irwin and A. H. Miller, "Depressive disorders and immunity: 20 years of progress and discovery," *Brain, Behavior, and Immunity*, vol. 21, no. 4, pp. 374–383, 2007.
[65] B. E. Leonard and A. Myint, "The psychoneuroimmunology of depression," *Human Psychopharmacology*, vol. 24, no. 3, pp. 165–175, 2009.
[66] M. A. Rosenkranz, D. C. Jackson, K. M. Dalton et al., "Affective style and in vivo immune response: neurobehavioral mechanisms," *Proceedings of the National Academy of Sciences of the United States of America*, vol. 100, no. 19, pp. 11148–11152, 2003.
[67] A. H. Miller, "Neuroendocrine and immune system interactions in stress and depression," *Psychiatric Clinics of North America*, vol. 21, no. 2, pp. 443–463, 1998.

[68] J. K. Kiecolt-Glaser, K. J. Preacher, R. C. MacCallum, C. Atkinson, W. B. Malarkey, and R. Glaser, "Chronic stress and age-related increases in the proinflammatory cytokine IL-6," *Proceedings of the National Academy of Sciences of the United States of America*, vol. 100, no. 15, pp. 9090–9095, 2003.

[69] M. B. Howren, D. M. Lamkin, and J. Suls, "Associations of depression with c-reactive protein, IL-1, and IL-6: a meta-analysis," *Psychosomatic Medicine*, vol. 71, no. 2, pp. 171–186, 2009.

[70] K. A. Hestad, S. Tonseth, C. D. Stoen, T. Ueland, and P. Aukrust, "Raised plasma levels of tumor necrosis factor alpha in patients with depression: normalization during electroconvulsive therapy," *Journal of Electroconvulsive Therapy*, vol. 19, pp. 183–188, 2003.

[71] C. Tuglu, S. H. Kara, O. Caliyurt, E. Vardar, and E. Abay, "Increased serum tumor necrosis factor-alpha levels and treatment response in major depressive disorder," *Psychopharmacology*, vol. 170, no. 4, pp. 429–433, 2003.

[72] B. E. Leonard and A. Myint, "The psychoneuroimmunology of depression," *Human Psychopharmacology*, vol. 24, no. 3, pp. 165–175, 2009.

[73] S. J. Schleifer, S. E. Keller, and A. T. Meyerson, "Lymphocyte function in major depressive disorder," *Archives of General Psychiatry*, vol. 41, no. 5, pp. 484–486, 1984.

[74] S. J. Schleifer, S. E. Keller, R. N. Bond, J. Cohen, and M. Stein, "Major depressive disorder and immunity. Role of age, sex, severity, and hospitalization," *Archives of General Psychiatry*, vol. 46, no. 1, pp. 81–87, 1989.

[75] M. Irwin, T. L. Smith, and J. C. Gillin, "Electroencephalographic sleep and natural killer activity in depressed patients and control subjects," *Psychosomatic Medicine*, vol. 54, no. 1, pp. 10–21, 1992.

[76] R. W. Bartrop, E. Luckhurst, and L. Lazarus, "Depressed lymphocyte function after bereavement," *The Lancet*, vol. 1, no. 8016, pp. 834–836, 1977.

[77] E. P. Zorrilla, L. Luborsky, J. R. McKay et al., "The relationship of depression and stressors to immunological assays: a meta-analytic review," *Brain, Behavior, and Immunity*, vol. 15, no. 3, pp. 199–226, 2001.

[78] K. A. Hestad, S. Tonseth, C. D. Stoen, T. Ueland, and P. Aukrust, "Raised plasma levels of tumor necrosis factor alpha in patients with depression: normalization during electroconvulsive therapy," *Journal of Electroconvulsive Therapy*, vol. 19, pp. 183–188, 2003.

[79] C. Tuglu, S. H. Kara, O. Caliyurt, E. Vardar, and E. Abay, "Increased serum tumor necrosis factor-alpha levels and treatment response in major depressive disorder," *Psychopharmacology*, vol. 170, no. 4, pp. 429–433, 2003.

[80] N. Castanon, B. E. Leonard, P. J. Neveu, and R. Yirmiya, "Effects of antidepressants on cytokine production and actions," *Brain, Behavior, and Immunity*, vol. 16, no. 5, pp. 569–574, 2002.

[81] M. H. Antoni, D. G. Cruess, N. Klimas et al., "Increases in a marker of immune system reconstitution are predated by decreases in 24-h urinary cortisol output and depressed mood during a 10-week stress management intervention in symptomatic HIV-infected men," *Journal of Psychosomatic Research*, vol. 58, no. 1, pp. 3–13, 2005.

[82] M. H. Antoni, S. Lechner, A. Diaz et al., "Cognitive behavioral stress management effects on psychosocial and physiological adaptation in women undergoing treatment for breast cancer," *Brain, Behavior, and Immunity*, vol. 23, no. 5, pp. 580–591, 2009.

[83] H. Van Middendorp, R. Geenen, M. J. Sorbi, L. J. P. Van Doornen, and J. W. J. Bijlsma, "Health and physiological effects of an emotional disclosure intervention adapted for application at home: a randomized clinical trial in rheumatoid arthritis," *Psychotherapy and Psychosomatics*, vol. 78, no. 3, pp. 145–151, 2009.

[84] L. S. Berk, S. Tan, and L. G. Tan, "Mirthful laughter, as adjunct therapy in diabetic care, increases HDL cholesterol and attenuates inflammatory cytokines and CRP and possible CVD risk," *The FASEB Journal*, 2009, Abstract no. 370.

[85] A. D. L. Roberts, A. S. Papadopoulos, S. Wessely, T. Chalder, and A. J. Cleare, "Salivary cortisol output before and after cognitive behavioural therapy for chronic fatigue syndrome," *Journal of Affective Disorders*, vol. 115, no. 1-2, pp. 280–286, 2009.

[86] L. H. Powell, L. Shahabi, and C. E. Thoresen, "Religion and spirituality. Linkages to physical health," *American Psychologist*, vol. 58, no. 1, pp. 36–52, 2003.

[87] Y. Chida, A. Steptoe, and L. H. Powell, "Religiosity/spirituality and mortality: a systematic quantitative review," *Psychotherapy and Psychosomatics*, vol. 78, no. 2, pp. 81–90, 2009.

[88] K. S. Seybold and P. C. Hill, "The role of religion and spirituality in mental and physical health," *Current Directions in Psychological Science*, vol. 10, no. 1, pp. 21–24, 2001.

[89] H. G. Koenig and H. J. Cohen, *The Link Between Religion and Health: Psychoneuroimmunology and the Faith Factor*, Oxford University Press, New York, NY, USA, 2002.

[90] J. Levin, "How faith heals: a theoretical model," *Explore*, vol. 5, no. 2, pp. 77–96, 2009.

[91] S. E. Sephton, C. Koopman, M. Schaal, C. Thoresen, and D. Spiegel, "Spiritual expression and immune status in women with metastatic breast cancer: an exploratory study," *Breast Journal*, vol. 7, no. 5, pp. 345–353, 2001.

[92] G. Ironson, R. Stuetzle, and M. A. Fletcher, "An increase in religiousness/spirituality occurs after HIV diagnosis and predicts slower disease progression over 4 years in people with HIV," *Journal of General Internal Medicine*, vol. 21, no. 5, pp. S62–S68, 2006.

[93] T. E. Woods, M. H. Antoni, G. H. Ironson, and D. W. Kling, "Religiosity is associated with affective and immune status in symptomatic HIV-infected gay men," *Journal of Psychosomatic Research*, vol. 46, no. 2, pp. 165–176, 1999.

[94] N. L. McCain, D. P. Gray, R. K. Elswick et al., "A randomized clinical trial of alternative stress management interventions in persons with HIV infection," *Journal of Consulting and Clinical Psychology*, vol. 76, no. 3, pp. 431–441, 2008.

[95] P. Lissoni, G. Messina, D. Parolini et al., "A spiritual approach in the treatment of cancer: relation between faith score and response to chemotherapy in advanced non-small cell lung cancer patients," *In Vivo*, vol. 22, no. 5, pp. 577–582, 2008.

[96] H. G. Koenig, H. J. Cohen, L. K. George, J. C. Hays, D. B. Larson, and D. G. Blazer, "Attendance at religious services, interleukin-6, and other biological parameters of immune function in older adults," *International Journal of Psychiatry in Medicine*, vol. 27, no. 3, pp. 233–250, 1997.

[97] S. K. Lutgendorf, P. Ullrich, R. Wallace, D. Russell, and T. B. Harris, "Religious participation, interleukin-6, and mortality in older adults," *Health Psychology*, vol. 23, no. 5, pp. 465–475, 2004.

[98] D. E. King, A. G. Mainous, and W. S. Pearson, "C-reactive protein, diabetes, and attendance at religious services," *Diabetes Care*, vol. 25, no. 7, pp. 1172–1176, 2002.

[99] E. A. Dedert, J. L. Studts, I. Weissbecker, P. G. Salmon, P. L. Banis, and S. E. Sephton, "Private religious practice: protection of cortisol rhythms among women with fibromyalgia," *International Journal of Psychiatry in Medicine*, vol. 34, pp. 61–77, 2004.
[100] J. Tartaro, L. J. Luecken, and H. E. Gunn, "Exploring heart and soul: effects of religiosity/spirituality and gender on blood pressure and cortisol stress responses," *Journal of Health Psychology*, vol. 10, no. 6, pp. 753–766, 2005.
[101] G. Ironson, G. F. Solomon, E. G. Balbin et al., "The Ironson-Woods Spirituality/Religiousness Index is associated with long survival, health behaviors, less distress, and low cortisol in people with HIV/AIDS," *Annals of Behavioral Medicine*, vol. 24, no. 1, pp. 34–48, 2002.
[102] A. W. Carrico, G. Ironson, M. H. Antoni et al., "A path model of the effects of spirituality on depressive symptoms and 24-h urinary-free cortisol in HIV-positive persons," *Journal of Psychosomatic Research*, vol. 61, no. 1, pp. 51–58, 2006.
[103] C. L. W. Chan, R. T. H. Ho, P. W. H. Lee et al., "A randomized controlled trial of psychosocial interventions using the psychophysiological framework for Chinese breast cancer patients," *Journal of Psychosocial Oncology*, vol. 24, no. 1, pp. 3–26, 2006.
[104] N. L. McCain, D. P. Gray, R. K. Elswick et al., "A randomized clinical trial of alternative stress management interventions in persons with HIV infection," *Journal of Consulting and Clinical Psychology*, vol. 76, no. 3, pp. 431–441, 2008.
[105] R. J. Davidson, J. Kabat-Zinn, J. Schumacher et al., "Alterations in brain and immune function produced by mindfulness meditation," *Psychosomatic Medicine*, vol. 65, no. 4, pp. 564–570, 2003.
[106] T. W. W. Pace, L. T. Negi, D. D. Adame et al., "Effect of compassion meditation on neuroendocrine, innate immune and behavioral responses to psychosocial stress," *Psychoneuroendocrinology*, vol. 34, no. 1, pp. 87–98, 2009.
[107] L. Witek-Janusek, K. Albuquerque, K. R. Chroniak, C. Chroniak, R. Durazo-Arvizu, and H. L. Mathews, "Effect of mindfulness based stress reduction on immune function, quality of life and coping in women newly diagnosed with early stage breast cancer," *Brain, Behavior, and Immunity*, vol. 22, no. 6, pp. 969–981, 2008.
[108] R. Sudsuang, V. Chentanez, and K. Veluvan, "Effect of Buddhist meditation on serum cortisol and total protein levels, blood pressure, pulse rate, lung volume and reaction time," *Physiology and Behavior*, vol. 50, no. 3, pp. 543–548, 1991.
[109] J. R. Infante, F. Peran, M. Martinez et al., "ACTH and beta-endorphin in transcendental medication," *Physiology & Behavior*, vol. 64, pp. 311–315, 1998.
[110] K. G. Walton, J. Z. Fields, D. K. Levitsky, D. A. Harris, N. D. Pugh, and R. H. Schneider, "Lowering cortisol and CVD risk in postmenopausal women: a pilot study using the transcendental meditation program," *Annals of the New York Academy of Sciences*, vol. 1032, pp. 211–215, 2004.
[111] P. Jin, "Efficacy of Tai Chi, brisk walking, meditation, and reading in reducing mental and emotional stress," *Journal of Psychosomatic Research*, vol. 36, no. 4, pp. 361–370, 1992.
[112] J. A. Curiati, E. Bocchi, J. O. Freire et al., "Meditation reduces sympathetic activation and improves the quality of life in elderly patients with optimally treated heart failure: a prospective randomized study," *Journal of Alternative and Complementary Medicine*, vol. 11, no. 3, pp. 465–472, 2005.
[113] J. Granath, S. Ingvarsson, U. von Thiele, and U. Lundberg, "Stress management: a randomized study of cognitive behavioural therapy and yoga," *Cognitive Behaviour Therapy*, vol. 35, no. 1, pp. 3–10, 2006.
[114] H. G. Koenig, *Medicine, Religion and Health*, Templeton Foundation Press, Philadelphia, Pa, USA, 2008.
[115] L. R. Propst, R. Ostrom, P. Watkins, T. Dean, and D. Mashburn, "Comparative efficacy of religious and nonreligious cognitive-behavioral therapy for the treatment of clinical depression in religious individuals," *Journal of Consulting and Clinical Psychology*, vol. 60, no. 1, pp. 94–103, 1992.
[116] R. Bowen, M. Baetz, C. D'Arcy, and R. Bowen, "Self-rated importance of religion predicts one-year outcome of patients with panic disorder," *Depression and Anxiety*, vol. 23, no. 5, pp. 266–273, 2006.
[117] L. R. Propst, "The comparative efficacy of religious and non-religious imagery for the treatment of mild depression in religious individuals," *Cognitive Therapy and Research*, vol. 4, no. 2, pp. 167–178, 1980.
[118] L. R. Propst, R. Ostrom, P. Watkins, T. Dean, and D. Mashburn, "Comparative efficacy of religious and nonreligious cognitive-behavioral therapy for the treatment of clinical depression in religious individuals," *Journal of Consulting and Clinical Psychology*, vol. 60, no. 1, pp. 94–103, 1992.
[119] D. H. Rosmarin, K. I. Pargament, S. Pirutinsky, and A. Mahoney, "A randomized controlled evaluation of a spiritually integrated treatment for subclinical anxiety in the Jewish community, delivered via the Internet," *Journal of Anxiety Disorders*, vol. 24, no. 7, pp. 799–808, 2010.
[120] M. Z. Azhar, S. L. Varma, and A. S. Dharap, "Religious psychotherapy in anxiety disorder patients," *Acta Psychiatrica Scandinavica*, vol. 90, no. 1, pp. 1–3, 1994.
[121] M. Z. Azhar and S. L. Varma, "Religious psychotherapy in depressive patients," *Psychotherapy and Psychosomatics*, vol. 63, no. 3-4, pp. 165–168, 1995.
[122] M. Z. Azhar and S. L. Varma, "Religious psychotherapy as management of bereavement," *Acta Psychiatrica Scandinavica*, vol. 91, no. 4, pp. 233–235, 1995.
[123] S. M. Razali, C. I. Hasanah, K. Aminah, and M. Subramaniam, "Religious-sociocultural psychotherapy in patients with anxiety and depression," *Australian and New Zealand Journal of Psychiatry*, vol. 32, no. 6, pp. 867–872, 1998.
[124] S. Xiao, D. Young, and H. Zhang, "Taoistic cognitive psychotherapy for neurotic patients: a preliminary clinical trial," *Psychiatry and Clinical Neurosciences*, vol. 52, supplement, pp. S238–S241, 1998.
[125] M. A. Stanley, A. L. Bush, M. E. Camp et al., "Older adults' preferences for religion/spirituality in treatment of anxiety and depression," *Aging and Mental Health*, vol. 15, no. 3, pp. 334–343, 2011.
[126] E. M. Rose, J. S. Westefeld, and T. N. Ansley, "Spiritual issues in counselling: clients' beliefs and preferences," *Journal of Counseling Psychology*, vol. 48, no. 1, pp. 61–71, 2001.
[127] E. W. Kelly Jr., "Spirituality and religion in counselor education: a national survey," *Counselor Education and Supervision*, vol. 33, pp. 227–237, 1995.
[128] N. Krause, "Religious involvement, gratitude, and change in depressive symptoms over time," *International Journal for the Psychology of Religion*, vol. 19, no. 3, pp. 155–172, 2009.
[129] K. M. Sheldon, "How to increase and sustain positive emotion: the effects of expressing gratitude and visualizing vest possible selves," *Journal of Positive Psychology*, vol. 1, pp. 73–82, 2006.
[130] S. J. Morris and F. H. Kanfer, "Altruism and depression," *Personality and Social Psychology Bulletin*, vol. 9, pp. 567–577, 1983.

[131] T. Fujiwara, "The role of altruistic behavior in generalized anxiety disorder and major depression among adults in the United States," *Journal of Affective Disorders*, vol. 101, no. 1–3, pp. 219–225, 2007.
[132] H. G. Koenig, D. E. King, and V. B. Carson, *Handbook of Religion and Health*, Oxford University Press, New York, NY, USA, 2nd edition, 2012.
[133] B. C. Post and N. G. Wade, "Religion and spirituality in psychotherapy: a practice-friendly review of research," *Journal of Clinical Psychology*, vol. 65, no. 2, pp. 131–146, 2009.
[134] B. J. Rounsaville, K. M. Carroll, and L. S. Onken, "A stage model of behavioral therapies research: getting started and moving on from stage I," *Clinical Psychology*, vol. 8, no. 2, pp. 133–142, 2001.
[135] K. Pargament, *Spiritually Integrated Psychotherapy: Understanding and Addressing the Sacred*, Guilford Press, New York, NY, USA, 2007.
[136] L. R. Propst, R. Ostrom, P. Watkins, T. Dean, and D. Mashburn, "Comparative efficacy of religious and nonreligious cognitive-behavioral therapy for the treatment of clinical depression in religious individuals," *Journal of Consulting and Clinical Psychology*, vol. 60, no. 1, pp. 94–103, 1992.
[137] B. C. Post and N. G. Wade, "Religion and spirituality in psychotherapy: a practice-friendly review of research," *Journal of Clinical Psychology*, vol. 65, no. 2, pp. 131–146, 2009.

8

Postpartum Depression: Screening, Diagnosis, and Management Programs 2000 through 2010

Barbara P. Yawn,[1] Ardis L. Olson,[2] Susan Bertram,[1] Wilson Pace,[3] Peter Wollan,[1] and Allen J. Dietrich[4]

[1] *Department of Research, Olmsted Medical Center, Rochester, MN 55904, USA*
[2] *Departments of Pediatrics and Community and Family Medicine, Dartmouth Medical School, Dartmouth Medical School, Hanover, NH 03755, USA*
[3] *National Research Network, American Academy of Family Physicians, Leawood, KS 66211, USA*
[4] *Department of Community and Family Medicine, Dartmouth Medical School, Hanover, NH 03735, USA*

Correspondence should be addressed to Barbara P. Yawn, byawn@olmmed.org

Academic Editor: Mark Williams

The value and appropriateness of universal postpartum depression (PPD) screening remains controversial in the United States. To date, several PPD screening programs have been introduced and a few have been evaluated. Among those programs that have been evaluated, most report screening rates, diagnosis rates, or treatment initiation rates. Only four studies included patient outcomes such as the level of depressive symptoms at 6 to 12 months postpartum, and only two reported success in improving outcomes. Program characteristics that appear to result in low rates of diagnosis and followup after PPD screening include requirements for a formal psychiatric evaluation, the need to refer women to another site for therapy, and failure to integrate the PPD screening into the care provided at the woman's or her child's medical home. The two programs that reported improved outcomes were both self-contained within primary care and included specific followup, management, and therapy procedures. Both resulted in the need for outside referrals in less than 10% of women diagnosed with postpartum depression. Future studies should be based on the successful programs and their identified facilitators while avoiding identified barriers. To affect policies, the future program must report maternal outcomes going beyond the often reported process outcomes of screening, referral, and therapy initiation rates.

1. Introduction

Postpartum depression (PPD) is common, reported to be experienced by 15% or more of women during the 12 months after they deliver [1–4]. Despite nearly universal health care encounters at some time during this period, only about 50% of women with significant depressive symptoms are recognized [4–6]. PPD occurs among women of all ages, parities, races, and socioeconomic groups [7, 8]. Untreated and unresolved PPD adversely affects the woman, her infant and her relationship with family members [9–12]. Therefore, universal screening for PPD is an attractive approach, and several groups have made recommendations regarding universal PPD screening in the maternity or early well child care setting [2, 13–19].

Many United States (US) as well as international programs have attempted to implement universal postpartum depression screening with or without followup care. Some programs have included formal evaluations, but few have resulted in improved patient outcomes [20–30]. Reviews by several evidence-based guideline groups have reported insufficient or inconclusive information regarding improved outcomes with PPD screening, preventing them from recommending universal PPD screening. While these reviews provide summary assessments, they fail to assess program design, context, setting, or components of the program as potential factors influencing success or failure [2–4, 15, 18, 25].

This paper also reviews the published evidence regarding PPD screening and follow up, describing the methods and outcomes reported for recent published PPD studies [20–24, 27–30]. Unlike the reviews completed for the guidelines panels, our goal is to summarize elements of program design, program setting, and program components as they may relate to program success in not only providing PPD screening but improving outcomes of women judged to have PPD.

2. Methods

We reviewed PPD screening programs described in the English language peer-reviewed literature between 1998 and 2011 [20–24, 27–32]. Studies were identified from Medline/PubMed, PsychINFO, and Cinahl using title, abstract and keyword searches for the terms "postpartum depression," "maternal depression," and "perinatal depression," each independently and then linked to "screening." We also identified work published in the same time frame from the references in the Institute of Medicine's (IOM's) report on parental depression [1]. Finally a Google search using the phrase "postpartum depression screening programs" was completed to identify reported puslihed in nonindexed health care and social science journals. Only programs that reported an intervention and some type of outcomes such as screening rates, rates of screen failure, diagnosis rates, or maternal depression outcomes were included. The programs described here vary from small studies done in three to seven clinics in a single city to regional, state, and national programs. The published reports of several US programs were supplemented by additional information from the first or senior author of the paper(s) describing the programs (personal communications Kim Yonkers, MD, Dwenda Gjerdigen, MD and Ardis Olson, MD).

3. Results

Overall, reports on 54 programs were identified but only eight of those had both clearly stated interventions and outcomes resulting in their inclusion in this report (Table 1). The total number of women included in these programs is difficult to ascertain since little data was provided on the number of potentially eligible women in some of the largest of the programs [22, 28–32]. All of the programs were designed to address postpartum women from less than a week after birth [20, 21] to 6 months postpartum [22]. Five programs were limited to patients literate in English. The Hong Kong program was limited to Chinese [26]. Two programs, the New Haven [22] and the family medicine program [27], allowed either English or Spanish. Characteristics of the women enrolled, such as insurance, marital and socioeconomic status (SES) were variably reported and when reported differed by program and country. In the US, Medicaid was the most common insurer and coverage often ended at 6 to 8 weeks postpartum [29]. The New Jersey program was open to all women, but only those with Medicaid insurance were included in the outcomes assessment [29]. In Australia and in Hong Kong, national health insurance assured that all enrolled women received insurance coverage for the entire prenatal and postpartum period [26, 28, 30].

4. Program Characteristics

4.1. Screening. All programs used the EPDS [21, 27, 33], the PHQ-9 [27, 34], or the PHQ-2 [35–38] for PPD screening. One program used a combination of the EPDS with all elevated scores being further assessed by the PHQ-9 [27, 39]. The cutoff scores for normal versus elevated were similar for all programs: an EPDS of 10 or greater or a PHQ-9 of 10 or greater [33, 34, 39].

Screening was most often reported to be initiated at the site of well child or maternal postpartum care [21, 23, 26–32]. The New Haven program was an exception. Designed as a community-based program, women were referred or self-referred to the community program office where they were screened and could be further evaluated [22]. Screening rates varied from a low of 33% to over 95% of eligible women in the US clinic-based programs [21, 27]. In Australia, the screening rate was estimated to be approximately 40% in one region of the country [31, 32]. The New Haven and New Jersey programs did not report screening rates [22, 29]. However, screening was assumed to be limited since participation in the physician educational offerings for these programs was low, with only 58% of obstetricians, 13% of pediatricians, and 12% of family physicians attending PPD education offered to support the New Jersey statewide program [29].

Procedures for further evaluation of elevated screening scores were not uniform across the programs and not all programs included plans for management or monitoring of women with diagnosed depression. For example, the screening programs in Australia, New Jersey, and Olmsted County, MN, US [23, 24, 28–32] did not report any specific follow-up procedures for further evaluation of elevated screening scores. In three programs procedures for evaluation of women with elevated screening scores required referral to an offsite mental health clinics or to delayed visits to staff at the screening site [20, 22, 33]. Those referrals were reported to include the Structured Clinical Interview for DSM Disorders (SCID) which is a formal interview that requires 30 to 45 minutes to complete and is usually administered by a psychologist or psychiatrist (http://www.SCID4.org/) [40]. Only two programs maintained screening and evaluation within the same site. Both of these programs also included specific procedures and support for PPD management and monitoring. Neither included evaluation with the SCID [26, 27].

5. Outcomes

All programs except the New Haven program reported one or more process outcomes such as screening rates (see above).

Table 1

Site	New Haven Healthy Start Program [22] (n = 1,336)	Minneapolis and St. Paul, MN, screening at well child programs [21] (n = 506)	Australia, universal PPD screening [28, 30–32] (n unknown)	US family medicine practices [27] (n = 1,263)	Olmsted County, MN universal PPD screening program [23] (n = 342)	New Hampshire, screening at all well child visits in pediatric practices [20, 33] (n = 1,398)	New Jersey State wide initiative [29] (30,955 analyzed)	Hong Kong Program [26] (n = 462)
Enrollment criteria	Low-income women within 6 months of delivery (i) self-referred (ii) referred by outreach worker	Women bringing children to 0-1 month to well child visits at family medicine or pediatric clinics	All postpartum women in all practices in the country	All women between 4 and 12 weeks PP coming for PP or well child visit to 28 enrolled practices	All women between 4 and 9 wks PP coming for PP visit to OB or FM to Olmsted County, MN provider	All women bringing children 0–18 years for well child visits for 6 month time period in three enrolled pediatric practices	All women with Medicaid insurance for during pregnancy and 1st yr PP were used in analyses, all women in state delivering an infant during time of interest were in program	All women visiting maternal and child health centers for 2 month well child check. Exclude if already receiving mental health care
	(English or Spanish)	(English only)	(English only)	(English or Spanish)	(English only)	(English only)	(Unknown)	(Mandarin only)
Site characteristics	New Haven Healthy Start initiative—a community-based program not within any clinic	Seven family clinics, 4 urban family medicine, and 3 suburban pediatric clinics	All clinics providing postpartum care in the country	28 US FM practices including rural, urban, and residency practices	All OB and FM postpartum care providers in the community	Rural Peds practices, all pediatric providers (pediatricians and nurse practitioners)	All maternity and well child practices in New Jersey	One maternal and child health clinic in Hong Kong, nurse run and staffed. Support from local psychiatrists
	Screening by staff	Screening by staff	Screening by staff	Screening by clinic staff and physician review	Screening by staff, review by physician	Screening by staff, review by clinicians	Screeners unknown	Screening by nurses
Screening tools	PHQ-9 (cutoff for followup 10), PTSD screener, anxiety and alcohol screener	PHQ-2 and then PHQ-9	EPDS	EPDS follow by PHQ-9 for all scores greater than 10 versus usual care with no formal screening	EPDS, score >9 considered high risk for PPD	PHQ-2, (scored 0–6) with cut point of 3 or more for positive screen	Left to the practice following an educational program to introduce screening and PPD management to physicians and other clinicians	EPDS, score >9 considered elevated compared to usual clinical assessment by nurse

Table 1: Continued.

Diagnostic methods	Telephone interview by master's level clinical social worker	Referral for SCID to mental health clinic	Unknown, primarily screening program	PHQ-9 and physician assessment	Physician or other clinician choice	Clinician discussed and offered referral resources	Physician or other clinician choice. Education covered both PPD care and referral	Onsite counseling by nurse trained with short program. Could go for additional referral
Followup program	Referral for therapy and calls by social worker at 1, 3, and 6 months for further referral suggestions Community education	As per mental health care professional to whom the patient is referred	Unknown	Detailed follow-up program and tools to support care, medication, and counseling use and schedule nurse calls	None provided	As per mental health professional to whom the patient is referred	Followup as determined by care providers	Followup was single session by trained nurse with optional additional counseling
Outcomes	Rates of therapy, levels of symptoms monthly after referral	Rates of screening completion including SCID	Rates of screening	Rates of screening, diagnosis, therapy initiation, levels of depressive symptoms at 6 and 12 months PP	Rates of PPD diagnosis and rates of PPD therapy initiated	Rates of screening completed and screen positive status, and rates of women willing to take action plus rates of pediatrician support offered	Rates of depression care initiation and continuation of care after 90 and 120 days	Levels of depressive symptoms at 6 and 18 months PP
Results	No change with program (before and after assessments)	Less than 33% completed screening and assessment with SCID	Rates of screening <40% in several regions	Increased rates of PPD diagnosis, therapy initiation, and lower levels of depressive symptoms at 12 months PP	Increased rates of PPD diagnosis and increased rates of PPD therapy initiated	Screening completed at 67% to 74% of well child visits. 6% of women had scores ≥ 3 Among screen + mothers: 47% thought might be depressed and willing to take action. 28% thought stressed, not PPD. Clinician action in 62%	No change in rates of care initiation or continuation (before and after the onset of the statewide program assessment)	Risk ratio of EPDS <10 was 0.50 for intervention versus usual care and NNS was 25 to prevent one EPDS of >10 at 12 months

Table 1: Continued.

Study design	Pre- and post-"open label"	RCT	Cohort	RCT	Pre- and post-cohort	Cohort	Pre- and post-study of Medicaid subset of population	RCT
Depression monitoring metrics	PHQ-9 score	Unknown	None	PHQ-9 score	None	N/A	None	None
Support systems and tools	Social worker phone calls, weekly drop in programs for behavioral health or pharmacological services, provided at no cost	None	None	IAP, medication table, nurse call scripts, self help tools, father's pamphlet, and monitoring schedule	None	N/A	Education attended by 38% of obstetrical care physicians and other clinicians and 16% of pediatricians and 12% of family physicians in New Jersey	Nurses doing counseling had 12 hours of training and could refer to psychiatrist if desired
Reported barriers to success	Adding mental health people into practice without integration may have decreased physician role as screener and evaluator, low SES population	Need to refer offsite for SCID	Unable to get EPDS screening integrated into many practices. A national program without incentives	Time barriers for clinic nurses to make calls, loss of insurance at 6 to 8 weeks PP for many of the women, failure to address PPD as chronic condition	No followup program included	Pediatrician role limited to screening, discussing impact on child, referral and short-term followup	Less than one-third of clinical care providers participated in the educational program	More than half of the women attending the clinic were ineligible including several who had already undergone PND screening

The Olmsted County, MN program reported increased rates of PPD diagnosis and treatment initiation following universal PPD screening [24]. The New Hampshire program, based in pediatricians' offices, reported "referral or maternal support from the pediatrician" in 67% of women with elevated screening scores. Buist et al. reported some increase in PPD diagnoses and therapy initiation in a subset of women screened in the Australian program [31, 32].

Four programs reported maternal outcome information [22, 26, 27, 29]. Both the New Haven Healthy Start and the New Jersey state programs reported no increases in any PPD-related clinical activities including no increases in rates of diagnoses or numbers of PPD related office visits [22, 29]. The Hong Kong and US primary care program reported both improved process outcomes and improved maternal outcomes at 6 or 12 months [26, 27]. Both reported declines in maternal depressive symptoms at either 6 or 12 months as well as high rates of screening, increased rates of PPD diagnosis and therapy initiation.

5.1. Reported Barriers to Success. In the New Haven [22] and Minneapolis and St. Paul studies [21], evaluation of women with elevated screening scores required an in-person or telephone-based referral to a mental health professional for an SCID assessment. The requirement for an SCID assessment appeared to be a major barrier [40, 41] for completion of PPD evaluation with a low percentage of women in the Minneapolis/St. Paul study program completing the referral visit for this SCID assessment. A similar pattern of failure to participate in the SCID evaluation was seen among the women in New Haven even though they could do the interview by telephone (personal communication Kim Yonkers, MD, February 21, 2012).

5.2. Possible Facilitators of Success. The Hong Kong and US family physician programs both introduced specific evaluation procedures to be completed with women with elevated screening scores and management and monitoring systems for those with diagnosed depression [26, 27]. In both cases, the procedures and care systems changes were based in the usual care site and usually began immediately after screening. To support the follow-up procedures and care system changes, the Hong Kong program provided a 12-hour educational experience for the nurses who completed screening in the well child visits. The nurses were taught some basics of supportive therapy and motivational interviewing [26]. In the US family medicine program short staff educational sessions (2 hours total), support tools for diagnosis, therapy selection and initiation, schedules of recommended management and monitoring visits, content outlines for nurse calls as well as an immediate action plan (IAP) to guide assessment of suicidal ideation [42] were provided to the practices. The PHQ-9 was used as a metric for assessing response to therapy and timing of remission in both the Hong Kong and US programs [26, 27]. Referral for complex problems occurred in about 6% of the women in each of the studies [26, 27].

6. Discussion

While the impact of PPD screening clearly differs among published studies, so do the programs that support that screening. To assess the reported results without considering the context in which screening was completed is likely to miss opportunities to identify parameters of successful translation of PPD screening into daily practice. It is important to recognize the complexity of the process of changing both clinician behavior and establishing effective office systems to consistently screen and intervene. In addition, the type of results reported must also be considered [43–47]. Screening rates, therapy initiation, or intent to treat are important preliminary results but must be followed by studies that assess and report patient outcomes [1, 12, 15, 16, 19]. Patient outcomes such as the level of depressive symptoms or rates of remission need to be assessed and reported in the context of the full program that achieved those outcomes [26, 27]. With a limited number of outcome studies published to date, the controversy surrounding the value of universal PPD screening continues.

Among the studies reviewed here, four programs reported screening at least two-thirds of eligible women and in all instances the programs were conducted within a woman's or her infant's usual care site [20, 23, 26, 27]. In these practices, PPD education was provided to the clinical and support staff within the practice site [20, 23, 26, 27]. In the largest programs, all of the state of New Jersey and all of Australia, plus the New Haven Healthy Start program, educational support for community physicians was not tailored to individual practices and only modestly attended. Providing education alone has been shown previously to not facilitate practice change [43–46, 48, 49].

Screening alone has not been shown to improve patient outcomes and may be unethical [13, 50]. Dealing with PPD is limited to adding ten questions to a patient care visit. Even a negative screening result requires some discussion. A positive screening result should trigger a cascade of events that change the visit content and practice work flow. Practice tools are required to facilitate these changes. Olson and her colleagues have developed a set of tools to facilitate the introduction and implementation of routine PPD and maternal depression screening into pediatric practices. The information is available on a website [51, 52] and has been widely disseminated through an American Academy of Pediatrics Task Force report [53]. Yawn et al. also developed primary care specific tools to support diagnosis, medication therapy initiation, and PPD followup and monitoring plan [27, 42]. Programs that support practice system changes such as universal PPD screening appear to benefit from local education and support for the practice change and its implementation. Without tools and support for system change, dissemination is likely to be slow with each practice reinventing similar work flow, education and support systems [45, 54].

Four studies did report patient outcomes, two without improvement (New Haven and New Jersey) [22, 29] and two with improved outcomes (Hong Kong and US family physicians) [26, 27]. Two important aspects that appear to differentiate successful and unsuccessful programs are the ability to provide the majority of care within the screening practice and the provision of education, tools and support for depression diagnosis and ongoing management to facilitate systems change. Primary care practices can provide care for major depressive disorder [47–49]. The Hong Kong and US family medicine studies suggest that this can include care of maternal depression [26, 27]. Referral to mental health specialists will continue to be necessary for the most complex patients and those who do not respond to primary care therapy. In both of the successful programs the referral rate to psychiatrists was 6% of screen positive women [26, 27]. However, with the worldwide shortage of mental health professionals [55] it is important that these resources be used for complex cases and that efforts are made to integrate mental health into primary care [42, 56, 57]. While some integration may mean bringing mental health professionals into primary care offices, an alternative may be to provide mental health services by the people already within the practice, the primary care physician supported by the primary care team [27, 43–45, 48, 49, 57, 58].

Requiring a SCID to diagnose PPD requires women to go outside their usual care sites and appears to be a major barrier to evaluation and diagnosis [21, 41]. Gjerdingen and others have similarly reported this potential barrier to PPD care [21, 57]. The need for the SCID assessment is based on results from studies of high-risk patients with complex mental health problems and who are referred to psychiatrists [1, 2]. These results may not be generalizable to a lower-risk primary care population being assessed within their continuity practices. The benefits of requiring a SCID for PPD diagnosis must be weighed against the risks of missing PPD and a chance to provide therapy and care to the women identified by screening without a SCID confirmation. Implementation of PPD care in primary care practices is feasible. Screening linked with appropriate and patient acceptable evaluation, monitoring, and depression management support can improve outcomes at 6 to 12 months postpartum. With education and support, primary care is likely to be able to provide the required evaluation and care for the majority of women with PPD leaving the limited numbers of mental health professionals to care for more complex cases. To date, the number of studies demonstrating positive patient outcomes is limited and additional studies and dissemination programs with careful evaluation will be required to confirm these results. In the future, primary care management of depression, including postpartum depression could be similar to primary care management of other chronic conditions such as hypertension, diabetes, and asthma where most patients can receive most of their care within the primary care setting and that care can meet the high standards of quality metrics [59].

References

[1] National Research Council and Institute of Medicine, "Depression in Parents, Parenting, and Children: Opportunities to Improve Identification, Treatment, and Prevention," Committee on Depression, Parenting Practices, and the Healthy Development of Children. Board on Children, Youth, and Families. Division of Behavioral and Social Sciences and Education. Washington, DC, USA, The National Academies Press, 2009.

[2] C. E. Hewitt and S. M. Gilbody, "Is it clinically and cost effective to screen for postnatal depression: a systematic review of controlled clinical trials and economic evidence," *An International Journal of Obstetrics & Gynaecology*, vol. 116, no. 8, pp. 1019–1027, 2009.

[3] C. E. Hewitt, S. M. Gilbody, S. Brealey et al., "Methods to identify postnatal depression in primary care: an integrated evidence synthesis and value of information analysis," *Health Technology Assessment*, vol. 13, no. 36, pp. 1–145, 2009.

[4] B. N. Gaynes, N. Gavin, S. Meltzer-Brody et al., "Perinatal depression: prevalence, screening accuracy, and screening outcomes," *Evidence Report/Technology Assessment*, no. 119, 2005, AHRQ Publications No. 05-E006-2.

[5] N. I. Gavin, B. N. Gaynes, K. N. Lohr, S. Meltzer-Brody, G. Gartlehner, and T. Swinson, "Perinatal depression: a systematic review of prevalence and incidence," *Obstetrics & Gynecology*, vol. 106, no. 5, part 1, pp. 1071–1083, 2005.

[6] M. W. O'Hara, "Postpartum depression: what we know," *Journal of Clinical Psychology*, vol. 65, no. 12, pp. 1258–1269, 2009.

[7] T. L. Bryan, A. M. Georgiopoulos, R. W. Harms, J. E. Huxsahl, D. R. Larson, and B. P. Yawn, "Incidence of postpartum depression in Olmsted County, Minnesota: a population-based, retrospective study," *Journal of Reproductive Medicine for the Obstetrician and Gynecologist*, vol. 44, no. 4, pp. 351–358, 1999.

[8] I. H. Bernstein, A. J. Rush, K. Yonkers et al., "Symptom features of postpartum depression: are they distinct?" *Depression and Anxiety*, vol. 25, no. 1, pp. 20–26, 2008.

[9] T. Field, "Prenatal depression effects on early development: a review," *Infant Behavior and Development*, vol. 34, no. 1, pp. 1–14, 2011.

[10] R. Feldman, A. Granat, C. Pariente, H. Kanety, J. Kuint, and E. Gilboa-Schechtman, "Maternal depression and anxiety across the postpartum year and infant social engagement, fear regulation, and stress reactivity," *Journal of the American Academy of Child and Adolescent Psychiatry*, vol. 48, no. 9, pp. 919–927, 2009.

[11] B. Avan, L. M. Richter, P. G. Ramchandani, S. A. Norris, and A. Stein, "Maternal postnatal depression and children's growth and behaviour during the early years of life: exploring the interaction between physical and mental health," *Archives of Disease in Childhood*, vol. 95, no. 9, pp. 690–695, 2010.

[12] L. Murray, A. Arteche, P. Fearon, S. Halligan, T. Croudace, and P. Cooper, "The effects of maternal postnatal depression and child sex on academic performance at age 16 years: a developmental approach," *Journal of Child Psychology and Psychiatry and Allied Disciplines*, vol. 51, no. 10, pp. 1150–1159, 2010.

[13] The Agency for Healthcare Research and Quality (AHRQ), "Recommendations of the U.S. Preventive Services Task Force. The Guide to Clinical Preventive Services," Pub No. 07-05100, September 2007, http://www.ahrq.gov/clinic/uspstf/uspstopics.htm.

[14] H. Mishina and J. I. Takayama, "Screening for maternal depression in primary care pediatrics," *Current Opinion in Pediatrics*, vol. 21, no. 6, pp. 789–793, 2009.

[15] NICE, http://guidance.nice.org.uk/CG90.

[16] Bright Futures, http://www.brightfutures.org/.

[17] J. Sheeder, K. Kabir, and B. Stafford, "Screening for postpartum depression at well-child visits: is once enough during the first 6 months of life?" *Pediatrics*, vol. 123, no. 6, pp. e982–e988, 2009.

[18] M. Paulden, S. Palmer, C. Hewitt, and S. Gilbody, "Screening for postnatal depression in primary care: cost effectiveness analysis," *British Medical Journal*, vol. 339, Article ID b5203, 2009.

[19] Committee Opinion No. 453, "Screening for depression during and after pregnancy," *Obstetrics & Gynecology*, vol. 115, no. 2, part 1, pp. 394–395, 2010.

[20] A. L. Olson, A. J. Dietrich, G. Prazar, and J. Hurley, "Brief maternal depression screening at well-child visits," *Pediatrics*, vol. 118, no. 1, pp. 207–216, 2006.

[21] D. Gjerdingen, W. Katon, and D. E. Rich, "Stepped care treatment of postpartum depression. A primary care based management model," *Women's Health Issues*, vol. 18, no. 1, pp. 44–52, 2008.

[22] K. A. Yonkers, M. V. Smith, H. Lin, H. B. Howell, L. Shao, and R. A. Rosenheck, "Depression screening of perinatal women: an evaluation of the healthy start depression initiative," *Psychiatric Services*, vol. 60, no. 3, pp. 322–328, 2009.

[23] A. M. Georgiopoulos, T. L. Bryan, P. Wollan, and B. P. Yawn, "Routine screening for postpartum depression," *Journal of Family Practice*, vol. 50, no. 2, pp. 117–122, 2001.

[24] A. M. Georgiopoulos, T. L. Bryan, B. P. Yawn, M. S. Houston, T. A. Rummans, and T. M. Therneau, "Population-based screening for postpartum depression," *Obstetrics & Gynecology*, vol. 93, no. 5, pp. 653–657, 1999.

[25] S. Gilbody, T. Sheldon, and A. House, "Screening and case-finding instruments for depression: a meta-analysis," *Canadian Medical Association Journal*, vol. 178, no. 8, pp. 997–1003, 2008.

[26] S. S. L. Leung, C. Leung, T. H. Lam et al., "Outcome of a postnatal depression screening programme using the Edinburgh Postnatal Depression Scale: a randomized controlled trial," *Journal of Public Health*, vol. 33, no. 2, pp. 292–301, 2011.

[27] B. P. Yawn, W. Pace, S. Bertram, P. Wollan, D. Graham, and A. Dietrich, "Translating PPD screening and management into primary care practice: An RCT," *The Annals of Family Medicine*, vol. 10, no. 2, pp. 320–329, 2012.

[28] S. Armstrong and R. Small, "Screening for postnatal depression: not a simple task," *Australian and New Zealand Journal of Public Health*, vol. 31, no. 1, pp. 57–61, 2007.

[29] K. B. Kozhimannil, A. S. Adams, S. B. Soumerai, A. B. Busch, and H. A. Huskamp, "New Jersey's efforts to improve postpartum depression care did not change treatment patterns for women on medicaid," *Health Affairs*, vol. 30, no. 2, pp. 293–301, 2011.

[30] M. P. Austin, N. Reilly, J. Milgrom, and B. Barnett, "A national approach to perinatal mental health in Australia: exercising caution in the roll-out of a public health initiative," *Medical Journal of Australia*, vol. 192, no. 2, p. 111, 2010.

[31] A. Buist, J. Condon, J. Brooks et al., "Acceptability of routine screening for perinatal depression," *Journal of Affective Disorders*, vol. 93, no. 1–3, pp. 233–237, 2006.

[32] A. Buist, D. Ellwood, J. Brooks et al., "National program for depression associated with childbirth: the Australian experience," *Best Practice & Research Clinical Obstetrics & Gynaecology*, vol. 21, no. 2, pp. 193–206, 2007.

[33] J. L. Cox, J. M. Holden, and R. Sagovsky, "Detection of postnatal depression: development of the 10-item Edinburgh postnatal depression scale," *British Journal of Psychiatry*, vol. 150, pp. 782–786, 1987.

[34] R. L. Spitzer, K. Kroenke, and J. B. W. Williams, "Validation and utility of a self-report version of PRIME-MD: the PHQ primary care study," *Journal of the American Medical Association*, vol. 282, no. 18, pp. 1737–1744, 1999.

[35] D. Gjerdincjen, S. Crow, P. McGovern, M. Miner, and B. Center, "Postpartum depression screening at well-child visits: validity of a 2-question screen and the PHQ-9," *Annals of Family Medicine*, vol. 7, no. 1, pp. 63–70, 2009.

[36] B. Löwe, K. Kroenke, W. Herzog, and K. Gräfe, "Measuring depression outcome with a brief self-report instrument: sensitivity to change of the patient health questionnaire (PHQ-9)," *Journal of Affective Disorders*, vol. 81, no. 1, pp. 61–66, 2004.

[37] I. M. Bennett, A. Coco, J. C. Coyne et al., "Efficiency of a two-item pre-screen to reduce the burden of depression screening in pregnancy and postpartum: an IMPLICIT network study," *Journal of the American Board of Family Medicine*, vol. 21, no. 4, pp. 317–325, 2008.

[38] K. Kroenke, R. L. Spitzer, and J. B. W. Williams, "The patient health questionnaire-2: validity of a two-item depression screener," *Medical Care*, vol. 41, no. 11, pp. 1284–1292, 2003.

[39] D. Lee, A. Yip, H. Chieu, and T. Chung, "Screening for postnatal depression using the double-test strategy," *Psychosomatic Medicine*, vol. 62, no. 2, pp. 258–263, 2000.

[40] D. Gjerdingen, P. McGovern, and B. Center, "Problems with a diagnostic depression interview in a postpartum depression trial," *Journal of the American Board of Family Medicine*, vol. 24, no. 2, pp. 187–193, 2011.

[41] M. V. Smith, L. Shao, H. Howell, H. Wang, K. Poschman, and K. A. Yonkers, "Success of mental health referral among pregnant and postpartum women with psychiatric distress," *General Hospital Psychiatry*, vol. 31, no. 2, pp. 155–162, 2009.

[42] B. Yawn, A. Dietrich, P. Wollan et al., "The IAP: a simple tool to guide assessment and immediate action for suicidal ideation," *Family Practice Management*, vol. 16, no. 5, pp. 17–20, 2009.

[43] D. Sit, C. Flint, D. Svidergol et al., "Best practices: an emerging best practice model for perinatal depression care," *Psychiatric Services*, vol. 60, no. 11, pp. 1429–1431, 2009.

[44] W. J. Katon, E. H. B. Lin, M. Von Korff et al., "Collaborative care for patients with depression and chronic illnesses," *The New England Journal of Medicine*, vol. 363, no. 27, pp. 2611–2620, 2010.

[45] A. J. Dietrich, T. E. Oxman, J. W. Williams et al., "Re-engineering systems for the treatment of depression in primary care: cluster randomised controlled trial," *British Medical Journal*, vol. 329, no. 7466, pp. 602–605, 2004.

[46] J. A. Horowitz, C. A. Murphy, K. E. Gregory, and J. Wojcik, "Best practices: community-based postpartum depression screening: results from the CARE study," *Psychiatric Services*, vol. 60, no. 11, pp. 1432–1434, 2009.

[47] M. Wiedmann and C. Garfield, "Perinatal Maternal Depression and Child Development Strategies for Primary Care Providers," 2007, http://www.iafp.com/pdfs/MaternalDepression.pdf.

[48] D. Castle, I. Schweitzer, and J. Tiller, "STAR*D: has it taught us anything about the management of depression?" *Australasian Psychiatry*, vol. 17, no. 5, pp. 360–364, 2009.

[49] K. L. Margolis, L. I. Solberg, A. L. Crain et al., "Prevalence of practice system tools for improving depression care among primary care clinics: the DIAMOND initiative," *Journal of General Internal Medicine*, vol. 26, no. 9, pp. 999–1004, 2011.

[50] I. Krantz, B. O. Eriksson, C. Lundquist-Persson, B. M. Ahlberg, and T. Nilstun, "Screening for postpartum depression with the Edinburgh Postnatal Depression Scale (EPDS): an ethical analysis," *Scandinavian Journal of Public Health*, vol. 36, no. 2, pp. 211–216, 2008.

[51] A. L. Olson, A. J. Dietrich, G. Prazar et al., "Two approaches to maternal depression screening during well child visits," *Journal*

of Developmental and Behavioral Pediatrics, vol. 26, no. 3, pp. 169–176, 2005.

[52] "CMWF website," http://www.commonwealthfund.org/Publications/Fund-Manuals/2007/Apr/Parental-Depression-Screening-for-Pediatric-Clinicians–An-Implementation-Manual.aspx.

[53] M. F. Earls and The Committee on Psychosocial Aspects of Child and Family Health, "Clincal report-incorporating recognition and management of perinaltaland postpartum depression into pediatric practice," *Pediatrics*, vol. 125, no. 5, pp. 1032–1039, 2010.

[54] L. I. Solberg, "Improving medical practice: a conceptual framework," *Annals of Family Medicine*, vol. 5, no. 3, pp. 251–256, 2007.

[55] "Mental health professional shortages," http://bhpr.hrsa.gov/shortage/.

[56] D. K. Gjerdingen and B. P. Yawn, "Postpartum depression screening: importance, methods, barriers, and recommendations for practice," *Journal of the American Board of Family Medicine*, vol. 20, no. 3, pp. 280–288, 2007.

[57] H. A. Flynn, E. Henshaw, H. O'Mahen, and J. Forman, "Patient perspectives on improving the depression referral processes in obstetrics settings: a qualitative study," *General Hospital Psychiatry*, vol. 32, no. 1, pp. 9–16, 2010.

[58] "A new direction in depression treatment in Minnesota: DIAMOND program, Institute for Clinical Systems Improvement, Bloomington, Minnesota," *Psychiatric Services*, vol. 61, no. 10, pp. 1042–1044, 2010.

[59] "IOM quality chasm," http://www.iom.edu/Reports/2001/Crossing-the-Quality-Chasm-A-New-Health-System-for-the-21st-Century.aspx.

9

Mental Health Outcomes in US Children and Adolescents Born Prematurely or with Low Birthweight

Gopal K. Singh, Mary Kay Kenney, Reem M. Ghandour, Michael D. Kogan, and Michael C. Lu

US Department of Health and Human Services, Health Resources and Services Administration, Maternal and Child Health Bureau, 5600 Fishers Lane, Room 18-41, Rockville, MD 20857, USA

Correspondence should be addressed to Gopal K. Singh; gsingh@hrsa.gov

Academic Editor: Michael Berk

We examined the effects of prematurity (<37 weeks of gestation) and low birthweight (<2500 g) on mental health outcomes among US children aged 2–17 years. The 2011-2012 National Survey of Children's Health (N = 95,677) was used to estimate prevalence of parent-reported mental health problems in children. Prevalence of mental disorders was 22.9% among children born prematurely, 28.7% among very-low-birth-weight (<1500 g) children, and 18.9% among moderately low-birth-weight (1500–2499 g) children, compared with 15.5% in the general child population. Compared to those born full term, children born prematurely had 61% higher adjusted odds of serious emotional/behavioral problems, 33% higher odds of depression, and 58% higher odds of anxiety. Children born prematurely had 2.3 times higher odds of autism/ASD, 2.9 times higher odds of development delay, and 2.7 times higher odds of intellectual disability than term children. Very-low-birth-weight children had 3.2 times higher odds of autism/ASD, 1.7 times higher odds of ADD/ADHD, 5.4 times higher odds of development delay, and 4.4 times higher odds of intellectual disability than normal-birth-weight children. Social factors were significant predictors of mental disorders in both premature/low-birth-weight and term/normal-birth-weight children. Neurodevelopmental conditions accounted for the relationship between prematurity and depression/anxiety/conduct problems. Prematurity and low birthweight are significant risk factors for mental health problems among children.

1. Introduction

Perinatal factors such as preterm birth and low birthweight (LBW) have significant impacts on the health and well-being of children and adolescents, which have been shown to persist well into adulthood and, indeed, throughout the life course [1–4]. Prematurity/LBW has long been the second leading cause of infant death in the United States after congenital malformations [5]. While US infant mortality rates due to prematurity and LBW (<2500 grams) have declined markedly over time, preterm (<37 weeks of gestation) infants are still 15 times more likely to die before their birthday than those born at term [5, 6]. Nearly two-thirds of all infant deaths in the USA occur among infants who are born preterm [5].

Nearly a quarter of all infants born with very low birthweight (<1500 grams) die during the first year of life [5]. The infant mortality rates for very-low-birth-weight (<1500 grams) and moderately low-birth-weight (1500–2499 grams) infants are, respectively, 105 and 6 times higher than the rate for normal-birth-weight infants [5, 6]. Despite the marked improvements in survival rates, preterm and LBW infants remain vulnerable to many physical and mental health problems, including respiratory distress syndrome, asthma and lung disease, cerebral palsy, visual, hearing, and cognitive impairments, and a range of behavioral and developmental disorders [1, 2, 4]. While physical health problems among premature and LBW children are well-documented, behavioral and mental health problems among them are less well studied [1]. Studies that do exist have reported increased risks of depression, anxiety, behavioral, and conduct disorders among preterm and LBW children, compared with the general population or children who are born at full term or with normal birthweight [2, 7–18]. Studies have also reported 2-to-4-fold higher rates of more serious neurodevelopmental conditions in premature/LBW populations, including autism spectrum disorders (ASD), ADHD, and learning difficulties [2, 19–23].

Most of the studies that have examined mental health problems among children born preterm or with LBW are small case-control studies, the findings of which may not be generalizable to the population at large or the US population [2, 7–23]. Moreover, such studies tend to assess mental health outcomes associated with prematurity/LBW at a specific age during late childhood or adolescence [2, 7–23]. Mental health assessment among preterm/LBW children during the entire age range, extending from early childhood to late adolescence, remains unexplored. Although several studies have focused on specific mental disorders, few studies have examined the association between prematurity/LBW and a wide range of mental health outcomes among both younger children and older adolescents in a comprehensive manner.

The 2011-2012 National Survey of Children's Health (NSCH), which is a large nationally representative sample of US children aged 0–17 years, allows us to explore the association between perinatal conditions and mental health outcomes in both childhood and adolescence, while controlling for current household socioeconomic status (SES), family environments, and other demographic variables. In this study, we examine (1) the prevalence of overall and specific mental health outcomes among US children by prematurity and LBW before and after controlling for household SES and sociodemographic characteristics, (2) whether mental health outcomes associated with prematurity and LBW vary by child's sex and age, (3) whether social factors are significant predictors of mental health problems in both preterm/LBW and general child populations, and (4) the extent to which neurodevelopmental conditions such as autism/ASD, ADHD, and developmental delay might account for the relationship between perinatal conditions and common emotional/behavioral disorders of depression, anxiety, and conduct problems.

2. Methods

Data for the present study came from the 2011-2012 NSCH [22, 23]. The survey was conducted by the National Center for Health Statistics (NCHS), with funding and direction from the Maternal and Child Health Bureau [24, 25]. The purpose of the NSCH was to provide national and state-specific prevalence estimates for a variety of children's health and well-being indicators [24, 25]. The survey included an extensive array of questions about children's health and the family, including parental health, stress and coping behaviors, family activities, and parental concerns about their children [24, 25]. Interviews were conducted with parents, and special emphasis was placed on factors related to children's well-being.

The 2011-2012 NSCH was a cross-sectional telephone survey conducted between February 2011 and June 2012 [24, 25]. The two previous rounds of the NSCH were conducted in 2003-2004 and 2007-2008 [25–28]. The 2011-2012 survey had a sample size of 95,677 children <18 years of age, including a sample of >1,800 children per state [24, 25]. In the survey, a random-digit-dial sample of households with children <18 years of age was selected from each of the 50 states and the District of Columbia. One child was selected from all children in each identified household to be the subject of the survey [24, 25]. Interviews were conducted in English, Spanish, and four Asian languages. The respondent was the parent or guardian who knew most about the child's health status and health care. All survey data were based on parental reports. The interview completion rate for the 2011-2012 NSCH, a measure of the response rate indicating the percentage of completed interviews among known households with children, was 54.1% for the landline sample and 41.2% for the cell phone sample [24, 25]. Substantive and methodological details of the 2011-2012 NSCH are described elsewhere [24]. The NCHS Research Ethics Review Board approved all data collection procedures for the survey.

The sample size for the present analysis was 85,535 children aged 2–17 years. Each of the 10 mental health outcomes studied is defined in Table 1. Eight specific mental health conditions were considered, with depression, anxiety, and conduct disorders combined into a composite emotional/behavioral problem variable. Additionally, we combined all eight disorders, including depression, anxiety, conduct disorders, autism/ASD, ADD/ADHD, developmental delay, learning disability, and intellectual disability, to define the total prevalence of mental disorders among children (Figure 1). Premature birth and birthweight were the primary covariates of interest. Premature birth is defined as a delivery before 37 completed weeks of gestation [5]. In the survey, prematurity was determined by asking the parents if their child was born prematurely, that is, more than 3 weeks before his/her due date [24]. Parents reported children's birthweight retrospectively. Children with birthweight <53 oz (<1,500 g) were classified as very-low-birth-weight (VLBW) children and those with birthweight between 53 and 88 oz (1500–2499) were classified as moderately low-birth-weight (MLBW) children. Children with birthweight <89 oz (<2500 g) were defined as low-birth-weight (LBW) children and those with ≥89 oz were considered as normal-birth-weight (NBW) children [5].

Using a life-course/social-determinants-of-health framework and past research as a guide, we considered, in addition to prematurity and birthweight, the following covariates of childhood mental disorders: child's age, sex, race/ethnicity, household composition, metropolitan/nonmetropolitan residence, household/parental education level, and household poverty status measured as a ratio of family income to the poverty threshold [25, 29–35]. These covariates were measured as shown in Tables 2–6.

Income was imputed for 9% of the observations by using a multiple imputation technique [24, 27]. Less than 1% of the observations had missing data on prematurity and 4.8% of the observations had missing data on birthweight. For all other covariates, there were few or no missing cases, which were excluded from the multivariate analyses, yielding an effective sample size of 84,685 for most of the analyses.

The χ^2 statistic was used to test the overall association between covariates and mental disorders. The t-statistic was used to test the difference in prevalence between any two

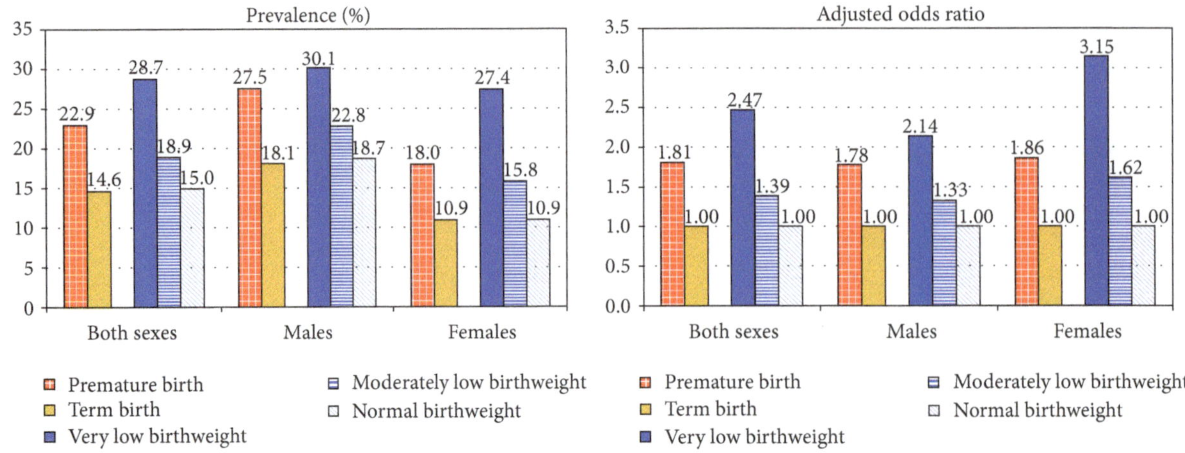

FIGURE 1: Prevalence (%) and adjusted odds of mental disorders (one or more of the eight conditions) among US children aged 3–17 years by prematurity and low birthweight. *Notes.* Differences in prevalence and odds between preterm and birthweight categories were all statistically significant at $P < 0.001$. Odds ratios were adjusted for child's age, sex, race/ethnicity, household composition, race/ethnicity, household composition, place of residence, household poverty, and education levels. Term birth and normal birthweight were the respective reference categories for the prematurity and birthweight variables. *Source.* The 2011-2012 National Survey of Children's Health ($N = 80{,}649$).

TABLE 1: Definitions of selected mental health indicators in the 2011-2012 National Survey of Children's Health.

Indicator	Definition
(1) Behavioral/emotional problem	Based on the questions, "Has a doctor or other health-care provider ever told you that the child had depression, anxiety, or behavioral or conduct problems, such as oppositional defiant disorder or conduct disorder? Does the child currently have depression, anxiety, or behavioral or conduct problems?" this composite, global mental health indicator is defined for children aged 2–17 years.
(2) Serious behavioral/emotional problem	This indicator is defined if the child's current depression, anxiety, and behavioral/conduct problems were described as moderate or severe. this indicator is defined for children aged 2–17 years.
(3) Depression	Based on the questions, "Has a doctor or other health-care provider ever told you that the child had depression? Does the child currently have depression?" this indicator is defined for children aged 2–17 years.
(4) Anxiety	Based on the questions, "Has a doctor or other health-care provider ever told you that the child had anxiety problems? Does the child currently have anxiety problems?" this indicator is defined for children aged 2–17 years.
(5) Oppositional defiant or conduct disorder	Based on the questions, "Has a doctor or other health-care provider ever told you that the child had behavioral or conduct problems, such as oppositional defiant disorder or conduct disorder? Does the child currently have behavioral or conduct problems?" this indicator is defined for children aged 2–17 years.
(6) Autism spectrum disorder	Based on the questions, "Has a doctor or other health-care provider ever told you that the child had autism, Asperger's Disorder, pervasive developmental disorder, or other autism spectrum disorder (ASD)? Does the child currently have autism or ASD?" this indicator is defined for children aged 3–17 years.
(7) ADD/ADHD	Based on the questions, "Has a doctor or other health-care provider ever told you that the child had attention deficit disorder (ADD) or attention deficit hyperactivity disorder (ADHD)? Does the child currently have ADD or ADHD?" this indicator is defined for children aged 2–17 years.
(8) Developmental delay	Based on the questions, "Has a doctor or other health-care provider ever told you that the child had any developmental delay that affects his/her ability to learn? Does the child currently have developmental delay problems?" this indicator is defined for children aged 2–17 years.
(9) Learning disability	Based on the questions, "Has a doctor, health-care provider, teacher, or school official ever told you that the child had a learning disability? Does the child currently have a learning disability?" this indicator is defined for children aged 3–17 years.
(10) Intellectual disability/mental retardation	Based on the questions, "Has a doctor or other health-care provider ever told you that the child had intellectual disability or mental retardation? Does the child currently have intellectual disability or mental retardation?" This indicator is defined for children aged 2–17 years.

TABLE 2: Descriptive statistics of the sample for children aged 2–17 years, according to perinatal and sociodemographic characteristics: the 2011-2012 National Survey of Children's Health (N = 85,535).

Sociodemographic characteristics	Unweighted number in sample	Weighted percent in sample
Child born prematurely (<37 weeks of gestation)		
Premature	9,590	11.45
Not premature	75,095	88.55
Child's birthweight		
Very low birthweight (<1,500 g)	1,255	1.68
Moderately low birthweight (1,500–2,499 g)	6,137	7.85
Normal birthweight (≥2,500 g)	73,626	90.47
Child's age (years)		
2–5	19,942	24.37
6–11	31,030	37.32
12–17	34,563	38.31
Child's sex		
Male	44,178	51.22
Female	41,357	48.78
Race/ethnicity		
Hispanic	11,136	22.55
Non-Hispanic white	55,235	51.58
Non-Hispanic black	8,073	13.43
Non-Hispanic mixed race	4,649	4.68
Other (Asians/Pacific Islanders and American Indians)	6,442	7.76
Household composition		
Two-parent biological	58,306	63.08
Two-parent stepfamily	6,517	9.64
Single mother	13,708	19.19
Other family type	7,004	8.10
Place of residence		
Metropolitan	62,845	84.35
Nonmetropolitan	21,486	15.65
Highest household or parental education level (years)		
<12	4,893	11.64
12	12,771	19.91
13–15	21,500	24.66
16+	44,186	43.79
Household poverty status (ratio of family income to poverty threshold)		
Below 100%	12,882	21.95
100–199%	15,347	21.72
200–399%	26,139	28.44
At or above 400%	31,167	27.90

groups. Logistic regression was used to examine the association between perinatal factors and mental health problems, after adjusting for the above covariates. To account for the complex sample design of the NSCH, SUDAAN software was used to conduct all statistical analyses [36].

3. Results

3.1. Descriptive Characteristics of the Study Sample. Descriptive characteristics of the study sample are shown in Table 2. Approximately 11.5% of the children aged 2–17 were born

Table 3: Weighted prevalence of selected mental health outcomes among US children aged 2–17 years by perinatal and sociodemographic characteristics: the 2011-2012 National Survey of Children's Health ($N = 84{,}685$).

Sociodemographic characteristics	Emotional/behavioral problem			Serious emotional/ behavioral problem			Depression			Anxiety			Oppositional defiant or conduct disorder		
	%	SE	*P* value	%	SE	*P* value	%	SE	*P* value	%	SE	*P* value	%	SE	*P* value
Child born prematurely			<0.001			<0.001			0.065			<0.001			<0.001
Premature	8.10	0.54		5.29	0.44		2.69	0.32		4.72	0.37		4.50	0.41	
Not premature	5.70	0.19		3.36	0.15		2.06	0.13		3.13	0.13		2.95	0.15	
Child's birthweight			0.086			0.293			0.555			0.242			0.044
Low birthweight	6.86	0.59		3.99	0.42		2.33	0.39		3.86	0.42		4.12	1.10	
Very low birthweight	7.30	1.31		5.01	1.21		2.12	0.60		4.05	0.81		4.12	1.10	
Moderately low birthweight	6.77	0.66		3.78	0.44		2.37	0.46		3.76	0.48		3.81	0.46	
Normal birthweight	5.80	0.20		3.52	0.16		2.08	0.13		3.29	0.14		2.96	0.15	
Child's age (years)			<0.001			<0.001			<0.001			<0.001			<0.001
2–5	2.03	0.23		1.22	0.17		0.26	0.08		0.83	0.14		1.50	0.20	
6–11	6.17	0.30		3.87	0.25		1.49	0.16		3.50	0.20		3.81	0.25	
12–17	8.46	0.35		4.95	0.26		4.00	0.26		4.81	0.25		3.65	0.24	
Child's sex			<0.001			<0.001			0.252			0.014			<0.001
Male	7.12	0.27		4.48	0.23		2.28	0.17		3.65	0.18		4.34	0.23	
Female	4.90	0.24		2.75	0.17		2.01	0.16		3.03	0.17		1.97	0.16	
Race/ethnicity			<0.001			<0.001			0.004			<0.001			<0.001
Hispanic	4.79	0.46		3.04	0.38		1.73	0.28		1.98	0.24		3.03	0.39	
Non-Hispanic white	6.79	0.24		4.01	0.19		2.32	0.16		4.37	0.2		3.07	0.17	
Non-Hispanic black	6.10	0.47		3.74	0.36		2.25	0.3		2.33	0.31		4.37	0.39	
Non-Hispanic mixed race	8.11	0.79		5.41	0.68		3.53	0.6		4.26	0.53		4.67	0.62	
Other	3.33	0.44		1.64	0.23		1.27	0.34		1.78	0.25		1.47	0.24	
Household composition			<0.001			<0.001			<0.001			<0.001			<0.001
Two-parent biological	3.83	0.18		2.10	0.14		0.97	0.09		2.51	0.14		1.65	0.13	
Two-parent stepfamily	9.99	0.82		6.04	0.65		4.66	0.62		4.98	0.52		5.95	0.72	
Single mother	9.74	0.50		6.43	0.42		3.97	0.34		4.92	0.34		5.63	0.39	
Other family type	9.82	0.85		6.14	0.67		4.08	0.62		4.22	0.48		6.05	0.64	
Place of residence			<0.001			<0.001			<0.001			<0.001			0.032
Metropolitan	6.04	0.21		3.63	0.16		2.08	0.13		3.37	0.14		3.19	0.16	
Non-metropolitan	6.56	0.38		4.08	0.31		2.77	0.28		3.59	0.28		3.39	0.24	
Highest household/parental education (years)			<0.001			<0.001			<0.001			<0.001			<0.001
<12	6.83	0.69		4.18	0.49		2.75	0.43		2.35	0.33		4.39	0.55	
12	7.11	0.43		4.30	0.34		2.79	0.28		3.01	0.24		4.72	0.37	
13–15	7.84	0.43		5.07	0.36		3.00	0.29		4.42	0.32		4.16	0.31	
16+	4.54	0.23		2.51	0.18		1.33	0.14		3.29	0.19		1.73	0.17	

TABLE 3: Continued.

Sociodemographic characteristics	Emotional/behavioral problem			Serious emotional/ behavioral problem			Depression			Anxiety			Oppositional defiant or conduct disorder		
	%	SE	P value	%	SE	P value	%	SE	P value	%	SE	P value	%	SE	P value
Household poverty status			<0.001			<0.001			<0.001			0.064			<0.001
Below 100%	9.05	0.50		5.82	0.40		3.48	0.32		3.83	0.28		5.94	0.43	
100–199%	6.66	0.41		4.01	0.31		2.50	0.25		3.65	0.31		3.68	0.29	
200–399%	5.18	0.36		3.15	0.30		1.95	0.24		2.99	0.24		2.52	0.27	
At or above 400%	4.06	0.24		2.13	0.17		1.03	0.13		3.11	0.21		1.32	0.16	

P values associated with chi-square tests for independence between each covariate and mental health outcome.

prematurely and 9.5% with LBW. Non-Hispanic white children were the largest racial/ethnic group (51.6%), followed by Hispanics (23.6%) and blacks (13.4%). Approximately 22.0% of children lived below the poverty line, and 11.6% of children had parents who had less than a high school education. Nearly one-fifth of children lived in single-mother households and 9.6% of children lived in stepfamily households.

3.2. Inequalities in Prevalence and Odds of Overall Mental Health Problems. The prevalence of mental health problems was higher in premature/LBW children than in term/normal-birth-weight children (Figure 1). The prevalence of mental disorders was 22.9% among children born prematurely, 28.7% among VLBW children, and 18.9% among MLBW children, all significantly higher than the prevalence for term/normal-birth-weight children (<15%) or for the general child population (15.5%) (Figure 1). The prevalence of mental disorders was much higher among prematurely born male than female children (27.5% versus 18.0%). Relative risks of mental disorders were largely unchanged after adjusting for socioeconomic and demographic covariates. Preterm children had 82% higher adjusted odds of mental disorders (OR = 1.81; 95% CI = 1.61–2.04) than term children. Male VLBW children had 2.1 times higher adjusted odds (OR = 2.14; 95% CI = 1.39–3.28) and female VLBW children 3.2 times higher odds (OR = 3.15; 95% CI = 2.05–4.85) than their normal-birth-weight counterparts (Figure 1).

3.3. Inequalities in Prevalence and Odds of Specific Mental Disorders. Tables 3 and 4 show prevalence of specific mental health problems according to perinatal and sociodemographic characteristics. Approximately 8.1% of children born prematurely had mental/emotional problems (depression, anxiety, or conduct disorders), compared with 5.7% of term children (Table 3). While prematurity and birthweight differentials in depression were not statistically significant, preterm children had significantly higher prevalence of anxiety (4.7%) and conduct disorder (4.5%) than term children. Both prematurity and birthweight were strongly associated with the prevalence of ASD and other neurobehavioral conditions (Table 4). Approximately 3.6% of premature children were diagnosed with autism/ASD, compared with 1.7% of term children. There was a birthweight gradient in the ASD prevalence, with 4.5% of VLBW, 2.3% of MLBW, and 1.8% of NBW children being diagnosed with ASD. Nearly 11% of VLBW or premature children had ADD/ADHD, compared with <8% of term/NBW children. The prevalence of development delay was 3–5 times higher among premature/VLBW children than that among term/NBW children. The prevalence rates of learning disability and intellectual disability among premature/LBW children were about two times higher than those among term/NBW children. More than 18% of VLBW children had learning disability, and 3.9% of VLBW children were diagnosed with intellectual disability (Table 4).

Adjustment for socioeconomic and demographic covariate did not attenuate the effects of prematurity and LBW on specific mental disorders. Compared to term children, children born prematurely had 61% higher adjusted odds of serious emotional/behavioral problems, 33% higher odds of depression, and 58% higher odds of anxiety (Table 5). Children born prematurely had 2.3 times higher odds of autism/ASD, 1.5 times higher odds of ADD/ADHD, 2.9 times higher odds of development delay, 2.1 times higher odds of learning disability, and 2.7 times higher odds of intellectual disability than those born at term (Table 6). The risk of several mental disorders increased significantly for very-low-birth-weight and moderately low-birth-weight children. VLBW children had 3.2 times higher odds of autism/ASD, 1.7 times higher odds of ADHD, 5.4 times higher odds of development delay, and 4.4 times higher odds of intellectual disability than normal-birth-weight children (Table 6). LBW was associated with increased risk of emotional/behavioral problems, particularly among female children, with the magnitude of the mental health effects being generally greater for females than males (Table 7).

3.4. Social Factors as Important Predictors of Mental Health Problems. SES, race/ethnicity, and household structure were significant predictors of mental health problems in the general population as well as among premature/LBW and term/normal-birth-weight children. Children living in poverty had 2.0–3.6 times higher odds of depression, anxiety, and conduct disorders than their most-affluent counterparts. Children in stepfamilies and single-mother households had

TABLE 4: Weighted prevalence of selected mental-health-related conditions among US children aged 2–17 years by perinatal and sociodemographic characteristics: the 2011-2012 National Survey of Children's Health (N = 84,685).

Sociodemographic characteristics	Autism spectrum disorder			ADD/ADHD			Developmental delay			Learning disability			Intellectual disability/mental retardation		
	%	SE	*P* value	%	SE	*P* value	%	SE	*P* value	%	SE	*P* value	%	SE	*P* value
Child born prematurely			<0.001			<0.001			<0.001			<0.001			<0.001
Premature	3.57	0.46		10.51	0.63		8.29	0.58		13.86	0.76		2.35	0.29	
Not premature	1.67	0.11		7.44	0.22		2.91	0.13		7.18	0.22		0.87	0.08	
Child's birthweight			0.053			0.201			<0.001			<0.001			<0.001
Low birthweight	2.67	0.42		8.52	0.60		7.53	0.60		12.84	0.81		2.25	0.34	
Very low birthweight	4.50	1.75		10.90	1.81		14.56	1.99		18.16	2.38		3.93	1.39	
Moderately low birthweight	2.28	0.34		8.01	0.62		6.02	0.59		11.68	0.85		1.89	0.29	
Normal birthweight	1.83	0.12		7.72	0.22		3.06	0.14		7.37	0.22		0.89	0.08	
Child's age (years)			0.095			<0.001			0.002			<0.001			<0.001
2–5	1.49	0.22		1.49	0.16		3.97	0.31		3.30	0.30		0.47	0.08	
6–11	2.14	0.19		9.19	0.37		3.87	0.23		8.16	0.35		1.11	0.14	
12–17	1.86	0.15		10.69	0.37		2.99	0.19		10.20	0.36		1.38	0.15	
Child's sex			<0.001			<0.001			<0.001			<0.001			<0.001
Male	3.04	0.20		10.73	0.33		4.63	0.21		10.04	0.32		1.33	0.13	
Female	0.69	0.08		4.91	0.24		2.43	0.16		5.87	0.27		0.78	0.09	
Race/ethnicity			<0.001			<0.001			<0.001			<0.001			0.006
Hispanic	1.57	0.31		4.83	0.46		2.69	0.32		7.19	0.55		0.94	0.23	
Non-Hispanic white	2.23	0.13		9.45	0.29		3.77	0.17		8.30	0.27		1.08	0.1	
Non-Hispanic black	1.46	0.25		8.73	0.60		4.53	0.44		9.62	0.63		1.39	0.22	
Non-Hispanic mixed race	2.55	0.41		9.53	0.8		3.99	0.48		8.73	0.77		1.25	0.28	
Other	1.01	0.18		3.91	0.41		2.73	0.35		5.16	0.52		0.58	0.13	
Household composition			0.459			<0.001			<0.001			<0.001			0.009
Two-parent biological	1.80	0.12		5.76	0.22		3.10	0.16		6.45	0.23		0.84	0.09	
Two-parent stepfamily	1.99	0.44		13.77	0.95		3.64	0.40		9.40	0.78		1.09	0.21	
Single mother	2.21	0.24		10.85	0.54		4.48	0.32		11.17	0.57		1.38	0.19	
Other family type	1.78	0.48		10.46	0.72		4.83	0.59		10.64	0.86		1.98	0.49	
Place of residence			<0.001			0.005			0.919			0.398			0.607
Metropolitan	2.00	0.13		7.69	0.23		3.55	0.15		7.97	0.24		1.06	0.09	
Non-metropolitan	1.55	0.16		9.22	0.45		3.61	0.27		8.43	0.45		1.10	0.14	
Highest household/parental education (years)			<0.001			<0.001			0.003			<0.001			0.007
<12	1.10	0.29		6.31	0.58		3.20	0.43		9.8	0.82		1.53	0.35	
12	1.36	0.16		9.87	0.53		3.95	0.30		10.65	0.57		1.26	0.17	
13–15	2.22	0.26		9.13	0.44		4.35	0.33		9.36	0.47		1.20	0.20	
16+	2.28	0.18		6.88	0.29		3.03	0.17		5.69	0.24		0.75	0.08	
Household poverty status			0.038			<0.001			<0.001			<0.001			<0.001
Below 100%	1.45	0.16		9.47	0.51		4.64	0.33		12.12	0.61		1.53	0.21	
100–199%	1.91	0.22		8.31	0.46		3.91	0.28		7.89	0.43		1.08	0.15	
200–399%	2.31	0.26		7.47	0.39		3.43	0.29		7.42	0.42		1.04	0.19	
At or above 400%	1.80	0.16		6.74	0.33		2.55	0.19		5.55	0.27		0.69	0.08	

P values associated with chi-square tests for independence between each covariate and mental health outcome.

TABLE 5: Adjusted odds ratios (AOR) and 95% confidence intervals for selected mental health outcomes among US children aged 2–17 years by perinatal and sociodemographic characteristics: the 2011-2012 National Survey of Children's Health (N = 84,685).

Sociodemographic characteristics	Emotional/behavioral problem		Serious emotional/behavioral problem		Depression		Anxiety		Oppositional defiant or conduct disorder	
	AOR	95% CI	AOR	95% CI	AOR	95% CI	AOR	95% CI	AOR	95% CI
Child born prematurely										
Premature	1.47	1.25–1.73	1.61	1.32–1.96	1.33	1.01–1.74	1.58	1.31–1.91	1.50	1.21–1.86
Not premature[1]	1.00		1.00		1.00		1.00		1.00	
Child's birthweight										
Low birthweight	1.25	1.03–1.52	1.18	0.93–1.49	1.13	0.79–1.62	1.32	1.04–1.68	1.28	1.00–1.63
Very low birthweight	1.31	0.88–1.96	1.47	0.87–2.48	0.98	0.54–1.80	1.49	0.97–2.30	1.26	0.73–2.19
Moderately low birthweight	1.24	0.99–1.54	1.12	0.86–1.44	1.16	0.77–1.74	1.29	0.98–1.70	1.28	0.98–1.67
Normal birthweight[1]	1.00		1.00		1.00		1.00		1.00	
Child's age (years)										
2–5[1]	1.00		1.00		1.00		1.00		1.00	
6–11	3.09	2.41–3.96	3.14	2.31–4.28	5.44	2.95–10.02	4.22	2.99–5.95	2.49	1.85–3.34
12–17	4.23	3.33–5.39	3.95	2.92–5.34	14.44	8.03–25.97	5.68	4.04–7.98	2.28	1.70–3.06
Child's sex										
Male	1.50	1.31–1.72	1.68	1.42–1.99	1.12	0.90–1.40	1.20	1.03–1.41	2.33	1.90–2.87
Female[1]	1.00		1.00		1.00		1.00		1.00	
Race/ethnicity										
Non-Hispanic white[1]	1.00		1.00		1.00		1.00		1.00	
Hispanic	0.54	0.42–0.68	0.58	0.42–0.81	0.60	0.40–0.89	0.42	0.32–0.57	0.66	0.48–0.92
Non-Hispanic black	0.50	0.41–0.61	0.49	0.38–0.62	0.48	0.35–0.67	0.33	0.24–0.44	0.74	0.59–0.93
Non-Hispanic mixed race	0.97	0.77–1.22	1.06	0.79–1.41	1.21	0.82–1.79	0.83	0.62–1.10	1.16	0.85–1.57
Other	0.48	0.35–0.66	0.42	0.30–0.60	0.73	0.41–1.28	0.42	0.30–0.59	0.42	0.28–0.64
Household composition										
Two-parent biological[1]	1.00		1.00		1.00		1.00		1.00	
Two-parent stepfamily	2.16	1.74–2.68	2.27	1.72–3.00	3.44	2.39–4.95	1.70	1.32–2.18	2.80	2.02–3.89
Single mother	2.26	1.91–2.68	2.60	2.09–3.23	3.25	2.42–4.35	2.08	1.69–2.57	2.42	1.92–3.07
Other family type	2.46	1.95–3.08	2.71	2.03–3.60	3.48	2.38–5.09	1.81	1.38–2.36	3.09	2.29–4.18
Place of residence										
Metropolitan	1.20	1.04–1.39	1.17	0.97–1.40	1.03	0.81–1.32	1.19	0.99–1.44	1.28	1.06–1.54
Non-metropolitan[1]	1.00		1.00		1.00		1.00		1.00	
Highest household/parental education (years)										
<12	0.93	0.70–1.25	0.91	0.64–1.31	1.08	0.68–1.71	0.56	0.38–0.81	1.20	0.81–1.78
12	0.99	0.81–1.21	0.99	0.76–1.29	1.11	0.79–1.56	0.66	0.52–0.84	1.38	1.02–1.88
13–15	1.25	1.04–1.50	1.36	1.07–1.72	1.36	0.98–1.89	1.08	0.87–1.35	1.43	1.07–1.90
16+[1]	1.00		1.00		1.00		1.00		1.00	
Household poverty status										
Below 100%	2.50	2.00–3.12	2.76	2.05–3.72	2.96	2.10–4.17	1.95	1.49–2.55	3.56	2.51–5.06
100–199%	1.63	1.32–2.01	1.72	1.32–2.26	2.01	1.42–2.84	1.46	1.13–1.88	2.21	1.57–3.09
200–399%	1.21	1.01–1.48	1.38	1.04–1.82	1.64	1.16–2.32	0.99	0.79–1.25	1.66	1.17–2.35
At or above 400%[1]	1.00		1.00		1.00		1.00		1.00	

The effects of prematurity and birthweight were estimated by separate logistic regression models that controlled for age, sex, race/ethnicity, household composition, place of residence, and household education and income levels. [1]Reference group.

TABLE 6: Adjusted odds ratios (AOR) and 95% confidence intervals for selected mental-health-related conditions among US children aged 2–17 years by perinatal and sociodemographic characteristics: the 2011-2012 National Survey of Children's Health (N = 84,685).

Sociodemographic characteristics	Autism spectrum disorder		ADD/ADHD		Developmental delay		Learning disability		Intellectual disability/ mental retardation	
	AOR	95% CI	AOR	95% CI	AOR	95% CI	AOR	95% CI	AOR	95% CI
Child born prematurely										
Premature	2.26	1.69–3.03	1.49	1.29–1.73	2.92	2.44–3.49	2.13	1.84–2.46	2.74	2.02–3.73
Not premature[1]	1.00		1.00		1.00		1.00		1.00	
Child's birthweight										
Low birthweight	1.80	1.28–2.53	1.23	1.04–1.46	2.64	2.18–3.20	1.95	1.66–2.30	2.62	1.84–3.72
Very low birthweight	3.16	1.42–7.04	1.67	1.13–2.47	5.43	3.93–7.50	2.88	2.04–4.06	4.40	2.07–9.36
Moderately low birthweight	1.53	1.10–2.11	1.14	0.95–1.37	2.09	1.67–2.62	1.76	1.47–2.11	2.23	1.58–3.15
Normal birthweight[1]	1.00		1.00		1.00		1.00		1.00	
Child's age (years)										
2–5[1]	1.00		1.00		1.00		1.00		1.00	
6–11	1.49	1.05–2.12	6.59	5.20–8.35	0.98	0.80–1.20	2.67	2.17–3.29	2.38	1.57–3.59
12–17	1.30	0.93–1.83	7.49	5.92–9.48	0.75	0.60–0.92	3.46	2.82–4.23	2.97	1.97–4.48
Child's sex										
Male	4.49	3.48–5.80	2.43	2.15–2.75	1.96	1.66–2.30	1.82	1.61–2.05	1.70	1.25–2.31
Female[1]	1.00		1.00		1.00		1.00		1.00	
Race/ethnicity										
Non-Hispanic white[1]	1.00		1.00		1.00		1.00		1.00	
Hispanic	0.85	0.53–1.36	0.42	0.33–0.54	0.60	0.44–0.81	0.65	0.53–0.80	0.65	0.36–1.19
Non-Hispanic black	0.61	0.41–0.92	0.64	0.53–0.77	0.90	0.71–1.15	0.80	0.67–0.94	0.87	0.60–1.26
Non-Hispanic mixed race	1.07	0.75–1.55	0.91	0.74–1.11	0.89	0.68–1.17	0.93	0.76–1.15	1.00	0.61–1.64
Other	0.60	0.40–0.89	0.33	0.25–0.43	0.60	0.43–0.83	0.54	0.41–0.71	0.41	0.23–0.76
Household composition										
Two-parent biological[1]	1.00		1.00		1.00		1.00		1.00	
Two-parent stepfamily	1.16	0.71–1.89	1.99	1.65–2.39	1.11	0.87–1.42	1.13	0.92–1.39	0.99	0.64–1.55
Single mother	1.53	1.15–2.04	1.79	1.54–2.08	1.23	1.00–1.51	1.36	1.17–1.58	1.19	0.78–1.83
Other family type	1.21	0.67–2.18	1.66	1.39–1.99	1.52	1.12–2.08	1.40	1.13–1.74	1.79	0.91–3.52
Place of residence										
Metropolitan	1.43	1.13–1.83	1.02	0.90–1.16	1.16	0.97–1.38	1.17	1.02–1.33	1.17	0.86–1.58
Non-metropolitan[1]	1.00		1.00		1.00		1.00		1.00	
Highest household/parental education (years)										
<12	0.44	0.24–0.81	0.81	0.62–1.06	0.81	0.58–1.15	1.35	1.07–1.72	1.59	0.90–2.81
12	0.52	0.38–0.71	1.17	0.98–1.38	0.97	0.77–1.21	1.53	1.28–1.84	1.30	0.87–1.96
13–15	0.86	0.63–1.18	1.11	0.95–1.30	1.16	0.93–1.45	1.44	1.22–1.68	1.32	0.84–2.06
16+[1]	1.00		1.00		1.00		1.00		1.00	
Household poverty status										
Below 100%	1.19	0.79–1.77	1.68	1.38–2.05	2.00	1.54–2.61	2.04	1.68–2.48	1.93	1.16–3.22
100–199%	1.41	1.01–1.97	1.27	1.06–1.52	1.59	1.24–2.03	1.24	1.04–1.48	1.37	0.90–2.07
200–399%	1.50	1.11–2.01	1.08	0.92–1.28	1.33	1.06–1.68	1.27	1.08–1.50	1.43	0.95–2.15
At or above 400%[1]	1.00		1.00		1.00		1.00		1.00	

The effects of prematurity and birthweight were estimated by separate logistic regression models that controlled for age, sex, race/ethnicity, household composition, place of residence, and household education and income levels. [1]Reference group.

TABLE 7: Sex differentials in adjusted odds of selected mental health outcomes among US children and adolescents according to premature birth and low birthweight status: the 2011-2012 National Survey of Children's Health (N = 84,685).

Mental health outcome	Adjusted odds for prematurity		Adjusted odds for LBW versus normal birthweight		Adjusted odds for VLBW versus normal birthweight		Adjusted odds for MLBW versus normal birthweight	
	AOR[a]	95% CI	AOR[a]	95% CI	AOR[a]	95% CI	AOR[a]	95% CI
Males								
Behavioral/emotional problem	1.48	1.20–1.82	1.04	0.81–1.33	1.29	0.72–2.31	0.98	0.75–1.29
Serious emotional health problem	1.50	1.18–1.91	0.96	0.71–1.31	1.38	0.63–3.01	0.87	0.65–1.18
Depression	1.35	0.95–1.90	0.92	0.62–1.38	0.95	0.39–2.33	0.92	0.60–1.42
Anxiety	1.59	1.24–2.02	1.02	0.76–1.37	1.06	0.57–1.99	1.02	0.74–1.40
Conduct problem	1.49	1.14–1.95	1.03	0.74–1.43	1.21	0.56–2.62	0.99	0.69–1.41
Autism spectrum disorder	2.18	1.54–3.08	1.49	0.96–2.31	3.41	1.35–8.61	1.09	0.75–1.60
ADD/ADHD	1.51	1.27–1.81	1.21	0.97–1.50	1.48	0.83–2.61	1.15	0.92–1.45
Developmental delay	2.65	2.10–3.33	2.29	1.77–2.95	4.44	2.75–7.17	1.85	1.38–2.46
Learning disability	1.94	1.62–2.33	1.73	1.41–2.14	2.30	1.42–3.73	1.61	1.29–2.03
Intellectual disability	2.58	1.73–3.85	2.10	1.24–3.54	4.77	1.66–13.71	1.53	1.01–2.31
Females								
Behavioral/emotional problem	1.47	1.14–1.91	1.53	1.14–2.05	1.36	0.80–2.31	1.56	1.12–2.17
Serious emotional health problem	1.79	1.28–2.49	1.47	1.02–2.10	1.62	0.85–3.09	1.44	0.97–2.15
Depression	1.29	0.83–2.00	1.32	0.77–2.25	1.04	0.46–2.34	1.38	0.76–2.52
Anxiety	1.58	1.18–2.12	1.64	1.14–2.35	1.99	1.10–3.59	1.57	1.04–2.37
Conduct problem	1.51	1.05–2.16	1.78	1.23–2.59	1.39	0.72–2.67	1.87	1.25–2.81
Autism spectrum disorder	2.54	1.54–4.21	2.97	1.73–5.10	2.18	0.99–4.78	3.11	1.73–5.59
ADD/ADHD	1.43	1.11–1.84	1.26	0.97–1.64	2.04	1.27–3.26	1.12	0.82–1.51
Developmental delay	3.50	2.64–4.64	3.25	2.40–4.41	7.41	4.83–11.38	2.51	1.74–3.62
Learning disability	2.45	1.94–3.11	2.25	1.75–2.89	3.56	2.19–5.80	1.98	1.50–2.62
Intellectual disability	3.00	1.87–4.82	3.53	2.17–5.73	3.82	1.88–7.75	3.47	2.00–6.00

[a]Adjusted by logistic regression for child's age, race/ethnicity, household composition, metro/nonmetro residence, household poverty, and education levels. LBW: low birthweight. VLBW: very low birthweight. MLBW: moderately low birthweight.

1.7–3.4 times higher odds of depression, anxiety, and conduct disorders than children from two-parent biological families. Black and Hispanic children had 46–50% lower adjusted odds of emotional/behavioral problems than non-Hispanic white children (Table 5). Although the association between social factors and neurodevelopmental conditions was less pronounced, poor children maintained 1.7–2.0 times higher adjusted odds of ADD/ADHD, intellectual disability, developmental delay, and learning disability than their affluent counterparts (Table 6). Although the income gradients in autism/ASD were not consistent, those with higher poverty levels had significantly higher risks than the most-affluent children. Non-Hispanic white children and those in single-mother households remained at significantly higher risk of all neurodevelopmental conditions even after controlling for SES (Table 6).

Social inequalities in mental health problems were smaller among premature/LBW children than among term/normal-birth-weight children (data not shown). For example, among premature/LBW children, 27.1% of children in step-families and 20.2% of children in single-mother households had mental health problems, compared with 17.2% of children in two-parent biological families. Among term/normal-birth-weight children, the respective prevalence rates were 21.8%, 20.2%, and 11.3%. Among premature/LBW children, 25.0% of poor children had mental health problems compared with 17.3% of affluent children (adjusted OR = 1.53; 95% CI = 1.11–2.12), whereas among term/normal-birth-weight children, 19.2% of poor children had mental health problems compared with 11.9% of affluent children (adjusted OR = 1.97; 95% CI = 1.66–2.35).

3.5. Regression Models with Comorbid Conditions. We estimated regression models of both the overall emotional/behavioral problem variable and specific conditions of depression, anxiety, and conduct disorder that included sociodemographic characteristics and prematurity, along with comorbid conditions of ASD, ADD/ADHD, development delay, learning disability, and intellectual disability. The increased risks of mental health problems associated with prematurity were accounted for by these neurodevelopmental conditions, whose effects on emotional/behavioral problems were quite marked (data not shown for brevity). Children diagnosed with autism, ADHD, developmental delay, and learning disability, respectively, had 4.4, 8.4, 3.0, and 2.4 times higher adjusted odds of emotional/behavioral problems than children without such neurodevelopmental conditions. Children diagnosed with autism had 2.1, 4.7, and 3.3 times higher adjusted odds of depression, anxiety, and conduct disorders than children without autism, respectively. Children with ADD/ADHD had 5.8, 4.9, and 14.0 times higher adjusted odds of depression, anxiety, and conduct disorders than children without ADD/ADHD, respectively. In each of the comorbidity models, SES, family structure, and race/ethnicity remained strong risk factors for mental health problems.

The prevalence of mental health problems increased with child's age. Approximately 19.6% of adolescents aged 12–17 had mental health problems, compared with 15.9% of children aged 6–11 and 6.7% of children aged 3–5 years. Given that the prevalence of overall mental health problems and of depression, anxiety, ADHD, learning disability, and intellectual disability were mostly concentrated among older children and adolescents, we explored age interactions by estimating prematurity and LBW models stratified by child's age. However, the age interactions were not statistically significant, and the effects of the prematurity and LBW on mental health problems were similar for younger and older children and adolescents (data not shown).

4. Discussion

Although the rates of preterm birth and LBW in the USA have declined slightly in recent years, the current rates remain fairly high and represent a 10–16% increase compared to the rates in 1990 [37, 38]. Growing economic, social, and healthcare costs associated with prematurity and LBW are a major public health concern in the USA [1], and their marked impact on mental health problems during childhood and adolescence, as reported here, adds to the overall health and societal burden associated with prematurity [1]. According to our study, approximately 23% or 1.6 million premature/LBW children and adolescents in the USA are estimated to have one or more mental health problems. In all, 15.5% or an estimated 9.6 million US children aged 3–17 have mental health problems.

To our knowledge, ours is the first large-scale population-based US study to examine the prevalence of several mental health problems among preterm and LBW children using a nationally representative sample of preschool and school-aged children and adolescents. The analysis of the large NSCH sample allowed us to study in detail age- and sex-specific variations in the prevalence of some of the rarer mental health conditions such as depression, ASD, and intellectual disability among premature and LBW children. The overall prevalence of mental health problems among premature, VLBW, and MLBW children in our study generally varied from 20% to 30%, which is consistent with the prevalence estimates from other smaller-scale studies using diagnostic evaluations despite their use of extremely low-birth-weight and gestational-age categories [2].

While our study adds to the current US and international research on mental disorders associated with perinatal conditions, additional research is needed to explain the substantial effects of social factors on mental health outcomes among both premature/LBW and term/normal-birth-weight children. Consideration of additional factors such as adverse neighborhood social conditions, built environments, parental health status, parental stress, family conflict, family cohesiveness, social support, child's exposure to environmental tobacco smoke, alcohol and substance use, excess television viewing or recreational computer use, and physical inactivity may further explain the role of social factors in mental health problems [29, 31–35].

Mental health effects of prematurity and LBW reported here are generally consistent with previous research that shows higher risks of mental disorders in children associated with these perinatal outcomes [2, 7–23]. Compatible with our findings, inverse gestational-age and birth-weight gradients in ADHD and ASD have been reported previously [2, 18, 19, 22]. Additionally, we found a birthweight specific gradient in overall mental health prevalence and in development delay, learning disability, and intellectual disability.

In our study, the association between prematurity/LBW and mental health problems was largely explained by the consideration of neurodevelopmental conditions of ASD, ADHD, and developmental delay. This appears to provide evidence in support of biological pathways through which prematurity and LBW might lead to increased risks of mental health problems [1, 2]. Brain injuries and changes in brain development associated with premature births have been implicated as the causal mechanism for the increased risk of mental disorders in premature/LBW children [2]. However, even in children diagnosed with neurodevelopmental conditions, socioeconomic circumstances, family structure, and race/ethnicity played an important role in determining mental health risks, albeit to a smaller degree than in term/normal-birth-weight children.

A major strength of our study includes estimating the effects of prematurity and LBW on a variety of mental health conditions across the entire age range of childhood and adolescence. Another important contribution of this study is the estimation of overall prevalence of mental disorders in the preterm/LBW and the general child populations. The other strengths of our study include the large sample size, the generalizability of our findings, and examination of whether the effects of prematurity/LBW and socioeconomic factors vary by sex, age, and mental health outcome.

Our study has limitations. Children's mental health conditions in the NSCH were based on parental reports and may not accurately reflect the true prevalence, particularly among older adolescents [32, 33]. However, the prevalence of mental health disorders reported here is consistent with that reported in other epidemiologic studies [2, 39, 40]. Second, the prematurity and birthweight measures in the NSCH may be subject to recall bias, particularly among mothers of older children and adolescents, which may underestimate the prevalence and mental health effects of prematurity/LBW among older adolescents. However, a comparison of rates of prematurity and LBW by child's age in the NSCH and those based on vital records over time shows a substantial agreement. For example, the proportion of children aged

1 year born prematurely in the 2011-2012 NSCH was 12.2%, compared with 12.0% in the 2010 national vital records [37, 38]. Approximately 10% of children aged 17 in the NSCH were premature, compared with 11.0% in the vital records in 1994 [37, 38]. Although LBW in NSCH is not as precisely measured (in grams) as in vital records and is slightly overestimated, the correspondence in birthweight appears to be good between the two data sources. While 9.7% of children aged <1 year in the NSCH were of LBW, the rate from the vital records in 2011 was 8.1% [38]. Approximately 7.8% of children aged 17 in the NSCH were LBW, compared with 7.3% in the vital records in 1994 [37]. Third, because of the cross-sectional nature of the NSCH, causal inferences about the relationships between more contemporary measures of the social and familial environments and childhood mental health problems cannot be drawn [32, 33]. Lastly, as with most sample surveys, the potential for nonresponse bias exists for the NSCH, implying that the sample interviewed differed from the targeted child population in a systematic fashion [25, 27]. Since response rates in the NSCH tend to be lower in urban areas and low-income and ethnic-minority populations, differential nonresponse bias might affect (most likely underestimate) the impact of social factors on mental health problems [27]. However, the nonresponse adjustment to the sampling weights in the NSCH might have reduced the potential magnitude of these biases [27].

In conclusion, the evidence presented here suggests that premature birth and LBW are significant risk factors for mental health problems among children and adolescents. The most prevalent disorders among premature/LBW children are ADHD, learning disability, developmental delay, and anxiety. Increased mental health surveillance and screening are recommended for children born prematurely and/or with LBW, providing the opportunity for early diagnosis and intervention [2]. Given the important role of social factors in overall and specific mental health problems, including neurodevelopmental conditions, improvements in contemporary social environments as well as socioeconomic circumstances during pregnancy can be vital in preventing and reducing mental health problems in children.

Ethical Approval

According to human subjects review, no IRB approval was required for this study, which is based on the secondary analysis of a public-use federal database.

Conflict of Interests

The authors declare that there is no conflict of interests.

Disclosure

The views expressed are the authors' and not necessarily those of the Health Resources and Services Administration or the US Department of Health and Human Services.

References

[1] R. E. Behrman and A. S. Butler, Eds., *Preterm Birth: Causes, Consequences, and Prevention*, Institute of Medicine; National Academies Press, Washington, DC, USA, 2007.

[2] S. Johnson and N. Marlow, "Preterm birth and childhood psychiatric disorders," *Pediatric Research*, vol. 69, no. 5, pp. 11R–8R, 2011.

[3] N. J. Wiles, T. J. Peters, D. A. Leon, and G. Lewis, "Birth weight and psychological distress at age 45–51 years: results from the Aberdeen children of the 1950s cohort study," *British Journal of Psychiatry*, vol. 187, pp. 21–28, 2005.

[4] D. Moster, R. T. Lie, and T. Markestad, "Long-term medical and social consequences of preterm birth," *The New England Journal of Medicine*, vol. 359, no. 3, pp. 262–273, 2008.

[5] T. J. Mathews and M. F. MacDorman, "Infant mortality statistics from the 2009 period linked birth/infant death data set," *National Vital Statistics Reports*, vol. 61, no. 8, pp. 1–28, 2013.

[6] G. K. Singh and M. D. Kogan, "Persistent socioeconomic disparities in infant, neonatal, and postneonatal mortality rates in the United States, 1969–2001," *Pediatrics*, vol. 119, no. 4, pp. e928–e939, 2007.

[7] A. T. Bhutta, M. A. Cleves, P. H. Casey, M. M. Cradock, and K. J. Anand, "Cognitive and behavioral outcomes of school-aged children who were born preterm: a meta-analysis," *Journal of the American Medical Association*, vol. 288, no. 6, pp. 728–737, 2002.

[8] M. C. McCormick, J. Brooks-Gunn, K. Workman-Daniels, J. Turner, and G. J. Peckham, "The health and developmental status of very low-birth-weight children at school age," *Journal of the American Medical Association*, vol. 267, no. 16, pp. 2204–2208, 1992.

[9] C. S. H. Aarnoudse-Moens, N. Weisglas-Kuperus, J. B. van Goudoever, and J. Oosterlaan, "Meta-analysis of neurobehavioral outcomes in very preterm and/or very low birth weight children," *Pediatrics*, vol. 124, no. 2, pp. 717–728, 2009.

[10] G. C. Patton, C. Coffey, J. B. Carlin, C. A. Olsson, and R. Morley, "Prematurity at birth and adolescent depressive disorder," *British Journal of Psychiatry*, vol. 184, pp. 446–447, 2004.

[11] M. Hack, E. A. Youngstrom, L. Cartar et al., "Behavioral outcomes and evidence of psychopathology among very low birth weight infants at age 20 years," *Pediatrics*, vol. 114, no. 4, pp. 932–940, 2004.

[12] M. Hack, H. G. Taylor, M. Schluchter, L. Andreias, D. Drotar, and N. Klein, "Behavioral outcomes of extremely low birth weight children at age 8 years," *Journal of Developmental and Behavioral Pediatrics*, vol. 30, no. 2, pp. 122–130, 2009.

[13] M. R. Potijk, A. F. de Winter, A. F. Bos, J. M. Kerstjens, and S. A. Reijneveld, "Higher rates of behavioural and emotional problems at preschool age in children born moderately preterm," *Archives of Disease in Childhood*, vol. 97, no. 2, pp. 112–117, 2012.

[14] L. K. Lund, T. Vik, S. Lydersen et al., "Mental health, quality of life and social relations in young adults born with low birth weight," *Health and Quality of Life Outcomes*, vol. 10, article 146, 2012.

[15] M. S. Indredavik, T. Vik, K. A. Evensen, J. Skranes, G. Taraldsen, and A. M. Brubakk, "Perinatal risk and psychiatric outcome in adolescents born preterm with very low birth weight or term small for gestational age," *Journal of Developmental and Behavioral Pediatrics*, vol. 31, no. 4, pp. 286–294, 2010.

[16] M. S. Indredavik, T. Vik, S. Heyerdahl, S. Kulseng, and A. M. Brubakk, "Psychiatric symptoms in low birth weight adolescents, assessed by screening questionnaires," *European Child and Adolescent Psychiatry*, vol. 14, no. 4, pp. 226–236, 2005.

[17] S. J. Bayless, I. M. Pit-ten Cate, and J. Stevenson, "Behaviour difficulties and cognitive function in children born very prematurely," *International Journal of Behavioral Development*, vol. 32, no. 3, pp. 199–206, 2008.

[18] H. G. Taylor, N. Klein, N. M. Minich, and M. Hack, "Middle-school-age outcomes in children with very low birthweight," *Child Development*, vol. 71, no. 6, pp. 1495–1511, 2000.

[19] K. M. Linnet, K. Wisborg, E. Agerbo, N. J. Secher, P. H. Thomsen, and T. B. Henriksen, "Gestational age, birth weight, and the risk of hyperkinetic disorder," *Archives of Disease in Childhood*, vol. 91, no. 8, pp. 655–660, 2006.

[20] N. Botting, A. Powls, R. W. I. Cooke, and N. Marlow, "Attention deficit hyper-activity disorders and other psychiatric outcomes in very low birthweight children at 12 years," *Journal of Child Psychology and Psychiatry and Allied Disciplines*, vol. 38, no. 8, pp. 931–941, 1997.

[21] H. J. Larsson, W. W. Eaton, K. M. Madsen et al., "Risk factors for autism: perinatal factors, parental psychiatric history, and socioeconomic status," *The American Journal of Epidemiology*, vol. 161, no. 10, pp. 916–925, 2005.

[22] K. Williams, M. Helmer, G. W. Duncan, J. K. Peat, and C. M. Mellis, "Perinatal and maternal risk factors for autism spectrum disorders in New South Wales, Australia," *Child: Care, Health and Development*, vol. 34, no. 2, pp. 249–256, 2008.

[23] J. A. Pinto-Martin, S. E. Levy, J. F. Feldman, J. M. Lorenz, N. Paneth, and A. H. Whitaker, "Prevalence of autism spectrum disorder in adolescents born weighing <2000 grams," *Pediatrics*, vol. 128, no. 5, pp. 883–891, 2011.

[24] National Center for Health Statistics, *The national survey of children's health (NSCH), 2011–2012: the public use data file and documentation*, US Department of Health and Human Services, Hyattsville, Md, USA, 2013, http://www.cdc.gov/nchs/slaits/nsch.htm.

[25] G. K. Singh and M. K. Kenney, "Rising prevalence and neighborhood, social, and behavioral determinants of sleep problems in US children and adolescents, 2003–2012," *Sleep Disorders*, vol. 2013, Article ID 394320, 15 pages, 2013.

[26] Health Resources and Services Administration, Maternal and Child Health Bureau, *The National Survey of Children's Health 2007: The Health and Well-Being of Children, A Portrait of States and the Nation*, US Department of Health and Human Services, Rockville, Md, USA, 2009.

[27] S. J. Blumberg, E. B. Foster, and A. M. Frasier, "Design and operation of the National Survey of Children's Health, 2007," *Vital and Health Statistics*, vol. 1, no. 55, pp. 1–149, 2012.

[28] S. J. Blumberg, L. Olson, M. R. Frankel, L. Osborn, K. P. Srinath, and P. Giambo, "Design and operation of the National Survey of Children's Health, 2003," *Vital and Health Statistics*, vol. 1, no. 43, pp. 1–124, 2005.

[29] R. Wilkinson and M. Marmot, Eds., *Social Determinants of Health: The Solid Facts*, World Health Organization, Regional Office for Europe, Copenhagen, Denmark, 2nd edition, 2003.

[30] P. Braveman and C. Barclay, "Health disparities beginning in childhood: a life-course perspective," *Pediatrics*, vol. 124, no. 3, pp. S163–S175, 2009.

[31] M. Fisher and F. Baum, "The social determinants of mental health: implications for research and health promotion," *Australian and New Zealand Journal of Psychiatry*, vol. 44, no. 12, pp. 1057–1063, 2010.

[32] G. K. Singh and S. M. Yu, "The impact of ethnic-immigrant status and obesity-related risk factors on behavioral problems among US children and adolescents," *Scientifica*, vol. 2012, Article ID 648152, 14 pages, 2012.

[33] G. K. Singh and R. M. Ghandour, "Impact of neighborhood social conditions and household socioeconomic status on behavioral problems among US children," *Maternal and Child Health Journal*, vol. 16, supplement 1, pp. S158–S169, 2012.

[34] Y. Xue, T. Leventhal, J. Brooks-Gunn, and F. J. Earls, "Neighborhood residence and mental health problems of 5- to 11-year-olds," *Archives of General Psychiatry*, vol. 62, no. 5, pp. 554–563, 2005.

[35] T. Leventhal and J. Brooks-Gunn, "The neighborhoods they live in: the effects of neighborhood residence on child and adolescent outcomes," *Psychological Bulletin*, vol. 126, no. 2, pp. 309–337, 2000.

[36] SUDAAN, "Software for the Statistical Analysis of Correlated Data, Release 10.0.1," Research Triangle Institute, Research Triangle Park, NC, USA, 2009.

[37] J. A. Martin, B. E. Hamilton, S. J. Ventura et al., "Births: final data for 2010," *National Vital Statistics Reports*, vol. 61, no. 1, pp. 1–72, 2012.

[38] B. E. Hamilton, J. A. Martin, and S. J. Ventura, "Births: preliminary data for 2011," *National Vital Statistics Reports*, vol. 61, no. 5, pp. 1–20, 2012.

[39] B. Bloom, R. A. Cohen, and G. Freeman, "Summary health statistics for U.S. children: National Health Interview Survey, 2011," *Vital and Health Statistics*, no. 254, pp. 1–80, 2012.

[40] R. Perou, R. H. Bitsko, S. J. Blumberg, P. Pastor, R. M. Ghandour, J. C. Gfroerer et al., "Mental health surveillance among children—United States, 2005–2011," *Morbidity and Mortality Weekly Report*, vol. 62, no. 2, pp. 1–35, 2013.

10

Trends of Postpartum Depression in Iran

Yousef Veisani,[1,2] Ali Delpisheh,[2,3] Kourosh Sayehmiri,[2,3] and Shahab Rezaeian[4]

[1] *Student Research Committee, Ilam University of Medical Sciences, P.O. Box 69311-57793, Ilam, Iran*
[2] *Department of Clinical Epidemiology, Faculty of Medicine, Ilam University of Medical Sciences, P.O. Box 69315-138, Ilam, Iran*
[3] *Prevention of Psychosocial Injuries Research Centre, P.O. Box 69311-57793, Ilam, Iran*
[4] *Department of Epidemiology, School of Health & Nutrition, Shiraz University of Medical Sciences, P.O. Box 71348-14366, Shiraz, Iran*

Correspondence should be addressed to Kourosh Sayehmiri; sayehmiri@razi.tums.ac.ir

Academic Editor: Klaus Ebmeier

Background. Postpartum depression (PPD) is a serious mental health disorder affecting 13% of women in developed communities. The present study reviews available epidemiological publications on PPD-related aspects in Iranian women to help policy makers and health workers to design preventative strategies and further researches. *Materials and Methods.* A systematic review was constructed based on the computerized literature valid database. The 95% confidence intervals were calculated by random effects models. Metaregression was introduced to explore and explain heterogeneity between studies. Data manipulation and statistical analyses were performed using Stata 11. *Results.* Overall, 41 studies met the inclusion criteria. The pooled prevalence of PPD in Iran was 25.3% (95% CI: 22.7%–27.9%). Amongst subgroups of unwanted delivery, illiterate, housewives, and having history of depression the prevalence was 43.4% (35.6–51.1), 31.6% (18.1–45.0), 30.7% (25.2–36.3), and 45.2% (35.4–53.1), respectively. *Conclusions.* Interventions that would specifically target women with a prior history of depression, illiterates, housewives, or women with unwanted pregnancies could be helpful to decrease the prevalence of postpartum depression in Iran.

1. Introduction

Postpartum depression (PPD) affects almost 13% of women in developed high income communities [1] and may be even more common in developing countries [2, 3]. According to the Diagnostic and Statistical Manual of Mental Disorders, Fourth Edition (DSM-IV), PPD is a major depression when symptoms have onset within 5 weeks of childbirth [4]. PPD presents with the same symptoms as for a major depressive episode occurring outside of the prenatal period, including core symptoms of depressed mood and/or loss of pleasure, together with additional symptoms, including changes in weight or sleep, fatigue or loss of energy, feelings of worthlessness or guilt, concentration difficulties, and suicidal ideation [4].

Majority of PPD researches in Iran have not utilized diagnostic assessments to identify cases. Alternatively, they have used the validated self-report depression screening instruments, such as the Edinburgh Postnatal Depression Scale (EPDS) [5]. Although this approach has been criticized, the EPDS has showed good sensitivity and specificity, particularly when used to detect both major and minor depressions [5].

In terms of etiology, PPD is a multifactorial disorder with biological, psychological, and sociological aspects interacting with woman's risk individually [6]. Sociological factors such as unwanted delivery, occupation, literacy, and history of depression have been more frequently reported throughout original researches and a meta-analysis [7]. However, they are not comprehensive as the present review is. Many of them drew incompatible or even contradictory conclusions, and the utilization of these statistics is therefore limited. The present study reviews available epidemiological publications on PPD-related aspects in Iranian women to help policy makers and health workers to design preventative strategies and further researches.

2. Methods and Materials

2.1. Literature Search. Our search strategy, selection of publications, and the reporting of results for the review will be conducted in accordance with the PRISMA guidelines [8]. Literature on the postpartum depression among Iranian women was acquired through searching the Scientific Information Databases (SID), Global Medical Article Limberly (Medlib), Iranian Biomedical Journal (Iran Medex), and Iranian Journal Database (Magiran) as well as international databases including PubMed/Medline, Scopus, and ISI Web of Knowledge. The search strategy was limited to the Persian and/or English language papers published until Feb 2012. All publications with medical subject headings (MeSh) and keywords in title, abstract, and text for words including postpartum depression were investigated. Iranian scientific databases were searched only using the keyword "postpartum depression," as these databases do not distinguish synonyms from each other and do not allow sensitive search operation using linking terms such as "AND," "OR," or "NOT." Consequently, this single keyword search was the most practical option. The postpartum depression, depression, and Iran MeSh combined with the Selection and Quality Assessment of Articles operator "OR" versus "AND."

2.2. Selection and Quality Assessment of Articles. All identified papers were critically appraised independently by two reviewers. Disagreements between reviewers were resolved by consensus. Appraisal was guided by a checklist assessing clarity of aims and research questions. The inclusion criteria were as follows: (1) studies in the mentioned databases with full text, despite the language of original text; (2) having a standardized assessment of depression (either self-report or observer rated), using Edinburgh Postnatal Depression Scale (EPDS) and Beck depression inventory (BDI) instruments and study conducting of between 2 and 52 weeks postpartum were the main inclusion criteria. Exclusion criteria were (1) studies upon women overlapping time intervals of sample collection from the same origin; (2) inappropriate study design; (3) inadequate reporting of results.

2.3. Data Extraction. Data were extracted using a standardized and prepiloted data extraction form. Data extraction will be undertaken by the first reviewer and checked by a second reviewer although the process will be discussed and piloted by both reviewers. All identified papers will be critically appraised independently by both reviewers. Disagreements were resolved through discussion. Appraisal will be guided by a checklist assessing clarity of aims and research questions. Information was extracted from each included study (including author, title, year and setting of study, methods of sample selection, sample size, study type, age, and prevalence). Therefore, risk of bias as an "Inadequate Reporting" reduced. These data-abstraction forms were reviewed, and eligible papers were entered into the meta-analysis. Besides, as with all meta-analyses, this study has potential limitation of publication bias. Many of our data were extracted from studies written in Persian (language bias). However, we have confidence in our results since the included literature was published in non-Persian language, which should reduce publication bias to some extent.

2.4. Statistical Analysis. The random effects model was used for combining results of studies in meta-analysis. Variance for each study was calculated using the binomial distribution formula. The presence of heterogeneity was determined by the Der Simonian-Laird (DL) approach [9]. Significance level was <0.1, and I^2 statistic was used for estimates of inconsistency within the meta-analyses. The I^2 statistic estimates the percent of observed between-study variability due to heterogeneity rather than to chance and ranges from 0 to 100 percent (values of 25%, 50%, and 75% were considered representing low, medium, and high heterogeneity resp.) [10]. A value of 0% indicates no observed heterogeneity whilst 100% indicates significant heterogeneity. For this review, we determined that I^2 values above 75 percent were indicative of significant heterogeneity warranting analysis with a random effect model as opposed to the fixed effects model to adjust for the observed variability. The I^2 is an estimate of the proportion of the total variation across studies that are beyond chance. In situations with high between-study heterogeneity, the use of random effects models is recommended as it produces study weights that primarily reflect the between-study variation and thus provide close to equal weighting. Univariate and multivariate metaregression analyses were used to explore possible sources of heterogeneity among studies [11]. We analyzed sources of heterogeneity by subgroup and metaregression analysis using dichotomous and continuous variables. Univariate and multivariate approaches were employed to assess the causes of heterogeneity among the selected studies. Metaregression was used to show the trend of variation of prevalence during time. Egger test was conducted to examine potential publication bias. Egger's test can reveal a symmetric or asymmetric funnel plot. The latter indicates the existence of a significant publication bias or a systematic heterogeneity between studies. Data manipulation and statistical analyses were done using STATA software, version 11.2. P values <0.05 were considered as statistically significant.

3. Results

According to the literature search strategies, 268 studies were identified, but 227 studies were excluded as they did not meet the inclusion criteria. There were 9 studies in English [5, 12–19] and 32 studies in Persian [20–51] of the finally adopted 41 studies, and they were published between 1995 and 2012. The pooled sample sizes included 21907 women (Table 1 and Figure 1).

The heterogeneity between studies was 94.5% with an I square (I^2) statistic ($P \leq 0.001$). The pooled prevalence of postpartum depression was 25% (95% CI: 22.7–27.9%) (Figure 2). Based on the Edinburgh Postnatal Depression Scale (EPDS) and Beck depression inventory (BDI), the PPD prevalence in Iran was 24.3% (95% CI: 21.0–27.7) and 25.3% (95% CI: 22.7–27.9), respectively.

TABLE 1: Feature of studies among women with postpartum depression at different regions.

Study number/author(s)	Place	No. of population	Assessment times	Instrument Assessment	Cut point	Prevalence of PPD (%)
(1) Kheirabadi et al. [12, 16]	Isfahan	6627	2–12 weeks	EPDS	13	30
(2) Khorramirad et al. [38]	Qom	300	6–12 weeks	EPDS	13	23.7
(3) Hosseini Sazi et al. [34]	Gorgan	180	2–14 weeks	BDI	16	23.3
(4) Zangeneh et al. [51]	Kermanshah	531	2–6 weeks	EPDS	13	40.7
(5) Azimi Lolati et al. [24]	Sari	442	6–8 weeks	EPDS	13	22
(6) Sehhatie Shafaei et al. [49]	Tabriz	600	10–20 weeks	EPDS	12	34.7
(7) Shobeiri et al. [50]	Hamadan	400	2–8 weeks	BDI	16	32
(8) Khodadadi et al. [36]	Rasht	350	6–8 weeks	EPDS	13	16
(9) Hosseini et al. [33]	Kermanshah	330	4–14 weeks	BDI	16	24.8
(10) Ghaffari et al. [31]	Ramsar	100	6–16 weeks	GHQ 28	22	36.6
(11) Foruzandeh and Dashtebozorgi [30]	Shahrekord	300	6–10 weeks	BDI	16	21.3
(12) Bahrami et al. [26]	Dezful	140	6–10 weeks	EPDS	13	31.4
(13) Dolatian et al. [28]	Tehran	285	2–6 weeks	EPDS	12	20.3
(14) Ajh et al. [22]	Astaneh	440	2–4 weeks	BDI	16	18.6
(15) Khooshemehry et al. [37]	Tehran	250	6–52 weeks	BDI	16	30
(16) Tabrizi et al. [52]	Hamadan	144	2–12 weeks	BDI	16	16.8
(17) Barekatain et al. [27]	Isfahan	1898	6–8 weeks	EPDS	13	24.4
(18) Rahmani et al. [45]	Tabriz	560	8–52 weeks	EPDS	12	32
(19) Jafarpour et al. [35]	Kermanshah	975	13–26 weeks	EPDS	12	17.5
(20) Mousavi et al. [42]	Kashan	204	9–13 weeks	BDI	13	34.7
(21) Bagherzadeh et al. [25]	Bushehr	400	2–12 weeks	EPDS	15	15.5
(22) Kiani et al. [39]	Astara	105	2–4 weeks	EPDS	12	25
(23) Kamranpour and Shakiba [20]	Rasht	310	2–8 weeks	EPDS	12	6.4
(24) Dolatian et al. [28, 29]	Marivan	204	2–6 weeks	EPDS	10	34.2
(25) Salary et al. [47]	Mashhad	60	2–4 weeks	EPDS	10	9.9
(26) Lashkaripour et al. [40]	Zahedan	300	4–18 weeks	BDI	15	33.7
(27) Nikpour et al. [43]	Amol	420	2–8 weeks	EPDS	12	10.3
(28) Asadi Sadeghi Azar et al. [13]	Zabol	408	2–8 weeks	BDI	16	40.4
(29) Aghapoor and Mohammadi [21]	Tabriz	300	6–12 weeks	BDI	16	28
(30) Ghaffari Nejad et al. [32]	Kerman	400	2–8 weeks	BDI	16	31.1
(31) Akbari et al. [53]	Hamadan	159	4–8 weeks	EPDS	13	26.4
(32) Salehi [48]	Hormozgan	164	2–8 weeks	EPDS	13	14.9
(33) Sadr et al. [46]	Tehran	300	2–8 weeks	EPDS	13	23.7
(34) Taavoni et al. [14]	Tehran	597	4–12 weeks	EPDS	13	22.6
(35) Alipour et al. [15]	Qom	160	4–12 weeks	EPDS	13	25
(36) Montazeri et al. [5]	Isfahan	100	12–14 wWeks	EPDS	13	22
(37) Kheirabadi et al. [12, 16]	Isfahan	1291	6–8 weeks	EPDS	13	26.3
(38) Iranfar et al. [17]	Kermanshah	163	2–8 weeks	BDI	10	48.7
(39) Abbaszadeh et al. [18]	Kerman	400	8–28 weeks	EPDS	13	45.8
(40) Tashakori et al. [19]	Ahvaz	210	8–28 weeks	EPDS	12	21.4
(41) Akbarzadeh et al. [23]	Shiraz	400	2–8 weeks	BDI	16	21.1

Amongst subgroups of unwanted delivery, illiterate, housewives, and having history of depression, the prevalence was 43.4% (35.6–51.1), 31.6% (18.1–45.0), 30.7% (25.2–36.3), and 45.2% (35.4–53.1), respectively (Table 2). A significant geographic difference in pooled PPD was observed.

The lowest PPD rate was observed in central, and the highest rate was observed in west and south-eastern border areas of Iran (Figure 3).

The metaregression of the prevalence PPD for each study on the interval sample size showed a negative and no statistically significant relationship ($\beta = -0.0003$, s.e. $(\beta) = 0.0002$, $P = 0.995$) and no statistically significant change in prevalence over the time ($\beta = -0.4539$, s.e. $(\beta) = 0.025$, $P = 0.536$) (Figure 4). Since 1995, the PPD rates showed an increasing trend (Figure 5).

4. Discussion

Comprehensiveness of available information and a large sample size made the present study representative. There have been recent systematic reviews of studies dealing with risk factors of PPD in Iranian women [7], but the present study aimed to determine prevalence of PPD by a systematic review and meta-analysis method. The psychometric properties of

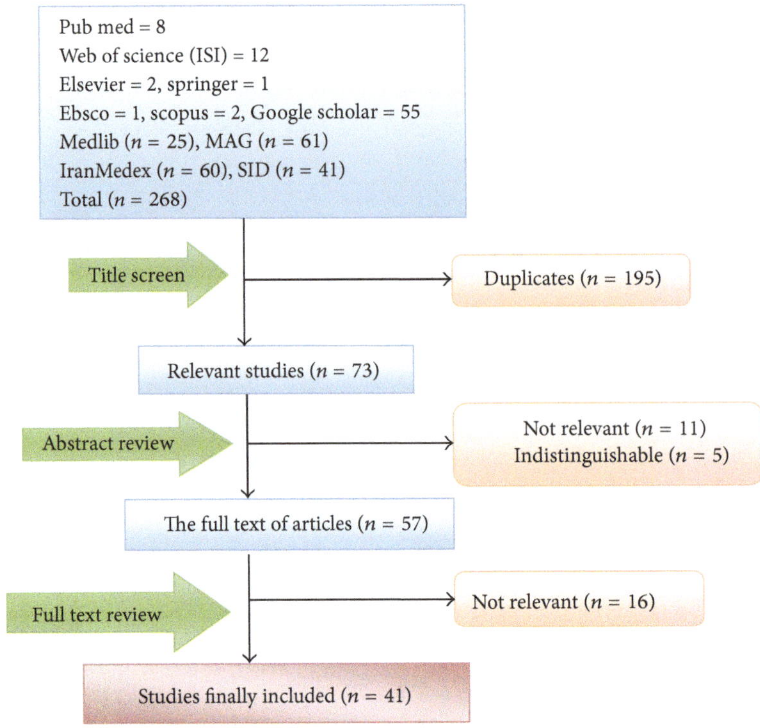

FIGURE 1: Results of the systematic literature search.

two main screening tools such as the Edinburgh Postnatal Depression Scale (EPDS) and Beck depression inventory (BDI) have been repeatedly assessed across the world.

The present study showed that the pooled prevalence of PPD among Iranian women was 25.3%, which is similar to the finding of a recent meta-analysis reported by Paulson and colleagues (25.6%) [54]. But it was not consistent with another meta-analysis of 15.6% [55]. This difference may be due to the assessment tools, geographic, and cut-off point differences. Prior studies that have noted the importance of recurrent PPD in women with a prior episode of postpartum affective psychosis may be at risk for recurrence postpartum 50–70% [56].

A significant geographic difference of the prevalence of PPD was also observed. Compared with other regions, west and south-eastern borders of Iran had relatively higher prevalence rates, accounting for 48.7% and 40.4%, respectively. Meanwhile, the lowest prevalence rate was found in north of Iran of 6.4%. Notably, during the period through 1995 and 2012, the prevalence rates were commonly at high level among different regions of Iran especially in border regions; the rates even reached nearly 50%. Possible reasons for this lack of reduction may include backwardness of border province to the central provinces, poor economic conditions, lack of program education in the sensitive groups, or limited sampling.

An extensive list of characteristics of PPD was examined among a diverse and representative sample of Iranian women. Conducting this study with a large sample size increased the statistical power. Sociological factors in Iran such as unwanted delivery as a result of the lack of family planning, illiterate result of gender discrimination, and carrier because most women are housewives have been more studied. The results of this study indicate that prevalence of PPD in illiterate women, unwanted delivery, and housewives women with a prior history of depression was 31.6%, 43.4%, 30.7%, 45.2%, respectively. Rates of relapse are particularly high in women with a prior history of depression with estimates ranging from 25%–50% [57]. Interventions that would specifically target women with a prior history of depression, illiterate women, housewives mothers, or women with unwanted pregnancy may help to decrease the prevalence of PPD among this population.

The strengths of this review include the large number of samples included and therefore the ability to examine prevalence in clinically relevant subgroups with some degree of precision. The I^2 is an estimate of the proportion of the total variation across studies that is beyond chance. In situations with high between-study heterogeneity, the use of random effects models is recommended as it produces study weights that primarily reflect the between-study variation and thus provides close to equal weighting. Univariate and multivariate metaregression analyses were used to explore possible sources of heterogeneity among studies [11]. Furthermore, we have examined heterogeneity using subgroup analyses and metaregression, which allowed us to investigate dichotomous and continuous variables such as age, sample size, and the date when the study was conducted. According to the metaregression analysis, none of the data were not statistically significant with changes of PPD prevalence. The high levels of heterogeneity between the studies are to be expected as the studies were conducted in different samples,

TABLE 2: Prevalence of postpartum depression among subgroups.

Variables	No. of studies	No. of patients	Prevalence % (95% CI)	Heterogeneity I^2	Heterogeneity P value	Model
Housewife	8	10756	30.7 (25.2–36.3)	96.4%	0.000	REM*
Employee	8	10756	29.3 (21.8–36.8)	96.4%	0.000	REM
History of depression	8	10787	45.2 (35.4–53.1)	97.9 %	0.000	REM
No history of depression	8	10787	27.3 (21.1–33.5)	97.3%	0.000	REM
Unwanted delivery	11	11702	43.4 (35.6–51.1)	98.3%	0.000	REM
Desired delivery	11	11702	29.0 (23.5–34.6)	97.1%	0.000	REM
Illiterate	4	7688	31.6 (18.1–45.0)	98.3%	0.000	REM
literate	4	7688	41.1 (25.1–57.1)	98.7%	0.000	REM
Pooled	41	21907	25.3 (22.7–27.9)	94.8%	0.000	REM

*Random effects model.

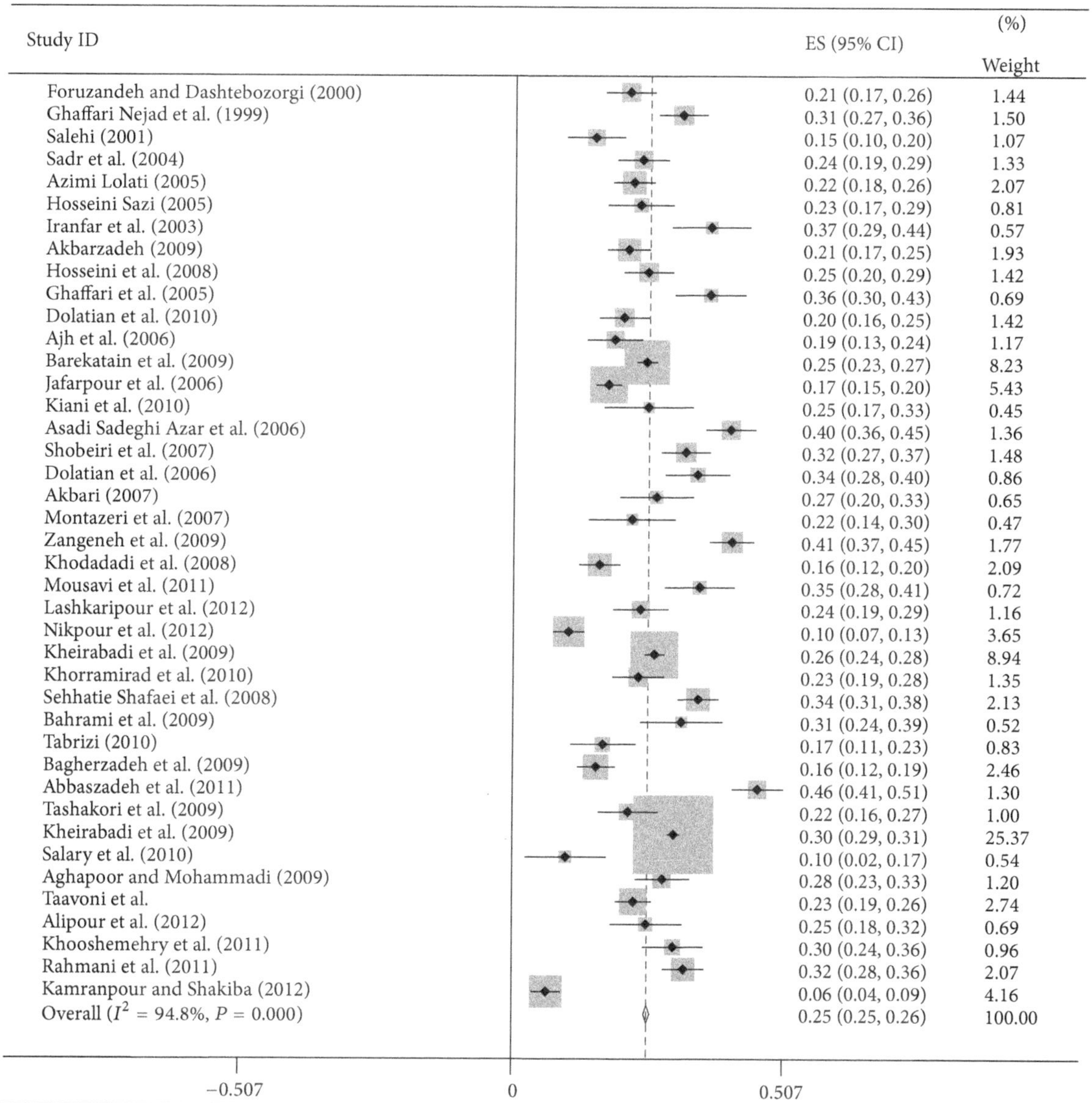

FIGURE 2: Forest plots for random effects meta-analyses. CI indicates confidence interval.

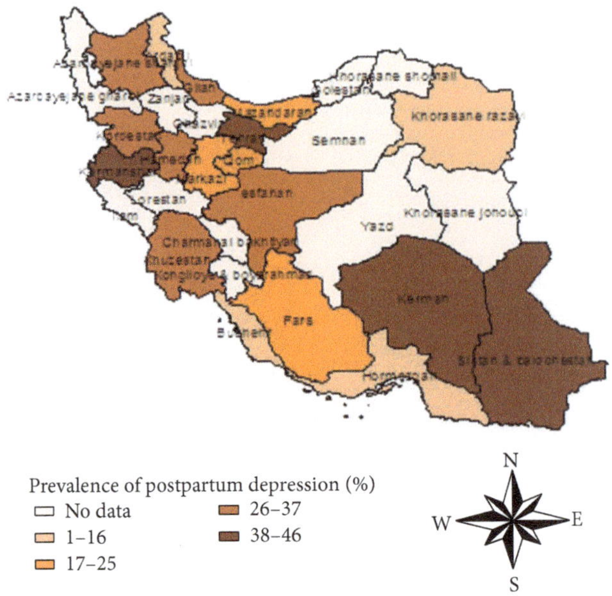

FIGURE 3: Regional distribution of pooled prevalence of postpartum depression in Iran.

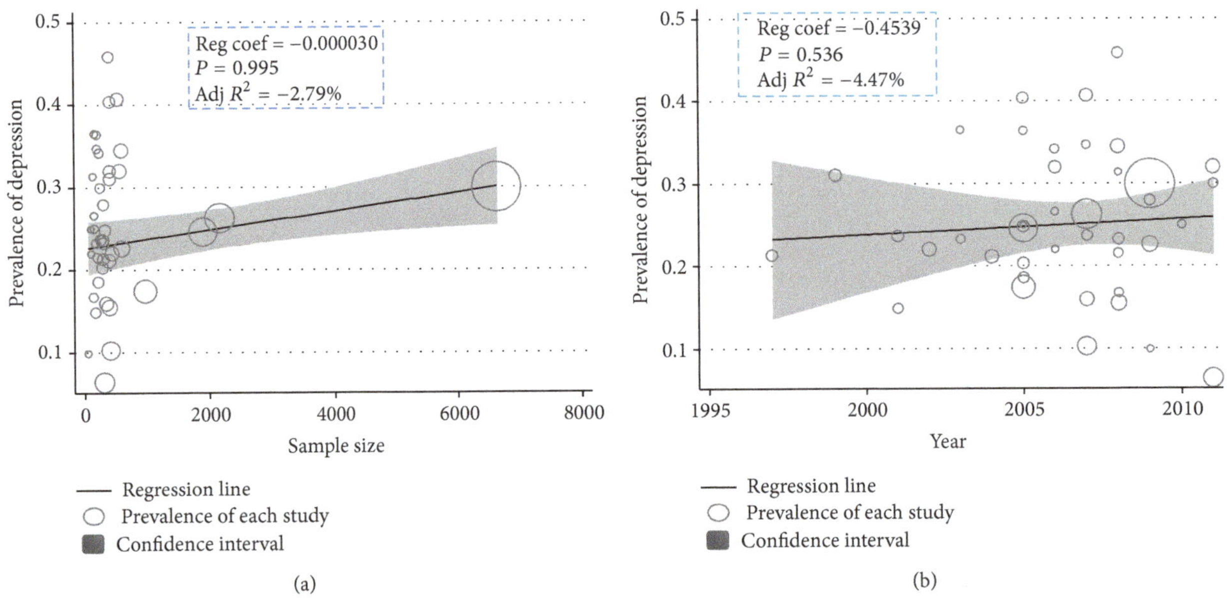

FIGURE 4: Metaregression plots of change in PPD according to changes in continuous study moderator's year and sample size.

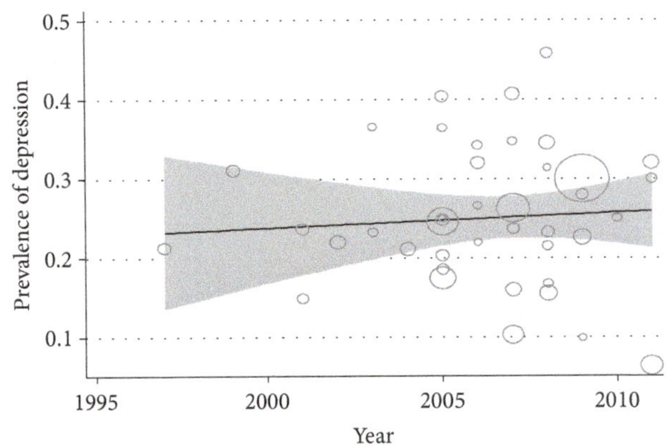

FIGURE 5: Prevalence of postpartum depression among Iranian women at different study periods.

and this may simply reflect real differences in prevalence over time and by region. Particular reasons for this difference in women are unclear. Our approach to this was to identify causes of heterogeneity, and two possible explanations were assessed. Possibilities include that in the diagnostic systems, fatigability is included in the core criteria for depression. In addition, it may be that the distinction between minor and major forms of depression is more important in women as the overlap between sadness and clinical depression is more difficult to determine.

There are some limitations in the present study which need to be addressed. First of all, more studies were observational and patients were not randomly chosen. Therefore, selection bias and confounding seem inevitable. Secondly, much of our data were extracted from the internal databases in Iran. Thirdly, our ability to assess study quality was limited by the fact that many studies failed to offer detailed information on selected subjects or valid data on important factors, and in the end timing of the administration of the EPDS and information bias may be present due to the self-report nature, and eventually in this review, there may be other explanations for the heterogeneity that we did not test, such as comorbidity with other mental disorders, but systematic data on this were lacking.

References

[1] B. N. Gaynes, N. Gavin, S. Meltzer-Brody et al., "Perinatal depression: prevalence, screening accuracy, and screening outcomes," *Evidence Report/Technology Assessment*, no. 119, pp. 1–8, 2005.

[2] H. M. Ahmed, S. K. Alalaf, and N. G. Al-Tawil, "Screening for postpartum depression using Kurdish version of Edinburgh postnatal depression scale," *Archives of Gynecology and Obstetrics*, vol. 285, no. 5, pp. 1249–1255, 2011.

[3] F. H. Al Dallal and I. N. Grant, "Postnatal depression among Bahraini women: prevalence of symptoms and psychosocial risk factors," *Eastern Mediterranean Health Journal*, vol. 18, no. 5, pp. 439–445, 2012.

[4] American Psychiatric Association, *Diagnostic and Statistical Manual of Mental Disorders*, American Psychiatric Press, Washington, DC, USA, 1994.

[5] A. Montazeri, B. Torkan, and S. Omidvari, "The edinburgh postnatal depression scale (EPDS): translation and validation study of the Iranian version," *BMC Psychiatry*, vol. 7, no. 11, pp. 1–6, 2007.

[6] P. Klainin and D. G. Arthur, "Postpartum depression in Asian cultures: a literature review," *International Journal of Nursing Studies*, vol. 46, no. 10, pp. 1355–1373, 2009.

[7] P. Bahadoran, S. S. Foroushani, S. Ehsanpour, and A. Abedi, "A meta-analysis on studies about obstetric risk factors of postpartum depression in Iran within 1995–2005," *Iranian Journal of Nursing and Midwifery Research*, vol. 13, no. 4, pp. 129–133, 2008.

[8] P. Grossman, L. Niemann, S. Schmidt, and H. Walach, "Mindfulness-based stress reduction and health benefits: a meta-analysis," *Journal of Psychosomatic Research*, vol. 57, no. 1, pp. 35–43, 2004.

[9] R. DerSimonian and N. Laird, "Meta-analysis in clinical trials," *Controlled Clinical Trials*, vol. 7, no. 3, pp. 177–188, 1986.

[10] A. E. Ades, G. Lu, and J. P. T. Higgins, "The interpretation of random-effects meta-analysis in decision models," *Medical Decision Making*, vol. 25, no. 6, pp. 646–654, 2005.

[11] M. Borenstein, L. V. Hedges, J. P. T. Higgins, and H. R. Rothstein, *Introduction to Meta-Analysis*, John Wiley & Sons, 2009.

[12] G.-R. Kheirabadi, M.-R. Maracy, M. Barekatain et al., "Risk factors of postpartum depression in rural areas of Isfahan Province, Iran," *Archives of Iranian Medicine*, vol. 12, no. 5, pp. 461–467, 2009.

[13] I. Asadi Sadeghi Azar, Z. Hashemi, and F. Forghani, "Postpartum depression and its correlates among women living in zabol (Iran)," *Iranian Journal of Psychiatry*, vol. 1, no. 4, pp. 140–147, 2006.

[14] S. Taavoni, P. Zarea, and H. Haghani, "P-532—postpartum depression: related factors in clients, whom had been visited in clinics of tehran university of medical sciences," *European Psychiatry*, vol. 27, Supplement 1, article 1.

[15] Z. Alipour, M. Lamyian, and E. Hajizadeh, "Anxiety and fear of childbirth as predictors of postnatal depression in nulliparous women," *Women and Birth*, vol. 25, no. 3, pp. e37–e43, 2012.

[16] G. R. Kheirabadia and M. R. Maracy, "Perinatal depression in a cohort study on Iranian women," *Journal of Research in Medical Sciences*, vol. 15, no. 1, pp. 41–49, 2010.

[17] S. Iranfar, J. Shakeri, M. Ranjbar, P. NazhadJafar, and M. Razaie, "Is unintended pregnancy a risk factor for depression in Iranian women?" *Eastern Mediterranean Health Journal*, vol. 11, no. 4, pp. 618–624, 2005.

[18] A. Abbaszadeh, F. P. Kermani, H. Safizadeh, and N. Nakhee, "Violence during pregnancy and postpartum depression," *Pakistan Journal of Medical Sciences*, vol. 27, no. 1, pp. 177–181, 2011.

[19] A. Tashakori, A. Shanesaz, and A. Rezapour, "Assessment of some potential risk factors of postpartum depression," *Pakistan Journal of Medical Sciences*, vol. 25, no. 2, pp. 261–264, 2009.

[20] S. B. Kamranpour and M. Shakiba, "Cesarean section and post partum depression," *Iranian Journal of Obstetrics, Gynecology and Infertility*, vol. 15, no. 1, part 41, pp. 56–62, 2012.

[21] M. Aghapoor and A. Mohammadi, "Comparing postpartum depression of working women and housewives and its relationship with social support and marital adjustment," *Women & Study of Family*, vol. 1, no. 4, pp. 9–32, 2009.

[22] N. Ajh, M. Unesian, A. Fili, and A. Abasi Motejaded, "The study of supportive activities during pregnancy on postpartum depression," *Journal of Nursing and Midwifery*, vol. 12, no. 3, pp. 73–80, 2006.

[23] M. Akbarzadeh, F. Sharif, N. Zare, and F. Ghodrati, "Prevalence of symptoms post-partum anxiety and baby blues and factors effective uponit in women with high risk pregnancies," *Journal of Family Research*, vol. 5, no. 1, pp. 57–71, 2009.

[24] H. Azimi Lolati, M. M. Danesh, S. H. Hosseini, A. R. Khalilian, and M. Zarghami, "Postpartum depression in clients at health care centers in Sari," *Iranian Journal of Psychiatry and Psychology*, vol. 111, no. 40, pp. 31–42, 2005.

[25] R. Bagherzadeh, N. Zahmatkeshan, N. Moatamed, R. Khorramroudi, and M. Ganjoo, "Prevalence of maternal blues, postpartum depression and their correlation with premenstrual syndrome in women refferred to health centers affiliated to bushehr university of medical sciences," *Iranian Journal of Obstetric, Gynecology and Infertility*, vol. 12, no. 3, pp. 9–15, 2009.

[26] N. Bahrami, M. Araban, and S. Bahrami, "The Impact of antenatal education on postpartum," *Journal of Hormozgan University of Medical Sciences*, vol. 13, no. 14, pp. 277–283, 2009.

[27] M. Barekatain, M. Tavakkoli, G. Kheirabadi, and M. R. Maracy, "The relationship between life-time prevalence of bipolar spectrum disorders and incidence of postnatal depression," *Iranian Journal of Psychiatry and Clinical Psychology*, vol. 15, no. 2, pp. 183–192, 2009.

[28] M. Dolatian, K. Hesami, J. Shams, and H. A. Majd, "Relationship between violence during pregnancy and postpartum depression," *Iranian Red Crescent Medical Journal*, vol. 12, no. 4, pp. 377-383, 2010.

[29] M. Dolatian, P. Maziar, H. Alavi-Majd, and M. Yazdjerdi, "The relationship between mode of delivery and postpartum depression," *Journal of Reproduction and Infertility*, vol. 7, no. 328, pp. 260–268, 2006.

[30] N. Foruzandeh and B. Dashtebozorgi, "Prevalence and predisposing factors of post-partum depression among women referred to the health care centers of Shahrekord, 1996," *Journal of Shahrekord University of Medical Sciences*, vol. 2, no. 1, pp. 43–51, 2000.

[31] F. Ghaffari, T. Pourghaznain, and R. Mazlom, "A mental health of women and their husbands during pregnancy and postpatrum in health center of ramsar," *Journal of Gorgan University of Medical Sciences*, vol. 5, no. 5, pp. 74–80, 2005.

[32] A. R. Ghaffari Nejad, F. Khobyari, and F. F. P, "Prevalence of postpartum depression in Kerman," *Quarterly Journal of Mentality & Behavior*, vol. 5, article 1, 1999.

[33] H. Hosseini, A. H. Naghibi, and M. Khademloo, "Postpartum depression and relaship with some related factors," *Journal of Babol University of Medical Sciences*, vol. 10, no. 2, pp. 76–81, 2008.

[34] F. Hosseini Sazi, A. Poor Reza, M. Hosseini, and D. Shojaei Zadeh, "Depression during pregnancy," *Journal of Gorgan University of Medical Sciences*, vol. 7, no. 1, pp. 60–65, 2005.

[35] M. Jafarpour, M. Esfandyari, Mokhtarsahi sh, and F. Hoseini, "The effect of stressful life events on postpartum depression," *University of Medical Sciences, Kermanshah*, vol. 10, no. 4, pp. 320–331, 2006.

[36] N. Khodadadi, H. Mahmoudi, and N. Mir hagh jo, "Postpartum depression relationship with some psychosocial effects in mothers," *Journal of Ardabil University of Medical Sciences*, vol. 8, no. 2, pp. 142–148, 2008.

[37] G. Khooshemehry, A. Shariati Feizabady, V. Naserkhaki, and V. Naserkhak, "Prevalence of postpartum depression and the factors that decides in clinics in the North of Tehran," *Journal of Nursing and Midwifery*, vol. 19, no. 1, pp. 59–64, 2011.

[38] A. Khorramirad, M. Mousavi Lotfi, and A. Shoori Bidgol, "Prevalence of postpartum depression and related factors in qom," *Pejohandeh*, vol. 15, no. 2, part 74, pp. 62–66, 2010.

[39] F. Kiani, T. Khadivzadeh, M. R. Sargolzaee, and H. Behnam, "Relationship between marital satisfaction during Pregnancy and Postpartum Depression (PPD)," *Iranian Journal of Obstetrics, Gynecology and Infertility*, vol. 13, no. 5, pp. 37–44, 2010.

[40] K. Lashkaripour, N. Bakhshani, S. Hokmabadi, A. R. Sajjadi-Ameneh, and A. Safarzadeh Sarasiyab, "Postpartum depression and related factors: a 4.5 months study," *Journal of Fundamentals of Mental Health*, vol. 134, no. 52, pp. 404–412, 2012.

[41] M. J. Modabernia, H. Shodjaei tehrani, and S. Heydari Nezhad, "Survey the frequency of depression in the last third months of pregnancy," *Journal of Guilan University of Medical Sciences*, vol. 18, no. 71, pp. 19–25, 2009.

[42] G. A. Mousavi, S. Sabahi Bidgoli, A. Omidi et al., "Prevalence of postpartum depression and its relation to some psychosocial factors in mothers referred to health centers of Kashan during 2007-8," *Faiz*, vol. 15, no. 3, pp. 247–253, 2011.

[43] M. Nikpour, Z. Abedian, N. Mokhber, S. Ebrahimzadeh, and S. Khani, "Relationship between delivery method and postpartum depression," *Journal of Fundamentals of Mental Health*, vol. 14, no. 1, part 53, pp. 46–53, 2012.

[44] F. Pazande, J. Tominas, F. Valai, and N. Afshar, "Prevalence of depression and its associated factors in women's centers martyr Beheshti University of Medical Sciences, 1999," *Faiz*, no. 28, pp. 66–70, 2002.

[45] F. Rahmani, N. Seyedfatemi, M. Asadollahi, and A. Seyedrasooli, "Predisposing factors of postpartum depression," *Iran Journal of Nursing*, vol. 24, no. 72, pp. 78–87, 2011.

[46] S. S. Sadr, M. Dowlatian, and Z. Behboudi Moghadam, "Prevalence of postpartum depression and factors affecting it in Tehran," *Journal of Medical Council of IRI*, vol. 22, no. 3, pp. 189–193, 2004.

[47] P. Salary, E. Banafshe, P. Hebrani, and J. Jabbari Nooghabi, "On the relationship between maternal fatigue and postpartum depression," *Journal of Fundamentals of Mental Health*, vol. 114, no. 14, pp. 302–311, 2010.

[48] L. Salehi, "Postpartum depression prevalence in primiparous and multiparous women," *Journal of Hormozgan University of Medical Sciences*, vol. 5, no. 2, pp. 22–25, 2001.

[49] F. Sehhatie Shafaei, F. Ranjbar Koochaksariie, M. Ghojazadeh, and Zh. Mohamadrezaei, "Study of relationship between some predisposing factors and postpartum depression," *Journal of Ardabil University of Medical Sciences*, vol. 81, no. 27, pp. 54–61, 2008.

[50] F. Shobeiri, A. Farhadi Nasab, and M. Nazar, "Detecting postpartum depression in referents to medical and health centers in hamadan city," *Scientific Journal of Hamadan University of Medical Sciences and Health Services*, vol. 14, no. 3, pp. 24–28, 2007.

[51] M. Zangeneh, N. S. Alizadeh, M. Kaamrvamanesh, M. Rezaie, and S. Pormehr, "Postpartum depression and its relation to baby gender and unplanned pregnancy," *Scientific Journal of Kurdistan University of Medical Sciences*, vol. 14, no. 2, pp. 65–71, 2009.

[52] M. Tabrizi and K. H. Lorestani, "Eclectic effectiveness of interventions to reduce depression in pregnancy and prevention of Postpartum Depression," *Thought and Behavior in Clinical Psychology*, vol. 5, no. 17, pp. 19–26, 2010.

[53] S. Amir Ali Akbari, M. Toghiri, N. Karimian, and H. Alavi-Majd, "Association between anemia during pregnancy and postpartum depression," *Journal of Nursing and Midwifery*, vol. 16, no. 54, pp. 19–26, 2007.

[54] J. F. Paulson and S. D. Bazemore, "Prenatal and postpartum depression in fathers and its association with maternal depression: a meta-analysis," *Journal of the American Medical Association*, vol. 303, no. 19, pp. 1961–1969, 2010.

[55] J. Fisher, M. C. de Mello, V. Patel et al., "Prevalence and determinants of common perinatal mental disorders in women in low-and lower-middle-income countries: a systematic review," *Bulletin of the World Health Organization*, vol. 90, no. 2, pp. 139–149, 2012.

[56] L. S. Cohen, "Pharmacologic treatment of depression in women: PMS, pregnancy, and the postpartum period," *Depression and Anxiety*, vol. 8, no. 1, pp. 18–26, 1998.

[57] K. L. Wisner, J. M. Perel, and R. L. Findling, "Antidepressant treatment during breast-feeding," *American Journal of Psychiatry*, vol. 153, no. 9, pp. 1132–1137, 1996.

Temperament, Character, and Depressive Symptoms during Pregnancy

Mariko Minatani,[1,2] Sachiko Kita,[1,2] Yukiko Ohashi,[2] Toshinori Kitamura,[2,3] Megumi Haruna,[1] Kyoko Sakanashi,[4] and Tomoko Tanaka[5]

[1] *Division of Health Sciences & Nursing, Department of Midwifery and Women's Health, Graduate School of Medicine, University of Tokyo, 7-3-1 Hongo, Bunkyo, Tokyo 113-0033, Japan*
[2] *Kitamura Institute of Mental Health Tokyo, 101 Akasaka 8-5-13, Minato, Tokyo 107-0052, Japan*
[3] *Nagoya University, 65 Tsurumai-cho, Showa, Nagoya, Aichi 466-8550, Japan*
[4] *Department of Women's Health and Mother-Child Nursing, Faculty of Life Sciences, Kumamoto University, 4-24-1 Kuhonji, Chuo, Kumamoto 862-0976, Japan*
[5] *Aso Health Center, 1204 Uchimaki, Aso, Kumamoto 869-2301, Japan*

Correspondence should be addressed to Toshinori Kitamura; kitamura@institute-of-mental-health.jp

Academic Editor: Claude Robert Cloninger

Background. To examine the effects of temperament and character domains on depression during pregnancy. *Methods.* We examined 601 pregnant women using a questionnaire that included the Edinburgh Postnatal Depression Scale (EPDS), the Temperament and Character Inventory (TCI), and demographic variables. *Results.* In a hierarchical regression analysis, severity of depression during pregnancy was predicted by the women's negative response towards the current pregnancy, low self-directedness, and high harm avoidance, persistence, and self-transcendence. *Conclusion.* Depression during pregnancy is predicted by personality traits as well as women's negative attitudes towards the current pregnancy.

1. Introduction

The World Mental Health Survey [1], conducted in 17 countries, found that on average about one in 20 people reported having had an episode of depression. The prevalence of depression among women is two to three times higher than that among men. Depression is one of the most serious health problems among women [2], with younger women affected more frequently than middle-age women [3].

Personality is one of the major factors associated with depression [4–7]. Personality traits predict the course and treatment response of depression [8]. Cloninger et al. [9] proposed a psychobiological model that included both temperament and character domains. According to their theory, the temperament domain consists of four dimensions: harm avoidance (HA), novelty seeking (NS), reward dependence (RD), and persistence (PS). The character domain consists of three dimensions: self-directedness (SD), cooperativeness (CO), and self-transcendence (ST). As a measure of these dimensions, they developed the Temperament and Character Inventory (TCI) [10].

Many studies have used the TCI to explore the relationship between depression on the one hand and temperament and character dimensions on the other. Most of these studies demonstrated that individuals with depressive disorder or depression were more likely to have high HA and low SD and CO [6, 7, 11–16]. No consensus, however, has been reached regarding the relationship between PS and depression. While some researchers [12, 17–19] have reported *high* PS among those with depression, others have found *low* PS among those with depression [7, 20, 21], depressive disorder [22, 23], and bipolar disorder [22, 24–26]. It is of interest to us that PS was reported to be low among individuals with postpartum depression [27].

Depression that appears during pregnancy is called antenatal depression. The prevalence of this condition has been reported to be between 4% and 29% [28, 29], and it has been associated with unwanted and unplanned pregnancy, high neuroticism, attitudes towards the present pregnancy, lack of social support, and pregnancy complications [28, 30, 31].

Depression and depressive symptoms during pregnancy impact several perinatal health outcomes, including preterm delivery [32], low birth weight, intrauterine growth restriction [33], diabetes [34], and postpartum depression [35]. It is therefore of clinical as well as research importance to identify pregnant women with depression.

However, unlike depression in general and postnatal depression, antenatal depression has been infrequently studied with regard to its association with personality traits. Andriola and colleagues [36] found that antenatal depression was significantly related to high HA and low SD, but this study enrolled only 65 pregnant women. The present study aimed to explore the associations between antenatal depression and temperament and character dimensions in a large population of pregnant Japanese women.

2. Methods

2.1. Participants. All 55 obstetric clinics in Kumamoto Prefecture were solicited to participate in this multiwave study on perinatal mental health. Eighteen (33%) clinics responded to our request. There were one university hospital (the only academia-affiliated hospital in the prefecture), public and private hospitals ($N = 12$), and private clinics ($N = 5$). Hence we obtained a mixture of different types of antenatal institutions. We then invited pregnant women of at least 28 weeks' gestation who attended one of these antenatal clinics during the whole month of November 2011. It is of note that the gestational age in Japan is calculated as week since the first day of the last menstruation. Women were eligible for the study if they were above 20 years old. Pregnant women who were illiterate, who had severe mental illness, or who had been hospitalized with pregnancy complications were excluded. Of 1442 eligible women, 601 (42%) returned the questionnaire while still pregnant.

2.2. Measures

2.2.1. Depression. We used the Edinburgh Postnatal Depression Scale (EPDS) [37]. This is a self-report of postnatal depression with 10 items rated on a 4-point scale (from 0 to 3). Its psychometric properties have been reported [37]. The total score ranges from 0 to 30 with higher scores indicating more severe depressive symptoms. The Japanese version of the EPDS was made available by Okano and colleagues [38] who also verified its reliability and validity.

Temperament and character dimensions: we used the 130-item Temperament and Character Inventory [39]. This is based on the original 125-item TCI [10] with the addition of five more PS items in order to increase the internal reliability of the scale, as suggested by Kijima and colleagues [40]. The TCI measures the four temperament dimensions (NS, HA, RD, and PS) and the three character dimensions (SD, CO, and ST). The original true-false response scale was modified into a 4-point scale, which has better internal consistency among Japanese populations [39]; the 4-point scale ranges from 0 (strongly disagree) to 3 (strongly agree). Reliability and factor validity of the Japanese version of the TCI were reported by Kijima and colleagues [40] and Takeuchi and colleagues [41].

2.2.2. Demographic Data. We measured age, partner's age, number of children, complications of pregnancy (such as threatened labour, pregnancy hypertension, placenta previa, and anomaly of the fetus), gestational week, response to the present pregnancy (from very displeased: 1 to very pleased: 5), and desire for baby (from not desired: 1 to very desired: 5).

2.3. Statistical Analysis. After examining the means and standard deviations of the variables used in this study, we calculated bivariate correlations between the EPDS scores and the TCI subscale scores and the demographic variables.

In order to identify the relative magnitude of each predictor of depression during pregnancy, we regressed the EPDS scores on predictor variables using the following four steps. First we entered the ages of the participants and their partners. Then we entered the demographic variables that showed significant correlation with the EPDS scores. In the third step, we entered the scores of the character domain scales. This is because we presumed, based on Cloninger and colleagues' [9, 10] assumption, that character domain develops on the basis of temperament domain. Finally, in the fourth step, we entered the scores of the temperament scales.

The criterion for statistical significance was set at $P < .05$. All statistical analyses were conducted using the Statistical Package for Social Science (SPSS) Version 20.

2.4. Procedure. All the questionnaires were distributed at the clinics. The participants were asked to bring the questionnaire home, fill it in, and return it to the researcher (T.K.) using a stamp-added envelope. The present study was approved by the Ethical Committee of Kumamoto University Graduate School of Life Sciences.

3. Results

The EPDS scores were significantly correlated with NS, HA, ST, and negative response to the current pregnancy. They were significantly negatively correlated with SD, CO, the woman's age, the partner's age, and desire for a baby (Table 1).

In the regression analysis, the EPDS scores were predicted by the woman's and partner's ages, negative response to the current pregnancy, low SD, high ST, high HA, and high PS (Table 2).

Because the Cloninger theory dictates that character develops on the basis of temperament, we entered into a regression analysis the temperament scales before character scales. However, the results were virtually the same (table not shown).

4. Discussion

As in Andriola and colleagues' [36] study on postnatal depression as well as other studies on depression in general [6, 7, 13, 15], our study showed that severity of depression

TABLE 1: Means, SDs, and correlations of the variables used in this study ($N = 608$ to 633).

	1	2	3	4	5	6	7	8	9	10	11	12	13	14	15
(1) EPDS	—														
(2) NS	0.15***	—													
(3) HA	0.35***	−0.25***	—												
(4) RD	−0.08	0.3	−0.01	—											
(5) PS	0.08	−0.16***	−0.03	0.11**	—										
(6) SD	−0.56***	−0.23***	−0.48***	0.14**	0.05	—									
(7) CO	−0.29***	−0.22***	−0.25***	0.45***	0.18***	0.50***	—								
(8) ST	0.14**	0.21***	−0.22***	0.01	0.21	−0.11**	0.07	—							
(9) Age	−0.13**	−0.01	−0.11**	−0.07	0.03	0.12**	0.11*	0.07	—						
(10) Partner's age	−0.09*	−0.03	−0.13**	−0.13**	0.03	0.12**	0.05	0.09*	0.68***	—					
(11) No. of children	0.05	−0.04	0.4	−0.03	0.04	−0.02	0.03	−0.03	0.21***	0.14**	—				
(12) Pregnancy complications	0.04	−0.06	−0.01	0.03	0.04	−0.01	0.09*	0.07	0.11**	0.11**	−0.01	—			
(13) Gestational week	−0.02	−0.00	−0.11**	−0.05	0.01	0.03	−0.03	0.04	0.06	−0.00	−0.02	−0.05	—		
(14) Response to pregnancy	0.16***	0.04	0.03	−0.12**	−0.06	−0.11**	−0.09*	−0.08	−0.03	0.01	0.26***	−0.01	0.05	—	
(15) Desire for baby	−0.13**	−0.05	0.00	0.08*	0.02	0.06	0.05	0.01	0.21***	0.15***	−0.18***	0.6	−0.04	−0.47***	—
Mean	4.5	25.5	33.1	29.0	16.3	43.7	50.0	17.2	30.0	32.1	0.7	0.2	34.1	1.3	3.3
SD	4.1	6.0	7.2	4.6	3.0	8.1	6.4	5.8	4.9	5.9	0.8	0.5	3.6	0.6	1.0
Skewness	1.5	−0.1	−0.2	−0.01	0.1	−0.4	−0.1	0.3	0.1	0.7	1.1	2.5	−1.4	2.4	−0.3
Cronbach's alpha									—	—	—	—	—	—	—

Because pregnancy complications and response to pregnancy were more 2.0 positively skewed, both of them were log-transformed for correlations with other variables. $^{*}P < 0.05$, $^{**}P < 0.01$, and $^{***}P < 0.001$.

Table 2: Hierarchical multiple regression analyses predicting EPDS score during pregnancy.

	R^2	R^2 increase	Standardised beta	t
Step 1: demographics	0.01	0.01*		
Age			−0.07	−1.4
Partner's age			0.03	0.7
Step 2: psychological response	0.04	0.03***		
Response to pregnancy			0.13	3.1**
Desire for baby			−0.02	0.6
Step 3: character	0.33	0.29***		
SD			−0.41	−8.5***
CO			−0.01	0.3
ST			0.11	3.0**
Step 4: temperament	0.37	0.03***		
NS			0.08	1.9
HA			0.19	4.2***
RD			−0.01	−0.3
PS			0.12	3.2**
Standardised R^2	0.353			

*$P < 0.05$, **$P < 0.01$, and ***$P < 0.001$.

during pregnancy was associated with high HA and low SD. Because the effects of the temperament domain on depression remained statistically significant after controlling for the effects of character domains, we could eliminate the possibility that the effects of temperament on depression were wholly explained by mediation of the effects of character domains.

In addition to personality, it was the woman's negative response to the current pregnancy ("I was very displeased") that significantly predicted the severity of depression during pregnancy. We are not aware of any studies examining the association between such negative psychological attitudes and depression during pregnancy. Much remains to be investigated regarding the temporal sequence of depression during pregnancy and negative psychological reactions towards pregnancy.

Like Cloninger and colleagues' [12] study, our research showed a link between high ST and depression. High ST has reported to be characteristic of individuals with bipolar disorder [13, 42]. Because this study used a self-report of depressive symptoms, we were unable to distinguish individuals with bipolar depression from those with unipolar depression. It is likely that our participants who scored highly on the EPDS included individuals who had previously experienced manic or hypomanic episodes.

As in some studies [12, 13, 18, 19], our results showed a link between high PS and depression during pregnancy. This is, however, in contrast with other studies reporting the reverse association of depression with PS [7, 20–27]. People high in PS are hardworking, persistent, and stable, even in frustrating situations [10]. Coupled with high HA, high PS is associated with obsessive compulsive personality traits [43]. About one-third of people with obsessive compulsive disorder were found to have had current or previous episodes of major depressive disorder [44], and, in about 40% of women with children, obsessive compulsive symptoms had their onset during pregnancy [45]. Depression during pregnancy may be associated with obsessive compulsive traits. Because, however, we failed to measure obsessive compulsive traits or symptoms, our speculation awaits reports in future studies.

Despite the strengths of the present study, including its use of a large community population of pregnant women, its limitations should be discussed. First, caution should be exercised because of the cross-sectional study design. HA is likely to be influenced by the individual's mood at the time of examination [46]. Hence studies with longitudinal follow-up are necessary before firm conclusions can be made regarding the association between personality traits and depression during pregnancy. Alternatively, we could conduct unique statistical analysis applying a nonrecursive model with a "statistical anchor" to fix the effects of an otherwise correlational relationship [47]. Second, the use of a self-report measure of depression made it impossible to distinguish between depressive symptoms and the nosological entity of major depression and allowed for the possible inclusion of individuals with bipolar depression. Another drawback of this study was a low participation rate (42%) though such a high nonparticipation rate was not a rare phenomenon in mental health epidemiologic studies in Japan. For example, in one of the first community studies of mental disorders in Japan [48], the participation rate was 41%. Although it is desirable, we are unaware even of the demographic data such as age and parity of those women who refrained.

Taking these limitations into consideration, the present preliminary study suggests that depression during pregnancy is predicted by high HA, PS, and ST as well as by low SD and women's negative attitudes towards the current pregnancy.

Conflict of Interests

The authors declare that they have no conflict of interests.

References

[1] World Health Organization, Mental Health World Mental Health Day, 2012, http://www.who.int/mental_health/management/depression/wfmh_paper_depression_wmhd_2012.pdf.

[2] L. S. Goldman, N. H. Nielsen, and H. C. Champion, "Awareness, diagnosis, and treatment of depression," *Journal of General Internal Medicine*, vol. 14, no. 9, pp. 569–580, 1999.

[3] S. Kasen, P. Cohen, H. Chen, and D. Castille, "Depression in adult women: age changes and cohort effects," *American Journal of Public Health*, vol. 93, no. 12, pp. 2061–2066, 2003.

[4] H. S. Akiskal, R. M. A. Hirschfeld, and B. I. Yerevanian, "The relationship of personality to affective disorders. A critical review," *Archives of General Psychiatry*, vol. 40, no. 7, pp. 801–810, 1983.

[5] R. M. A. Hirschfeld, G. L. Klerman, P. J. Clayton, and M. B. Keller, "Personality and depression. Empirical findings," *Archives of General Psychiatry*, vol. 40, no. 9, pp. 993–998, 1983.

[6] P. Jylhä and E. Isometsä, "Temperament, character and symptoms of anxiety and depression in the general population," *European Psychiatry*, vol. 21, no. 6, pp. 389–395, 2006.

[7] T. Matsudaira and T. Kitamura, "Personality traits as risk factors of depression and anxiety among Japanese students," *Journal of Clinical Psychology*, vol. 62, no. 1, pp. 97–109, 2006.

[8] D. N. Klein, R. Kotov, and S. J. Bufferd, "Personality and depression: explanatory models and review of the evidence," *Annual Review of Clinical Psychology*, vol. 7, pp. 269–295, 2011.

[9] C. R. Cloninger, D. M. Svrakic, and T. R. Przybeck, "A psychobiological model of temperament and character," *Archives of General Psychiatry*, vol. 50, no. 12, pp. 975–990, 1993.

[10] C. R. Cloninger, T. R. Przybeck, D. M. Svrakic, and R. D. Wetzel, *The Temperament and Character Inventory (TCI): A Guide to Its Development and Use*, Center for Psychobiology of Personality, Washington University, St. Louis, Mo, USA, 1994.

[11] F. C. Celikel, S. Kose, B. E. Cumurcu et al., "Cloninger's temperament and character dimensions of personality in patients with major depressive disorder," *Comprehensive Psychiatry*, vol. 50, no. 6, pp. 556–561, 2009.

[12] C. R. Cloninger, D. M. Svrakic, and T. R. Przybeck, "Can personality assessment predict future depression? A twelve-month follow-up of 631 subjects," *Journal of Affective Disorders*, vol. 92, no. 1, pp. 35–44, 2006.

[13] R. F. Farmer and J. R. Seeley, "Temperament and character predictors of depressed mood over a 4-year interval," *Depression and Anxiety*, vol. 26, no. 4, pp. 371–381, 2009.

[14] K. Furumura, T. Koide, T. Okada et al., "Prospective study on the association between harm avoidance and postpartum depressive state in a maternal cohort of Japanese women," *PLoS ONE*, vol. 7, no. 4, Article ID e34725, 2012.

[15] F. G. Nery, J. P. Hatch, M. A. Nicoletti et al., "Temperament and character traits in major depressive disorder: influence of mood state and recurrence of episodes," *Depression and Anxiety*, vol. 26, no. 4, pp. 382–388, 2009.

[16] E. Tanaka, N. Kijima, and T. Kitamura, "Correlations between the temperament and character inventory and the self-rating depression scale among Japanese students," *Psychological Reports*, vol. 80, no. 1, pp. 251–254, 1997.

[17] L. Evans, H. S. Akiskal, P. E. Keck Jr. et al., "Familiality of temperament in bipolar disorder: support for a genetic spectrum," *Journal of Affective Disorders*, vol. 85, no. 1-2, pp. 153–168, 2005.

[18] A. Farmer, A. Mahmood, K. Redman, T. Harris, S. Sadler, and P. McGuffin, "A sib-pair study of the temperament and character inventory scales in major depression," *Archives of General Psychiatry*, vol. 60, no. 5, pp. 490–496, 2003.

[19] M. Hansenne, J. Reggers, E. Pinto, K. Kjiri, A. Ajamier, and M. Ansseau, "Temperament and character inventory (TCI) and depression," *Journal of Psychiatric Research*, vol. 33, no. 1, pp. 31–36, 1999.

[20] M. Ghazinour, J. Richter, and M. Eisemann, "Personality related to coping and social support among Iranian refugees in Sweden," *Journal of Nervous and Mental Disease*, vol. 191, no. 9, pp. 595–603, 2003.

[21] D. M. Goncalves and C. R. Cloninger, "Validation and normative studies of the Brazilian Portuguese and American versions of the Temperament and Character Inventory—Revised (TCI-R)," *Journal of Affective Disorders*, vol. 124, no. 1-2, pp. 126–133, 2010.

[22] P. Jylhä, O. Mantere, T. Melartin et al., "Differences in temperament and character dimensions in patients with bipolar I or II or major depressive disorder and general population subjects," *Psychological Medicine*, vol. 41, no. 8, pp. 1579–1591, 2011.

[23] O. Minaya and A. Fresán, "Anxiety disorders comorbidity in first-episode depressed patients: personality differences based on the temperament and character inventory," *Personality and Individual Differences*, vol. 47, no. 5, pp. 522–526, 2009.

[24] Y. Osher, C. R. Cloninger, and R. H. Belmaker, "TPQ in euthymic manic-depressive patients," *Journal of Psychiatric Research*, vol. 30, no. 5, pp. 353–357, 1996.

[25] Y. Osher, E. Lefkifker, and M. Kotler, "Low persistence in euthymic manic-depressive patients: a replication," *Journal of Affective Disorders*, vol. 53, no. 1, pp. 87–90, 1999.

[26] R. Tillman, B. Geller, J. L. Craney et al., "Temperament and character factors in a prepubertal and early adolescent bipolar disorder phenotype compared to attention deficit hyperactive and normal controls," *Journal of Child and Adolescent Psychopharmacology*, vol. 13, no. 4, pp. 531–543, 2003.

[27] A. Josefsson, C. Larsson, G. Sydsjö, and P.-O. Nylander, "Temperament and character in women with postpartum depression," *Archives of Women's Mental Health*, vol. 10, no. 1, pp. 3–7, 2007.

[28] T. Kitamura, S. Shima, M. Sugawara, and M. A. Toda, "Clinical and psychosocial correlates of antenatal depression: a review," *Psychotherapy and Psychosomatics*, vol. 65, no. 3, pp. 117–123, 1996.

[29] B. M. Y. Leung and B. J. Kaplan, "rinatal depression: prevalence, risks, and the nutrition link—a review of the literature," *Journal of the American Dietetic Association*, vol. 109, no. 9, pp. 1566–1575, 2009.

[30] R. Bunevicius, L. Kusminskas, A. Bunevicius, R. J. Nadisauskiene, K. Jureniene, and V. J. M. Pop, "Psychosocial risk factors for depression during pregnancy," *Acta Obstetricia et Gynecologica Scandinavica*, vol. 88, no. 5, pp. 599–605, 2009.

[31] A. M. Wangel, B. Schei, and E. L. Ryding, "Mental health status in pregnancy among native and non-native Swedish-speaking women: a Bidens study," *Acta Obstetricia et Gynecologica Scandinavica*, vol. 91, no. 12, pp. 1395–1401, 2012.

[32] S. Grigoriadis, E. H. VonderPorten, L. Mamisashvili et al., "The impact of maternal depression during pregnancy on perinatal outcomes: a systematic review and meta-analysis," *The Journal of Clinical Psychiatry*, vol. 74, no. 4, pp. 321–341, 2013.

[33] N. K. Grote, J. A. Bridge, A. R. Gavin, J. L. Melville, S. Iyengar, and W. J. Katon, "A meta-analysis of depression during pregnancy and the risk of preterm birth, low birth weight, and intrauterine growth restriction," *Archives of General Psychiatry*, vol. 67, no. 10, pp. 1012–1024, 2010.

[34] M. A. Byrn and S. Penckofer, "Antenatal depression and gestational diabetes: a review of maternal and fetal outcomes," *Nursing for Women's Health*, vol. 17, pp. 22–33, 2013.

[35] T. Kitamura, K. Yoshida, T. Okano et al., "Multicentre prospective study of perinatal depression in Japan: incidence and correlates of antenatal and postnatal depression," *Archives of Women's Mental Health*, vol. 9, no. 3, pp. 121–130, 2006.

[36] E. Andriola, M. di Trani, A. Grimaldi, and R. Donfrancesco, "The relationship between personality and depression in expectant parents," *Depression Research and Treatment*, vol. 2011, Article ID 356428, 5 pages, 2011.

[37] J. L. Cox, J. M. Holden, and R. Sagovsky, "Detection of postnatal depression. Development of the 10-item Edinburgh Postnatal Depression Scale," *British Journal of Psychiatry*, vol. 150, pp. 782–786, 1987.

[38] T. Okano, M. Murata, F. Masuji et al., "Validation and reliability of Japanese version of EPDS (Edinburgh Postnatal Depression Scale)," *Archives of Psychiatric Diagnostics and Clinical Evaluation*, vol. 7, pp. 525–533, 1996 (Japanese).

[39] N. Kijima, R. Saito, M. Takeuchi et al., "Cloninger's seven-factor model of temperament and character and Japanese version of Temperament and Character Inventory (TCI)," *Archives of Psychiatric Diagnostics and Clinical Evaluation*, vol. 7, pp. 379–399, 1996 (Japanese).

[40] N. Kijima, E. Tanaka, N. Suzuki, H. Higuchi, and T. Kitamura, "Reliability and validity of the Japanese version of the temperament and character inventory," *Psychological Reports*, vol. 86, no. 3, pp. 1050–1058, 2000.

[41] M. Takeuchi, H. Miyaoka, A. Tomoda, M. Suzuki, X. Lu, and T. Kitamura, "Validity and reliability of the Japanese version of the Temperament and Character Inventory: a study of university and college students," *Comprehensive Psychiatry*, vol. 52, no. 1, pp. 109–117, 2011.

[42] J. A. Harley, J. E. Wells, C. M. A. Frampton, and P. R. Joyce, "Bipolar disorder and the TCI: higher self-transcendence in bipolar disorder compared to major depression," *Depression Research and Treatment*, vol. 2011, Article ID 529638, 6 pages, 2011.

[43] C. Maggini, P. Ampollini, C. Marchesi, S. Gariboldi, and C. R. Cloninger, "Relationships between tridimensional personality questionnaire dimensions and DSM-III-R personality traits in Italian Adolescents," *Comprehensive Psychiatry*, vol. 41, no. 6, pp. 426–431, 2000.

[44] M. Zimmerman and W. Coryell, "DSM-III personality disorder diagnoses in a nonpatient sample. Demographic correlates and comorbidity," *Archives of General Psychiatry*, vol. 46, no. 8, pp. 682–689, 1989.

[45] F. Neziroglu, R. Anemone, and J. A. Yaryura-Tobias, "Onset of obsessive-compulsive disorder in pregnancy," *American Journal of Psychiatry*, vol. 149, no. 7, pp. 947–950, 1992.

[46] S. L. Brown, D. M. Svrakic, T. R. Przybeck, and C. R. Cloninger, "The relationship of personality to mood and anxiety states: a dimensional approach," *Journal of Psychiatric Research*, vol. 26, no. 3, pp. 197–211, 1992.

[47] R. Klein, *Principles and Practice of Structural Equation Modeling*, Guilford Press, New York, NY, USA, 2nd edition, 2005.

[48] T. Kitamura, S. Fujihara, N. Iwata, A. Tomoda, and N. Kawakami, "Epidemiology of psychiatric disorders in Japan," in *Images in Psychiatry: Japan*, Y. Nakane and M. Radford, Eds., pp. 37–46, NHA Communications, World Psychiatric Association, Paris, France, 1999.

12

Does Personality Predict Depression and Use of an Internet-Based Intervention for Depression among Adolescents?

Hans Christian B. Vangberg, Kjersti R. Lillevoll, Knut Waterloo, and Martin Eisemann

Department of Psychology, University of Tromsø, 9037 Tromsø, Norway

Correspondence should be addressed to Hans Christian B. Vangberg, hans.christian.vangberg@uit.no

Academic Editor: Toshinori Kitamura

Background. Focus upon depression and prevention of its occurrence among adolescents is increasing. Novel ways of dealing with this serious problem have become available especially by means of internet-based prevention and treatment programs of depression and anxiety. The use of Internet-based intervention programs among adolescents has revealed some difficulties in implementation that need to be further elucidated. The aim of this study is to investigate the association between personality and adolescent depression and the characteristics of users of an Internet-based intervention program. *Method.* The Junior Temperament and Character Inventory (JTCI), the General Self-Efficacy scale (GSE) and the Centre for Epidemiological Studies-Depression scale (CES-D) have been administered to a sample ($n = 1234$) of Norwegian senior high-school students. *Results.* Multiple regression analysis revealed associations between depression and gender, and several JTCI domains and facets. In line with previous findings in adults, high Harm Avoidance and low Self-Directedness emerged as the strongest predictors of adolescent depressive symptoms. Further, in logistic regression analysis with the covariates JTCI, GSE and CES-D, the only significant variables predicting use/non-use were the CES-D and the temperament domain Reward Dependence. *Conclusion.* The results in this study revealed level of depressive symptoms as the strongest predictor of the use of the Internet based intervention and that personality might provide useful information about the users.

1. Introduction

The prevalence of depression in childhood is low, whereas adolescence is a period of life characterized by a substantial vulnerability to depression [1]. Accordingly, adolescent depression is highly prevalent [2], with a considerable risk of recurrence and is often followed by poor psychosocial functioning and scholastic outcome [3].

Factors affecting development and predisposition to depression are numerous [4]. Grant and colleagues [5] point to the importance of stressful negative life events in understanding the development of depression, while others [6] indicate the importance of genetic factors. Interpersonal vulnerabilities have also been investigated for significant factors that can contribute in the explanation of adolescent depression [4]. Cognitive vulnerability concerns mostly about how an individual perceives, interprets, and reasons about experiences and relationships. Cognitive factors receiving most attention are negative inferential styles [7], dysfunctional attitudes [8], tendencies towards rumination [9], and self-criticism [10]. Based on various vulnerabilities, Hankin [4] suggested a multifactorial approach to the study of depression.

There is increasing evidence that psychiatric disorders have specific associations with underlying temperament and character traits among children and adolescents [11–13]. The interrelationships between personality, depression and anxiety have been studied over the last decades in adult populations [14–22], and several personality traits have been identified affecting mood disorders, such as neuroticism [23–25], tendencies towards rumination [25], immature personality styles, and personality disorders [26, 27].

A model to assess temperament and character to describe underlying biogenic structures of personality had been developed by Cloninger et al. [28] resulting in the Temperament Character Inventory (TCI) that measures personality by two higher-order dimensions: temperament and character. Temperament varies on an individual basis and reflects the fundamental organization of brain systems responsible for activating, maintaining and/or inhibiting behavior in response to stimuli [14, 28]. The four derived temperament dimensions are *novelty seeking (NS), harm avoidance (HA), reward dependence (RD),* and *persistence (P)*. On the other hand, character refers to self-concepts and individual differences in goals and values, which in turn affect voluntary choices and intentions. According to Cloninger [29], character is moderately influenced by sociocultural learning and matures gradually throughout life. The three described character dimensions are *self-directedness (SD), cooperativeness (C),* and *self-transcendence (ST)*. These aspects of personality interact to allow for adaptation to life experiences and also influence the vulnerability for emotional and behavioral disorders.

Scores on the TCI have shown to be variant between depressed individuals and nondepressed [28]. Elevated scores on HA and lower scores on SD and C have often been found associated with depression or depressed mood in adult populations [30–32].

Since the adult version of the TCI might be unsuitable for use in an adolescent population, Luby et al. [33] developed the Junior Temperament and Character Inventory (JTCI).

So far, research on the relationship between JTCI and depression among adolescents is sparse. A few studies have reported associations between JTCI and psychopathology in adolescents [34–38]. Schmeck and colleagues [34] reported a negative correlation between several forms of psychopathology, including anxiety and depression and SD. Others [37] have found high scores on NS and HA, while low on RD and P among dysregulated children. Elevated levels of HA have also been reported among depressed adolescents [36].

Different relationships between temperament and character traits and mental health are suggested to exist in adolescents and adults [39]. Therefore, more research is needed to improve our understanding of the relationship between adolescent depression and personality.

One might expect that many depressed adolescent individuals will never formally seek help or contact with health services [40], rendering many with an unmet need for treatment [41]. This is a strong argument for finding novel approaches to reach adolescents struggling with mental health problems. Internet-based interventions like computerized cognitive behavior therapy (cCBT) is one way to reach a broader spectrum of troubled youth. One of these interventions is the MoodGYM, which is a self-help program developed at the Australian National University based on the principles of cognitive behavioral therapy (CBT) [42–44]. It consists of a set of five training modules aimed at increasing the users' knowledge about their symptoms, negative automatic thoughts, dysfunctional attitudes, emotions, and coping strategies with regard to stress and interpersonal relationships. Furthermore, the MoodGYM comprises a personal workbook that records and updates the user's responses and a feedback evaluation form.

The use of internet-based interventions among adolescent samples has revealed some difficulties in implementation [45]. Motivating young people to seek help for mental health problems also emerged as a challenge. One reason for low adherence might be that cCBT applications allow the users to enter and leave a treatment program and thus resulting in a lack of commitment to the treatment. Determining those using and benefiting from Internet interventions is an important issue. The identification of their characteristics could be useful for increasing adherence and for the prediction of treatment outcome [46–48]. Several hypotheses about possible relationship between different JTCI domains the use of MoodGYM can be formulated. It can be expected that high scores on SD and CO, and low scores on RD predict more use due to the nature of these domains [28]. It is reasonable to assume that a high score on SD to some degree reflects the internal drive and goal-orientation necessary to engage in a self-directed program such as MoodGYM. High scorers on CO might be more motivated to fulfill their commitment as participants in a research project and therefore be more likely to make use of the intervention. Individuals scoring low on RD are characterized as practical, socially distant, and independent. They might find this sort of intervention appealing because of the practical, socially independent nature of Internet-based interventions.

The concept of self-efficacy refers to a person's "conviction, that one can successfully execute the behavior required to produce the outcomes" (Bandura, 1977, p. 193 [49]) and thus is related to motivation and behavior. Self-efficacy has been found to be a significant predictor of motivation for learning-directed behavior [50]. With regards to help-seeking behavior in adolescents, Barker et al. [51] claim that research evidence on the influence of self-efficacy is conflicting. Nonetheless, it might represent a factor promoting help-seeking behavior and affecting the intervention outcome in mental health prevention programs. Contrary to their hypothesis, Pössel et al. [52] found students low on self-efficacy to benefit more from a depression prevention program. The current study will investigate whether self-efficacy can predict self-directed use of MoodGYM when presented to students in a school-based setting.

Being able to depict the role of personality and adolescent depression in this context it is important to understand fundamental and underlying mechanisms in order to get a better understanding and treatment of it. If researchers can understand what underlies the development and vulnerability towards depression among youth, treatment can be modified to better target key factors. Internet-based interventions for depression are, compared to traditional face-to-face treatment, easy to present and to implement.

2. Aims

The aims of the current study are twofold: firstly, to assess the predictive power of gender, age, and personality aspects

(Junior Temperament Character Inventory, JTCI) for the severity of depressive symptoms (Centre for Epidemiologic Studies Depression scale, CES-D), and secondly, to explore the characteristics of users versus nonusers of an Internet-based intervention program (MoodGYM) using the variables JTCI (domain and facets), GSE, gender, and CES-D.

3. Method

3.1. Procedure. Participants were recruited from four senior high schools in Troms County in Northern Norway as a part of a larger study with a four-arm randomized controlled trial design with repeated measures (pre- and post- intervention). Members of our research group visited the four participating schools for recruiting the participants. The recruitment process involved the delivery of a short informative lecture about mental health in general and a presentation of the MoodGYM program, followed by an invitation to the students to participate in the study. Students volunteering to participate signed a written consent form. If the students did not want to participate in the MoodGYM trial, they had the choice of participating in the preintervention survey only. As an incentive for becoming a participant, a lottery drawing was announced. There was an additional lottery for those participating in the MoodGYM trial.

The data collection for the current study was part of the preintervention survey, which was conducted by computer in a classroom setting on the day of the information session. The students without access to a computer completed a paper version.

Students willing to participate in the MoodGYM trial received username and passwords on e-mail within a week of recruitment for registration in the program. The use of MoodGYM was self-directed, without personal followup, and no time was allocated during school hours. Within 6–8 weeks, the research team returned to collect postintervention data.

The regional medical research ethics committee approved the study. Data of use of MoodGYM were securely stored on a server at the Australian National University and were retrieved for information about use/nonuse for participants in the trial.

3.2. MoodGYM. MoodGYM is an internet-based self-help program based on the principles of cognitive behavior therapy (CBT). It has been developed at the Centre for Mental Health Research at the Australian National University in Canberra. The aim of this program is prevention and treatment of depression by means of five modules and a personal workbook [53]. Each module has a specific theme and is designed for increasing the users' knowledge about their own symptoms, negative automatic thoughts, dysfunctional attitudes, emotions, and coping strategies with regard to stress and interpersonal relationships. Each module takes between 30–45 minutes to be completed.

4. Outcome Measures

4.1. Depressive Symptoms. Level of depression was measured using a Norwegian version of the Centre for Epidemiologic Studies-Depression scale (CES-D) [54], developed to measure depressive symptomatology in the general population. This 20-item self-report scale yields scores ranging from 0 to 60 (scores given from 0 to 3), with a score of 16 or above indicating a clinical level of depression. However, we used a cutoff score above 24 was used which is assumed to detect more accurately clinically cases among adolescents [55, 56]. The CES-Ds Cronbach alpha in the current study was .884.

4.2. Self-Efficacy (GSE). Self-efficacy was measured using the Norwegian version of the General Self-Efficacy Scale (GSE) [57]. The scale consists of 10 items and assesses the ability of an individual's beliefs in handling difficult situations in an appropriate way. Responses are reported on a four-point scale ranging from "not at all true" to "exactly true." Its Cronbach alpha in the current study was .882.

4.3. Junior Temperament and Character Inventory (JTCI). The JTCI is a self-administered questionnaire containing 106 items scored on a five-point scale (1 to 5) ranging from "totally agree" to "totally disagree." The Norwegian version of the JTCI was developed according to established guidelines following several steps based on the German version of the JTCI [58]. This procedure included translation, backtranslation by independent native speakers, and linguistic revision of items [59].

The Cronbach alpha for the current study were for NS = .795, HA = .846, RD = .792, P = .793, SD = .846, CO = .803, and for ST = .796.

4.4. Demographics. Demographic parameters were gender, age, and grade in high school.

4.5. Statistical Analysis. All statistical analyses were performed with the SPSS version 18 and 19 for Macintosh. To identify unique JTCI correlates and predictors of depressed mood, hierarchical regression methods were used. For the domain-level analysis, all JTCI domains were subjected to forced entry in the same analytic step and their unique contributions simultaneously evaluated. In the facet-level analysis all of the 29 facets scales were entered in the same model using forward entry.

Bonferroni adjustment was applied to the critical α level and for significance tests involving the seven domains and the 29 facet scores on the JTCI. This adjustment resulted in a critical α level of .0071 (.05/7) and .0017 (.05/29), respectively.

Direct logistic regression was run to assess the impact of nine independent variables (CES-D, GSE, and the JTCI subscales) on the likelihood that participants in the study would use MoodGYM or not.

Another direct logistic regression assessed in more detail the impact of JTCI facets on users versus nonusers of MoodGYM. The model contained thirty-two independent

TABLE 1: Mean scores and standard deviations for male and female (n = 1239).

	Male (n = 604)		Female (n = 635)	
	$\bar{x}$	SD	$\bar{x}$	SD
CES-D	10.996	8.334	15.776	9.845
GSE	29.842	5.119	29.001	4.234
NS	47.200	8.433	46.106	7.877
HA	36.480	8.473	40.962	8.832
RD	56.551	9.201	60.243	9.092
P	47.124	7.500	45.847	7.591
SD	51.940	9.408	49.230	9.341
CO	62.810	8.721	65.984	7.984
ST	26.204	7.098	28.224	7.256

CES-D: Centre for Epidemiological studies-Depression Scale; JTCI: The Junior Temperament and Character Inventory; NS: novelty seeking; HA: harm avoidance; RD: reward dependence; P: persistence; SD: self-directedness; CO: cooperativeness; ST: self-transcendence.

variables (CES-D, GSE, gender, and the twenty-nine JTCI facets).

5. Results

This study was conducted on adolescents from Norwegian senior high schools. The sample comprised 604 males (48.7%) and 635 females (51.3%) with a mean age of 16.8 (range = 15–20). Women scored significantly higher on CES-D than men $F(1, 1233) = 84.32$, $P < .001$ with a mean of 15.78 and 11.00, respectively (Table 1). The total mean score for CES-D in this sample was 13.45. The percentage scoring above the cut-off of 16 was 30.7%, whereas the percentage above the cut-off of 24 was 14.3%.

When CES-D scores were correlated with the seven JTCI domains all coefficients emerged as significant (Table 2). HA ($r = .56$, $P < .01$) and SD ($r = -.64$, $P < .01$) yielded the strongest association with depressed mood. Somewhat lower significant associations were obtained for $P(r = -.34, P < .01)$, while small ones emerged with NS ($r = .09$, $P < .01$), RD ($r = -.14$, $P < .01$), CO ($r = -.12$, $P < .01$), and ST ($r = .16$, $P < .01$).

5.1. Regression. A hierarchical multiple regression analysis was applied to assess the power of gender, age and personality to predict depressive symptoms (CES-D). A preliminary analysis was conducted to disclose any violations of assumptions. Gender and age were entered into step one, explaining 6.5% of the variance in depression (Table 3). After the entry of the JTCI at step two, the total variance explained totaled to 46.3%, $F(9, 1221) = 118.88$, $P < .001$. The JTCI explained an additional 40.2% of the variance in depression, R square change = .402, F change (7,1221) = 131.42, $P < .001$. In the final model the following measures were statistically significant: gender ($P < .001$, beta = .144), and after Bonferroni correction: NS ($P < .001$, beta = .109), HA ($P < .001$, beta = .181), RD ($P < .001$, beta = −.089), SD ($P < .001$, beta = −.487), and CO ($P < .001$, beta = .110).

5.2. Facet-Level Analyses. A more detailed analysis was performed on facet level of the JTCI domains to check for their ability to predict depression. For this analysis, facet scale scores were entered into the hierarchical regression analysis at the second step in the model using forward selection after age and gender were forcedly entered in step one. Nine of the 29 facet scales emerged as unique and significant predictors. Together with gender and age, they explained 52.8% of the variance in CES-D scores (Table 4). Gender was found significant ($P < .001$). Significant facets, after Bonferroni correction, were SD4 (self-striving) (beta = .24, $t = -8.06$, $P < .001$), SD2 (lack of goal direction) (beta = −.277, $t = -10.72$, $P < .001$), HA1 (anticipatory worry) (beta = .16, $t = 5.56$, $P < .001$), and RD4 (independence) (beta = −.80, $t = -3.76$, $P < .001$).

5.3. Logistic Regression of the JTCI Domains. Direct logistic regression was performed to assess the impact of a number of factors on the likelihood that participants in the study would use MoodGYM or not. The number of users in this sample was not optimal, with only 51 (7.3%) participants actually logging in and using the MoodGYM program.

The model contained ten independent variables (CES-D, GSE, gender, and the JTCI subscales). The overall model was significant $\chi^2(10, n = 691) = 20.71$, $P < .05$, indicating that the model was able to distinguish between participants that used and those who did not use MoodGYM. The model as a whole explained between 3.2 (Cox and Snell R square) and 7.9% (Nagelkerke R square) of the variance in use/nonuse and correctly classified 45.2% (an improvement of 37.8% from the model where only the constant is included) of the cases. Further, the Hosmer and Lemeshow test has a significance level of .584, thus indicating that the model prediction does not significantly differ from the observed. The Wald criterion showed (Table 5) that only two of the independent variables made a unique statistically significant contribution to the model (CES-D and the subscale RD on the JTCI). Gender, GSE, and six of the JTCI domains were not significant predictors. The strongest predictor of use/nonuse was CES-D, yielding an odds ratio of 1.05 ($P < .05$), and indicated that those who reported a higher level on CES-D were more likely to use MoodGYM than those who scored lower on CES-D, controlling for all the other factors in the model. This means that for every point a participant increased on the CES-D score, the odds of using MoodGYM increased with 5% (O.R. = 1.05). The odds ratio of .953 for RD (reward dependence) indicates that for every additional point on RD the odds were 4.7% less for the participants to use MoodGYM, controlling for other factors in the model.

5.4. Logistic Regression on the JTCI Facets. To investigate in more detail the traits of MoodGYM users, a direct logistic regression was performed to assess the impact of the JTCI facets on the likelihood that participants in the study would use MoodGYM or not.

The model contained thirty-two independent variables (CES-D, GSE, gender, and the twenty-nine facets of the JTCI). The overall model was significant $\chi^2(31, n = 691)$

TABLE 2: Correlation table of the variables in the hierarchical multiple regression ($n = 1231$).

	CES-D	Age	NS	HA	RD	P	SD	CO	ST
CES-D	—	.026	.093**	.559**	−.140**	−.339**	−.642**	−.115**	.155**
Age		—	−.037*	−.007	−.026	.018	.025	.079**	−.031
NS			—	−.059*	.216**	−.210**	−.109**	−.253**	.208**
HA				—	−.178**	−.427**	−.711**	−.153**	.261**
RD					—	.204**	.231**	.450**	.182**
P						—	.494**	.478**	−.001
SD							—	.305**	−.183**
CO								—	.111**
ST									—

CES-D: Center for Epidemiological studies-Depression Scale; JTCI: The Junior Temperament and Character Inventory; NS: novelty seeking; HA: harm avoidance; RD: reward dependence; P: persistence; SD: self-directedness; CO: cooperativeness; ST: self-transcendence. **$P < .01$, *$P < .05$.

TABLE 3: Hierarchical multiple regression analysis of CES-D as a function of JTCI domain scales after controlling for gender and age ($n = 1230$).

Correlates	Standardized beta coefficients	
	Model 1	Model 2
Gender	.254***	.144***
Age	.032	.036
NS		.109****
HA		.181****
RD		−.089****
P		−.023
SD		−.487****
CO		.110****
ST		−.017
$_{\text{Adj}}R^2$	.064	.463
ΔF	42.76*	131.42*
ΔR^2	.065	.402

CES-D: Centre for Epidemiological studies-Depression Scale; JTCI: The Junior Temperament and Character Inventory; NS: Novelty Seeking; HA: Harm Avoidance; RD: Reward Dependence; P: Persistence; SD: Self-Directedness; CO: Cooperativeness; ST: Self-Transcendence. For age, gender, and the evaluation of the ΔF statistic: ***$P \leq .001$, and **$P < .01$, and *$P < .05$. For the JTCI domains where Bonferroni adjustments were made on the critical α, ****$P < .0071$.

$= 59.92$, $P \leq .001$, indicating its ability to distinguish between participants who used versus not used MoodGYM. The model as a whole explained between 8.3 (Cox and Snell R square) and 20.3% (Nagelkerke R square) of the variance in use/nonuse and correctly classified 60.9% (an improvement of 53.5% from the model where only the constant is included) of the cases. Furthermore, the Hosmer and Lemeshow test yielded a significance level of .241, thus indicating that the model prediction does not significantly differ from the observed. The Wald criterion demonstrated (Table 6) that seven of the independent variables made a unique statistically significant contribution to the model (CES-D, gender, the JTCI facets ns4, ha1, ha4, rd4, p4, and sd3). The strongest predictor of use/nonuse was gender, yielding an odds ratio of 2.65 ($P < .05$) indicating that female students have a 26.5% increase of odds for using MoodGYM. Findings are reported in Table 6.

6. Discussion

The findings from this study underline the potential importance of personality in adolescent depression. The JTCI factors harm avoidance and self-directedness, yielded the strongest associations. In the regression model, JTCI domains explained additional 40.2% of the variance in CES-D after having controlled for age and gender. NS, HA, RD, SD, and CO emerged as significant correlates in explaining depression among adolescents, which is slightly different from an adult population [15, 16, 23]. Cloninger et al. [28] have described individuals with high scores on the temperament domain NS as exploratory and curious, impulsive and disordered while high scores on HA are associated with being worried and pessimistic, fearful, shy, and fatigable. Further, low scores on RD reflect a cold personality, detached and independent from others. Another association was found between CES-D and the character domains of SD and CO. Scoring low on SD is found to be associated with being immature and fragile, blaming, unreliable, ineffective, and having problems working towards long-term goals. Individuals scoring high on CO are described as socially tolerant, empathic, compassionate, and ethical. Studies report a significant negative correlation between depression and CO [15, 16, 23], which is confirmed in the current study. However, when included in the final regression model and considered together with other domains the negative correlation between CES-D and CO turns into a positive beta coefficient. This suppression effect seems to be due to variations of positive and negative correlations between the other personality domains and CES-D, but leaving the true direction of the association between CO and CES-D for this sample in a positive direction. As shown above, the strongest correlations toward CES-D occurred between SD and HA, which is in line with previous findings [15, 23]. Cloninger et al. [15] found that HA functions as a marker for vulnerability to depression, while SD was a marker of a central protective function towards depression. The current findings exhibit depressed individuals as

Table 4: Hierarchical multiple regression analysis of CES-D scores as a function of JTCI facet scales after controlling for age and gender (n = 1236).

Correlates	Standardized beta coefficients											
	Model 1	Model 2	Model 3	Model 4	Model 5	Model 6	Model 7	Model 8	Model 9	Model 10	Model 11	Model 12
Gender	.254***	.112***	.119***	.087***	.094***	.115***	.109***	.101***	.112***	.115***	.115***	.115***
Age	.032	.044*	.021	.025	.024	.023	.018	.015	.020	.020	.020	.014
SD4: self-striving		−.608***	−.427****	−.310****	−.285****	−.273****	−.272****	−.259****	−.258****	−.241****	−.240****	−.243****
SD2: lack of goal direction			−.306****	−.298****	−.296****	−.285****	−.297****	−.291****	−.283****	−.278****	−.268****	−.277****
HA1: anticipatory worry				.214****	.189****	.202****	.196****	.191****	.193****	.167****	.164****	.157****
ST1: self-forgetfulness					.099****	.092****	.087****	.080****	.068	.061	.068	.066
RD4: independence						−.080****	−.088****	−.089****	−.086****	−.089****	−.084****	−.080****
CO2: empathy							.057	.071	.067	.069	.083****	.061
HA4: fatigability								.065	.065	.061	.056	.063
NS4: disorderliness									.048	.056	.058	.060
HA2 fear of uncertainty										.067	.077	.089
ST2: transpersonal identification											−.055	−.054
SD3: resourcefulness												.057
$_{Adj}R^2$	.064	.413	.474	.502	.509	.514	.517	.520	.552	.524	.526	.528
ΔF	42.76	732.00	143.05	68.93	19.81	14.41	7.64	8.61	4.91	6.78	6.38	5.71
ΔR^2	.065	.349	.061	.028	.008	.006	.003	.003	.002	.002	.002	.002

CES-D: Centre for Epidemiological studies-Depression Scale; JTCI: The Junior Temperament and Character Inventory. For age, Gender, and the evaluation of ΔF statistics, $^{***}P < .001$; $^{**}P < .01$; $^{*}P < .05$. For the JTCI facets Bonferroni adjustments were made on the critical α level, $^{****}P < .0017$.

TABLE 5: Logistic regression predicting the likelihood of using MoodGYM (n = 691).

	B	SE	Wald	df	P	Odds ratio	95% CI for odds ratio	
							Lower	Upper
CES-D	.046	.019	5.67	1	.017*	1.047	1.008	1.087
GSE	−.039	.033	1.39	1	.239	.962	.901	1.026
Gender	.477	.346	1.90	1	.168	1.611	.817	3.175
Novelty seeking	−.019	.022	.780	1	.377	.981	.940	1.024
Harm avoidance	−.047	.025	3.57	1	.059	.954	.909	1.002
Reward dependence	−.048	.018	6.87	1	.009*	.953	.920	.988
Persistence	.014	.025	.33	1	.564	1.015	.966	1.066
Self directedness	.021	.026	.64	1	.425	1.021	.970	1.074
Cooperativeness	.017	.023	.54	1	.461	1.017	.973	1.063
Self-transcendence	.016	.022	.55	1	.460	1.016	.974	1.060
Constant	−.214	2.654	.01	1	.936	.807		

Significant $P < .05$*.

anxiety-prone and immature. The reason for the positive relationship between CO and depression might be due to being very empathic and considerate, thus experiencing an emotionally oversensitivity, leading to lowered mood states.

The facet level analysis reveals a more detailed picture of traits affecting depressed mood. The second regression model shows that the JTCI facets explain 46.4% of the variance in CES-D. The following facets emerged as significant associations with CES-D: SD4 (self-striving), SD2 (lack of goal direction), HA1 (anticipatory worry), and RD4 (independence). Cloninger et al. [28] described individuals low on SD4 as self-striving people, never accepting nor enjoying their actual mental and physical features. They also have severe problems adjusting perceptions of themselves when corrected by the environment. High scores on SD2 characterize persons having difficulties in finding direction and meaning in their lives and instead react to current situations and immediate needs. Scoring high in HA1 indicates two types of behavioral tendencies. Such individuals are pessimistic, expecting failure and harm, especially in adverse and unfamiliar situations. Further, these individuals have difficulties in forgetting embarrassment and a tendency to ruminate about stressful situations for long periods of time. And finally, scoring low on RD4 describes individuals who are independent and accordingly do not seek emotional support and approval from the environment. They appear insensitive to social pressure, criticism and rarely give in to the wishes of others.

The present study was conducted among a younger sample that might affect which domains and facets emerge as specific. The results from the facet level analysis reflect adolescents with elevated depressive symptoms as individuals lacking the ability to work towards long-term goals, which in addition, worry and expect the worse in situations even when there is support and assurance available. They resemble withdrawn, independent individuals, who apparently are insensitive to social pressure, which at first glance might display them with a strong personality, not vulnerable to depression. This finding might be a combined effect of the other facets and seems like a natural response when individuals struggle with their self-image at the same time as they worry and expect negative outcomes and do not cope adequately with embarrassment. A subject with such a personality will most likely not express true feelings.

The challenges concerning adherence of online CBT users deserve further investigations [46, 47]. Describing the users of Internet interventions will probably increase the ability to predict adherence and intervention outcome. The results from the logistic regression used in the current study revealed that the only predictors for the use of MoodGYM were depression and RD (reward dependence). This is both in accordance with findings of some studies [47] but also contrasts others [48]. The indication that higher scores on CES-D predictive use of this online intervention tells us that presenting this kind of intervention to the population will most likely facilitate use among individuals with elevated symptoms on depression. This highlights the importance of finding effective strategies to maintain adherence among those who decide to use the program. Another significant predictor was reward dependence. Cloninger et al. [28] described individuals scoring low on this temperament trait as cold, socially insensitive, preferring to keep distance to others, and having objective views that are not romanticized by a desire to please others or wishful thinking. A possible explanation for this domain being a significant predictor for use might be that these individuals prefer a self-help approach to deal with their problems, rather than seek help from others.

In order to give a more detailed description of the users of MoodGYM, a second logistic regression was done including the same predictors, but based on the JTCI facets. Here, gender was the strongest predictor, indicating that female students are more likely than male students to use this kind of intervention. The level of depressive symptomatology also predicted its use, reflecting that depressed individuals might actively use this kind of program. The facet sd3 (resourcefulness) also emerged as a strong predictor of use, indicating that the users are resourceful and effective

Table 6: Logistic regression predicting the likelihood of using MoodGYM ($n = 691$).

	B	SE	Wald	df	P	odds ratio	95% CI for odds ratio Lower	Upper
CESD	.052	.023	5.01	1	.025*	1.054	1.007	1.103
GSE	−.057	.038	2.22	1	.136	.945	.877	1.018
Gender	.973	.415	5.50	1	.019*	2.646	1.173	5.969
ns1 (exploratory excitability)	.027	.071	.14	1	.704	1.027	.894	1.181
ns2 (impulsiveness)	.000	.072	.00	1	.999	1.000	.869	1.151
ns3 (extravagance)	.037	.067	.31	1	.580	1.038	.911	1.182
ns4 (regimentation)	−.154	.069	4.98	1	.026*	.858	.749	.981
ha1(anticipatory worry)	−.163	.082	3.91	1	.048*	.850	.723	.999
ha2 (fear of uncertainty)	−.017	.068	.06	1	.804	.983	.861	1.123
ha3 (shyness with strangers)	.035	.081	.18	1	.671	1.035	.883	1.214
ha4 (vigor)	−.153	.075	4.22	1	.040*	.858	.741	.993
rd1 (sentimentality)	−.082	.064	1.65	1	.198	.921	.813	1.044
rd2 (openness to warm communication)	.049	.045	1.16	1	.281	1.050	.961	1.147
rd3 (detachment)	−.152	.091	2.80	1	.094	.859	.719	1.026
rd4 (independence)	−.124	.063	3.92	1	.048*	.883	.781	.999
p1 (eagerness to effort)	−.047	.082	.33	1	.563	.954	.812	1.120
p2 (work hardened)	.090	.081	1.26	1	.263	1.094	.935	1.282
p3 (ambitious)	.004	.071	.00	1	.958	1.004	.874	1.153
p4 (perfectionist)	−.230	.111	4.30	1	.038*	.795	.640	.987
sd1 (blaming)	−.034	.076	.20	1	.653	.966	.833	1.121
sd2 (purposefulness)	.003	.089	.00	1	.974	1.003	.842	1.194
sd3 (resourcefulness)	.373	.113	10.87	1	.001**	1.453	1.163	1.814
sd4 (self-striving)	−.018	.059	.09	1	.764	.982	.875	1.103
co1 (social acceptance)	.087	.092	.90	1	.342	1.091	.912	1.305
co2 (social disinterest)	−.152	.091	2.77	1	.096	.859	.719	1.027
co3 (helpfulness)	.111	.089	1.56	1	.212	1.117	.938	1.331
co4 (compassion)	.075	.097	.60	1	.438	1.078	.892	1.303
co5 (self-serving advantage)	−.081	.081	.99	1	.320	.922	.786	1.082
st1 (self-forgetfulness)	.011	.065	.03	1	.865	1.011	.890	1.148
st2 (transpersonal identification)	.173	.089	3.79	1	.052	1.188	.999	1.414
st3 (rational materialism)	−.056	.051	1.21	1	.271	.945	.856	1.045
Constant	2.017	3.28	.38	1	.539	7.513	—	—

Significant $P < .05$* and $P \leq .001$.

individuals, focused on solving problems and are perceived by others as competent and productive. On the other hand, they score lower on p4 (pragmatic) [29], describing them as somewhat lazy underachieving individuals who can be seen as pragmatics accepting compromises easily [28]. Further, they obtain low scores on rd4 (independence) implying that they rarely seek emotional support from others, rather impress others as self-sufficient and they are not reacting to social pressure. Another significant facet, ha1 (anticipatory worry) describes individuals as worried and anticipating harm. Ha4 (vigor) also emerged as specific. Low scores on this facet depict individuals as energetic and dynamic, with less need for rest, who rarely have to push themselves. Further, ns4 (regimentation) emerged significant in predicting use, identifying individuals who tend to be organized, methodical, and systematic. They prefer activities with strict rules and are able to postpone gratification longer than most of us.

This gives a picture of the MoodGYM users as effective and strict rule-followers, working effectively in order to achieve goals, at the same time as they seem similar to independent individuals reluctant to take into account what others do or mean. These individuals' worry of failure might function as worry of failure might function as a facilitator towards goal-directed behavior, at the same time as it reflects their vulnerability to depression. They also seem to be like resourceful individuals who are underachieving, holding a pragmatic view upon what they are doing. These aspects, together with the level of depression symptoms and gender, moderately predict use of MoodGYM, indicating that there could exist other important factors that will better predict its use.

The assessment of the characteristics of internet-based intervention users is an intriguing aspect of online delivery healthcare research that needs further investigation. The fact that only a few students used the MoodGYM program might indicate that this kind of intervention is most appealing to and effective in individuals with specific characteristics. The delineated characteristics of MoodGYM users might aid us in the further development of internet-based programs, their implementation and last but not least facilitate uptake and adherence.

7. Limitations

Data collection occurred in a classroom environment, not ensuring sufficient privacy for the participants. Further, the effect sizes reported are small. Also the variables failed to explain a larger portion of the variance, indicating that definite conclusions of both predicting use/nonuse and depression cannot be drawn. A relatively small number of MoodGYM users (7.3%) also compromise the study. Further, the large sample size also raises concern about unreliable responses. To minimize the possible effect, repeated "data-washing" was made, and this effect is assumed to be minimal. Finally, this group of adolescents had not been specifically asked to take part in a treatment intervention, which may also affect the outcome and possibly the low rate of adherence to the intervention. Since this investigation represents part of a larger study on identifying and exploring different aspects of MoodGYM after its introduction in Norway, its results should be regarded as preliminary.

References

[1] B. L. Hankin, L. Y. Abramson, T. E. Moffitt, P. A. Silva, R. McGee, and K. E. Angell, "Development of depression from preadolescence to young adulthood: emerging gender differences in a 10-year longitudinal study," *Journal of Abnormal Psychology*, vol. 107, no. 1, pp. 128–140, 1998.

[2] J. L. Rushton, M. Forcier, and R. M. Schectman, "Epidemiology of depressive symptoms in the National Longitudinal Study of Adolescent Health," *Journal of the American Academy of Child & Adolescent Psychiatry*, vol. 41, no. 2, pp. 199–205, 2002.

[3] P. Cuijpers, P. Boluijt, and A. van Straten, "Screening of depression in adolescents through the Internet: sensitivity and specificity of two screening questionnaires," *European Child & Adolescent Psychiatry*, vol. 17, no. 1, pp. 32–38, 2008.

[4] B. L. Hankin, "Adolescent depression: description, causes, and interventions," *Epilepsy & Behavior*, vol. 8, no. 1, pp. 102–114, 2006.

[5] K. E. Grant, B. E. Compas, A. F. Stuhlmacher, A. E. Thurm, S. D. McMahon, and J. A. Halpert, "Stressors and child and adolescent psychopathology: moving from markers to mechanisms of risk. [review]," *Psychological Bulletin*, vol. 129, no. 3, pp. 447–466, 2003.

[6] W. R. Beardslee, E. M. Versage, and T. R. Gladstone, "Children of affectively Ill parents: a review of the past 10 years," *Journal of the American Academy of Child & Adolescent Psychiatry*, vol. 37, no. 11, pp. 1134–1141, 1998.

[7] L. Y. Abramson, L. B. Alloy, and G. I. Metalsky, "Hopelessness depression: a theory-based subtype of depression," *Psychological Review*, vol. 96, no. 2, pp. 358–372, 1989.

[8] A. Beck, N. Epstein, and R. Harrison, "Cognitions, attitudes and personality dimensions in depression," *British Journal of Cognitive Psychotherapy*, vol. 1, pp. 1–16, 1983.

[9] S. Nolen-Hoeksema and J. Morrow, "A prospective study of depression and posttraumatic stress symptoms after a natural disaster: The 1989 Loma Prieta Earthquake," *Journal of Personality and Social Psychology*, vol. 61, no. 1, pp. 115–121, 1991.

[10] S. J. Blatt and D. C. Zuroff, "Interpersonal relatedness and self-definition: two prototypes for depression," *Clinical Psychology Review*, vol. 12, no. 5, pp. 527–562, 1992.

[11] J. Csorba, E. Dinya, E. Ferencz, P. Steiner, G. Bertalan, and A. Zsadon, "Novelty seeking: difference between suicidal and non-suicidal Hungarian adolescent outpatients suffering from depression," *Journal of Affective Disorders*, vol. 120, no. 1–3, pp. 217–220, 2010.

[12] Z. Tamás, M. Kovacs, A. L. Gentzler et al., "The relations of temperament and emotion self-regulation with suicidal behaviors in a clinical sample of depressed children in Hungary," *Journal of Abnormal Child Psychology*, vol. 35, no. 4, pp. 640–652, 2007.

[13] C. E. Schwartz, N. Snidman, and J. Kagan, "Adolescent social anxiety as an outcome of inhibited temperament in childhood," *Journal of the American Academy of Child & Adolescent Psychiatry*, vol. 38, no. 8, pp. 1008–1015, 1999.

[14] C. R. Cloninger, "A unified biosocial theory of personality and its role in the development of anxiety states," *Psychiatric Developments*, vol. 4, no. 3, pp. 167–226, 1986.

[15] C. R. Cloninger, D. M. Svrakic, and T. R. Przybeck, "Can personality assessment predict future depression? A twelve-month follow-up of 631 subjects," *Journal of Affective Disorders*, vol. 92, no. 1, pp. 35–44, 2006.

[16] M. Hansenne, J. Reggers, E. Pinto, K. Kjiri, A. Ajamier, and M. Ansseau, "Temperament and character inventory (TCI) and depression," *Journal of Psychiatric Research*, vol. 33, no. 1, pp. 31–36, 1999.

[17] T. Matsudaira and T. Kitamura, "Personality traits as risk factors of depression and anxiety among Japanese students," *Journal of Clinical Psychology*, vol. 62, no. 1, pp. 97–109, 2006.

[18] H. Eysenck, "Personality and behaviour therapy," *Proceedings of the Royal Society of Medicine*, vol. 53, pp. 504–508, 1960.

[19] P. Boyce, G. Parker, B. Barnett, M. Cooney, and F. Smith, "Personality as a vulnerability factor to depression," *British Journal of Psychiatry*, vol. 159, pp. 106–114, 1991.

[20] K. S. Kendler, M. Gatz, C. O. Gardner, and N. L. Pedersen, "Personality and major depression: a Swedish longitudinal, population-based twin study," *Archives of General Psychiatry*, vol. 63, no. 10, pp. 1113–1120, 2006.

[21] R. T. Mulder, "Personality pathology and treatment outcome in major depression: a review," *American Journal of Psychiatry*, vol. 159, no. 3, pp. 359–371, 2002.

[22] M. Halvorsen, C. E. Wang, J. Richter et al., "Early maladaptive schemas, temperament and character traits in clinically depressed and previously depressed subjects," *Clinical Psychology and Psychotherapy*, vol. 16, no. 5, pp. 394–407, 2009.

[23] R. F. Farmer and J. R. Seeley, "Temperament and character predictors of depressed mood over a 4-year interval," *Depression and Anxiety*, vol. 26, no. 4, pp. 371–381, 2009.

[24] M. V. Christensen and L. V. Kessing, "Do personality traits predict first onset in depressive and bipolar disorder?" *Nordic Journal of Psychiatry*, vol. 60, no. 2, pp. 79–88, 2006.

[25] R. M. Hirschfeld, G. L. Klerman, P. Lavori, M. B. Keller, P. Griffith, and W. Coryell, "Premorbid personality assessments of first onset of major depression," *Archives of General Psychiatry*, vol. 46, no. 4, pp. 345–350, 1989.

[26] S. Nystrom and B. Lindegard, "Predisposition for mental syndromes: a study comparing predisposition for depression, neurasthenia and anxiety state," *Acta Psychiatrica Scandinavica*, vol. 51, no. 2, pp. 69–76, 1975.

[27] R. Farmer and R. O. Nelson-Gray, "Personality disorders and depression: hypothetical relations, empirical findings, and methodological considerations," *Clinical Psychology Review*, vol. 10, no. 4, pp. 453–476, 1990.

[28] C. R. Cloninger, T. R. Przybeck, D. M. Svakic, and R. D. Wetzel, *The Temperament and Character Inventory (TCI): A Guide to its Development and Use*, Center for Psychology of Personality, St. Louis, Mo, USA, 1994.

[29] C. R. Cloninger, "The psychobiological theory of temperament and character: comment on Farmer and Goldberg," *Psychological Assessment*, vol. 20, no. 3, pp. 292–299, 2008.

[30] J. Richter, T. Polak, and M. Eisemann, "Depressive mood and personality in terms of temperament and character among the normal population and depressive inpatients," *Personality and Individual Differences*, vol. 35, no. 4, pp. 917–927, 2003.

[31] J. Richter, M. Eisemann, and G. Richter, "Temperament and character during the course of unipolar depression among inpatients," *European Archives of Psychiatry and Clinical Neuroscience*, vol. 250, no. 1, pp. 40–47, 2000.

[32] C. R. Cloninger, C. Bayon, and D. M. Svrakic, "Measurement of temperament and character in mood disorders: a model of fundamental states as personality types," *Journal of Affective Disorders*, vol. 51, no. 1, pp. 21–32, 1998.

[33] J. L. Luby, D. M. Svrakic, K. McCallum, T. R. Przybeck, and C. R. Cloninger, "The junior temperament and character inventory: preliminary validation of a child self-report measure," *Psychological Reports*, vol. 84, no. 3, part 2, pp. 1127–1138, 1999.

[34] K. Schmeck, K. Goth, F. Poustka, and R. C. Cloninger, "Reliability and validity of the Junior Temperament and Character Inventory," *International Journal of Methods in Psychiatric Research*, vol. 10, no. 4, pp. 172–182, 2001.

[35] L. Poustka, P. Parzer, R. Brunner, and F. Resch, "Basic symptoms, temperament and character in adolescent psychiatric disorders," *Psychopathology*, vol. 40, no. 5, pp. 321–328, 2007.

[36] E. Dinya, J. Csorba, and Z. Grósz, "Are there temperament differences between major depression and dysthymic disorder in adolescent clinical outpatients?" *Comprehensive Psychiatry*, vol. 53, no. 4, pp. 350–354, 2012.

[37] R. Althoff, L. Ayer, E. Crehan, D. Rettew, J. Baer, and J. Hudziak, "Temperamental profiles of dysregulated children," *Child Psychiatry & Human Development*, vol. 43, no. 4, pp. 511–522, 2012.

[38] E. Dinya, J. Csorba, and Z. Grosz, "Differential characteristics of anxiety syndromes in clinical adolescents," *Central European Journal of Medicine*, vol. 7, no. 1, pp. 45–50, 2012.

[39] E. Yamano, S. Fukuda, T. Joudoi et al., "Temperament and character as predictors of fatigue-induced symptoms among school children in Japan: a 1-year follow-up study," *Comprehensive Psychiatry*, vol. 51, no. 3, pp. 256–265, 2010.

[40] E. J. Costello, H. Egger, and A. Angold, "10-Year research update review: the epidemiology of child and adolescent psychiatric disorders: I. Methods and public health burden," *Journal of the American Academy of Child & Adolescent Psychiatry*, vol. 44, no. 10, pp. 972–986, 2005.

[41] I. Gasquet, M. Chavance, S. Ledoux, and M. Choquet, "Psychosocial factors associated with help-seeking behavior among depressive adolescents," *European Child and Adolescent Psychiatry*, vol. 6, no. 3, pp. 151–159, 1997.

[42] H. Christensen, K. M. Griffiths, and A. F. Jorm, "Delivering interventions for depression by using the Internet: randomised controlled trial," *British Medical Journal*, vol. 328, no. 7434, pp. 265–269, 2004.

[43] H. Christensen, K. M. Griffiths, A. E. Korten, K. Brittliffe, and C. Groves, "A comparison of changes in anxiety and depression symptoms of spontaneous users and trial participants of a cognitive behavior therapy website," *Journal of Medical Internet Research*, vol. 6, no. 4, article e46, 2004.

[44] O. K. Lintvedt, K. M. Griffiths, K. Sørensen et al., "Evaluating the effectiveness and efficacy of unguided internet-based self-help intervention for the prevention of depression: a randomized controlled trial," *Clinical Psychology & Psychotherapy*. In press.

[45] H. Christensen, J. Reynolds, and K. M. Griffiths, "The use of e-health applications for anxiety and depression in young people: challenges and solutions," *Early Intervention in Psychiatry*, vol. 5, no. 1, pp. 58–62, 2011.

[46] L. M. Ritterband, G. Andersson, H. M. Christensen, P. Carlbring, and P. Cuijpers, "Directions for the International Society for Research on Internet Interventions (ISRII)," *Journal of Medical Internet Research*, vol. 8, no. 3, p. 6, 2006.

[47] P. J. Batterham, A. L. Neil, K. Bennett, K. M. Griffiths, and H. Christensen, "Predictors of adherence among community users of a cognitive behavior therapy website," *Patient Preference and Adherence*, vol. 2, pp. 97–105, 2008.

[48] A. Yildiz, D. K. Pauler, and G. S. Sachs, "Rates of study completion with single versus split daily dosing of antidepressants: a meta-analysis," *Journal of Affective Disorders*, vol. 78, no. 2, pp. 157–162, 2004.

[49] A. Bandura, "Self-efficacy: toward a unifying theory of behavioral change," *Psychological Review*, vol. 84, no. 2, pp. 191–215, 1977.

[50] J. A. Colquitt, J. A. LePine, and R. A. Noe, "Toward an integrative theory of training motivation: a meta-analytic path analysis of 20 years of research," *Journal of Applied Psychology*, vol. 85, no. 5, pp. 678–707, 2000.

[51] G. Barker, A. Olukoya, and P. Aggleton, "Young people, social support and help-seeking," *International Journal of Adolescent Medicine and Health*, vol. 17, no. 4, pp. 315–335, 2005.

[52] P. Pössel, C. Baldus, A. B. Horn, G. Groen, and M. Hautzinger, "Influence of general self-efficacy on the effects of a school-based universal primary prevention program of depressive symptoms in adolescents: a randomized and controlled follow-up study," *Journal of Child Psychology and Psychiatry and Allied Disciplines*, vol. 46, no. 9, pp. 982–994, 2005.

[53] H. Christensen, K. M. Griffiths, and A. Korten, "Web-based cognitive behavior therapy: analysis of site usage and changes in depression and anxiety scores," *Journal of Medical Internet Research*, vol. 4, no. 1, article e3, 2002.

[54] L. Radloff, "The CES-D Scale: A Self Report Depression Scale for Research in the General," Applied Psychological Measurement, 1977.

[55] R. E. Roberts, P. M. Lewinsohn, and J. R. Seeley, "Screening for adolescent depression: a comparison of depression scales," *Journal of the American Academy of Child & Adolescent Psychiatry*, vol. 30, no. 1, pp. 58–66, 1991.

[56] L. S. Radloff, "The use of the Center for Epidemiologic Studies Depression Scale in adolescents and young adults," *Journal of Youth and Adolescence*, vol. 20, no. 2, pp. 149–166, 1991.
[57] E. Røysamb, R. Schwarzer, and M. Jerusalem, "Norwegian version of the general perceived self-efficacy scale, 2008," 1998, http://userpage.fu-berlin.de/~health/norway.htm.
[58] K. Goth and K. Schmeck, *Das Junior Temperament und Charakter Inventar (JTCI)*, Göttingen, Germany, 2009.
[59] N. Sartorius and W. Kuyken, *Translation of Health Status Instruments In Quality Life Assessment: International Perspectives*, Springer, Berlin, Germany, 1994.

13

Using Self-Guided Treatment Software (*ePST*) to Teach Clinicians How to Deliver Problem-Solving Treatment for Depression

James A. Cartreine,[1,2] Trina E. Chang,[2,3] Janette L. Seville,[4] Luis Sandoval,[5] John B. Moore,[2] Shuai Xu,[2] and Mark T. Hegel[4]

[1] *Department of Psychiatry, Brigham and Women's Hospital, Harvard Medical School, 1249 Boylston Avenue 3rd floor, Boston, MA 02215, USA*
[2] *Harvard Medical School, Boston, MA 02215, USA*
[3] *Department of Psychiatry, Massachusetts General Hospital, Harvard Medical School, Boston, MA 02114, USA*
[4] *Department of Psychiatry, Dartmouth-Hitchcock Medical Center, Dartmouth Medical School, Lebanon, NH 03756, USA*
[5] *Department of Educational Psychology, University of Texas at Austin, Austin, TX 72705, USA*

Correspondence should be addressed to James A. Cartreine, jcartreine@partners.org

Academic Editor: Amy Kilbourne

Problem-solving treatment (PST) offers a promising approach to the depression care; however, few PST training opportunities exist. A computer-guided, interactive media program has been developed to deliver PST electronically (*ePST*), directly to patients. The program is a six-session, weekly intervention modeled on an evidence-based PST protocol. Users are guided through each session by a clinician who is presented via hundreds of branching audio and video clips. Because expert clinician behaviors are modeled in the program, not only does the *ePST* program have the potential to deliver PST to patients but it may also serve as a training tool to teach clinicians how to deliver PST. Thirteen social workers and trainees used *ePST* self-instructionally and subsequently attended a day-long workshop on PST. Participants' PST knowledge level increased significantly from baseline to post-*ePST* (P = .001) and did not increase significantly further after attending the subsequent workshop. Additionally, attending the workshop did not significantly increase the participants' skill at performing PST beyond the use of the *ePST* program. Using the *ePST* program appears to train novices to a sufficient level of competence to begin practicing PST under supervision. This self-instructional training method could enable PST for depression to be widely disseminated, although follow-up supervision is still required.

1. Introduction

Effective treatments have been developed for depression, including antidepressant medications and psychotherapies. Many patients prefer counseling or psychotherapy to taking medications, if it is available [1], and matching treatment (medication or therapy) to patient preference has been demonstrated to improve outcomes, independent from depression severity [2, 3]. Unfortunately, many mental healthcare providers lack training in evidence-based treatments [4] or fail to implement them properly [5], making evidence-based psychotherapy unavailable to many persons with depression in the United States. One way to increase access to evidence-based psychotherapies is to develop more cost-efficient and accessible training methods.

Problem-solving treatment (PST; also known as problem-solving therapy) has emerged as an effective treatment for depression [6–8]. The basis of PST is that enhancing problem-solving skills and attitudes and working to solve concrete problems in one's life can reduce depression. PST breaks the problem-solving process into steps and teaches participants to go through these steps systematically and effectively, targeting parts of the process that are particularly challenging for depressed patients. PST has been found to produce outcomes comparable to antidepressant medications [9, 10] and better than treatment as usual [11, 12].

PST has great potential for dissemination because it can be delivered by mental health as well as nonmental health specialists in a wide range of healthcare settings, including primary care [13]. Healthcare professionals, such as nurses and social workers are trained in a one- to two-day seminar that includes didactics, demonstrations, and roleplay with feedback [14]. They are then supervised on PST by a recognized expert over the course of three to five cases. For each case, the supervisor listens to and critiques a recording of three PST sessions, sometimes providing this supervision via the telephone.

Automating PST training could improve the ability to further disseminate PST and potentially result in cost savings. Although the supervision portion of the training requires the involvement of a live clinician, it is conceivable that some or all of the workshop could be automated. Self-instructional training is not a new concept; self-instructional books have existed for centuries and self-instructional videos for decades. These could be good starting points to learn PST. However, it has been demonstrated that the more interactive a training experience is, the more effective it is [15–18]. Since the skill at hand, PST, is a highly interactive process, developing a highly interactive self-guided training approach should enhance PST skill building.

1.1. ePST Software. An interactive media-based computer program has been developed to provide PST electronically (*ePST*) in an entirely automated manner [19]. In this self-help program, users are guided through six sessions of PST by a master clinician (M. T. Hegel) who is an expert in the intervention and conveys the "nonspecific" characteristics of effective therapists, such as warmth, genuineness, compassion, and the ability to provide support when the patient experiences setbacks [20]. Users interact with the program by entering text via the keyboard or by clicking on answers to questions, and hundreds of branching audio and video clips are used to tailor the program to users' inputs. The program tracks the user's depression via the Patient Health Questionnaire-9 (PHQ-9; [21]) and the on-camera host provides feedback and recommendations. The program reviews the user's work across sessions and across problems to provide guidance on how to improve his or her problem-solving success, through the use of failure analyses [22–24] algorithms. Although the program was originally developed for astronauts to treat their own depression on long-duration space missions, it was designed for use by the public.

Because the program models best practices for providing PST, it may be useful not only as an intervention but also as a teaching tool, to demonstrate how to deliver PST. The purpose of this study was to obtain pilot data on the feasibility and efficacy of using this program to teach PST to therapists unfamiliar with the intervention. Primary research questions addressed were as follows.

(1) Is use of *ePST* associated with change in knowledge of the steps and process of PST?

(2) Is live training associated with change in skill at performing PST, for persons who have already been trained via *ePST*?

Secondary research questions were as follows.

(1) Is use of *ePST* associated with change in self-efficacy for performing PST-specific skills, and for doing counseling in general?

(2) How acceptable and easy to use is *ePST* for training?

2. Methods

2.1. Participants. The subject population consisted of clinical staff and trainees from a human services organization in Framingham, MA, with no prior training in PST. All participants volunteered for the study and received no compensation for participation. Training was offered to all clinicians and trainees working at the site.

2.2. Procedure. The study was approved by the Massachusetts General Hospital's Institutional Review Board, and consent to participate in the study was implied by voluntary completion of the study questionnaires. Receiving training was not contingent on participation in the evaluation component, and participants were not required to participate as part of their employment.

Training consisted of participants using the *ePST* program for four sessions *as if they were patients*. Participants were encouraged to work on real problems in their own lives via *ePST* as a means of learning how PST works. They were also asked to view the on-camera therapist as a model for delivering PST. Although a full course of treatment via *ePST* involves six sessions, the investigators judged *a priori* that using the program for only four sessions would provide sufficient exposure to the model for trainees to learn PST. At no point in this study did the participants interact with actual patients using the PST approach.

Assessments were conducted at three time points and trainings were conducted at two points. At baseline (before beginning training), participants completed a test of their knowledge of PST and a measure of self-efficacy to do counseling (regarding both general and PST-specific skills). Following completion of their training using *ePST*, participants again completed questionnaires on their knowledge of PST and self-efficacy as well as the acceptability and usability of the computer program. They also participated in audiotaped roleplay sessions as a PST therapist treating a standardized patient (a research assistant trained to portray a depression patient). After the workshop, participants completed the knowledge and self-efficacy questionnaires for the third time and then conducted another taped roleplay session with a different standardized patient. Three standardized patient cases of similar difficulty were written for the roleplay. Subjects were randomly assigned to different cases for their roleplay sessions.

2.3. Measures

Knowledge of PST. This was a primary measure, which consisted of one open-ended essay-format question: "Please describe the process of problem-solving therapy in detail, including all steps and the criteria for successfully completing each one." Essays were scored using criteria developed for the study (see Appendix A). The possible range of scores was 0 to 120, with higher scores indicating greater knowledge. The essays were rated by M. T. Hegel and J. L. Seville, blind to the time point of each essay.

Skill Implementing PST. The standardized patient roleplay was a primary measure. The audiotaped roleplay sessions were scored using the Problem-Solving Treatment in Primary Care Adherence and Competence Scale (PST-PAC) [25, 26] which evaluates trainees' performance on nine dimensions of PST, each on a six-point scale (0–5; worst to best performance) (see Appendix B). Because each standardized patient was being seen for an initial PST session, the first rating dimension, "Defining the outcome" (of the previous session's action plan) was not included. Therefore, participants were rated on dimensions two through eight of the PST-PAC. The possible range of scores was 0 to 40, with higher scores indicating better performance.

Scoring was performed by J. A. Cartreine and J. L. Seville, who were blind to the time point of each roleplay. One of the raters (J. L. Seville) had been trained in the use of the PST-PAC previously; the other (J. A. Cartreine) was trained to rate roleplays by rating audio recordings of sample cases.

Self-Efficacy for Implementing PST and Doing Counseling, in General. The *PST and Counseling Self-Estimate Inventory* (PCSEI) was created for this study, it consists of 30 items that measure different aspects of a therapist's perception of his or her ability to perform specific PST skills and general counseling skills (see Appendix C). It was adapted from the Counseling Self-Estimate Inventory (CSEI) [27]. To reduce the length of the measure, some items from the CSEI less relevant to the study were dropped, while several new items pertinent to performing PST-specific skills were added, using similar language. Items were scored on a six-point scale (1 = "strongly disagree"; 6 = "strongly agree"), with a possible range of 30 to 180 for the total measure, a range of 16 to 96 for the "PST-specific" subscale and 14 to 84 for the "General" subscale. Some items are reverse scored to avoid acquiescence bias; higher scores reflect higher self-efficacy.

Acceptability of Using ePST to Learn PST. The Program Acceptability Questionnaire (PAQ) was written for this study and consisted of six questions on various aspects of the acceptability of the PST computer program, such as how much the program helped the trainee learn PST and whether the subject would recommend its use to other prospective trainees (see Appendix D). Items were rated on a six-point scale as above (1 = "strongly disagree"; 6 = "strongly agree").

Usability of the ePST Program. The System Usability Scale (SUS) [28, 29] was used to assess ease of using the software. The SUS is a ten-item questionnaire that is widely used for assessing software usability, such as whether a system is excessively complex or cumbersome to use, or whether the trainee needs technical support to use it. Statements about the software are rated on a six-point scale (0 = "strongly disagree"; 6 = "strongly agree").

2.4. Analytic Methods

Score Calculations. Scores for the PST-PAC were obtained using the following procedures: for each standardized patient interview, all eight scores given by each rater were averaged, yielding two scores (one for each rater). For items where the raters' scores differed by more than one point, the raters discussed the item and arrived at a consensus score for that item. Then, the average was taken of the two raters' scores, yielding one final score per standardized patient interview.

PST knowledge essays were scored on 27 items that map onto seven subscales, which correspond to the steps of PST. Because the seven subscales contain different numbers of items, an average of the scores for each subscale, for each rater, was calculated. The seven scores were then summed, yielding one score per essay for each rater. Finally, an average was calculated between scores awarded by each rater, to obtain a full-scale score for each participant on each essay written.

Self-efficacy scores were calculated by summing the responses to individual items (with some questions reverse scored). Additionally, subscales were calculated by summing the items measuring general self-efficacy and those measuring PST-specific self-efficacy.

Analyses. Due to the small sample size, nonparametric analyses were used to answer the research questions. The Wilcoxon signed ranks test was used to compare skill levels between Assessment 2 and 3 (no skill test was administered in Assessment 1). The same test was also used to gauge change in knowledge and self-efficacy at Assessment 1 compared to 2, and Assessment 2 compared to 3. Because multiple comparisons were made, a Bonferroni correction was used, which set the P cutoff for significance at $P = .0125$ for the primary outcomes of skill and knowledge. The Bonferroni correction was not used for the secondary outcome of self-efficacy.

Descriptive statistics were used to characterize the sample and results of the SUS and PAQ. Because the PAQ was created for this study, an insufficient quantity of data has been collected to support a factor analysis and the reporting of a composite score. Therefore, results on this questionnaire are reported by item.

3. Results

Thirteen participants (11 female and 2 male) enrolled, with a mean age of 37.5 (±12.9); 11 self-identified as Caucasian and the other 2 as racial minorities. Six were licensed clinical social workers, with an average of 2 years in practice (±1.4, range 2 to 6 years); the other 7 were social work graduate students. No participants who inquired about the study subsequently refused to participate or dropped out.

Interrater reliability for both the essay and roleplay scoring was calculated using percent agreement between raters. For the skill measure, interrater agreement per item (defined as agreement on the rating plus or minus 1 point) between the two raters averaged 79.6%. To increase concordance between raters, consensus scores (as described in the methods section) were obtained for items in which raters

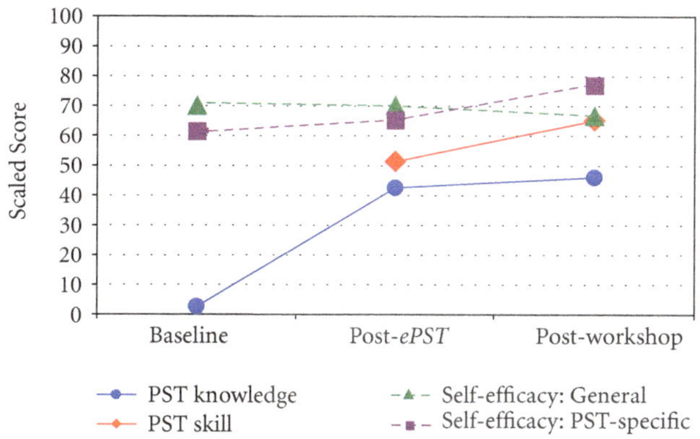

Figure 1: Scaled scores for skill, knowledge, and self-efficacy. Scaled Score = Median converted to percent of maximum possible score.

differed by >1 point. For the knowledge (essay) measure, the percent agreement (within one point) between the raters across items was 87.5%. Because agreement between raters on the knowledge measure was high from the outset, a consensus process was not needed to improve concordance.

Summary results of the knowledge, skill, self-efficacy, and usability measures are presented in Table 1.

3.1. Primary Outcomes. Knowledge scores significantly increased from pretraining to post-using *ePST* ($Z = 3.18$, $P = .001$) but did not increase significantly more after attending the live workshop ($Z = 1.363$, $P = .173$). No significant difference was found in skill level after using *ePST* versus after the live workshop, using either nonparametric (Wilcoxon signed ranks test $Z = -2.040$; $P = .041$) or parametric ($t = -2.346$; $df = 12$; $P = .037$) statistics. This suggests that the workshop did not substantially increase the knowledge or skill of the participants beyond what they learned using the *ePST* program. On an item-level analysis of the roleplay ratings, only skill at helping patients identify pros and cons of solutions changed before to versus after attending the live workshop. On this item, before attending the workshop (but after completing *ePST*) the median score was 2.5 on a scale of 0 to 5 (range .5 to 4.5; mean of 2.5 ± 1); and after the workshop, the median increased to 3.5 (range .5 to 5.0; mean 3.81 ± .9; Wilcoxon signed ranks test $Z = -2.599$; $P = .009$). Also, across outcome measures and time points, there were no significant correlations between participants' knowledge, skill, or self-efficacy levels.

To facilitate comparisons between knowledge and skill levels, scaled scores of 0 to 100 were calculated by converting the median to the percentage of the maximum score possible on each scale (see Figure 1). Both knowledge and skill were near the midpoint after using *ePST* (42.46 and 51.25, resp.) and remained near that point after completing the workshop (45.97 and 65).

3.2. Secondary Outcomes

Self-Efficacy for PST and Counseling, Overall. Five items were unanswered in the PCSEI data set. Values for these missing data points were imputed by calculating the mean of the participant's responses to the other items from the same subscale on that administration of the PCSEI. Composite self-efficacy scores, which included all items on the PCSEI, remained stable from pretraining to post-*ePST* training to post-live workshop, although there was a significant increase in composite self-efficacy from pre-training to post-workshop ($P = .028$). The Wilcoxon signed ranks test Z-score for self-efficacy at pretest compared to post-*ePST* was -1.014; $P = .311$ ($t = -1.365$; $df = 12$; $P = .199$) and the Z-score for post-*ePST* compared to post-live training was -1.751; $P = .080$ ($t = -1.977$; $df = 12$; $P = .071$). On the PST-specific subscale, there was a significant improvement from post-*ePST* and post-live workshop training (Z-score $= -2.033$; $P = .042$). No significant difference was found for the subscale of general counseling self-efficacy between pretest and post-*ePST* training, or between post-*ePST* and post-live workshop training.

3.3. Usability and Acceptability. The median SUS score was 67.5 (range 60 to 87.5; mean = 69.23 ± 7.8) on a scale of 0 to 100. On the PAQ, the medians for all but one item were 5 (means ranged from 4.54 to 5.23) on a scale of 0 to 6 (see Table 2).

4. Discussion

PST is an evidence-based intervention for depression; however, few providers have training in it. A novel approach to teaching PST is the use of a computer-automated treatment, *ePST*. Users are guided through it via branching videos to simulate the experience of being in treatment with a master clinician (M. T. Hegel). As such, best practices for delivering PST are modeled and the program may serve as a training tool for practitioners, in addition to a treatment for patients.

Thirteen persons with no prior experience delivering PST (6 licensed clinical social workers and 7 social work graduate students) used the *ePST* interactive media program for four sessions over the course of two weeks. They were instructed to work on a real problem in their own lives, to make the training more meaningful. After the self-guided instruction, all 13 attended a standard PST training workshop presented by a veteran PST trainer (also M. T. Hegel), which is the standard method to train new practitioners.

It was found that live training does not add knowledge or skill beyond what *ePST* provides. Trainees were assessed on knowledge at three points: once at baseline, again after using *ePST* for four sessions, and again after completing the live day-long workshop. They were also assessed on PST skill via roleplays with standardized patients after completing *ePST* and again after completing the workshop. Knowledge about how to conduct PST went from a near-zero level (1.5 on a scale of 0 to 35) at baseline to a significantly higher level after using *ePST* (mean score 14.1) and did not significantly improve following the workshop (mean score 16.7).

PST skill was not assessed at baseline due to logistical constraints; however, it is likely that it would also have been very low before training, since none of the subjects had received prior training. After completing 4 sessions of *ePST*,

TABLE 1: Assessments of knowledge, skill, self-efficacy, and *ePST* program usability.

	Pre-training			Post-*ePST* (computerized) Training			Post-live training		
	Median (range)	Mean ± SD	Scaled score (0 to 100)[a]	Median (range)	Mean ± SD	Scaled score (0 to 100)[a]	Median (range)	Mean ± SD	Scaled score (0 to 100)[a]
Knowledge of PST	0.9 (0 to 6.45)	1.53 ± 2.04	2.57	14.86[b] (3.33 to 24.49)	14.06 ± 6.74	42.46	16.09 (8.74 to 24.63)	16.74 ± 5.17	45.97
Skill implementing PST	—	—	—	20.5 (7 to 28)	19.65 ± 6.70	51.25	26 (11 to 34)	25.23 ± 7.16	65.00
Self-efficacy (Composite)	126 (106 to 162)	129.54 ± 14.64	64.00	133 (112 to 156)	134.31 ± 13.81	67.33	145[c] (106 to 168)	143.31 ± 17.36	76.67
Self-efficacy (General)	63 (54 to 76)	63.31 ± 6.29	70.00	65 (52 to 73)	64.23 ± 6.10	70.00	66 (54 to 78)	66.54 ± 8.23	74.29
Self-efficacy (PST-specific)	65 (50 to 86)	66.23 ± 9.59	61.25	68 (52 to 86)	70.08 ± 9.21	65.00	77[d,e] (52 to 90)	76.77 ± 10.52	76.25
Usability of *ePST*	—	—	—	67.5 (60 to 87.5)	69.23 ± 7.8	—	—	—	—

[a]Median converted to percent of maximum possible score.
[b]Compared to pre-training ($P = 0.001$).
[c]Compared to pre-training ($P = 0.028$).
[d]Compared to pretraining ($P = .023$).
[e]Compared to post-*ePST* ($P = .042$).

Table 2: Program Acceptability Questionnaire (scale range 0 to 6).

Item	Mean ± SD	Median (range)
I felt comfortable using the PST program for training	5.23 ± 0.73	5 (4 to 6)
Doing training using this program was acceptable to me	4.92 ± 0.76	5 (4 to 6)
Using the program helped me understand how to do PST	4.69 ± 0.75	5 (4 to 6)
I enjoyed using the program to learn PST	4.62 ± 1.12	4 (3 to 6)
I would rather do training in a live workshop than with the computer	4.54 ± 1.05	5 (3 to 6)
I would recommend this program to a colleague who is interested in learning how to do PST	4.54 ± 1.13	5 (2 to 6)

mean skill was 19.7 (on a scale of 0 to 40) and was 25.2 following the live workshop. This change was not statistically significant. Composite self-efficacy for performing PST skills and for doing counseling in general gradually increased from baseline to post-live training. This appears to be due to a significant improvement in self-efficacy for performing PST skills after the workshop and one standardized patient interview. Therefore, confidence in one's ability to conduct PST increased significantly as a result of the live workshop and/or standardized patient interview, even though actual skill and knowledge did not.

The only specific areas of improvement found after completing the workshop were knowledge and implementation of decision-making guidelines (i.e., evaluation of pros and cons in problem solving). Both skill and knowledge regarding decision-making guidelines improved following the workshop, suggesting that *ePST* could be strengthened in this regard. No significant change in either direction was noted for other content areas following the live workshop.

A key ingredient in clinical training is supervision while treating actual patients, and it is unrealistic to expect that use of a self-instructional training program or a one-day workshop would produce fully competent PST clinicians. However, after using *ePST,* social workers and social work trainees possessed a sufficient level of skill to begin providing PST under supervision. As such, *ePST* may be a convenient and low-cost alternative to the in-person PST workshops that are the standard of practice. As the number of PST practitioners increases, the number of persons with sufficient experience to serve as supervisors will also increase. Moreover research has already supported PST supervision via telephone [12], meaning the supervisor need not be in the same room—or the same time zone—as the trainee. Together, *ePST* plus telephone-based supervision could support the diffusion of PST throughout the medical and mental health communities.

Regarding the usability of *ePST*, an analysis of all published studies that used the SUS to evaluate software of all types found that the mean score was 70.14 [28]. The mean SUS score for *ePST* was 69.23; however, this may underestimate the program usability. Because *ePST* is designed for weekly sessions, to run the program more than once per week (as was done in this study), participants had to manually advance the system date on their computers, which can be challenging. A training version of *ePST* could readily overcome this limitation.

Acceptability of *ePST* appeared high. That said results of the Program Acceptability Questionnaire, written for this study, may have been subject to response set, as the means and standard deviations were very similar between items. For example, on a scale of 1 to 6, the mean of "I would recommend the program to a colleague" was 4.54 (±1.13); similarly, "I would rather do training in a live workshop than with the computer" was also 4.54 (±1.05).

ePST appears to be only the second computer program to evaluated the potential of a computer-automated treatment to train clinicians, and this appears to be the first study to use a behavioral outcome measure (i.e., standardized patient roleplays). The researchers identified one other computer-automated treatment program that has been used to teach clinicians how to perform a skill. *FearFighter*, a UK program for these treatment of panic and phobias [30], was used to teach the process of exposure therapy in two studies [31, 32]. Both studies used written measures to assess instructional gains, and both concluded that educational gains were equivalent to classroom training.

This study advances the literature on self-instructional training of therapists, and of clinicians in general, by using an e-therapy program as a training tool to teach clinicians an evidence-based treatment. Research on self-directed/computer-automated/online training has reported mixed training outcomes, likely because the pedagogies of the tools vary widely, from passively viewed didactics to written manuals to interactive programs [33]. Highly interactive training experiences, such as using *ePST*, have been demonstrated to produce superior outcomes regarding therapists' skill and actual behavior in the implementation of evidence-based treatments [33].

4.1. Limitations and Future Directions. This study has several limitations, including the mixed educational background of the sample and the lack of a comparison group design, which limit generalizability. Without a comparison group, it is impossible to say for certain what trainees learned from *ePST* versus from the live workshop. This study also had a relatively small sample size; however, we have noted that training studies often enroll fewer participants than treatment studies. Additionally, the use of standardized patients is a well-accepted measure of clinician skill [34, 35]; however, participants' performance might have been different with actual patients. Confidence in these results would be strengthened if interrater reliability of participant skill (in the roleplays) were higher. Finally, trainees may have learned from participating in the roleplay (the first of which happened after the post-*ePST* assessment and before the workshop); this effect might have artificially inflated the estimates of learning from the workshop, thus leading to an underestimate of the full effect of *ePST* training.

Regarding modifications to the *ePST* software, many trainees suggested the inclusion of a modeling video demonstrating the use of PST with a patient. Such a video has already been recorded and can be incorporated into a training version of *ePST*. Also, there exists a wealth of print training material for PST that could augment the computer-based training. Finally, supervision of new PST therapists is a necessary component of PST training [25, 26] and is unlikely to be automated.

Several national and statewide initiatives are implementing evidence-based treatments for depression and could benefit from cost-effective training, such as those by the National Network of Depression Centers [36], The University of Washington's Improving Mood: Promoting Access to Collaborative Treatment (IMPACT) [37] and its Program to Encourage Active, Rewarding Lives for Seniors (PEARLS) [38] programs, and Depression Improvement Across Minnesota, Offering a New Direction (DIAMOND) [39]. *ePST* opens the door to a new training method that could promote the mass dissemination of PST among healthcare providers in order to improve patient access to care and ultimately reduce the impact of depression in the population.

Appendices

A. PST Knowledge

A.1. Problem-Solving Treatment Knowledge Assessment

Authors. James A. Cartreine, Brigham and Women's Hospital/Harvard Medical School, Boston, MA.

Janette L. Seville, Geisel School of Medicine at Dartmouth, Hanover, NH.

Trina E. Chang, Massachusetts General Hospital/Harvard Medical School, Boston, MA.

Mark T. Hegel, Geisel School of Medicine at Dartmouth, Hanover, NH.

Instructions. In the space below, please answer the following essay question. You have 10 minutes.

> *Please describe the process of problem-solving therapy in detail, including all steps and the criteria for successfully completing each one.*

Scoring Criteria. Assess whether the written response addresses each element below, on a scale of 0–5.

0	1	2	3	4	5
Very Poor	Poor	Borderline	Satisfactory	Good	Very Good

Number	Element	Subscale
(1)	Problem should be observable	Problem
(2)	Problem should be under client's control	Problem
(3)	Goal should be behavioral (something client does)	Goal
(4)	Goal should be general (more than one way to reach it)	Goal
(5)	Goal should be observable (or countable)	Goal
(6)	Goal should be achievable (or short term, i.e., 2 weeks)	Goal
(7)	Goal should not just be the converse of the problem	Goal
(8)	Brainstorming should include multiple ideas/solutions	Brainstorming
(9)	Do not prejudge solutions	Brainstorming
(10)	Pros are identified for each idea/solution (or what makes each unique)	Solutions
(11)	Multiple cons are assessed for each idea/solution	Solutions
(12)	Effort to implement solution is assessed	Solutions
(13)	Time to implement solution is assessed	Solutions
(14)	Cost of solution is assessed	Solutions
(15)	Need for other people to implement solution is assessed	Solutions
(16)	Negative impact on others is assessed	Solutions
(17)	One or more solutions must be chosen	Solutions
(18)	Action plan can be implemented soon	Action plan
(19)	Action plan is step by step, detailed	Action plan
(20)	Action plan includes Who, What, Where, and When are the steps to be taken	Action plan
(21)	Anticipate obstacles and plan around them	Action plan
(22)	Plan B's (backup plans) are created	Action plan
(23)	Enjoyable activities should be scheduled for each week	Pleasant events
(24)	Clinician checks whether action plan was implemented and goal was reached	Progress check

(25)	Clinician checks client's satisfaction with his or her effort	Progress check
(26)	Clinician helps clients troubleshoot how to improve their problem solving	Progress check

B. PST Skill

B.1. Problem-Solving Treatment in Primary Care Therapist Adherence and Competence Scale. Version 8-13-09

Authors. Mark T. Hegel, Ph.D., Geisel School of Medicine at Dartmouth, Hanover, NH.

Laurence Mynors-Wallis, M.D., University of Southampton, UK.

Rater Instructions. For each item, assess the therapist on a scale of 0–5 and record the rating on the line next to the item number.

0	1	2	3	4	5
Very Poor	Poor	Borderline	Satisfactory	Good	Very Good

(1) Evaluating the outcome

Review of all current tasks
Praise success
Exploration of failure
Rate Satisfaction and Mood
Reinforce PST-PC Model
Review previous problem areas

(2) Defining the problem

Specific, feasible problem chosen
Described in objective terms
Problem explored, clarified
Identify barriers

(3) Establishing a realistic goal

Goal is objective
Described in behavioral terms
Goal is achievable
Goal is general
Follows directly from problem statement
Addresses barriers identified in problem

(4) Generating solutions

Prime for brainstorming
Brainstorming facilitated
Solutions from patient
Withhold judgment

(5) Implementing Decision-Making Guidelines and Choosing the Solution(s)

Consider "pros" and "cons" for one's self/others
Rate each theme
Compare solutions
Solution(s) satisfies the goals
Negative impact is limited

(6) Implementing the preferred solution(s)

Specific tasks identified
Realistic behavior requirements
Plan B
Plan pleasant activities for the week

(7) Process tasks

Clear demarcation of PST-PC stages
Kept session near a 30-minute timeframe
Cue and review for stages
Summarize process at end of session
Facilitate a positive problem orientation
Facilitate independence in guiding PST process

(8) Communication and interpersonal effectiveness

Facilitates communication (supportive vocalizations/nonverbals)
Use of patient's own language and phrases
Warm/confident/professional
Tactful limiting of peripheral and unproductive discussion

(9) Global rating

How would you rate the problem-solving therapist overall in this session? (does not need to approach a mathematical average of previous eight items)

C. Self-Efficacy

C.1. PST and Counseling Self-Estimate Inventory

Authors. Based on Larson et al. [27]. (PST-specific questions added by the authors.)

Instructions. This is not a test. There are no right or wrong answers. Rather, this is an inventory that attempts to measure how you think you behave doing problem-solving therapy. Please respond to the items as honestly as you can to most accurately portray how you think you behave as a PST therapist. Do not respond with how you wish you could perform each item, or think you might in the future. Rather, answer in a way that reflects your actual estimate of how you perform as a counselor at the present time.

1	2	3	4	5	6
Strongly Disagree					Strongly Agree

	Item	Subscale
(1)	I can effectively redirect clients who choose to work on problems over which they have limited control	PST
(2)	I am likely to impose my values on the client during the interview	General
(3)	When I initiate the end of a session, I am positive it is in a manner that is neither abrupt nor brusque, and I end sessions on time	General
(4)	I can help clients construct action plans that meet the criteria of problem-solving therapy	PST
(5)	I feel that I will not be able to respond to the client in a nonjudgmental way with respect to the client's values, beliefs, and so forth	General
(6)	I feel that I can respond to the client in an appropriate amount of time (neither interrupting the patient nor waiting too long to respond)	General
(7)	I anticipate that the type of response I use at a particular time may not fit with the problem-solving therapy approach	PST
(8)	I can help clients with the brainstorming step of problem-solving therapy	PST
(9)	I feel confident that I have resolved conflicts in my personal life so that they will not interfere with my counseling abilities	General
(10)	I feel that I have enough fundamental knowledge to do effective problem-solving therapy	PST
(11)	I am able to respond in a helpful way when clients report that they have not worked on a problem since last session	PST
(12)	I may not be able to maintain the intensity and energy level needed to produce client confidence and active participation	General
(13)	I am not sure that when doing problem-solving therapy I will express myself in a way that is natural without deliberating over every response or action	PST
(14)	I am confident that I can conduct problem-solving therapy, adhering to the guidelines set out in the PST therapy manual	PST
(15)	My assessments of client problems may not be as accurate as I would like them to be	PST
(16)	I am confident that I can help patients define their problems in a manner suitable for problem solving	PST
(17)	I do not feel I possess a large enough repertoire of techniques to deal with the different problems my client may present	General
(18)	I am uncomfortable about dealing with clients who appear unmotivated to work toward their goals	PST
(19)	I have difficulty dealing with clients who do not verbalize their thoughts during the counseling session	General
(20)	I am unsure how to deal with clients who appear noncommittal and indecisive	General
(21)	I am an effective counselor with clients of a different socioeconomic status	General
(22)	I am unsure how to lead my client to work toward concrete goals	PST
(23)	I am confident that I can assess my client's readiness and commitment to work on a given problem	PST
(24)	When working with ethnic minority clients I am confident that I will be able to bridge cultural differences in the counseling process	General

(25)	I am confident that I can help my patients evaluate the pros and cons of their solutions and choose a feasible solution in an efficient and helpful manner	PST
(26)	I am confident that I can support the client in choosing his or her own problems on which to work	PST
(27)	I feel I may give advice	General
(28)	In working with culturally different clients, I have a difficult time viewing situations from their perspective	General
(29)	I anticipate having difficulty helping clients write goal statements that meet all of the problem-solving therapy criteria	PST
(30)	I am afraid that I may not be able to effectively relate to someone of lower socioeconomic status than me	General

D. Acceptability

D.1. Program Acceptability Questionnaire

Author. James A. Cartreine, Brigham and Women's Hospital/Harvard Medical School, Boston, MA.

Instructions. Please read each item carefully and circle a number to show how much you agree or disagree with the statement.

1	2	3	4	5	6
Strongly Disagree					Strongly Agree

(1) I felt comfortable using the PST program for training

(2) Doing training using this program was acceptable to me

(3) Using the program helped me understand how to do PST

(4) I enjoyed using the program to learn PST

(5) I would rather do training in a live workshop than with the computer

(6) I would recommend this program to a colleague who is interested in learning how to do PST

Disclosures

The *ePST* software was designed by Cartreine (née Carter). When this study was conducted, the *ePST* software was owned by Beth Israel Deaconess Medical Center and Dartmouth Medical School. The *ePST* software is now owned by Cognitive Behavioral Technologies, LLC, which was founded by Cartreine and Hegel. Data analysis was conducted by another author (TC) in consultation with a statistical analyst, both who have no financial interest in *ePST*.

Acknowledgments

Development of the *ePST* software was supported by the National Space Biomedical Research Institute through NASA NCC 9–58. The authors wish to thank Ms. Rie Maurer for her statistical assistance and Ms. Lynn Kerner of Advocates, Inc., Framingham Massachusetts, and Mr. Steven Corso of Baypath Elder Services, Marlborough, Massachusetts, for their assistance in the recruitment and administration of this study. They also wish to thank Mr. Fred Connors and the Staff of The Troupe Modern Media (http://www.thetroupe.com/), of Windham, New Hampshire, which produced the *ePST* software and research assistants Kate Bentley, Elizabeth Dalton, Tracie Goodness, Irene Shyu, Jessica Sousa, Soo Youn, and Carrie Brintz.

References

[1] M. Dwight-Johnson, C. D. Sherbourne, D. Liao, and K. B. Wells, "Treatment preferences among depressed primary care patients," *Journal of General Internal Medicine*, vol. 15, no. 8, pp. 527–534, 2000.

[2] P. Lin, D. G. Campbell, E. F. Chaney et al., "The influence of patient preference on depression treatment in primary care," *Annals of Behavioral Medicine*, vol. 30, no. 2, pp. 164–173, 2005.

[3] R. Mergl, V. Henkel, A. K. Allgaier et al., "Are treatment preferences relevant in response to serotonergic antidepressants and cognitive-behavioral therapy in depressed primary care patients? Results from a randomized controlled trial including a patients' choice arm," *Psychotherapy and Psychosomatics*, vol. 80, no. 1, pp. 39–47, 2010.

[4] S. R. Woody, J. Weisz, and C. McLean, "Empirically supported treatments: 10 years later," *The Clincical Psychologist*, vol. 58, no. 4, pp. 5–11, 2005.

[5] F. Azocar, B. Cuffel, W. Goldman, and L. McCarter, "The impact of evidence-based guideline dissemination for the assessment and treatment of major depression in a managed behavioral health care organization," *Journal of Behavioral Health Services and Research*, vol. 30, no. 1, pp. 109–118, 2003.

[6] A. C. Bell and T. J. D'Zurilla, "Problem-solving therapy for depression: a meta-analysis," *Clinical Psychology Review*, vol. 29, no. 4, pp. 348–353, 2009.

[7] P. Cuijpers, A. van Straten, and L. Warmerdam, "Problem solving therapies for depression: a meta-analysis," *European Psychiatry*, vol. 22, no. 1, pp. 9–15, 2007.
[8] J. M. Malouff, E. B. Thorsteinsson, and N. S. Schutte, "The efficacy of problem solving therapy in reducing mental and physical health problems: a meta-analysis," *Clinical Psychology Review*, vol. 27, no. 1, pp. 46–57, 2007.
[9] L. M. Mynors-Wallis, D. H. Gath, A. Day, and F. Baker, "Randomised controlled trial of problem solving treatment, antidepressant medication, and combined treatment for major depression in primary care," *British Medical Journal*, vol. 320, no. 7226, pp. 26–30, 2000.
[10] L. M. Mynors-Wallis, D. H. Gath, A. R. Lloyd-Thomas, and D. Tomlinson, "Randomised controlled trial comparing problem solving treatment with amitriptyline and placebo for major depression in primary care," *British Medical Journal*, vol. 310, no. 6977, pp. 441–445, 1995.
[11] T. E. Oxman, M. T. Hegel, J. G. Hull, and A. J. Dietrich, "Problem-solving treatment and coping styles in primary care for minor depression," *Journal of Consulting and Clinical Psychology*, vol. 76, no. 6, pp. 933–943, 2008.
[12] P. A. Arean, M. Hegel, S. Vannoy, M. Y. Fan, and J. Unuzter, "Effectiveness of problem-solving therapy for older, primary care patients with depression: results from the IMPACT project," *Gerontologist*, vol. 48, no. 3, pp. 311–323, 2008.
[13] M. T. Hegel and P. A. Arean, "Problem-solving Treatment for Primary Care (PST-PC): A Treatment Manual for Depression," 2003, http://impact-uw.org/tools/pst_manual.html .
[14] M. T. Hegel, J. Imming, M. Cyr-Provost, P. H. Noel, P. A. Arean, and J. Unutzer, "Role of behavioral health professionals in a collaborative stepped care treatment model for depression in primary care: project IMPACT," *Families, Systems and Health*, vol. 20, no. 3, pp. 265–277, 2002.
[15] D. A. Eckerman, C. A. Lundeen, A. Steele, H. L. Fercho, T. A. Ammerman, and W. K. Anger, "Interactive training versus reading to teach respiratory protection," *Journal of Occupational Health Psychology*, vol. 7, no. 4, pp. 313–323, 2002.
[16] R. E. Mayer, "The promise of multimedia learning: using the same instructional design methods across different media," *Learning and Instruction*, vol. 13, no. 2, pp. 125–139, 2003.
[17] R. E. Mayer, G. T. Dow, and S. Mayer, "Multimedia learning in an interactive self-explaining environment: what works in the design of agent-based microworlds?" *Journal of Educational Psychology*, vol. 95, no. 4, pp. 806–813, 2003.
[18] H. H. Teo, L. B. Oh, C. Liu, and K. K. Wei, "An empirical study of the effects of interactivity on web user attitude," *International Journal of Human Computer Studies*, vol. 58, no. 3, pp. 281–305, 2003.
[19] J. A. Carter, J. C. Buckey, L. Greenhalgh, A. W. Holland, and M. T. Hegel, "An interactive media program for managing psychosocial problems on long-duration spaceflights," *Aviation Space and Environmental Medicine*, vol. 76, no. 6, pp. B213–B223, 2005.
[20] D. F. Peck, "The therapist-client relationship, computerized self-help and active therapy ingredients," *Clinical Psychology and Psychotherapy*, vol. 17, no. 2, pp. 147–153, 2010.
[21] K. Kroenke and R. L. Spitzer, "The PHQ-9: a new depression diagnostic and severity measure," *Psychiatric Annals*, vol. 32, no. 9, pp. 509–515, 2002.
[22] T. T. Hewett, "Importance of failure analysis for human-computer interface design," *Interacting with Computers*, vol. 3, no. 1, pp. 3–8, 1991.
[23] S. I. Nishida, *Failure Analysis in Engineering Applications, Materials and Corrosion*, vol. 43, Butterworth-Heinemann, Oxford, UK, 1992.
[24] A. Sutcliffe and G. Rugg, "A taxonomy of error types for failure analysis and risk assessment," *Plastics, Rubber and Composites Processing and Applications*, vol. 10, no. 4, pp. 381–405, 1998.
[25] M. T. Hegel, J. E. Barrett, and T. E. Oxman, "Training therapists in problem-solving treatment of depressive disorders in primary care: lessons learned from the 'treatment effectiveness project'," *Families, Systems and Health*, vol. 18, no. 4, pp. 423–435, 2000.
[26] M. T. Hegel, A. J. Dietrich, J. L. Seville, and C. B. Jordan, "Training residents in problem-solving treatment of depression: a pilot feasibility and impact study," *Family Medicine*, vol. 36, no. 3, pp. 204–208, 2004.
[27] L. M. Larson, L. A. Suzuki, K. N. Gillespie, M. T. Potenza, M. A. Bechtel, and A. L. Toulouse, "Development and validation of the counseling self-estimate inventory," *Journal of Counseling Psychology*, vol. 39, no. 1, pp. 105–120, 1992.
[28] A. Bangor, P. T. Kortum, and J. T. Miller, "An empirical evaluation of the system usability scale," *International Journal of Human-Computer Interaction*, vol. 24, no. 6, pp. 574–594, 2008.
[29] J. Brooke, "SUS: a quick and dirty usability scale," in *Usability Evaluation in Industry*, P. W. Jordan et al., Ed., pp. 189–194, Taylor & Francis, London, UK, 1996.
[30] M. Kenwright, S. Liness, and I. Marks, "Reducing demands on clinicians by offering computer-aided self-help for phobia/panic. Feasibility study," *British Journal of Psychiatry*, vol. 179, pp. 456–459, 2001.
[31] L. Gega, I. J. Norman, and I. M. Marks, "Computer-aided vs. tutor-delivered teaching of exposure therapy for phobia/panic: randomized controlled trial with pre-registration nursing students," *International Journal of Nursing Studies*, vol. 44, no. 3, pp. 397–405, 2007.
[32] M. McDonough and I. M. Marks, "Teaching medical students exposure therapy for phobia/panic—randomized, controlled comparison of face-to-face tutorial in small groups vs. solo computer instruction," *Medical Education*, vol. 36, no. 5, pp. 412–417, 2002.
[33] R. S. Beidas and P. C. Kendall, "Training therapists in evidence-based practice: a critical review of studies from a systems-contextual perspective," *Clinical Psychology*, vol. 17, no. 1, pp. 1–30, 2010.
[34] L. A. H. Erby, D. L. Roter, and B. B. Biesecker, "Examination of standardized patient performance: accuracy and consistency of six standardized patients over time," *Patient Education and Counseling*, vol. 85, no. 2, pp. 194–200, 2011.
[35] M. Shirazi, M. Sadeghi, A. Emami et al., "Training and validation of standardized patients for unannounced assessment of physicians' management of depression," *Academic Psychiatry*, vol. 35, no. 6, pp. 382–387, 2011.
[36] The National Network of Depression Centers, "About Us, The National Network of Depression Centers, Ann Arbor, MI," 2012, http://www.nndc.org/about-us .
[37] University of Washington, "IMPACT Evidence-based Depression Care, Seattle, WA: University of Washington," 2011, http://impact-uw.org/.
[38] Harborview Medical Center, "PEARLS: Together We Create Active and Rewarding Lives, Seattle, WA: Harborview Medical Center," 2011, http://www.pearlsprogram.org/ .
[39] Institute for Clinical Systems Improvement, "DIAMOND, Bloomington, MN: Institute for Clinical Systems Improvement," 2011, http://www.icsi.org/health_care_redesign_/diamond_35953/.

14

Psychometric Properties of the Attitudes toward Self-Revised in Italian Young Adults

Marco Innamorati,[1,2,3] Stella Tamburello,[1,2] Anna Contardi,[1,2] Claudio Imperatori,[1] Antonino Tamburello,[1,2] Aristide Saggino,[3] and Michela Balsamo[3]

[1] *Università Europea di Roma, 00163 Rome, Italy*
[2] *Istituto Skinner, 00184 Rome, Italy*
[3] *DISPUTer, Dipartimento di Scienze Psicologiche, Umanistiche e del Territorio, "G. d'Annunzio" University, 66100 Chieti, Italy*

Correspondence should be addressed to Michela Balsamo; michela.balsamo@libero.it

Academic Editor: Klaus Ebmeier

Objectives and Methods. Several researchers have provided support for the critical role of cognitive vulnerabilities in the development of depression. The Attitudes toward Self-Revised (ATS-R) was designed to assess three potential self-regulatory vulnerabilities to depression: High Standards (HS), Self-Criticism (SC), and Negative Generalization (NG). The aim of the study was to assess the psychometric properties of the ATS-R in the Italian young adult population. The ATS-R, the Beck Depression Inventory-II (BDI-II), the Beck Hopelessness Scale (BHS), and the Teate Depression Inventory (TDI) were administered to 857 (320 men and 537 women) young adults. *Results.* The best-fitting solution for the ATS-R was a 2-factor model, which obtained satisfactory homogeneity of content (HS/SC: Cronbach $\alpha = 0.81$; mean interitem correlation = 0.46. NG: Cronbach $\alpha = 0.75$; mean interitem correlation = 0.43) and significant correlation with the BDI-II (NG: Pearson $r = 0.29$, $P < 0.01$), the TDI (HS/SC: Pearson $r = -0.26$, $P < 0.01$), and the BHS (HS/SC: Pearson $r = -0.29$, $P < 0.01$; NG: Pearson $r = 0.22$, $P < 0.01$). *Conclusions.* The Italian version of the ATS-R seems to be a valid instrument for the study of the role of cognitive tendencies as potential vulnerability for depression.

1. Introduction

Depression involves a wide variety of pathological conditions which vary along a continuum from more mild to more severe and persistent forms, such as major depressive disorder (MDD). MDD is the most widespread psychiatric disorder in the world [1–4], although its prevalence differs between countries around the world [5].

At the end of the eighties, the Epidemiological Catchment Area (ECA) study investigated the prevalence of MDD in the US general population and reported 30-day prevalence rates ranging between 1.7% and 3.4% [6]. More recently, the National Comorbidity Survey Replication (NCS-R) estimated a 12-month prevalence of 6.6% [7]. In Italy, the European study on the Epidemiology of Mental Disorders (ESEMeD) estimated rates of 3.0% and 10.0%, respectively, for the 12-month and lifetime MDD prevalence [8].

MDD is one of the major causes of disability, currently estimated as the fourth cause for the global burden of diseases [9, 10], and expected to become the second one within the year 2020 [9].

Numerous etiological models have been proposed and studied to explain how individuals become depressed. Cognitive theories of depression postulate that the dysfunctional interpretation of a life event may lead the individual to be vulnerable to depression following the occurrence of the stressful event. The most renowned cognitive theories of depression are the hopelessness theory [11] and the Beck's theory [12, 13]. Abramson et al. [11] focused on three maladaptive depressogenic inferential styles which predispose individuals to the development of depression: (1) the tendency to attribute negative events to global and stable causes; (2) the tendency to perceive negative events as having many disastrous consequences; and (3) the tendency to view the self as flawed or deficient following negative events. Beck [12, 13] hypothesized that depressed people have unrealistical and dysfunctional beliefs about the self, the world, and the future, a set of faulty cognitive processes known as the "cognitive triad."

Several researches have provided support for the critical role of cognitive vulnerability (i.e., a trait-like tendency to interpret information in negative and distorted ways in face of subjectively perceived stressful events [14]) in the development of depressive disorders [15–18]. For example, Evans et al. [18] found that holding a negative self-schema is an independent risk factor for the onset of depression in women, whereas Alloy et al. [16] reported that a negative inferential style increases the risk for the initial onset and recurrence of depressive episodes.

According to Carver and Ganellen [19], self-punitiveness is a salient feature of depression, associated with the holding of overly high standards, the tendency to be too critical with the self for failing to attain a standard, and the tendency to generalize from a single failure to the broader sense of self-worth. In order to confirm their hypothesis and to assess the relationship among these three processes and depression, the authors developed the Attitudes toward Self (ATS). The ATS was composed of 18 items divided into three subscales: Negative Generalization, High Standards, and Self-Criticism. In 1988, the authors elaborated a revised version of the measure (ATS-R) with a reduced number of items, focusing more explicitly on the cognitive tendencies than the original items [20]. Several studies indicated that, among the three tendencies, negative generalization was the only one reliably related to depression and mediating the relationship between life events and depression [20, 21] and between negative events and self-esteem [22]. Studies constantly indicated that homogeneity of content of the three factors was sufficient (Cronbach alpha > 0.70), except for self-criticism [20–24].

This analysis of the literature suggests the importance to assess cognitive vulnerabilities (CV) to depression and the utility of the ATS-R in measuring three tendencies potentially associated with a higher risk to develop depression. Thus, the aim of the study was to assess the psychometric properties of the ATS-R [20] in the Italian young adult population.

2. Materials and Methods

2.1. Participants. Participants were 857 (320 men and 537 women) Italian young adults recruited between January 2011 and May 2011 in Central Italy. Mean age of the sample was 22.41 years (SD = 4.36; range: 18–34 years). Inclusion criteria included age between 18 and 34 years and the ability to read and write in Italian. Exclusion criteria included the presence of any condition affecting the ability to complete the assessment, including illiteracy and denial of informed consent.

The sample was nonrandomly recruited through attendants of adult education classes and advertisement posted to established community groups. More than 89% of the respondents had completed high school at the time of the assessment, and 55.5% of them were university students. Educational attainment in our sample was higher than the national average (according to the National Institute of Statistics (http://www.istat.it/) in Central Italy around 80% of people 20–24 years old complete secondary school, and 40% of people 19–25 years old attend university), and our sample should not be considered representative of the Italian young adult population.

All participants took part voluntarily in the study, gave informed consent, and completed the assessment anonymously.

2.2. Measures. All participants were administered the ATS-R, the BDI-II, the Teate Depression Inventory (TDI) [25], and the Beck Hopelessness Scale (BHS) [26]. The assessment protocol was self-administered; the questionnaires were delivered to participants in a group setting or individually and completed in the presence of a researcher, who possibly helped with the compilation.

The ATS-R [20] is a 10-item scale measuring three potential self-regulatory vulnerabilities to depression (holding overly high standards, the tendency to be self-critical at any failure to perform well, and the tendency to generalize from a single failure to the broader sense of self-worth). Compared to the previous version [27] ATS-R is characterized by new items focused more explicitly on the cognitive tendencies than the originals, and its shortness reflects the straightforwardness of each cognitive tendency [21, 23].

Respondents are asked to rate the degree to which they agree/disagree with each statement on a 5-point Likert-type scale (ranging from "*I agree a lot*" to "*I disagree a lot*"). The Italian version of the ATS-R was translated from the original English version into Italian by two authors of the present study (Marco Innamorati and Michela Balsamo); then, the Italian version was independently and blindly back-translated by a native English speaking researcher.

The BDI-II is a well-known self-report inventory composed of 21 items designed to assess the presence and severity of depressive symptoms, according to DSM-IV [28] criteria. Respondents endorse specific statements reflecting their feelings over the last two weeks, including today. Each statement is rated on a 4-point Likert-type scale ranging from 0 to 3, based on the severity of depressive symptoms. Importantly, the extensive literature has supported the psychometric properties of the scale in clinical and nonclinical samples [29, 30]. In the current study, Cronbach alpha index was 0.87.

The BHS is a 20-item scale for measuring negative attitudes about the future [26]. When responding to the 20 true-false items on the BHS, individuals either endorse a pessimistic statement or deny an optimistic statement. Research has consistently supported a positive significant relationship between BHS scores and measures of depression, suicidal intent, and suicidal ideation [31–35]. Studies on the Italian population have been carried out successfully [36] and have led to validation of the scale [37]. In the present study, Cronbach alpha was 0.84.

The TDI is a new 21-item self-report instrument designed to assess the *Diagnostic and Statistical Manual of Mental Disorders*, fourth edition, text revision (DSM-IV-TR) [28], criteria for major depression [25]. It was developed via Rasch logistic analysis of responses [38, 39], in order to overcome psychometric inherent weaknesses of existing measures of depression [30]. Each item is rated on a 5-point Likert-type scale ranging from 0 (always) to 4 (never). The total score ranges from 0 to 84, with higher scores indicating more severe depressive symptoms. In the standardization samples, the TDI displayed very good psychometric properties (with an excellent Person separation index, equal to 0.95), no evidence of bias due to item-trait interaction, high sensitivity and specificity, and control of major response sets [25]. In our study, Cronbach's alpha was 0.92. Pearson r for the correlation between the TDI and the BDI-II was 0.65 ($P < 0.01$).

2.3. Statistical Analysis. We used Velicer's Minimum Average Partial (MAP) test [40, 41] and structural equation modeling (SEM) to determine the factor model which best fitted the data.

The Velicer's MAP test has been proposed as a rule to find the best solution in exploratory factor analysis. It is accurate under many conditions, although, under certain conditions, it may have a tendency to underestimate the number of factors [42]. SEM was performed with a Robust Diagonally Weighted Least Squares Estimator (DWLSE) on a polychoric correlational matrix using the statistical package Lisrel 8.8 [43]. We evaluated the fit of the model by means of the following indexes: (a) the Root Mean Square Error of Approximation (RMSEA) [44, 45]; (b) the Incremental Comparative Fit Index (CFI) [45]; (c) the Satorra-Bentler scaled chi-square (SB χ^2); and (d) the Standardized Root Mean Square Residual (SRMSR) [45]. In the design and planning phase, we set a target recruitment size of 800 participants, greater than the standard of 10 participants per parameter estimated and a minimum of 300 participants reported in the literature [46, 47]. This sample size was set to have adequate power to have stability of the factorial solution.

According to the results from the SEM and the Velicer's MAP test, we performed an exploratory factor analysis using ordinary least squares to find minimum residual (MINRES). We used an oblique rotation method (ProMAX) because we expected that the ATS-R factors are correlated.

We reported Cronbach alphas, interitem mean correlations, and corrected item-total indices (i.e., discrimination indices) for the best-fitting factor model. Also, the convergent validity of the ATS-R with the BDI-II and the BHS was investigated by means of Pearson correlation coefficients. To test whether scores on the ATS-R dimensions were independently associated with depressive severity, we performed a generalized linear model with the BDI-II as dependent variable and the ATS-R factors and the BHS as independent variables. We reported odds ratio and their 95% confidence interval (CI) as indices of association. In addition, multivariate general linear model (GLM) was used to assess whether scores on the ATS-R factors were associated with the respondent's sex.

3. Results

3.1. Depression and Hopelessness Severity. One hundred twelve respondents (13.1% of the sample) had scores of 20 and higher on the BDI-II, indicative of moderate to severe depression, and 136 respondents (15.9% of the sample) had scores between 14 and 19, indicative of mild depression. Finally, 29.7% of the respondents reported scores of 9 or higher on the BHS, indicating severe hopelessness.

3.2. Factorial Validity. The Velicer's MAP test indicated that the best number of factors to extract was two. Furthermore, the three factor model proposed by Carver et al. [20] had poor fit (SB $\chi^2_{32} = 321.04$; $P < 0.01$; RMSEA = 0.10; 90% CI for RMSEA = 0.093/0.11; CFI = 0.94; SRMR = 0.075).

As a result, we performed a MINRES factor analysis which indicated that items no. 1, no. 3, no. 4, no. 6, and no. 7 load on the first factor ("High Standards/Self-Criticism"), while items no. 2, no. 8, no. 9, and no. 10 load on the second factor ("Negative Generalization") (see Table 1). The item no. 5, which originally was included in the Negative Generalization factor, did not load on any factor, while items no. 3, no. 6, and no. 9, which originally were included in the Self-Criticism factor, loaded sparsely on the "High Standards/Self-Criticism" (items no. 3, no. 6) and Negative Generalization (item no. 9) factors.

3.3. Reliability and Convergent Validity. Factors had satisfactory homogeneity of content (High Standards/Self-Criticism: Cronbach $\alpha = 0.81$; mean interitem correlation = 0.46. Negative Generalization: Cronbach $\alpha = 0.75$; mean interitem correlation = 0.43) (see Table 1) and correlated significantly with the BHS (High Standards/Self-Criticism: Pearson $r = -0.29$; $P < 0.01$. Negative Generalization: Pearson $r = 0.22$; $P < 0.01$). The pattern of correlations with measures of depression was less clear: Negative Generalization correlated significantly with the BDI-II (Pearson $r = 0.29$; $P < 0.01$), and nonsignificantly with the TDI (Negative Generalization: Pearson $r = 0.01$; $P = 0.99$), while High Standards/Self-Criticism correlated significantly with the TDI (Pearson $r = -0.26$; $P < 0.01$) and nonsignificantly with the BDI-II (Pearson $r = 0.01$; $P = 0.67$).

The GLM indicated that both the ATS-R factors were independently associated with the BDI-II even when controlling for the severity of hopelessness. Young adults with higher depressive symptoms severity were (1) 1.23 times more likely to have higher High Standards/Self-Criticism scores (95% confidence interval: 1.08/1.39; $P < 0.01$); (2) 1.36 times more likely to have higher Negative Generalization scores (95% confidence interval: 1.17/1.58; $P < 0.001$); and (3) 2.66 times more likely to have higher BHS scores (95% confidence interval: 2.28/3.11; $P < 0.001$).

The GLM analysis indicated that sex had a significant effect (Wilks $\lambda = 0.97$; $P < 0.001$): men and women differed for High Standards/Self-Criticism mean scores (17.78 ± 3.99 and 16.38 ± 5.02, resp., for males and females; $F = 18.08$; $P < 0.001$) but not for Negative Generalization scores (11.29 ± 3.80 and 11.78 ± 4.09, resp., for males and females; $F = 3.01$; $P = 0.08$).

4. Discussion

Our results indicated that the three-factor solution obtained by Carver et al. [20] did not fit well the structure of the

TABLE 1: Factor loadings and reliability indices.

	Factor loadings	Corrected item-total correlation	Cronbach's alpha if item deleted
High Standards/Self-Criticism			
ATS-R no. 1	0.77	0.62	0.77
ATS-R no. 3	0.61	0.63	0.77
ATS-R no. 4	0.76	0.56	0.79
ATS-R no. 6	0.62	0.64	0.76
ATS-R no. 7	0.69	0.54	0.79
Cronbach $\alpha = 0.81$; mean interitem correlation = 0.46			
Negative Generalization			
ATS-R no. 2	0.77	0.58	0.68
ATS-R no. 8	0.61	0.51	0.71
ATS-R no. 9	0.52	0.46	0.74
ATS-R no. 10	0.85	0.64	0.64
Cronbach $\alpha = 0.75$; mean interitem correlation = 0.43			

Italian version of the ATS-R. In our sample of Italian young adults, the ATS-R seems to measure two self-regulatory attitudes toward the self: the tendency to generalize from a single failure to a broader sense of personal inadequacy ("Negative Generalization") and one dimension assessing the tendency to hold overly high standards and to be self-critical ("High Standards/Self-Criticism"). Furthermore, the pattern of loadings was partly discordant from that reported by Carver et al. [20]. Nonetheless, the pattern of loadings resulting from the factor analysis is consistent with the results reported by Carver [21]: in their research, the authors reported that Self-Criticism was significantly associated with the dimensions High Standards ($r = 0.33$; $P < 0.01$) and Negative Generalization ($r = 0.52$; $P < 0.01$), while the High Standards factor was almost unrelated to Negative Generalization ($r = 0.05$; $P =$ n.s.) factor. In fact, in our sample, Negative Generalization and High Standards resulted in two independent factors, while the items originally loading on Self-Criticism loaded sparsely on the two remaining factors.

Our findings about the convergent validity of the ATS-R are only partially consistent with those reported by Carver et al. [20] and Carver [21]. While in the bivariate analyses, only the dimension of Negative Generalization correlated significantly with depression as measured with the BDI-II; at the multivariate level also the dimension High Standards/Self-Criticism resulted independently associated with depression, and not only the BHS and the Negative Generalization factor. These results suggest that a tendency to generalize from a single failure to a broader sense of personal inadequacy, a pessimistic view of the future, the holding of overly high standards, and the tendency to be self-critical are all important in the phenomenology of depression. However, there could be some differences between sexes. For example, while male and female Italian young adults did not differ in their tendency to generalize from a single failure to a broader sense of personal inadequacy, male young adults reported to hold more overly high standards and the tendency to be more self-critical at any failure to perform well. Furthermore, the effect sizes of the correlations between Negative Generalization, hopelessness, and depression were stronger in men than in women. This is discordant with Carver [21], who investigated the role of the ATS-R dimensions as prospective predictors of depressive symptoms in 336 US undergraduates. In their sample, the author reported that women had higher tendency toward Negative Generalization than did men, but the groups did not differ for the tendency to be self-critical or the holding of overly high standards. However, the author did not investigate whether the size of the associations between the ATS-R dimensions and depression may differ between sexes.

Reliability indices for the ATS-R factors were satisfactory but not good (Cronbach alphas between 0.75 and 0.81), due to a good homogeneity of content (mean interitem correlation >0.40 for both the factors), but the low number of items included in each factor. For Carver et al. [20], the brevity of the scale is a strength of the ATS-R, reflecting the fact that the essence of the cognitive tendencies measured with the ATS-R is "relatively straightforward." However, from a psychometric point of view, scale's brevity might be a limitation for the use of the instrument in clinical settings [48].

Our findings have some limitations in their generalizability. First, we examined cognitive diatheses for depression in a sample of young adults recruited from the general population, a population in which the level of depression is generally low. Second, we used only self-report measures potentially biased by social desirability. Third, we did not assess other important psychometric characteristics of the ATS-R, such as the test-retest reliability. On the other hand, to our knowledge, this is the first study examining psychometric properties of the ATS-R in a sample of Italian young adults.

In conclusion, the Italian version of the ATS-R seems to be a valid instrument for the study of the role of cognitive tendencies as potential diathesis in the development of depression. Further research is needed to verify whether the psychometric properties and the factor structure of the ATS-R obtained in our sample are also replicable in clinical samples and in samples of adolescents and older adults.

Conflict of Interests

The authors declare that they have no conflict of interests for this research.

Authors' Contribution

All authors have made substantial contributions to conception and design or acquisition of data or analysis and interpretation of data, have been involved in drafting the paper or revising it critically for important intellectual content, and have given final approval of the version to be published.

References

[1] D. S. Hasin, R. D. Goodwin, F. S. Stinson, and B. F. Grant, "Epidemiology of major depressive disorder: results from the National Epidemiologic Survey on Alcoholism and Related Conditions," *Archives of General Psychiatry*, vol. 62, no. 10, pp. 1097–1106, 2005.

[2] C. Blanco, M. Okuda, J. C. Markowitz, S.-M. Liu, B. F. Grant, and D. S. Hasin, "The epidemiology of chronic major depressive disorder and dysthymic disorder: results from the national epidemiologic survey on alcohol and related conditions," *Journal of Clinical Psychiatry*, vol. 71, no. 12, pp. 1645–1656, 2010.

[3] V. Lehtinen and M. Joukamaa, "Epidemiology of depression: prevalence, risk factors and treatment situation," *Acta Psychiatrica Scandinavica*, vol. 89, no. 377, pp. 7–10, 1994.

[4] M. M. Ohayon, "Epidemiology of depression and its treatment in the general population," *Journal of Psychiatric Research*, vol. 41, no. 3-4, pp. 207–213, 2007.

[5] M. M. Weissman, R. C. Bland, G. J. Canino et al., "Cross-national epidemiology of major depression and bipolar disorder," *Journal of the American Medical Association*, vol. 276, no. 4, pp. 293–299, 1996.

[6] D. A. Regier, J. H. Boyd, J. D. Burke Jr. et al., "One-month prevalence of mental disorders in the United States, based on five epidemiologic catchment area sites," *Archives of General Psychiatry*, vol. 45, no. 11, pp. 977–986, 1988.

[7] R. C. Kessler, P. Berglund, O. Demler et al., "The epidemiology of major depressive disorder: results from the National Comorbidity Survey Replication (NCS-R)," *Journal of the American Medical Association*, vol. 289, no. 23, pp. 3095–3105, 2003.

[8] G. de Girolamo, G. Polidori, P. Morosini et al., "La prevalenza dei disturbi mentali in italia. Il progetto ESEMED-WMH," Una sintesi. Roma: Centro Nazionale di Epidemiologia, Sorveglianza e Promozione della Salute, 2005.

[9] World Health Organisation, "Depression. What is depression?" World Health Organisation, Geneva, Switzerland, 2011, http://www.who.int/mental_health/management/depression/definition/en/index1.html.

[10] T. B. Üstün, J. L. Ayuso-Mateos, S. Chatterji, C. Mathers, and C. J. L. Murray, "Global burden of depressive disorders in the year 2000," *British Journal of Psychiatry*, vol. 184, pp. 386–392, 2004.

[11] L. Y. Abramson, G. I. Metalsky, and L. B. Alloy, "Hopelessness depression: a theory-based subtype of depression," *Psychological Review*, vol. 96, no. 2, pp. 358–372, 1989.

[12] A. T. Beck, *Depression: Clinical, Experimental, and Theoretical Aspects*, Harper & Row, New York, NY, USA, 1967.

[13] A. T. Beck, "Cognitive models of depression," *Journal of Cognitive Psychotherapy*, vol. 1, pp. 5–37, 1987.

[14] M. Zhong, X. Wang, J. Xiao et al., "Amygdala hyperactivation and prefrontal hypoactivation in subjects with cognitive vulnerability to depression," *Biological Psychology*, vol. 88, no. 2-3, pp. 233–242, 2011.

[15] L. Y. Abramson, L. B. Alloy, B. L. Hankin et al., "Cognitive vulnerability-stress models of depression in a self-regulatory and psychobiological context," in *Handbook of Depression*, I. H. Gotlib and C. L. Hammen, Eds., pp. 268–294, The Guilford Press, New York, NY, USA, 2002.

[16] L. B. Alloy, L. Y. Abramson, W. G. Whitehouse, M. E. Hogan, C. Panzarella, and D. T. Rose, "Prospective incidence of first onsets and recurrences of depression in individuals at high and low cognitive risk for depression," *Journal of Abnormal Psychology*, vol. 115, no. 1, pp. 145–156, 2006.

[17] B. M. Iacoviello, L. B. Alloy, L. Y. Abramson, W. G. Whitehouse, and M. E. Hogan, "The course of depression in individuals at high and low cognitive risk for depression: a prospective study," *Journal of Affective Disorders*, vol. 93, no. 1–3, pp. 61–69, 2006.

[18] J. Evans, J. Heron, G. Lewis, R. Araya, and D. Wolke, "Negative self-schemas and the onset of depression in women: longitudinal study," *British Journal of Psychiatry*, vol. 186, pp. 302–307, 2005.

[19] C. S. Carver and R. J. Ganellen, "Depression and components of self-punitiveness: high standards, self-criticism, and overgeneralization," *Journal of Abnormal Psychology*, vol. 92, no. 3, pp. 330–337, 1983.

[20] C. S. Carver, L. La Voie, J. Kuhl et al., "Cognitive concomitants of depression: a further examination of the roles of generalization, high standards, and self-criticism," *Journal of Social and Clinical Psychology*, vol. 7, pp. 350–365, 1988.

[21] C. S. Carver, "Generalization, adverse events, and development of depressive symptoms," *Journal of Personality*, vol. 66, no. 4, pp. 606–619, 1998.

[22] A. M. Hayes, M. S. Harris, and C. S. Carver, "Predictors of self-esteem variability," *Cognitive Therapy and Research*, vol. 28, no. 3, pp. 369–385, 2004.

[23] L. R. Eisner, S. L. Johnson, and C. S. Carver, "Cognitive responses to failure and success relate uniquely to bipolar depression versus mania," *Journal of Abnormal Psychology*, vol. 117, no. 1, pp. 154–163, 2008.

[24] C. S. Carver and S. L. Johnson, "Tendencies toward mania and tendencies toward depression have distinct motivational, affective, and cognitive correlates," *Cognitive Therapy and Research*, vol. 33, no. 6, pp. 552–569, 2009.

[25] M. Balsamo and A. Saggino, *Il Teate Depression Inventory—Manuale di Standardizzazione*, Hoegrefe, Berne, Germany.

[26] A. T. Beck, A. Weissman, D. Lester, and L. Trexler, "The measurement of pessimism: the hopelessness scale," *Journal of Consulting and Clinical Psychology*, vol. 42, no. 6, pp. 861–865, 1974.

[27] C. S. Carver, R. J. Ganellen, and V. Behar-Mitrani, "Depression and cognitive style. Comparisons between measures," *Journal of Personality and Social Psychology*, vol. 49, no. 3, pp. 722–728, 1985.

[28] American Psychiatric Association, *Diagnostic and Statistical Manual of Mental Disorders*, American Psychiatric Association, Washington, DC, USA, 4th edition, 2000.

[29] P. A. Arbisi, "Review of the beck depression inventory-II," in *The 14th Mental Measurements Yearbook*, B. S. Plake and J. C. Impara, Eds., Buros Institute of Mental Measurements, Lincoln, Neb, USA, 2001.

[30] M. Balsamo and A. Saggino, "Test per l'assessment della depressione nel contesto italiano: un'analisi critica," *Psicoterapia Cognitiva e Comportamentaie*, vol. 13, pp. 167–199, 2007.

[31] A. T. Beck, G. Brown, R. J. Berchick, B. L. Stewart, and R. A. Steer, "Relationship between hopelessness and ultimate suicide: a replication with psychiatric outpatients," *American Journal of Psychiatry*, vol. 147, no. 2, pp. 190–195, 1990.

[32] E. David Klonsky, R. Kotov, S. Bakst, J. Rabinowitz, and E. J. Bromet, "Hopelessness as a predictor of attempted suicide among first admission patients with psychosis: a 10-year cohort study," *Suicide and Life-Threatening Behavior*, vol. 42, no. 1, pp. 1–10, 2012.

[33] M. Bouvard, S. Charles, J. Guerin, G. Aimard, and J. Cottraux, "Study of Beck's hopelessness scale. Validation and factor analysis," *L'Encephale*, vol. 18, no. 3, pp. 237–240, 1992.

[34] M. Innamorati, M. Pompili, X. Gonda et al., "Psychometric properties of the Gotland Scale for Depression in Italian psychiatric inpatients and its utility in the prediction of suicide risk," *Journal of Affective Disorders*, vol. 132, no. 1-2, pp. 99–103, 2011.

[35] M. Innamorati, M. Pompili, G. Serafini et al., "Psychometric properties of the suicidal history self-rating screening scale," *Archives of Suicide Research*, vol. 15, no. 1, pp. 87–92, 2011.

[36] M. Pompili, R. Tatarelli, J. R. Rogers, and D. Lester, "The hopelessness scale: a factor analysis," *Psychological Reports*, vol. 100, no. 2, pp. 375–378, 2007.

[37] M. Pompili, P. Iliceto, D. Lester et al., *BHS Beck Hopelessness Scale: Manuale*, Giunti O.S. Organizzazioni Speciali, Firenze, Italy, 2009.

[38] G. Rasch, *Probabilistic Models for Some Intelligence and Attainment Tests*, University of Chicago Press, Chicago, Ill, USA, 1980.

[39] D. Andrich, "Models for measurement, precision, and the nondichotomization of graded responses," *Psychometrika*, vol. 60, no. 1, pp. 7–26, 1995.

[40] B. P. O'Connor, "SPSS and SAS programs for determining the number of components using parallel analysis and Velicer's MAP test," *Behavior Research Methods, Instruments, and Computers*, vol. 32, no. 3, pp. 396–402, 2000.

[41] W. F. Velicer, "Determining the number of components from the matrix of partial correlations," *Psychometrika*, vol. 41, no. 3, pp. 321–327, 1976.

[42] R. D. Ledesma and P. Valero-Mora, "Determining the number of factors to retain in EFA: an easy-to-use computer program for carrying out Parallel Analysis," *Practical Assessment, Research & Evaluation*, vol. 12, pp. 1–11, 2007.

[43] K. G. Jöreskog and D. Sörbom, "LISREL for Windows [Computer software]," Lincolnwood, Ill, USA, Scientific Software International, 2006.

[44] M. W. Browne and R. Cudek, "Alternative ways of assessing model fit," in *Testing Structural Equation Models*, J. S. Long, Ed., pp. 136–162, Sage, Newbury Park, Calif, USA, 1993.

[45] L.-T. Hu and P. M. Bentler, "Cutoff criteria for fit indexes in covariance structure analysis: conventional criteria versus new alternatives," *Structural Equation Modeling*, vol. 6, no. 1, pp. 1–55, 1999.

[46] K. G. Joreskog and D. Sorbom, *LISREL 7: User's Reference Guide*, Scientific Software, Mooresville, Ind, USA, 1989.

[47] F. J. Floyd and K. F. Widaman, "Factor analysis in the development and refinement of clinical assessment instruments," *Psychological Assessment*, vol. 7, no. 3, pp. 286–299, 1995.

[48] J. C. Nunnally and I. H. Bernstein, *Psychometric Theory*, McGraw-Hill, New York, NY, USA, 3rd edition, 1994.

Cognitive Vulnerabilities and Depression in Young Adults

Michela Balsamo,[1] Claudio Imperatori,[2] Maria Rita Sergi,[1]
Martino Belvederi Murri,[3] Massimo Continisio,[2,4] Antonino Tamburello,[2,4]
Marco Innamorati,[1,2,4] and Aristide Saggino[1]

[1] *DISPUTer, Dipartimento di Scienze Psicologiche, Umanistiche e del Territorio, "G. d'Annunzio" University, 66100 Chieti, Italy*
[2] *Università Europea di Roma, 00163 Rome, Italy*
[3] *Division of Psychiatry, Department of Neurosciences, University of Parma, 43100 Parma, Italy*
[4] *Istituto Skinner, 00184 Rome, Italy*

Correspondence should be addressed to Michela Balsamo; michela.balsamo@libero.it

Academic Editor: H. Grunze

Objectives and Methods. The aim of the present study was to evaluate, by means of receiver operating characteristic (ROC) curves, whether cognitive vulnerabilities (CV), as measured by three well-known instruments (the Beck Hopelessness Scale, BHS; the Life Orientation Test-Revised, LOT-R; and the Attitudes Toward Self-Revised, ATS-R), independently discriminate between subjects with different severities of depression. Participants were 467 young adults (336 females and 131 males), recruited from the general population. The subjects were also administered the Beck Depression Inventory-II (BDI-II). *Results.* Four first-order (BHS Optimism/Low Standard; BHS Pessimism; Generalized Self-Criticism; and LOT Optimism) and two higher-order factors (Pessimism/Negative Attitudes Toward Self, Optimism) were extracted using Principal Axis Factoring analysis. Although all first-order and second-order factors were able to discriminate individuals with different depression severities, the Pessimism factor had the best performance in discriminating individuals with moderate to severe depression from those with lower depression severity. *Conclusion.* In the screening of young adults at risk of depression, clinicians have to pay particular attention to the expression of pessimism about the future.

1. Introduction

Major depressive disorder (MDD) is one of the most widespread psychiatric disorder [1–4] and the leading cause of disability as measured by years lived with disability (YLDs) [5–9]. Currently, MDD is estimated to be the fourth leading cause of global disease burden [10, 11], and, by the year 2020, it is projected to reach the second place in the ranking of the major causes of Disability Adjusted Life Years (DALYs). Today, depression is already the second cause of DALYs in the age category 15–44 years [11]. The estimated 12-month prevalence of MDD was 6.6% in the USA [12] and 3.0% in Italy [13].

Many approaches have been taken in attempts to explain the origins of depression [14]. Whereas some of these theories involved genetics and biological functioning, other approaches focused on the study of personal characteristics of individuals who are believed to be vulnerable to experiencing depressive episodes. A large body of research examining cognitive models of vulnerability for depression hypothesized that the way the individual interprets his/her experiences represents a protective or risk factor for the development of depressive disorders when negative stressful life events occur [15]. Depressed people engage in prolonged and repetitive thinking about the self, the world, and the future in a negative way with detrimental effects on mood [16–18]. Cognitive vulnerability (CV) for depression may be defined as a trait-like tendency to interpret information in a negative and distorted way when facing a subjectively perceived stressful event [19]. The literature indicated that CV may play a crucial role in the development and maintenance of depressive disorders not only in adulthood but also in childhood and adolescence (for a review see [20]).

Despite similarities, currently there are several different theories which hypothesize the cognitive processes to be a diathesis for the development of depressive disorders. Two of the most renowned theories are the hopelessness theory [21] and Beck's theory [22, 23]. According to the hopelessness theory, three kinds of maladaptive inferences that people may make when confronted with negative events contribute to the development of hopelessness and, in turn, depressive symptoms: causal attributions, inferred consequences, and inferred characteristics about the self. Hopelessness and depressive symptoms are likely to occur when negative life events are (1) attributed to stable (i.e., likely to persist over time) and global (i.e., likely to affect many areas of life) causes; (2) viewed as likely to lead to further negative consequences; and (3) construed as implying that the person is unworthy or deficient. Similarly, Beck [22, 23] and Beck et al. [24] hypothesized depressogenic self-schemata, activated by the occurrence of negative life events, that take the form of overly pessimistic views of the self, the world, and the future (the *negative cognitive triad*). Also, Carver and Ganellen [25] considered self-punitiveness as a salient feature of depression, associated with the holding of overly high standards, the tendency to be too critical with the self for failing to attain a standard, and the tendency to generalize from a single failure to the broader sense of self-worth. To measure these three potential self-regulatory vulnerabilities to depression, Carver and colleagues developed the Attitudes Toward Self (ATS).

Several researches have provided support for the critical role of CV in the origin and course of depressive disorders [26–30]. For example, Beckham et al. [26] reported that all the cognitive triad components are significantly associated with the severity of depressive symptoms in depressed patients. Evans et al. [28] indicated that holding a negative self-schema is an independent risk factor for the onset of depression in women. Furthermore, pessimistic views about the future have been found to be highly predictive of suicide behaviors [31, 32] and worse health and social functioning [33] in psychiatric patients. Again, in a longitudinal study, it was reported that undergraduate students with a more generalized negative cognitive style were 3.5–6.8 times more likely to report more depressive episodes compared to students with a less generalized negative cognitive style [29]. Some studies also indicated a partial overlap between the hopelessness and Beck's theories [34, 35].

Our literature review suggests that investigating the role of CV in the development of depression may be beneficial for a better understanding and treatment of depressive disorders. What is more is that research has failed to investigate the role of CV for depression in discriminating different levels of severity of depression. Thus, the aim of the present study was to evaluate, by means of ROC curves, whether some dimensions of CV for depression, as measured by three well-known instruments, that are the Beck Hopelessness Scale (BHS) [24], the Life Orientation Test-Revised (LOT-R) [36], and the Attitudes Toward Self-Revised (ATS-R) [37], discriminate independently between subjects with different severities of depression.

2. Materials and Methods

2.1. Participants. Participants were 467 young adults (131 males, 28.1%; 336 females, 71.9%). Mean age of the sample was 23.58 ± 5.03 years (range 18–39). Subjects were included if they had an age between 18 and 40 years old. Exclusion criteria were the presence of any condition affecting the ability to complete the assessment, including illiteracy and denial of informed consent.

All participants were nonrandomly recruited in Central Italy between February 2012 and June 2012. They accepted to participate voluntarily and gave their informed consent.

2.2. Measures. The Beck Depression Inventory-II (BDI-II) [38], the BHS, the LOT-R, and the ATS-R were administered to all subjects.

The BDI-II is a well-known self-report inventory composed of 21 items designed to assess the presence and severity of depressive symptoms, according to DSM-IV [39] criteria. Respondents endorse specific statements reflecting their feelings over the last two weeks, including today. Each statement is rated on a 4-point Likert-type scale ranging from 0 to 3, based on the severity of depressive symptoms. Importantly, extensive literature has supported the psychometric properties of the scale in clinical and nonclinical samples [40, 41]. In the current sample, Cronbach alpha was 0.86.

The BHS [24] is a 20-item scale for measuring the cognitive component of the depression. The scale assesses three major aspects of hopelessness: feelings about the future, loss of motivation, and expectations. Responding to the 20 true or false items, individuals have to either endorse a pessimistic statement or deny an optimistic statement. Research consistently have supported a positive relationship between BHS scores and measures of depression, suicidal intent, and current suicidal ideation [31, 42–44]. The Italian version of the BHS has reported good psychometric properties [45, 46].

The LOT-R is a 6-item scale measuring optimism: three items are positively worded (e.g., *"I'm always optimistic about my future"*), and the other three items are negatively worded (e.g., *"If something can go wrong for me, it will"*). Each item is rated on a five-point Likert-type scale (from 1—"I agree a lot"—to 5—"I disagree a lot"). Sum scores range between 6 and 30 with higher scores indicating higher optimism.

The ATS-R is a self-report measure designed to measure three potential self-regulatory vulnerabilities to depression. One of them is the holding of overly high standards, the second is the tendency to be self-critical at any failure to perform well, and the third is the tendency to generalize from a single failure to the broader sense of self-worth. The negative generalization scale has been found to be the dimension more strongly associated with depression [37, 47, 48]. Items are rated on a Likert-type scale, ranging from 1 (*"I agree a lot"*) to 5 (*"I disagree a lot"*). A study assessing the psychometric properties of the Italian version of the ATS-R has been recently published, indicating that

TABLE 1: Characteristics of the sample.

	%
Men	28.2
Age—M ± SD	23.59 ± 5.03
Job	
Employed	32.9
Students	63.7
Unemployed	3.4
Marital status	
Not married	87.8
Married	10.8
Divorced	1.4
Education	
5 years	0.6
8 years	12.3
13 years	72.0
16+ years	15.1
BDI-II—M ± SD	10.40 ± 8.36
BDI ≥ 20	12.5

the measure is a valid instrument for the study of the role of cognitive tendencies as potential diathesis in the development of depression [49].

2.3. Statistical Analysis. The BHS, LOT-R, and ATS-R items were subjected to Principal Axis Factoring in order to obtain common factors of vulnerability for depression. The number of latent factors to retain was selected using the scree test [50] and confirmed by means of Velicer's Minimum Average Partial (MAP) test [51]. Promax rotation with Kaiser Normalization was used in order to produce correlated factors. According to Kline [52], items were retained if they had a factor loading of 0.40 and higher and if they were loaded on a single factor. Then, factor scores for all subjects were calculated and used to assess the presence of possible higher-order factors.

A generalized linear model with robust estimator was used to assess independent associations between depression severity and factors of vulnerability for depression. Associations were reported as odds ratio and their 95% confidence intervals (95% CI).

In order to assess the performance of the dimensions of vulnerability for depression in categorizing individuals on the basis of depression severity, a series of ROC test procedures were performed [53].

All analyses were performed with the Statistical Package for the Social Sciences (SPSS 17.0 for Windows).

TABLE 2: Factor solution (Principal Factor Analysis, Promax rotation with Kaiser Normalization).

	Factor			
	BHS Optimism	BHS Pessimism	Generalized Self-Criticism	LOT Optimism
BHS no. 1	0.67	—	—	—
BHS no. 2	—	0.53	—	—
BHS no. 3	0.75	—	—	—
BHS no. 4	—	—	—	—
BHS no. 5	0.53	—	—	—
BHS no. 6	0.82	—	—	—
BHS no. 7	—	0.69	—	—
BHS no. 8	—	—	—	—
BHS no. 9	—	0.61	—	—
BHS no. 10	0.66	—	—	—
BHS no. 11	—	0.68	—	—
BHS no. 12	—	0.49	—	—
BHS no. 13	0.70	—	—	—
BHS no. 14	—	0.43	—	—
BHS no. 15	0.55		—	—
BHS no. 16	—	0.74	—	—
BHS no. 17	—	0.75	—	—
BHS no. 18	—	—	—	—
BHS no. 19	0.88		—	—
BHS no. 20	—	0.70	—	—
ATS no. 1	−0.74	—	—	—
ATS no. 2	—	—	0.69	—
ATS no. 3	−0.55	—	0.47	—
ATS no. 4	—	—	—	—
ATS no. 5	—	—	—	—
ATS no. 6	−0.50	—	0.53	—
ATS no. 7	—	—	—	—
ATS no. 8	—	—	0.66	—
ATS no. 9	—	—	0.62	—
ATS no. 10	—	—	0.75	—
LOT no. 1	—	—	—	−0.62
LOT no. 3	—	—	—	—
LOT no. 4	—	—	—	−0.69
LOT no. 7	—	—	—	—
LOT no. 9	—	—	—	—
LOT no. 10	—	—	—	−0.51
Cronbach alpha	0.84	0.84	0.78	0.70

Extraction method: Principal Axis Factoring. Rotation method: Promax with Kaiser Normalization.

3. Results

Descriptive statistics are listed in Table 1. The mean BDI-II score was 10.40 ± 8.36 (quartiles [25°/50°/75°]: 4/9/15), and 12.5% of the sample had scores of 20 and higher indicating moderate to severe depressive symptoms, consistent with the nonclinical nature of the sample.

The scree test and Velicer's MAP test indicated a factorial solution with four factors, explaining 47% of the variability of the data (Table 2). Nine items were loaded on the first factor (BHS Optimism), which explained 19.2% of the variance (eigenvalue = 6.92), with loadings ranging from 0.53

Table 3: Generalized linear model (criterion: BDI-II).

Parameter	Beta	Std. error	OR	95% Wald confidence interval for OR		$P<$
				Lower	Upper	
BHS Optimism	0.12	0.36	1.13	0.55	2.31	0.74
BHS Pessimism	3.96	0.56	52.35	17.31	158.37	**<0.001**
Generalized Self-Criticism	0.33	0.47	1.39	0.56	3.47	0.48
LOT Optimism	2.21	0.44	9.13	3.87	21.56	**<0.001**

Likelihood Ratio $\chi^2_4 = 200.03$; $P < 0.001$; AIC = 3013.74; AICC = 3013.93; Pearson $\chi^2_{448} = 20017.73$; value/DF = 44.68.

[BHS item no. 5] to 0.88 [BHS item no. 19]: 8 items from the BHS endorsing an optimistic statement and 1 item from the ATS-R denying higher standard for the self. On the second factor (BHS Pessimism), which explained 15.7% of the total variance (eigenvalue = 5.65), 9 items presented loadings ranging from 0.43 [BHS item no. 14] to 0.75 [BHS item no. 17]: all items were from the BHS and endorsed a pessimistic statement. On the third factor (Generalized Self-Criticism), which explained 7.3% of the variance (eigenvalue = 2.61), 4 items had loadings ranging from 0.62 [ATS-R item no. 9] to 0.75 [ATS-R item no. 10]: all items were extracted from the original Generalization and Self-Criticism factors of the ATS-R. On the fourth factor (LOT-R Optimism), which explained 4.8% of the variance (eigenvalue = 1.74), 3 items had loadings ranging from −0.51 [LOT-R item no. 10] to −0.69 [LOT-R item no. 4]: the items were from the LOT-R, and the individual had to endorse an optimistic statement. ATS-R items no. 3 and no. 6 loaded on two factors (factors no. 1 and no. 3) and were excluded from the solution. All factors were rated so that higher scores measured the presence of pessimism or negative attitudes toward the self or denied the presence of optimism. Correlation between factors ranged between −0.18, for the association between BHS Optimism and Generalized Self-Criticism, and 0.45, for the association between BHS Optimism and LOT-R Optimism.

Factor scores were entered in a second-order factor analysis to extract higher-order common factors. The analysis resulted in two factors with eigenvalues >1. On the first factor (Optimism), which explained 43.3% of the variance (eigenvalue = 1.73), first-order factors LOT-R Optimism (0.80) and BHS Optimism (0.72) loaded. On the second factor (Pessimism/Negative attitudes toward self), which explained 34.0% of the variance (eigenvalue = 1.36), first-order factors BHS Pessimism (0.62) and Generalized Self-Criticism (0.69) loaded. The factors were weakly correlated with each other ($r = 0.20$).

A generalized linear model with robust estimator was performed to assess whether the factors measuring CV for depression were independently associated with the BDI-II (Table 3). The model fitted the data well (Likelihood Ratio $\chi^2_4 = 200.03$; $P < 0.001$). The four factors were inserted as independent variables in the analysis and the BDI-II as criterion. Only the BHS Pessimism and the LOT-R Optimism were independently associated with BDI-II scores, indicating that (1) subjects with higher scores on the BHS Pessimism were 52.4 times more likely to have higher BDI-II scores (95% CI: 17.3/158.4; $P < 0.001$) compared with those reported having lower scores and (2) people with higher scores on the LOT-R Optimism were 9.1 times more likely to have higher BDI-II scores (95% CI: 3.9/21.6; $P < 0.001$) compared with people having higher scores. A second generalized linear model was performed with higher order factors as independent variables (not reported in the tables). The model fitted the data well (Likelihood Ratio $\chi^2_2 = 170.31$; $P < 0.001$). Both the higher-order factors were independently associated with the BDI-II: (1) subjects with higher scores on Optimism were 10.1 times more likely to have higher BDI-II scores (95% CI: 4.7/21.5; beta = 2.31 [std. error = 0.39]; $P < 0.001$) compared with those having lower scores; and (2) people with higher scores on Pessimism/Negative Attitudes Toward Self were 91.1 times more likely to have higher BDI-II scores (95% CI: 32.7/254.3; beta = 4.51 [std. error = 0.52]; $P < 0.001$) than people reported having lower scores.

A series of ROC curves indicated that first-order and second-order factors of vulnerability for depression were able to discriminate individuals with different depression severities (Table 4). The performance of the BHS Optimism was quite stable at any level of depression. A randomly chosen individual had 57%–60% of probability to have higher scores on the BHS Optimism compared with a randomly chosen individual with lower levels of depression. Generalized Self-Criticism performance was the best when discriminating individuals with moderate to severe depression from other individuals: at these levels of depression, a randomly chosen individual with moderate to severe depression (BDI-II ≥ 20) had 67% of probability to have higher scores on Generalized Self-Criticism than a randomly chosen individual with lower levels of depression. The performance of the BHS Pessimism increased linearly from lower levels (BDI-II cutoffs of 5 and 9: AUC [area under the curve] = 0.72–0.74) to higher levels of depression (AUC of 0.81 and 0.87, resp., for BDI-II cutoffs of 15 and 19). The performance of the LOT-R Optimism was similar for lower cutoffs (AUC of 0.69 and 0.70, resp., for BDI-II cutoffs of 5 and 9) and higher cutoffs (AUC of 0.74 for BDI-II cutoffs of 15 and 19). When analyzing the performance of the second-order factors, a randomly chosen individual had 66%–72% of probability to have higher scores on Optimism than a randomly chosen individual with lower levels of depression, while a randomly chosen individual had 68%–81% of probability to have higher scores on Pessimism/Negative Attitudes Toward Self than a randomly chosen individual with lower levels of depression. Thus, the presence of Pessimism and Negative Attitudes Toward Self was more useful in discriminating individuals with

Table 4: ROC curves.

Variables	Area under the curve	Std. error	Asymptotic sig.
BDI-II > 5			
BHS Optimism	0.57	0.03	0.05
BHS Pessimism	0.72	0.03	<0.001
Generalized Self-Criticism	0.58	0.03	0.01
LOT Optimism	0.69	0.03	<0.001
Optimism	0.66	0.03	<0.001
Pessimism/Negative Attitudes Toward Self	0.68	0.03	<0.001
BDI-II > 9			
BHS Optimism	0.58	0.03	0.01
BHS Pessimism	0.74	0.02	<0.001
Generalized Self-Criticism	0.59	0.03	0.001
LOT Optimism	0.70	0.02	<0.001
Optimism	0.67	0.03	<0.001
Pessimism/Negative Attitudes Toward Self	0.70	0.03	<0.001
BDI-II > 15			
BHS Optimism	0.60	0.03	0.01
BHS Pessimism	0.81	0.02	<0.001
Generalized Self-Criticism	0.60	0.04	0.01
LOT Optimism	0.74	0.03	<0.001
Optimism	0.72	0.03	<0.001
Pessimism/Negative Attitudes Toward Self	0.75	0.03	<0.001
BDI-II > 19			
BHS Optimism	0.59	0.03	0.05
BHS Pessimism	0.87	0.02	<0.001
Generalized Self-Criticism	0.67	0.04	<0.001
LOT Optimism	0.74	0.03	<0.001
Optimism	0.71	0.03	<0.001
Pessimism/Negative Attitudes Toward Self	0.81	0.03	<0.001

moderate to severe depression than denying an optimistic one. However, the BHS Pessimism appeared to have the best performance in discriminating individuals at any level of depression severity.

4. Discussion

The aim of the present study was to evaluate, by means of ROC curves, whether CV for depression, as measured by three well-known instruments, may independently discriminate between subjects with different depression severities.

Our results indicated that the instruments we administered measure four common vulnerabilities for depression: (1) denying optimism/endorsing high standards (BHS/ATS-R); (2) endorsing pessimism (BHS); (3) generalizing self-criticism (ATS-R); and (4) denying optimism (LOT-R). These dimensions are loaded on two second-order factors: (1) denying optimism and (2) endorsing pessimism and generalizing self-criticism.

In our sample of young adults, the assessment of pessimism with the BHS, compared with other factors, had the best performance in discriminating individuals with different levels of depression severity, and its performance improved from lower cutoffs to higher cutoffs of depression. A randomly chosen individual with moderate to severe depression had 87% of probability to have higher BHS Pessimism compared with a randomly chosen individual with lower levels of depression.

Pessimism was also independently associated with depression severity while controlling for other dimensions of vulnerability for depression. People having more severe pessimism were above 52 times more at risk to have higher depression compared with people with milder pessimism. This finding is consistent with the studies indicating a strong link between negative beliefs about the future and depression [54–58]. For example, Strunk et al. [56], investigating the relationship between depressive symptoms and bias in future event prediction, documented that individuals with elevated depressive symptoms showed a pessimistic bias in making predictions about the outcomes of future life events by overpredicting that undesirable events would happen to them and underpredicting that desirable events would happen to them. Alford et al. [59], in a sample of university students, found that in males hopelessness may predict specifically future depression severity but not anxiety.

From a psychometric point of view, our results may be related to the differences in the methods employed in the three scales we administered to measure CV for depression: (1) the BHS uses dichotomous format of response, while for the LOT-R and the ATS-R the respondents are asked to rate each item on a Likert-type scale; (2) both the BHS and LOT-R ask the individuals to rate positive items which are directly associated with the construct they measure and negative statements which are negatively associated with these constructs. Furthermore, while the BHS is considered a measure of pessimism, the LOT-R is generally considered a measure of optimism [60].

Scheier and Carver [60], investigating construct validity of the LOT-R, reported the fit of a two-factor model: one factor contained positively worded items and the other included negatively worded items. The authors considered that the two-factor solution was probably due to item wording rather than content item [60]. Indeed, responses, particularly to the positively and negatively worded items, reflected a complicated combination of substantively meaningful trait effects and apparently idiosyncratic method effects associated with the wording of particular items [61–63].

Nevertheless, in the last decades several authors reported results supporting the hypothesis that Optimism and Pessimism are two distinct constructs with different patterns of correlations with other psychological constructs [64–70]. Recently, similar results have been found for the BHS: in a sample of medical patients, a bifactor model was the best-fitting solution and the most parsimonious among models evaluated [71]. Results from the higher-order factor analysis we performed support the hypothesis that the two factors often extracted from factorizing LOT-R and BHS items are not an artifact due to item wording and may have different roles as factors of vulnerability for depression.

Finally, our study has some limitations. First, above 60% of our sample were composed of university students and may not be representative of the Italian population, so that generalizability of the results to older people and to individuals with low school attainment is not suggested. Second, our sample is nonclinical and only 12.5% of the subjects reported having moderate to severe depression at the BDI-II, so that our results may not be replicable in clinical samples, even though cognitive theories of depression did not predict differences in the associations of cognitive variables with depressive symptoms between clinical and nonclinical samples [21, 72, 73]. Third, the measures used in the present study were limited to only paper-and-pencil self-report instruments and we did not administered clinician-rated scales to measure depression, as recommended elsewhere [74]. Thus, our results may be biased by social desirability [75, 76]. Fourth, we did not assess participants for family history of mood disorders, which may have predisposed individuals to develop future depression and negative cognitive biases. Nevertheless, there are several noteworthy strengths, including the large size of sample and the use of three different measures often used to assess cognitive vulnerability for depression.

In conclusion, when screening young adults at risk for depression, clinicians have to pay particular attention to expressions of pessimism about the future, which may discriminate well individuals with moderate to severe depression from individuals reported having lower depression severity. Furthermore, at these levels of depression severity, Generalized Self-Criticism is less effective in discriminating individuals at risk for depression compared not only with statements of pessimism but also with statements denying optimism.

Conflict of Interests

The authors declare that they have no conflict of interests for this research.

Authors' Contribution

All authors have made substantial contributions to conception and design or acquisition of data or analysis and interpretation of data, have been involved in drafting the paper or revising it critically for important intellectual content, and have given final approval of the version to be published.

References

[1] C. Blanco, M. Okuda, J. C. Markowitz, S.-M. Liu, B. F. Grant, and D. S. Hasin, "The epidemiology of chronic major depressive disorder and dysthymic disorder: results from the national epidemiologic survey on alcohol and related conditions," *Journal of Clinical Psychiatry*, vol. 71, no. 12, pp. 1645–1656, 2010.

[2] D. S. Hasin, R. D. Goodwin, F. S. Stinson, and B. F. Grant, "Epidemiology of major depressive disorder: results from the National Epidemiologic Survey on Alcoholism and Related Conditions," *Archives of General Psychiatry*, vol. 62, no. 10, pp. 1097–1106, 2005.

[3] V. Lehtinen and M. Joukamaa, "Epidemiology of depression: prevalence, risk factors and treatment situation," *Acta Psychiatrica Scandinavica, Supplement*, vol. 89, no. 377, pp. 7–10, 1994.

[4] M. M. Ohayon, "Epidemiology of depression and its treatment in the general population," *Journal of Psychiatric Research*, vol. 41, no. 3-4, pp. 207–213, 2007.

[5] C. Haslam, S. Atkinson, S. S. Brown, and R. A. Haslam, "Anxiety and depression in the workplace: effects on the individual and organisation (a focus group investigation)," *Journal of Affective Disorders*, vol. 88, no. 2, pp. 209–215, 2005.

[6] N. D. Shippee, N. D. Shah, M. D. Williams, J. P. Moriarty, M. A. Frye, and J. Y. Ziegenfuss, "Differences in demographic composition and in work, social, and functional limitations among the populations with unipolar depression and bipolar disorder: results from a nationally representative sample," *Health and Quality of Life Outcomes*, vol. 9, article 90, 2011.

[7] P. S. Wang, A. L. Beck, P. Berglund et al., "Effects of major depression on moment-in-time work performance," *American Journal of Psychiatry*, vol. 161, no. 10, pp. 1885–1891, 2004.

[8] S. W. Whitton and M. A. Whisman, "Relationship satisfaction instability and depression," *Journal of Family Psychology*, vol. 24, no. 6, pp. 791–794, 2010.

[9] J.-M. Woo, W. Kim, T.-Y. Hwang et al., "Impact of depression on work productivity and its improvement after outpatient treatment with antidepressants," *Value in Health*, vol. 14, no. 4, pp. 475–482, 2011.

[10] T. B. Ustun, J. L. Ayuso-Mateos, S. Chatterji, C. Mathers, and C. J. L. Murray, "Global burden of depressive disorders in the year 2000," *British Journal of Psychiatry*, vol. 184, pp. 386–392, 2004.

[11] World Health Organisation, "Depression. What is depression?" 2011, http://www.who.int/mental_health/management/depression/en/.

[12] R. C. Kessler, P. Berglund, O. Demler et al., "The epidemiology of major depressive disorder: results from the National Comorbidity Survey Replication (NCS-R)," *Journal of the American Medical Association*, vol. 289, no. 23, pp. 3095–3105, 2003.

[13] G. de Girolamo, G. Polidori, P. Morosini et al., "La prevalenza dei disturbi mentali in italia. Il progetto ESEMED-WMH. Una sintesi," Centro Nazionale di Epidemiologia, Sorveglianza e Promozione della Salute, Roma, Italia, 2005.

[14] I. H. Gotlib and C. L. Hammen, *Handbook of Depressioned*, Guilford Press, New York, NY, USA, 2nd edition, 2010.

[15] L. B. Alloy, L. Y. Abramson, W. G. Whitehouse et al., "Depressogenic cognitive styles: predictive validity, information processing and personality characteristics, and developmental origins," *Behaviour Research and Therapy*, vol. 37, no. 6, pp. 503–531, 1999.

[16] E. R. Watkins, "Constructive and unconstructive repetitive thought," *Psychological Bulletin*, vol. 134, no. 2, pp. 163–206, 2008.

[17] M. Balsamo, "Anger and depression: evidence of a possible mediating role for rumination," *Psychological Reports*, vol. 106, no. 1, pp. 3–12, 2010.

[18] E. H. W. Koster, E. De Lissnyder, N. Derakshan, and R. De Raedt, "Understanding depressive rumination from a cognitive science perspective: the impaired disengagement hypothesis," *Clinical Psychology Review*, vol. 31, no. 1, pp. 138–145, 2011.

[19] M. Zhong, X. Wang, J. Xiao et al., "Amygdala hyperactivation and prefrontal hypoactivation in subjects with cognitive vulnerability to depression," *Biological Psychology*, vol. 88, no. 2-3, pp. 233–242, 2011.

[20] R. H. Jacobs, M. A. Reinecke, J. K. Gollan, and P. Kane, "Empirical evidence of cognitive vulnerability for depression among children and adolescents: a cognitive science and developmental perspective," *Clinical Psychology Review*, vol. 28, no. 5, pp. 759–782, 2008.

[21] L. Y. Abramson, G. I. Metalsky, and L. B. Alloy, "Hopelessness depression: a theory-based subtype of depression," *Psychological Review*, vol. 96, no. 2, pp. 358–372, 1989.

[22] A. T. Beck, *Depression: Clinical, Experimental, and Theoretical Aspects*, Harper & Row, New York, NY, USA, 1967.

[23] A. T. Beck, "Cognitive models of depression," *Journal of Cognitive Psychotherapy*, vol. 1, pp. 5–37, 1987.

[24] A. T. Beck, A. Weissman, D. Lester, and L. Trexler, "The measurement of pessimism: the hopelessness scale," *Journal of Consulting and Clinical Psychology*, vol. 42, no. 6, pp. 861–865, 1974.

[25] C. S. Carver and R. J. Ganellen, "Depression and components of self-punitiveness: high standards, self-criticism, and overgeneralization," *Journal of Abnormal Psychology*, vol. 92, no. 3, pp. 330–337, 1983.

[26] E. E. Beckham, W. R. Leber, J. T. Watkins, J. L. Boyer, and J. B. Cook, " Development of an instrument to measure Beck's cognitive triad: the Cognitive Triad Inventory," *Journal of Consulting and Clinical Psychology*, vol. 54, no. 4, pp. 566–567, 1986.

[27] L. Y. Abramson, L. B. Alloy, B. L. Hankin, G. J. Haeffel, D. G. MacCoon, and B. E. Gibb, "Cognitive vulnerability-stress models of depression in a self-regulatory and psychobiological context," in *Handbook of Depression*, I. H. Gotlib and C. L. Hammen, Eds., pp. 268–294, The Guilford Press, New York, NY, USA, 2002.

[28] J. Evans, J. Heron, G. Lewis, R. Araya, and D. Wolke, "Negative self-schemas and the onset of depression in women: longitudinal study," *British Journal of Psychiatry*, vol. 186, pp. 302–307, 2005.

[29] L. B. Alloy, L. Y. Abramson, W. G. Whitehouse, M. E. Hogan, C. Panzarella, and D. T. Rose, "Prospective incidence of first onsets and recurrences of depression in individuals at high and low cognitive risk for depression," *Journal of Abnormal Psychology*, vol. 115, no. 1, pp. 145–156, 2006.

[30] J. R. Z. Abela, C. Aydin, and R. P. Auerbach, "Operationalizing the "vulnerability" and "stress" components of the hopelessness theory of depression: a multi-wave longitudinal study," *Behaviour Research and Therapy*, vol. 44, no. 11, pp. 1565–1583, 2006.

[31] A. T. Beck, R. A. Steer, M. Kovacs, and B. Garrison, "Hopelessness and eventual suicide: a 10-year prospective study of patients hospitalized with suicidal ideation," *American Journal of Psychiatry*, vol. 142, no. 5, pp. 559–563, 1985.

[32] A. T. Beck, G. Brown, R. J. Berchick, B. L. Stewart, and R. A. Steer, "Relationship between hopelessness and ultimate suicide: a replication with psychiatric outpatients," *American Journal of Psychiatry*, vol. 147, no. 2, pp. 190–195, 1990.

[33] M. Pompili, M. Innamorati, X. Gonda et al., "Affective temperaments and hopelessness as predictors of health and social general functioning in mood disorders patients: a prospective follow-up study," *Journal of Affective Disorders*, 2013.

[34] G. I. Metalsky and T. E. Joiner Jr., "Vulnerability to depressive symptomatology: a prospective test of the diathesis-stress and causal mediation components of the hopelessness theory of depression," *Journal of Personality and Social Psychology*, vol. 63, no. 4, pp. 667–675, 1992.

[35] P. Pössel and S. D. Thomas, "Cognitive triad as mediator in the hopelessness model? a three-wave longitudinal study," *Journal of Clinical Psychology*, vol. 67, no. 3, pp. 224–240, 2011.

[36] M. F. Scheier, C. S. Carver, and M. W. Bridges, "Distinguishing optimism from neuroticism (and trait anxiety, self-mastery, and self-esteem): a reevaluation of the Life Orientation Test," *Journal of Personality and Social Psychology*, vol. 67, no. 6, pp. 1063–1078, 1994.

[37] C. S. Carver, L. La Voie, J. Kuhl, and R. J. Ganellen, "Cognitive concomitants of depression: a further examination of the roles of generalization, high standards, and self-criticism," *Journal of Social and Clinical Psychology*, vol. 7, pp. 350–365, 1988.

[38] A. T. Beck, R. A. Steer, and G. K. Brown, *Manual for the Beck Depression Inventory-II*, Psychological Corporation, San Antonio, Tex, USA, 1996.

[39] American Psychiatric Association, *Diagnostic and Statistical Manual of Mental Disorders*, American Psychiatric Association, Washington, DC, USA, 4th edition, 2000.

[40] P. A. Arbisi, "Review of the Beck depression inventory-II," in *The Fourteenth Mental Measurements Yearbook*, B. S. Plake and J. C. Impara, Eds., Buros Institute of Mental Measurements, Lincoln, Neb, USA, 2001.

[41] M. Balsamo and A. Saggino, "Test per l'assessment della depressione nel contesto italiano: un'analisi critica," *Psicoterapia Cognitiva e Comportamentale*, vol. 13, pp. 167–199, 2007.

[42] A. T. Beck, R. A. Steer, J. S. Beck, and C. F. Newman, "Hopelessness, depression, suicidal ideation, and clinical diagnosis of

depression," *Suicide and Life-Threatening Behavior*, vol. 23, no. 2, pp. 139–145, 1993.

[43] E. D. Klonsky, R. Kotov, S. Bakst, J. Rabinowitz, and E. J. Bromet, "Hopelessness as a predictor of attempted suicide among first admission patients with psychosis: a 10-year cohort study," *Suicide and Life-Threatening Behavior*, vol. 42, no. 1, pp. 1–10, 2012.

[44] M. Innamorati, M. Pompili, X. Gonda et al., "Psychometric properties of the Gotland Scale for Depression in Italian psychiatric inpatients and its utility in the prediction of suicide risk," *Journal of Affective Disorders*, vol. 132, no. 1-2, pp. 99–103, 2011.

[45] M. Pompili, P. Iliceto, D. Lester et al., *BHS Beck Hopelessness Scale*, O.S. Organizzazioni Speciali, Florence, Italy, 2009.

[46] M. Pompili, R. Tatarelli, J. R. Rogers, and D. Lester, "The hopelessness scale: a factor analysis," *Psychological Reports*, vol. 100, no. 2, pp. 375–378, 2007.

[47] C. S. Carver, "Generalization, adverse events, and development of depressive symptoms," *Journal of Personality*, vol. 66, no. 4, pp. 606–619, 1998.

[48] L. R. Eisner, S. L. Johnson, and C. S. Carver, "Cognitive responses to failure and success relate uniquely to bipolar depression versus mania," *Journal of Abnormal Psychology*, vol. 117, no. 1, pp. 154–163, 2008.

[49] M. Innamorati, S. Tamburello, A. Contardi et al., "Psychometric properties of the attitudes toward self-revised in Italian young adults," *Depression Research and Treatment*, vol. 2013, Article ID 209216, 6 pages, 2013.

[50] R. B. Cattell, "The scree test for the number of factors," *Multivariate Behavioral Research*, vol. 1, pp. 245–276, 1966.

[51] W. F. Velicer, "Determining the number of components from the matrix of partial correlations," *Psychometrika*, vol. 41, no. 3, pp. 321–327, 1976.

[52] P. Kline, *A Handbook of Test Construction: Introduction to Psychometric Design*, Methuen, London, UK, 1986.

[53] H. Gleitman, *Psychologyed*, W.W. Norton, New York, NY, USA, 2nd edition, 1986.

[54] L. B. Alloy and A. H. Ahrens, "Depression and pessimism for the future: biased use of statistically relevant information in predictions for self versus others," *Journal of Personality and Social Psychology*, vol. 52, no. 2, pp. 366–378, 1987.

[55] A. Lavender and E. Watkins, "Rumination and future thinking in depression," *British Journal of Clinical Psychology*, vol. 43, no. 2, pp. 129–142, 2004.

[56] D. R. Strunk, H. Lopez, and R. J. DeRubeis, "Depressive symptoms are associated with unrealistic negative predictions of future life events," *Behaviour research and therapy*, vol. 44, no. 6, pp. 861–882, 2006.

[57] A. T. Beck, J. H. Riskind, G. Brown, and R. A. Steer, "Levels of hopelessness in DSM-III disorders: a partial test of content specificity in depression," *Cognitive Therapy and Research*, vol. 12, no. 5, pp. 459–469, 1988.

[58] D. R. Strunk and A. D. Adler, "Cognitive biases in three prediction tasks: a test of the cognitive model of depression," *Behaviour Research and Therapy*, vol. 47, no. 1, pp. 34–40, 2009.

[59] B. A. Alford, J. M. Lester, R. J. Patel, J. P. Buchanan, and L. C. Giunta, "Hopelessness predicts future depressive symptoms: a prospective analysis of cognitive vulnerability and cognitive content specificity," *Journal of Clinical Psychology*, vol. 51, no. 3, pp. 331–339, 1995.

[60] M. F. Scheier and C. S. Carver, "Optimism, coping, and health: assessment and implications of generalized outcome expectancies," *Health Psychology*, vol. 4, no. 3, pp. 219–247, 1985.

[61] M. Balsamo, R. Romanelli, M. Innamorati, G. Ciccarese, L. Carlucci, and A. Saggino, "The state-trait anxiety inventory: shadows and lights on its construct validity," *Journal of Psychopathology and Behavioral Assessment*, 2013.

[62] L. J. Cronbach, "Response sets and test validity," *Educational and Psychological Measurement*, vol. 6, pp. 475–494, 1946.

[63] J. Millham and R. W. Kellogg, "Need for social approval: impression management or self-deception?" *Journal of Research in Personality*, vol. 14, no. 4, pp. 445–457, 1980.

[64] G. N. Marshall, C. B. Wortman, J. W. Kusulas, L. K. Hervig, and R. R. Vickers Jr., "Distinguishing optimism from pessimism: relations to fundamental dimensions of mood and personality," *Journal of Personality and Social Psychology*, vol. 62, no. 6, pp. 1067–1074, 1992.

[65] D. K. Mroczek, A. Spiro III, C. M. Aldwin, D. J. Ozer, and R. Bossé, "Construct validation of optimism and pessimism in older men: findings from the normative aging study," *Health Psychology*, vol. 12, no. 5, pp. 406–409, 1993.

[66] J. C. Lai, "Differential predictive power of the positively versus the negatively worded items of the Life Orientation Test," *Psychological Reports*, vol. 75, no. 3, pp. 1507–1515, 1994.

[67] S. Robinson-Whelen, C. Kim, R. C. MacCallum, and J. K. Kiecolt-Glaser, "Distinguishing optimism from pessimism in older adults: is it more important to be optimistic or not to be pessimistic?" *Journal of Personality and Social Psychology*, vol. 73, no. 6, pp. 1345–1353, 1997.

[68] P. Y. Herzberg, H. Glaesmer, and J. Hoyer, "Separating optimism and pessimism: a robust psychometric analysis of the revised Life Orientation Test (LOT-R)," *Psychological Assessment*, vol. 18, no. 4, pp. 433–438, 2006.

[69] M. Kivimäki, M. Elovainio, A. Singh-Manoux, J. Vahtera, H. Helenius, and J. Pentti, "Optimism and pessimism as predictors of change in health after death or onset of severe illness in family," *Health Psychology*, vol. 24, no. 4, pp. 413–421, 2005.

[70] K. Räikkönen, K. A. Matthews, J. D. Flory, J. F. Owens, and B. B. Gump, "Effects of optimism, pessimism, and trait anxiety on ambulatory blood pressure and mood during everyday life," *Journal of Personality and Social Psychology*, vol. 76, no. 1, pp. 104–113, 1999.

[71] M. Innamorati, D. Lester, M. Balsamo et al., "Factor validity of the Beck Hopelessness Scale in Italian medical patients," *Journal of Psychopathology and Behavioral Assessment*. In press.

[72] A. T. Beck, "Beyond belief: a theory of modes, personality, and psychopathology," in *Frontiers of Cognitive Therapy*, P. M. Salkovskis, Ed., Guildford Press, New York, NY, USA, 1996.

[73] A. T. Beck, *Cognitive Therapy of Depression*, Guilford Press, New York, NY, USA, 1979.

[74] D. T. Campbell and D. W. Fiske, "Convergent and discriminant validation by the multitrait-multimethod matrix," *Psychological Bulletin*, vol. 56, no. 2, pp. 81–105, 1959.

[75] H. J. Arnold and D. C. Feldman, "Social desirability response bias in self-report choice situations," *Academy of Management Journal*, vol. 24, pp. 377–385, 1981.

[76] E. E. Maccoby and N. A. Maccoby, "The interview: a tool of social science," in *Handbook of Social Psychology*, G. Lindzey, Ed., pp. 449–487, Addison-Wesley, Cambridge, Mass, USA, 1954.

16

Exercise for Adolescents with Depressive Disorders

Richard R. Dopp,[1] Ann J. Mooney,[1] Roseanne Armitage,[2,3] and Cheryl King[2]

[1] *Child and Adolescent Psychiatry Section, Department of Psychiatry, University of Michigan, 4250 Plymouth Road, Ann Arbor, MI 48109-2700, USA*
[2] *Departments of Psychiatry and Psychology, University of Michigan, 4250 Plymouth Road, Ann Arbor, MI 48109-2700, USA*
[3] *Sleep and Chronophysiology Laboratory, University of Michigan, 4250 Plymouth Road, Ann Arbor, MI 48109-2700, USA*

Correspondence should be addressed to Richard R. Dopp, dopp@umich.edu

Academic Editor: Amy Kilbourne

Objectives. Adolescence is associated with increased depressive symptoms and decreased aerobic exercise, yet the relationship between exercise and clinical depression among adolescents requires further examination. This study assessed the feasibility of a 12-week intervention designed to increase exercise for adolescents with depressive disorders: Will a teenager with depression exercise? *Methods.* Participants were 13 adolescents with depression reporting low levels of aerobic exercise. They completed a 12-week intervention (15 supervised exercise sessions and 21 independent sessions). Exercise was measured through the aerobic exercise Questionnaire, actigraphy, and heart-rate monitoring. Depression was measured with the Children's Depression Rating Scale, Revised, and Quick Inventory of Depressive Symptomatology, Self-Report. *Results.* All participants who started the intervention completed the protocol, attending all supervised exercise sessions. Actigraphy verified 81% adherence to the protocol's independent sessions. Analysis of secondary outcomes showed a significant increase in exercise levels and a significant decrease in depression severity. Initially, ten participants were overweight or obese, and three were healthy weight. After 12 weeks of exercise, the number of participants in the healthy-weight category doubled. *Conclusions.* Adolescents suffering from depression can complete a rigorous protocol requiring structured increases in aerobic exercise. Participants showed significant increases in exercise, and significant decreases in depressive symptoms.

1. Introduction

Adolescent depression has long-term consequences and is often associated with additional depressive episodes in adulthood [1]. The presence of a major depressive disorder (MDD) in adolescents can negatively affect academic, social, and family functioning [2]. Evidence-based psychotherapies and medication are indicated for children and adolescents with moderate-to-severe depression [3], but greater than one-third of adolescents with depression do not show an adequate clinical response to antidepressant medications [4]. In the Treatment for Adolescents with Depression Study, the response rates after 12 weeks of treatment were 35% for placebo, 43% for cognitive behavioral therapy (CBT), 61% for fluoxetine, and 71% for combination treatment. However, the rates of full remission after 12 weeks of treatment were only 17% for placebo, 16% for CBT, 23% for fluoxetine, and 37% for combination treatment [5].

In addition to low rates of response and remission, there is concern regarding the safety of antidepressant medications. In 2005, the Food and Drug Administration issued a black-box warning stating that antidepressants may increase the risk for suicidal thinking and behavior in children and adolescents. This regulatory decision was based on a meta-analysis of 24 trials involving over 4,500 patients which indicated an increased risk of suicidality (risk ratio = 1.95; 95% CI = 1.28–2.98) during the first few months of initiating antidepressant medication treatment [6]. This warning has been associated with a decline in youth and young adults seeking treatment with antidepressant medications, prompting patients and parents to consider alternative, nonpharmacologic interventions [7].

One alternative treatment option currently under investigation is exercise. A randomized controlled trial (RCT) of older adults with mild-to-moderate depression compared supervised exercise, home-based exercise, sertraline, and pill placebo [8]. In this study, Blumenthal and colleagues demonstrated that exercise was as effective as medication for decreasing depressive symptoms. In a study of young adults with MDD, Dunn et al. assigned participants to one of five treatment conditions that varied by intensity (public health dose exercise, low-dose exercise, stretching control) and frequency (three or five times per week) [9]. In this DOSE study, all exercise sessions were conducted individually in a structured, supervised setting. After the intervention, an intent-to-treat analysis of participants' scores on the 17-item Hamilton Rating Scale for Depression ($HRSD_{17}$) showed a reduction of 47% for participants in the public health dose exercise condition compared with 30% for the participants in the low dose condition and 29% for those in the stretching control condition.

While vigorous exercise appears to be an effective treatment for depression in adults, a Cochrane Review suggests that the effect of exercise as treatment for depression in children and adolescents requires further investigation, as evidence-based research is lacking [10]. In nonclinical samples of adolescents, there is evidence to support that increases in leisure-time physical activity are associated with decreases in depressive symptoms [11]. Intervention research targeting health behavior change in the areas of physical activity and nutrition among adolescents in primary care has shown a positive impact on several health behaviors with the exception of vigorous physical activity [12]. Meanwhile, the strength of evidence in the use of exercise as treatment for depression in adults supports an emphasis on higher levels of aerobic activity [13]. Based upon these research findings showing that exercise is effective as treatment for adults with major depressive disorders, we chose to examine the feasibility of conducting similar research in adolescents with depression. We began by designing an intervention that required aerobic exercise three times per week.

There are multiple challenges encountered when investigating exercise as treatment for depression in adolescents, including: (1) the adolescent desire for autonomy versus authoritarian demands of adults such as parents and medical professionals [14]; (2) the time commitments of adolescents with academic, social, and family demands; (3) expectations in society for quick-fix solutions to complicated medical illnesses like depression; (4) limited access to exercise facilities or safe environments for some youth [15]; and (5) sociocultural factors that may undermine some adolescents' efforts to change activity levels [16, 17]. There are additional challenges for the many adolescents who struggle with both depression and obesity. In children, depression is a risk factor for the development of obesity [18]. At the same time, obesity in childhood increases risk for later depression [19]. The factors that predispose individuals to depression, such as sleep disturbance and decreased activity levels, are some of the same factors that predispose individuals to obesity. Exercise may be more difficult to initiate and maintain for youth with both depression and weight issues.

A major concern in this area of research is the potential drop-out rate due to adolescents' many time commitments and potential loss of motivation. In reviewing the drop-out rates using exercise as treatment for adults with depression, Dunn's 2005 DOSE study reported that of the 80 randomized participants, 72 began exercise treatment and 53 completed 12 weeks, representing a drop-out rate of 34% [9]. In Blumenthal's 2007 SMILE study, supervised exercise and home-based exercise participants had drop-out rates of 20% and 6%, respectively [8]. Other research on exercise and depression in adults has proposed a combination of supervised and independent exercise sessions to reduce participant burden [20]. In designing our study protocol, we felt that requiring a combination of independent and supervised exercise sessions would encourage our adolescent participants to incorporate exercise into their lives. At the same time, we expected that adherence to, and completion of, our intervention protocol would still be potential challenges.

The primary aim of this research study was to assess the feasibility of participant recruitment and retention in an exercise intervention for adolescents with depressive disorders. We hypothesized that there would be approximately a 25% drop-out rate during the study. Secondary outcomes included changes in levels of exercise and depression severity. Increases in exercise, as measured by actigraphy, heart rate monitoring during supervised sessions, and self-report, would suggest compliance with the protocol's requirements. Our corresponding secondary outcomes' hypotheses were that the frequency of exercise would increase and that depression severity would decrease for all participants.

2. Materials and Methods

2.1. Study Design. This study required adolescent participants with depressive disorders to complete a 12-week exercise intervention. The intervention included three supervised exercise sessions in the first week, two supervised exercise sessions in the second week, and one supervised exercise session in weeks 3 through 12. Participants were expected to complete one independent exercise session in week 2 and two independent exercise sessions in weeks 3 through 12. A final assessment was conducted three months following the conclusion of the exercise intervention. Beginning with the baseline appointment for the first participant and continuing through the three-month followup for the final participant, this study took 11 months to complete.

2.2. Participants. Institutional Review Board (IRB) approval was obtained to recruit participants through flyers distributed in local mental health clinics and high schools. Telephone screens were conducted with 25 adolescents to assess their levels of depression severity and physical activity, using the Quick Inventory of Depressive Symptomatology and the Physical Activity Questionnaire. If the adolescent reported symptoms of clinical depression and low levels of physical activity, he or she was invited to come in for a clinical baseline screening, at which the Children's Depression Rating

Scale, Revised (CDRS-R) interview was conducted. A raw score of 36 or greater (T-Score of 61 or greater) on the CDRS-R was required for acceptance into the study. Screening took place over a four-month period to recruit 14 participants who met study eligibility. Eleven screened adolescents were excluded due to the following: elevated activity levels ($n = 4$), lack of willingness to exercise at required level ($n = 2$), failure to respond to research staff's attempts to set up initial interviews ($n = 2$), lack of depression ($n = 1$), unwillingness to ask parent for consent ($n = 1$), and diagnosis of bipolar disorder ($n = 1$). The adolescent with a prior diagnosis of bipolar disorder was excluded in order to maintain diagnostic homogeneity and due to a lack of published data regarding the effects of exercise on youth with bipolar disorder.

Adolescent assent and parental consent were obtained from 14 adolescents and basic demographic information was collected. One participant sustained a major orthopedic injury prior to initiating the exercise intervention. Thus, the intervention phase was initiated with 13 participants (see Table 1).

These 13 participants included nine females (69%) and four males (31%) who ranged in age from 13 to 17 years ($M = 15.2$, SD = 2.4). Ethnicity and race were consistent with regional demographics: Caucasian (54%), African American (23%), biracial or multiethnic (15%), and Hispanic (8%). Eleven participants met criteria for MDD (85%), and two for Depressive Disorder, Not Otherwise Specified (15%). Four participants had MDD and a comorbid diagnosis: one with Attention-Deficit/Hyperactivity Disorder (ADHD); one with Anxiety Disorder, Not Otherwise Specified; two with both ADHD and Anxiety Disorder, Not Otherwise Specified.

At baseline, nine of the 13 participants (69%) were in psychotherapy and/or medication treatment for their depression. Seven participants (54%) were taking no psychotropic medications during the study. Five participants (38.5%) were on selective serotonin reuptake inhibitors (SSRI) at the beginning of the intervention (four on fluoxetine and one on sertraline) and continued on them throughout the intervention. Three of the five participants on SSRIs at baseline were also taking stimulants. During the intervention, two participants initiated psychotherapy, and one participant began taking an SSRI (sertraline) during the intervention at approximately the week 3 time point. Two unmedicated participants terminated their psychotherapy treatment for depression during the intervention, both citing an improvement in mood as the reason for termination.

TABLE 1: Demographic characteristics of participants at baseline.

Baseline demographics	($N = 13$)
Age	13–17 years, $M = 15.2$, SD = (1.4)
Sex	
Males	4
Females	9
Race	
Caucasian	7 (54%)
African American	3 (23%)
Biracial/MultiEthnic	2 (15%)
Hispanic	1 (8%)
Medical diagnoses	
Major depressive disorder	11 (85%)
Depressive disorder NOS	2 (15%)
Co-morbid diagnoses	
Attention deficit/hyperactivity disorder	2 (15%)
Anxiety disorder, NOS	2 (15%)
Medications	
None	7 (54%)
Selective serotonin reuptake inhibitor	5 (38.5%)
Fluoxetine	4 (30%)
Sertraline	1 (8%)
Stimulants (also on SSRIs)	3 (23%)
Body mass index—CDC category	
Healthy weight	2 (23%)
Overweight	5 (38.5%)
Obese	5 (38.5%)

2.3. Measures

2.3.1. Physical Activity Questionnaire for Older Children (PAQ-A) [21]. The PAQ-A is a self-administered questionnaire which asks informants to recall activities which made them "sweat or make your legs feel tired, or games that make you breath hard" in the past seven days. A score of 1 on the PAQ-A is equivalent to no exercise in the last seven days. A score of 5 is equivalent to exercise greater than five times in the last seven days. The questionnaire assesses participation in specific activities and sports (e.g., walking, running, football, and basketball) as well as specific times (e.g., physical education classes, after school, evenings, and weekends). The PAQ-A was modified to include common types of physical activity in the study region. The PAQ-A has good internal consistency [22], and it has been shown to have convergent validity with concurrently used physical activity measures, including self-report questionnaires and motion sensors [23].

2.3.2. Children's Depression Rating Scale, Revised (CDRS-R) [24]. The CDRS-R consists of a semistructured interview with strong concurrent validity, demonstrated by associations with other measures of child and adolescent depressive symptoms. It has shown high internal consistency (alpha = 0.85) in cross-sectional samples and good interrater reliability [25]. In this study, two staff participated in the administration of the CDRS-R at all time points and recorded their ratings separately. Interrater reliability proved to be high. Across 17 items with a possible total raw score ranging from 17 to 113, total ratings within five points of each other were considered as being in agreement. Interrater agreement was 89.7% over all three time points. After each clinical assessment, the clinicians compared ratings, discussed differences, and determined a consolidated score. Raw score ratings are 30–42 for mild depression, 43–57 for moderate, 58–72 for severe, and 73 or higher for very severe depression [26].

2.3.3. Quick Inventory of Depressive Symptomatology (QIDS) [27]. The QIDS has highly acceptable psychometric properties which support the usefulness of this brief rating of depressive symptom severity in both clinical and research settings. Internal consistency is high for the self-report version, the QIDS-SR (Cronbach's alpha = 0.86). In a 2010 study of 140 adolescent outpatients, all versions of the QIDS (except the parent interview) were shown to have high reliability in use with adolescents [28]. Ratings on the QIDS-SR are 6–10 for mild depression, 11–15 for moderate, 16–20 for severe, and greater than 21 for very severe depression[27].

2.3.4. Actigraphy (Actiwatch-LTM, Mini Mitter Co., Inc., Bend, OR) [29]. The actigraphs are worn on the wrist like a watch and electronically measure the number of movements that exceed 0.01 g (gravitation force per minute of recording). Data were downloaded from the actigraphs at the end of each recording period. Initial data analyses were conducted with on-board Mini-Mitter software.

2.3.5. Body Mass Index (BMI). The Center for Disease Control and Prevention promotes using BMI as a way of assessing body fat for children and adolescents. The CDC Teen BMI Calculator was used to determine categories for participants pre- and post-intervention. A healthy weight for a teen is indicated by being in the 5th to 84th percentile; one is considered overweight if in the 85th to the 94th percentile; and an adolescent is considered obese if he or she is in the 95th percentile or above [30].

2.4. Procedures

2.4.1. Pre-Intervention Assessment. Baseline interviews were conducted with eligible adolescents and a parent or legal guardian. Self-report measures were completed by the participants, and clinical staff conducted the CDRS-R interview. Height and weight were measured at baseline, week 12, and three months post-intervention. The same scale (Scaletronix Model #5002) was used for all weight measurements.

The participants wore an actigraph for one week to document activity levels and sleep schedules prior to the intervention. Participants were told to keep the actigraph on 24/7 for this week, as well as weeks 3 and 12. Those subsequent weeks of actigraphy provided us with data to confirm compliance with planned independent exercise sessions. This was conducted by reviewing the actogram and verifying the independent exercise sessions as reported by the participant.

2.4.2. Intervention. Medical clearance was obtained from each participant's primary care physician prior to initiating exercise. In the first week of the exercise intervention, the adolescents came to the exercise laboratory three times for supervised sessions using a treadmill, an elliptical, and/or a stationary bike. These were individual sessions with only study staff present to collect self-report measures, monitor safety, and record heart rate. Participants were allowed to listen to music; many brought MP3 players or iPods, and a radio and CD player were provided for those without their own electronic devices. All pieces of exercise equipment had surfaces on which to put a book or magazine, so reading was allowed. One participant brought his laptop and watched online television programs during his exercise session. Listening to music was the most common activity.

Participants were encouraged to warm up slowly, to try all exercise equipment and develop their own preferences, and to increase the length of their workouts gradually. Each participant was asked to exercise for at least 30 minutes in the first supervised session and to exercise for 45 to 60 minutes by the second or third session and thereafter. Heart rates were recorded every 10 minutes using the Polar F55 BRO model heart rate monitor. Both the elliptical and the treadmill also had cardiogrip readings which helped the participants to be aware of their heart rate throughout the session.

Initially in this study, there was an expectation that working out on the available equipment (treadmill, elliptical, and stationary bike) would lead to an aerobic exercise session for participants. However, after six participants completed the 12-week intervention, it became apparent that the intensity of the supervised exercise varied greatly among the adolescents. It was determined that a target heart rate would be established for each participant. The algorithm used was 220 minus age, multiplied by 0.85. From that point forward, participants were told their target heart rate and were encouraged to hit that rate multiple times during their session. If that was accomplished easily within the first 10 to 15 minutes, they were encouraged to maintain that heart rate for as long as possible. The emphasis was on aerobic exercise. If participants hit and maintained their target heart rate during the first 40 minutes of the session, they were allowed to exercise using free weights for the last 10 minutes of their session. For participants who expressed interest in using the weights, this was used as an incentive to maintain aerobic levels in the first 40 minutes of their session.

In the second week, the participants had two supervised sessions at the exercise laboratory, and completed one exercise session independently. Suggestions were made for independent workouts, including using available equipment (at home, school, local gyms), jogging in safe neighborhoods or on tracks at school, or working out with exercise videos. Some participants made suggestions of their own: jumping rope, dancing with friends, and working out with exercise shows on cable television stations.

In weeks 3 through 12 of the intervention, the staff reviewed with the participant what exercise sessions had been accomplished independently in the past week, and assisted the participant in planning the independent sessions for the following week. For each of the next 10 weeks, the participants had one supervised session at the exercise laboratory and exercised twice on their own.

2.4.3. Post-Intervention Assessment. Three months after the intervention, participants wore an actigraphy watch for one more week before returning for a final clinical assessment. They then had an interview during which the CDRS-R was administered and completed measures assessing levels of exercise and depression.

Participants received five $25 cash payments at baseline; weeks 4, 8, 12, and at the three-month post-intervention time point.

2.5. Statistical Analysis. Paired samples *t*-tests were conducted to compare baseline and post-intervention outcomes. Pearson's two-tailed correlations were used for the analysis of exercise level and depression severity. Cohen's *d* was computed to evaluate the effect size of changes in exercise and depression severity [31].

3. Results and Discussion

3.1. Results

3.1.1. Feasibility. Every participant completed this exercise intervention. On average, it took 14.25 (SD = 3.1) weeks to complete the 15 supervised exercise sessions and the 21 independent sessions. Six participants completed the intervention in 12 consecutive weeks. Other participants took extra time to complete the study due to transportation problems, illness, vacations, and demands of high school academics. Adverse events which were reported to the IRB included minor orthopedic injuries and one suicide attempt. Additional negative life events also impacted time to completion, including temporary homelessness, parental separations (two participants), and a police arrest.

Consistent with our aim to assess feasibility of participant retention, the adolescents were asked to give reasons for their participation so that we might better understand the motivational factors involved in getting adolescents with depression to exercise. The request was verbal, no menu of options was offered, and multiple answers were allowed. Reasons given by participants were to have structured exercise ($n = 5$), to lose weight ($n = 5$), for incentive money ($n = 5$), to fight their depression ($n = 4$), to be involved in research ($n = 2$), and to help other people ($n = 1$). In four cases, either parents or participants stated that they initiated participation in this research project as an alternative to antidepressant medication.

3.1.2. Exercise Outcomes. In our study, heart rates were monitored every 10 minutes during the supervised exercise sessions, with averages ranging from 124 to 181 beats per minute. For participants exercising prior to the establishment of a heart rate goal (220 − age × 0.85), target heart rates were achieved in 39% of the supervised exercise sessions. After target heart rates were calculated and participants were encouraged to hit those rates, in the remaining supervised sessions of the study, they hit their targets in 79% of those sessions. As seen in Figure 1, scores on the adapted PAQ-A increased significantly during the intervention phase

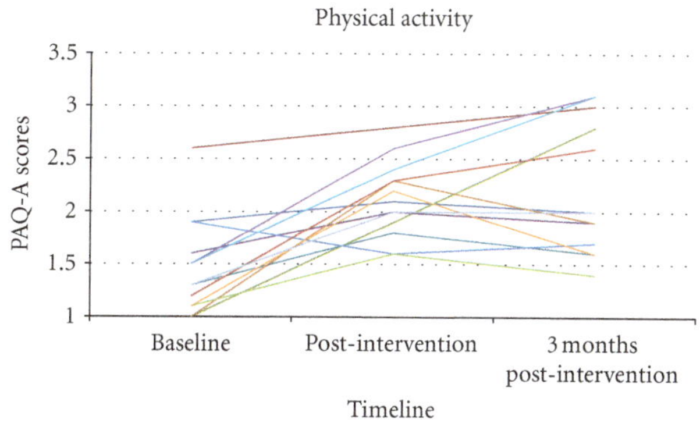

FIGURE 1: Adapted Physical Activity Questionnaire for Older Children scores at baseline, post-intervention, and three-month post-intervention time point.

($P = 0.001$). At baseline, the mean score on the adapted PAQ-A was 1.46 (SD = 0.48) with an increase to 2.10 (SD = 0.37) as measured during the final week of the intervention. The effect size based on Cohen's $d = 1.6$ was large, indicating robust effects. At the three-month post-intervention assessment, the mean score for the total sample on the adapted PAQ-A continued to rise to 2.21 (SD = 0.62).

Actigraphy recordings during weeks 3 and 12 were used to verify independent exercise sessions for those two weeks. Of the 52 expected independent physical activity sessions during those weeks, 42 sessions (81%) were verified by actigraphy. Of our 13 participants, one showed no actigraph data for both weeks 3 and 12; another had no actigraphy recorded for one of the two expected weeks. Absence of data was due to either technological malfunction of the actigraph or participant noncompliance (i.e., not wearing the actigraph as requested). Excluding the missing actigraphy, 91% of the expected independent exercise sessions were verified.

3.1.3. Depression Outcomes. The depression outcome measure was change in the CDRS-R score from baseline to completion of the exercise intervention, as seen in Figure 2. Depressive symptoms decreased significantly during the period of supported exercise ($P < 0.001$).

The mean score on the CDRS-R for these 13 participants was 48.9 (SD = 9.7) at baseline, and 28.5 (SD = 10.4) post-intervention, a decrease of more than 20 points. The effect size associated with depression improvement was also large, indicating robust effects on depression (Cohen's d = 2.0). Remission (CDRS-R < 28) was achieved by 62% of participants at the conclusion of the intervention. Three months after their final supervised exercise session, nine of the 13 participants had either maintained the same CDRS-R score or had a further decrease in depressive symptoms; mean score three months post-intervention was 25.9 (SD = 6.5). In this study, the mean score on the QIDS-SR was 10.2 (SD = 4.5) pre-intervention, 7.8 (SD = 5.5) post-intervention, and 6.2 (SD = 2.2) at the follow-up assessment three months after the intervention.

3.1.4. Body Mass Index. At baseline, five participants (38.5%) were obese, five (38.5%) were overweight, and only three

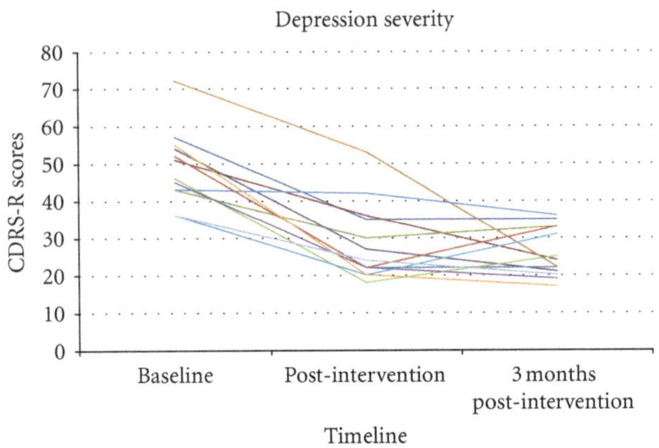

Figure 2: Children's Depression Rating Scale scores at baseline, post-intervention and three-month post-intervention time point.

(23%) were at a healthy weight. Between the baseline assessment and the conclusion of the exercise intervention, eight participants had a reduction in BMI while five participants had an increase in BMI. Following the intervention, three of the participants who had been in the overweight category were in the healthy-weight category. Of the three participants who moved to the healthy weight category, their mean BMI scores changed from 24.4 (SD = 1.4) pre-intervention to 23.6 (SD = 1.4) at 12 weeks.

Baseline BMI values ($r = -0.66$, $P = 0.03$) and post-intervention BMI values ($r = -0.75$, $P < 0.01$) were negatively correlated with average heart rates recorded during the supervised exercise sessions. Higher heart rates were positively correlated with change in BMI ($r = 0.75$, $P < 0.01$); the overweight adolescents who reached higher heart rates showed greater reductions in BMI.

3.2. Discussion. In this exercise intervention, adolescents with clinically significant depression were capable of completing a rigorous protocol requiring structured increases in exercise. Despite adopting a combination of supervised and independent exercise sessions, we expected that compliance with, and completion of, our intervention protocol would still be major challenges. However, 100% of these adolescent participants completed the 15 individual, supervised sessions required in our intervention protocol. Furthermore, adolescents reported ongoing exercise at the three-month post-intervention assessment, with six participants reporting an increase in exercise beyond the level reported at the conclusion of the intervention. This suggests the acceptability of incorporating exercise into their daily lives.

Given that our participants' compliance exceeded expectations, we reviewed the feasibility challenges we had expected to encounter and sought to identify which parameters of our study may have positively impacted those compliance and completion rates. First, the adolescents' independence was encouraged throughout our study. While parents or guardians were required to be involved in the consent process, during the period of exercise intervention all research staff communicated directly with the adolescent whenever possible rather than with the parents or guardians. Each week, participants reported to staff how they had met the independent exercise requirements, and goals for the following week were discussed. If parents asked if they should supervise or encourage the participant's independent sessions, research staff told them they were "off duty" for the independent sessions and that the teen would deal directly with the research staff regarding completion and reporting of the independent exercise. This helped to avoid having research expectations become a control issue or power struggle between adolescents and parents. The adolescents came up with creative ways of completing their independent sessions and were often proud of their exercise.

Second, having the exercise facilities in the same building as the outpatient psychiatric clinic building made the supervised sessions convenient for those participants who were also patients at that clinic. Third, research staff were extremely flexible in accommodating appointment hours outside of school, offering times during afternoons, evenings and weekends. To implement exercise as treatment for adolescents with depression in real world clinical practice, attention must be paid to issues such as encouraging adolescent autonomy, keeping appointment options flexible and suited to adolescents' demanding schedules, and establishing equitable access to facilities (e.g., onsite equipment, discounted or free passes to local gyms). Lastly, our experience is consistent with other researchers who report that compliance with the protocol is developed and maintained through an excellent therapeutic alliance between research staff and participants [32].

In addition to examining the factors that made this research study feasible, we also examined our secondary outcomes to understand the changes in exercise levels and depression severity. These 13 participants significantly increased their aerobic exercise levels as evidenced by the monitoring of heart rates in the weekly supervised exercise sessions; heart rates were even higher when specific targets were set for the participants to achieve. Actigraphy was recorded during weeks 3 and 12, verifying 81% adherence to the protocol's independent exercise sessions. Actigraphs were downloaded following the week of recording and did not provide any feedback to the participants. However, in future studies, independent exercise sessions and other increases in exercise will be verified using data from pedometers to provide more consistent monitoring of activity levels. The use of pedometers may help to reinforce positive health behavior by providing real-time feedback regarding one's level of activity. Furthermore, adolescents wearing pedometers could make a connection between their level of activity and their mood state.

Changes in depression severity were also assessed as a secondary outcome. Recognizing that previous research investigating exercise for adolescents with depression had been inconclusive in part due to a lack of repeated measures of depression severity [13], the design of this feasibility study included both clinician-rated and self-report measures of depression at multiple time points. All participants had reductions in their depression on both self-report (QIDS-SR) and the clinician-administered measure (CDRS-R). Of note, there was no control group in this research study. There is no way to confirm that the changes in depression were directly related to the exercise intervention. At the same time, several of these adolescents with depression had been engaged in psychotherapy and medication treatment for many months and in some cases for several years. Some of the adolescent participants reported that the exercise intervention had been the reason for their reduction in depressive symptoms.

Although weight was not considered in our inclusion criteria, 10 of our 13 participants were either overweight or obese at baseline. Also, five participants reported that losing weight was a motivating factor for their participation in this research. In this study, we found it feasible to both recruit and retain participants in all weight categories. For most participants, weight and BMI did not show significant change. However, several participants reported changes in how their clothing fit and felt positively about their change in physical appearance irrespective of a change in weight or BMI.

Alternative and augmenting treatment options, such as exercise, should be explored for all adolescents with depression, especially those who are overweight or obese. Obesity alone predisposes individuals to coronary heart disease, type 2 diabetes, certain cancers, hypertension, dyslipidemia, stroke, sleep apnea, respiratory problems, osteoarthritis, gynecologic problems, and liver and gallbladder disease. For adolescents dealing with depression, a positive health behavior change such as increasing exercise could prove to promote self-management of depressive symptoms while also serving to prevent nonpsychiatric medical comorbidity.

In addition to including adolescents with a range of body mass indices, we allowed participants to continue concurrent treatment with medication and/or psychotherapy. By including participants with varying symptom profiles and at various stages of treatment, the results of this study suggest that it is feasible to consider exercise as a primary treatment for certain patients and as an adjunctive treatment for others. Of these 13 adolescents with depression, eight participants (62%) achieved remission of their depressive symptoms following the exercise intervention. However, one participant, with a minimal decrease in depression, showed a greater treatment response after fluoxetine was initiated during the three-month follow-up period. For this individual, exercise alone did not appear to be the most effective treatment, supporting the ongoing need to consider multiple modalities of treatment. Interestingly, the five participants who were on antidepressant medications at the start of the exercise intervention had impressive reductions in CDRS-R scores, with three achieving remission. This suggests that the exercise may have been a useful adjunctive treatment to pharmacotherapy in these individuals. Future studies, with efficacy as the primary focus, should consider starting with untreated adolescents with depression to more clearly delineate the antidepressant effects of exercise from those of medication and psychotherapy.

Research on exercise and depression in adolescents will also need to address the challenging issues associated with control conditions, considering both scientific and safety questions. What is an appropriate control or "sham" condition in exercise research? Is it ethical to enroll adolescents with depressive disorders in a research protocol that includes randomization to conditions with unproven effectiveness in treating depression (i.e., exercise or placebo)? Previous researchers have explored several strategies to address these questions. Some have chosen to use stretching as a control condition which showed antidepressant effects similar to those of low-dose exercise [9]. In Blumenthal's SMILE study comparing exercise and medication, one of the conditions was a placebo control [8]. It has been suggested that the prospect of direct benefit to the participant is present even in RCTs with placebo conditions, as "the randomized design offers a prospect of active treatment to each participant" [33]. Many adolescents show a response to placebo [5] and a consensus statement of depression researchers stressed that placebo should not be considered as an absence of treatment [34]. Furthermore, a meta-analysis of studies in depression concluded that up to one in five participants in a wait-list control may experience remission of depression [35]. In combination with these published articles, the results of our study, which included both medicated and unmedicated participants, suggest that research investigating exercise as treatment for depression in adolescents is feasible and that randomized controlled trial designs should be considered.

3.2.1. Study Limitations and Strengths. Methodological limitations included the lack of an objective measure of acceptability, the lack of a control group, and the lack of blinding for clinical staff administering assessments. We also acknowledge that these participants were self-selected and that these results may not be generalizable to all adolescents with depressive disorders. In addition, these data from 13 participants lack statistical power for additional analyses that might further explore gender differences and other questions about the relationships among exercise, depression, and obesity.

In this study, exercise was measured via self-report, through heart rate monitoring, and with intermittent actigraphy. Despite the periodic use of actigraphy, there was no objective measure of exercise for the majority of the independent exercise sessions. In future research, we will strengthen this element of our investigation with the use of pedometers throughout the study period, which can assess more continuous compliance with the protocol as well the intensity of exercise.

4. Conclusions

Our primary aim was to assess the feasibility of recruiting and retaining adolescents with depression in an exercise intervention. In short, can you get a teenager with depression to exercise? These adolescents with clinically significant depression completed a rigorous research protocol examining the role of exercise in the treatment of depression. The feasibility of research in this area is supported by the 100% completion of 15 supervised exercise sessions, and the strong adherence to the protocol's independent sessions. During supervised sessions, the documented heart rates confirmed the participants' ability to achieve elevated levels of aerobic activity. Examination of secondary outcome measures showed that these adolescents had a significant increase in their exercise levels and a significant decrease in their depressive symptoms.

Ongoing research on depressive disorders and exercise is urgently needed to address the emerging epidemics of adolescent depression and obesity. Once the effectiveness of exercise is established as a treatment for depression in adolescents, the research must then focus on strategies to facilitate the implementation of this knowledge in the adolescents' world (e.g., psychiatric settings, school environment), and making the research results a catalyst for real behavioral change. If regular exercise can be proven to decrease depressive symptoms in adolescents, the information can and should impact clinical practice, encouraging the inclusion of exercise as part of the treatment plan. The ultimate goal is to use evidence-based research on exercise to influence the course of depressive illness during this vulnerable developmental stage.

Acknowledgments

The authors would like to thank the following for the valuable funding support which made this research possible: the Klingenstein Third Generation Fellowship in Childhood and Adolescent Depression, the Rachel Upjohn Clinical Scholars Award, and the Todd Ouida Clinical Scholars Award.

References

[1] M. Kovacs, "Presentation and course of major depressive disorder during childhood and later years of the life span," *Journal of the American Academy of Child and Adolescent Psychiatry*, vol. 35, no. 6, pp. 705–715, 1996.

[2] J. Puig-Antich, J. Kaufman, N. D. Ryan et al., "The psychosocial functioning and family environment of depressed adolescents," *Journal of the American Academy of Child and Adolescent Psychiatry*, vol. 32, no. 2, pp. 244–253, 1993.

[3] B. Birmaher, D. Brent, W. Bernet et al., "Practice parameter for the assessment and treatment of children and adolescents with depressive disorders," *Journal of the American Academy of Child and Adolescent Psychiatry*, vol. 46, no. 11, pp. 1503–1526, 2007.

[4] D. Brent, G. Emslie, G. Clarke et al., "Switching to another SSRI or to venlafaxine with or without cognitive behavioral therapy for adolescents with SSRI-resistant depression: the TORDIA randomized controlled trial," *Journal of the American Medical Association*, vol. 299, no. 8, pp. 901–913, 2008.

[5] J. March, S. Silva, B. Vitiello et al., "The Treatment for Adolescents with Depression Study (TADS): methods and message at 12 weeks," *Journal of the American Academy of Child and Adolescent Psychiatry*, vol. 45, no. 12, pp. 1393–1403, 2006.

[6] T. A. Hammad, T. Laughren, and J. Racoosin, "Suicidality in pediatric patients treated with antidepressant drugs," *Archives of General Psychiatry*, vol. 63, no. 3, pp. 332–339, 2006.

[7] A. M. Libby, D. A. Brent, E. H. Morrato, H. D. Orton, R. Allen, and R. J. Valuck, "Decline in treatment of pediatric depression after FDA advisory on risk of suicidality with SSRIs," *American Journal of Psychiatry*, vol. 164, no. 6, pp. 884–891, 2007.

[8] J. A. Blumenthal, M. A. Babyak, P. M. Doraiswamy et al., "Exercise and pharmacotherapy in the treatment of major depressive disorder," *Psychosomatic Medicine*, vol. 69, no. 7, pp. 587–596, 2007.

[9] A. L. Dunn, M. H. Trivedi, J. B. Kampert, C. G. Clark, and H. O. Chambliss, "Exercise treatment for depression: efficacy and dose response," *American Journal of Preventive Medicine*, vol. 28, no. 1, pp. 1–8, 2005.

[10] L. Larun, L. V. Nordheim, E. Ekeland, K. B. Hagen, and F. Heian, "Exercise in prevention and treatment of anxiety and depression among children and young people," *Cochrane Database of Systematic Reviews*, vol. 3, Article ID CD004691, 2006.

[11] R. W. Motl, A. S. Birnbaum, M. Y. Kubik, and R. K. Dishman, "Naturally occurring changes in physical activity are inversely related to depressive symptoms during early adolescence," *Psychosomatic Medicine*, vol. 66, no. 3, pp. 336–342, 2004.

[12] K. Patrick, J. F. Sallis, J. J. Prochaska et al., "A multicomponent program for nutrition and physical activity change in primary care: PACE+ for adolescents," *Archives of Pediatrics and Adolescent Medicine*, vol. 155, no. 8, pp. 940–946, 2001.

[13] A. L. Dunn and P. Weintraub, "Exercise in the prevention and treatment of adolescent depression: a promising but little researched intervention," *American Journal of Lifestyle Medicine*, vol. 2, no. 6, pp. 507–518, 2008.

[14] S. M. Sawyer and R. A. Aroni, "Self-management in adolescents with chronic illness. What does it mean and how can it be achieved?" *Medical Journal of Australia*, vol. 183, no. 8, pp. 405–409, 2005.

[15] A. J. Romero, "Low-income neighborhood barriers and resources for adolescents' physical activity," *Journal of Adolescent Health*, vol. 36, no. 3, pp. 253–259, 2005.

[16] L. B. Robbins, N. J. Pender, and A. S. Kazanis, "Barriers to physical activity perceived by adolescent girls," *Journal of Midwifery and Women's Health*, vol. 48, no. 3, pp. 206–212, 2003.

[17] K. A. Henderson and B. E. Ainsworth, "A synthesis of perceptions about physical activity among older African American and American Indian women," *American Journal of Public Health*, vol. 93, no. 2, pp. 313–317, 2003.

[18] C. S. Duarte, A. Sourander, G. Nikolakaros et al., "Child mental health problems and obesity in early adulthood," *Journal of Pediatrics*, vol. 156, no. 1, pp. 93–97, 2010.

[19] S. Mustillo, C. Worthman, A. Erkanli, G. Keeler, A. Angold, and E. J. Costello, "Obesity and psychiatric disorder: developmental trajectories," *Pediatrics*, vol. 111, no. 4, pp. 851–859, 2003.

[20] M. H. Trivedi, T. L. Greer, B. D. Grannemann, H. O. Chambliss, and A. N. Jordan, "Exercise as an augmentation strategy for treatment of major depression," *Journal of Psychiatric Practice*, vol. 12, no. 4, pp. 205–213, 2006.

[21] P. R. E. Crocker, D. A. Bailey, R. A. Faulkner, K. C. Kowalski, and R. Mcgrath, "Measuring general levels of physical activity: preliminary evidence for the physical activity questionnaire for older children," *Medicine and Science in Sports and Exercise*, vol. 29, no. 10, pp. 1344–1349, 1997.

[22] K. F. Janz, E. M. Lutuchy, P. Wenthe, and S. M. Levy, "Measuring activity in children and adolescents using self-report: PAQ-C and PAQ-A," *Medicine and Science in Sports and Exercise*, vol. 40, no. 4, pp. 767–772, 2008.

[23] K. C. Kowalski, P. R. E. Crocker, and N. P. Kowalski, "Convergent validity of the physical activity questionnaire for adolescents," *Pediatric Exercise Science*, vol. 9, no. 4, pp. 342–352, 1997.

[24] E. O. Poznanski and H. Mokros, *Children's depression rating scale revised (CDRS-R)*, Western Psychological Services, Los Angeles, Calif, USA, 1996.

[25] S. Jain, T. J. Carmody, M. H. Trivedi et al., "A psychometric evaluation of the CDRS and MADRS in assessing depressive symptoms in children," *Journal of the American Academy of Child and Adolescent Psychiatry*, vol. 46, no. 9, pp. 1204–1212, 2007.

[26] E. O. Poznanski and H. Mokros, "Children's depression rating scale revised (CDRS-R)—manual (w-242)," 1996, http://portal.wpspublish.com/portal/page?_pageid=53,69676&_dad=portal&_schema=PORTAL.

[27] A. J. Rush, "The 16-item Quick Inventory of Depressive Symptomatology (QIDS), clinician rating (QIDS-C), and self-report (QIDS-SR): a psychometric evalution in patients with chronic major depression," *Biological Psychiatry*, vol. 54, no. 5, p. 585, 2003.

[28] I. H. Bernstein, A. J. Rush, M. H. Trivedi et al., "Psychometric properties of the Quick Inventory of Depressive Symptomatology in adolescents," *International Journal of Methods in Psychiatric Research*, vol. 19, no. 4, pp. 185–194, 2010.

[29] Actigraphy, http://www.healthcare.philips.com/main/home-health/sleep/actiwatch/default.wpd.

[30] CDC Teen BMI Calculator, http://www.cdc.gov/healthyweight/assessing/bmi/childrens_bmi/about_childrens_ bmi.html.

[31] J. Cohen, *Statistical Power Analysis for the Behavioral Sciences*, Lawrence Earlbaum Associates, Hillsdale, NJ, USA, 2nd edition, 1988.

[32] C. W. Hughes, G. J. Emslie, M. L. Crismon et al., "Texas children's medication algorithm project: update from Texas consensus conference panel on medication treatment of childhood major depressive disorder," *Journal of the American Academy of Child and Adolescent Psychiatry*, vol. 46, no. 6, pp. 667–686, 2007.

[33] B. Vitiello, "Ethical considerations in psychopharmacological research involving children and adolescents," *Psychopharmacology*, vol. 171, no. 1, pp. 86–91, 2003.

[34] D. S. Charney, C. B. Nemeroff, L. Lewis et al., "National depressive and manic-depressive association consensus statement on the use of placebo in clinical trials of mood disorders," *Archives of General Psychiatry*, vol. 59, no. 3, pp. 262–270, 2002.

[35] M. A. Posternak and I. Miller, "Untreated short-term course of major depression: a meta-analysis of outcomes from studies using wait-list control groups," *Journal of Affective Disorders*, vol. 66, no. 2-3, pp. 139–146, 2001.

17

Grounded Theory of Barriers and Facilitators to Mandated Implementation of Mental Health Care in the Primary Care Setting

Justin K. Benzer,[1,2] Sarah Beehler,[1] Christopher Miller,[1] James F. Burgess,[1,2] Jennifer L. Sullivan,[1,2] David C. Mohr,[1,2] Mark Meterko,[1,2] and Irene E. Cramer[1,2]

[1] *Center for Organization, Leadership, and Management Research, VA Boston Healthcare System, Boston, MA 02130, USA*
[2] *Boston University School of Public Health, Boston, MA, USA*

Correspondence should be addressed to Justin K. Benzer, justin.benzer@va.gov

Academic Editor: Mark Williams

Objective. There is limited theory regarding the real-world implementation of mental health care in the primary care setting: a type of organizational coordination intervention. The purpose of this study was to develop a theory to conceptualize the potential causes of barriers and facilitators to how local sites responded to this mandated intervention to achieve coordinated mental health care. *Methods.* Data from 65 primary care and mental health staff interviews across 16 sites were analyzed to identify how coordination was perceived one year after an organizational mandate to provide integrated mental health care in the primary care setting. *Results.* Standardized referral procedures and communication practices between primary care and mental health were influenced by the organizational factors of resources, training, and work design, as well as provider-experienced organizational boundaries between primary care and mental health, time pressures, and staff participation. Organizational factors and provider experiences were in turn influenced by leadership. *Conclusions.* Our emergent theory describes how leadership, organizational factors, and provider experiences affect the implementation of a mandated mental health coordination intervention. This framework provides a nuanced understanding of the potential barriers and facilitators to implementing interventions designed to improve coordination between professional groups.

1. Introduction

Recent years have seen increasing recognition that the integration of mental health services into the primary care arena is an essential step for improving quality of mental health care [1, 2]. Based on this evidence, the Veterans Health Administration of the Department of Veterans Affairs (VA) has undertaken one of the largest implementations of Primary Care Mental Health Integration (PC/MHI) in the world [3]. The purpose of this integration was to improve the coordinated identification and treatment of prevalent mental health and substance use disorders in the VA primary care context [4].

At its broadest level, PC/MHI involves the implementation of structural organizational changes to policies, procedures, and practices that are intended to promote collaboration between primary care and clinical mental health experts in the assessment, treatment, and management of common mental health conditions [4]. As such, PC/MHI constitutes an organizational intervention to improve the coordination of patient care by effecting changes in care processes. The systematic implementation of PC/MHI across VA began with the first large-scale request for proposals occurring in 2007 [4]. Since then, spread of PC/MHI has been swift: as of 2011, over 85% of the more than 140 VA medical centers nationwide report some level of integration of mental health services into primary care. A 2010 issue of *Families, Systems, and Health* described many aspects of this national mandate within VA [4, 5].

Along with the rapid spread of PC/MHI throughout VA medical centers, research has investigated the factors important for successful PC/MHI implementation. For example, recent studies have explored the challenges faced by providers and clinics (within and outside VA) in transitioning to a PC/MHI model. These challenges include clarifying the responsibilities of PC/MHI versus specialty mental health clinics [6], balancing the availability of different types of appointments within PC/MHI [7], adjusting the timing and length of PC/MHI sessions [8], and establishing guidelines for smooth coordination between providers [9]. In addition, others have investigated factors that are important to consider when implementing large-scale changes across networks of VA medical centers [10].

With a few exceptions, PC/MHI research has been conducted in the context of implementations aimed at maintaining fidelity to a specific model or form of PC/MHI [8, 10, 11]. For example, the St. Louis Initiative for Integrated Care Excellence or SLI^{2}CE [6] carried an explicit emphasis on the integrated-collaborative-care model (e.g., time-limited interventions for a broad spectrum of disorders). VA, however, did not mandate one way of accomplishing PC/MHI. Instead, VA provided initial funding and allowed local site discretion in the implementation of at least one of three foundational models of integrated care: colocated collaborative care [12] and two models of care management [13, 14]. These models were similar in the introduction of a multidisciplinary treatment team but differed with respect to format (e.g., phone versus in-person), scope (e.g., depression versus broad range of mental health conditions), and types of care emphasized (e.g., triage versus care management versus brief interventions) [5]. The majority of VA facilities implemented some form of colocated care, with some sites including elements of care management, but rarely with strict fidelity to a theoretical model [5]. Thus, the conceptual differences in models may not be as pronounced in the local adaptations of PC/MHI. Despite isolated case studies [7], little is known about locally varied implementation of PC/MHI in response to the 2007 nationwide VA mandate.

The potential conflict between top-down-planned organizational changes and the autonomy of local practices has long been a concern in integrated health care systems such as VA, but the question of how to balance local needs for adaptation to mandated organizational changes with standardizing pressures is also broadly important to the private sector. For example, the Systems of Care program for children's mental health is similar to PC/MHI in that both are national programs that provide funding and guidelines for integrated care, while granting considerable autonomy to local sites/communities in tailoring the organizational changes [15]. More broadly, as part of the accreditation process, The Joint Commission often mandates certain outcomes and allows sites to determine the appropriate structure and processes for achieving them [16]. In addition, medical home and accountable care organization innovations in the US health care system are creating environments where these kinds of interventions are highly likely to be more common, particularly for psychotherapy interventions that have been poorly translated into community settings and/or limited to specialist mental health clinical settings [17].

The present paper addresses this gap in knowledge about the ability of local sites to respond to mandated organizational changes regarding mental health coordination processes. Rather than focus on fidelity to a specific model of PC/MHI (e.g., SLI^{2}CE), this study extends the scope of extant PC/MHI research by investigating the factors that may affect the ability of local clinical leaders to implement the structures and processes needed to coordinate mental health care across different VA clinics. There are several implementation models that have been used in the VA context [18, 19], but none of these models provide guidance as to how organizational factors (e.g., leadership, communication, staffing, physical space) may affect the ability of local sites to respond to a mandated organizational intervention. The concept of organizational coordination in health care was used to explicate the operational processes in PC/MHI and examine how organizational barriers and facilitators affected the ability of local sites to respond to the PC/MHI mandate.

1.1. Organizational Coordination in Integrated Care. The current study used an organizational coordination framework to guide our inquiry. We conceptualized the coordination processes involved in managing interdependent tasks across professional and team/unit boundaries to achieve integrated care. Organizational coordination can be achieved through standardized or interpersonal coordination processes [20, 21]. Standardized coordination processes (e.g., referral systems) are used to manage common coordination needs and interpersonal coordination processes (e.g., communication between providers, curbside consults) are used to manage less predictable coordination needs. Research has shown that both coordination modalities are needed for high-quality care [20]. Organizational coordination theories are well suited to elucidate the relationship between organizational structures, processes of care, and health outcomes [22] because they provide opportunities to identify organizational factors relevant to the PC/MHI implementation without unnecessarily constraining the data to conform to existing organizational models/structures.

Effective integrated care must be clinically appropriate as well as financially and operationally viable [23].The current study only examines the operational factors that influence implementation of coordination procedures. However, we acknowledge that operational factors are only one dimension of integrated care. Regarding the clinical dimension, we conceptualize both patient experiences and quality of care as important clinical outcomes of integrated mental health care. Outcomes of integrated mental health care include clinical outcomes such as increased identification and treatment of mental health symptoms and patient subjective experiences such as perceived access to mental health care and reduced stigma [24], but it is possible for organizational changes intended to promote integrated care to be implemented in ways that serve the needs of providers and administrators more than patients. Regarding the financial dimension, we acknowledge that improvements in quality of care should be cost effective, and thus cost is an important criterion for judging PC/MHI [25]. We conceptualize PC/MHI as an organizational coordination intervention that has the potential to impact access to mental health care, patient experiences of their care, quality of patient care, and healthcare costs.

Table 1: Interview questions and specific probes.

Interview question	Specific probes
(1) Imagine that a patient with depression symptoms comes to the clinic. Can you walk me through a typical process of care	Referral process, differences between diagnoses?
(2) How has this process changed over the past 10 years? (or since you arrived in the clinic)?	Recent changes, challenges, failures, leadership support, referrals, interpersonal interactions, physical structure?
(3) Tell me about your sense of the need for coordination between PC and MH.	Examples of good and poor coordination?
(4) How would you change your clinic to better coordinate care?	Communication, collaboration, resource barriers?
(5) Have you or anyone you know had to develop your own coordination procedures to ensure that patients receive the best care?	Work-arounds, ad-hoc coordination procedures?
(6) Can you tell me about the relationship between the people in the PC and MH clinics?	Face to face contact, trust?
(7) In what situations would you say that teamwork is most important?	Coworkers back each other up

Table 2: Sampling of key informants across the sixteen sites.

	Leaders	Physician	Psychologist	Psychiatrist	Nurse	Social worker	Physician assistant
Hospital-based clinics							
Site 1	2	1	2				
Site 2	2	2	1				
Site 3	2	1	1				
Site 4	2	1	2				
Site 5	1	1	1				
Site 6	2	1		1			
Site 7	2	1	1				
Site 8	2	1	1				
Large outpatient clinics							
Site 9	2		1		1		
Site 10	2	1		1			
Site 11	2					1	1
Site 12	1				1	1	
Site 13	2	1				1	
Site 14	2			1	1		
Site 15	2			1	1		
Site 16	2	1		1			

Psychologists, psychiatrists, nurses, social workers and the physician assistant were all associated with the PC-MHI clinic. These providers represent 51% of PC/MHI staff at these sites.

Regarding the operational dimension, we conceptualized PC/MHI as an organizational coordination intervention because it involves planned changes to the task-based standardized and interpersonal interactions between healthcare staff across team or unit boundaries (i.e., primary care and mental health). These operational changes represent structural integration of services that are exogenous to our framework of PC/MHI. Structural integration has been identified as a mechanism to promote coordination of patient care, but as noted in recent reviews, organizational changes that are intended to integrate services may not translate into either improved patient experiences [26] or effective collaborative care [27]. In order to build theory regarding how structural integration may or may not impact coordinated care, we focused our study on the processes of coordination (i.e., standardized and interpersonal) and allowed the organizational factors to emerge from the interviews. As shown in Table 1, our interview questions and data reflect this conceptual framework.

2. Methods

2.1. Participants. Key informants included 30 clinic leaders (12 PC physicians, 10 psychologists, 5 psychiatrists, 4 nurses, 3 social workers, 1 physician assistant) who were recruited from 16 PC/MHI clinics across eight VA medical centers as shown in Table 2. Interviewees were recruited from a hospital-based clinic and up to two large outpatient clinics (more than 10,000 unique patients) in each of eight medical centers. Informants varied in their tenure both at VA and also in the current position. Tenure in VA ranged from 1 to 32 years (Mean = 10.03, SD = 7.40). Tenure in current position ranged from 1 to 23 years (Mean = 5.53, SD = 5.07). Leaders were predominantly male (i.e., 12 female, 16 male), whereas staff were predominantly female (23 female, 10 male). The interviews were conducted as part of a managerial evaluation of the implementation of PC/MHI in these medical centers. Institutional review board approval was obtained to report this managerial evaluation data.

2.2. Data Collection. Semistructured telephone interviews were conducted between July and August 2009 to measure influences of implementation progress and effectiveness. Stratified purposeful sampling was used by first interviewing both PC and MH leaders who then, respectively, identified primary care and colocated mental health staff. Leaders used their understanding of the local clinic contexts to select professionals representing different clinical backgrounds who could best speak to coordination procedures or who were most closely involved with mental health treatment based on their local context judgment. The purpose of these interviews was to understand the implementation of colocated, collaborative care in local sites. Although some sites also implement depression care management, these models are less common in VA. Interviews required up to 45 minutes with a note taker instructed to record responses verbatim where possible.

In-depth interviews allow for intensive exploration of a phenomenon with individuals who have experienced it [28]. The evaluation team developed seven interview questions and specific probes to gather information on the processes used to coordinate primary care and mental health staff, how those processes changed over time, and how processes could be further improved (Table 1). Questions were generated based on management literature on coordination and were designed so the conversation became progressively more focused on the important aspects of informants' experiences they chose to discuss in the initial open-ended questions. Interviewers first asked two "grand tour" questions [29] that allowed informants to describe the present and evolved/past processes of care used in their sites openly and without a researcher-imposed framework. These questions focused informants on the processes used to provide depression care in the primary care setting and in particular on the changes in those processes. Interviews then turned toward interviewer-driven topics related to characteristics of the intervention (e.g., interpersonal relationships and coordination procedures), and how the intervention could be improved (e.g., communication, collaboration, resource barriers). These follow-up questions allowed us to explore our research questions in more detail [30, 31].

2.3. Data Analysis. The data analysis methodology was chosen to elaborate extant theory regarding the role of organization and leadership factors in intervention implementation. Very little theory has been developed regarding how healthcare organizations react to mandated organizational changes; however, we recognized that research on intervention implementation [17, 32–34] and organizational coordination [22] would likely be relevant. We used grounded theory techniques to identify emergent concepts and specify relationships between these theoretical concepts [35]. Specifically, we used NVivo [36] to analyze the data iteratively in four stages.

The purpose of the first two stages was to immerse ourselves in the data. In the first stage, we read through the interviews in their entirety to develop site summaries in order to begin theorizing about the factors that impacted PC/MHI implementation and to understand the gestalt PC/MHI implementation. These site summaries were needed to ensure that coded data were interpreted within the specific context of each site. In the second stage, the first author coded the raw data without any preconceived framework, looking for similarities across our key informants and across our sites. The purpose of this step was to identify similar types of data that could be analyzed in more depth. The output of this step was a set of codes that represented descriptive characteristics of PC/MHI (e.g., types of referral processes).

The purpose of the last two stages was to develop conceptual codes that represented potential causal factors that might impact the PC/MHI implementation (see Table 3) and identify how these codes are connected. Our knowledge of theoretical concepts from implementation science as well as the leadership and organizational psychology literature served as a foundation for our analysis. The concepts and framework presented here, however, were grounded in and emerged from the data analyses [37]. In the third stage, we reanalyzed the raw data associated with each descriptive code. Two coders (one, [blinded], trained in the organization sciences and a second, [blinded], an expert in mental health services) sequentially recoded the evaluation data in NVivo (version 2) to identify potential causal relationships among the codes [38]. Each first coder identified the relevant concepts through an iterative process of coding emergent concepts, reviewing the concepts, revising the conceptual codes, and developing a coding guide for the second coder, who then also coded the emergent concepts. The two coders discussed all disagreements, referred to the overall site summaries as needed and reached consensus for the definitions and application of each code. Thus, the codes represented a consensus between these two disciplinary perspectives. The fourth stage of analysis focused on establishing the connections between the concepts represented in this set of codes. Specifically, the data were divided between four authors such that each author was responsible for the data associated with 4-5 conceptual codes (e.g., one author reviewed only comments in the leadership factor). The authors then individually analyzed their set of data to identify how their conceptual codes were related to the other conceptual codes listed in Table 3. The outcome of this process was a summary of each conceptual code that detailed the empirical support for causal links with other conceptual codes. With input from all other authors the first author then led a process of integrating these analyses to formulate the emergent theory presented in Figure 1. The first author created an initial path diagram that detailed all of the possible

TABLE 3: Emergent codes.

Code	Definition
(A) Leadership	Leadership does/does not provide direction, coordinate between different services, obtain needed resources, make timely decisions, communicate with staff.
(B1) Resources (space)	Lack of space includes barriers due to physical structure of facility, includes lack of space and distance barriers.
(B1) Resources (staffing)	Not enough staff available to provide coordinated mental health care.
(B1) Resources (knowledge and skills)	Specific mention of staff knowledge, skills, or abilities. It includes general comments such as "good staff"
(B2) Training	Training for MH procedures, including training of admin personnel
(B3) Work design	Intentional choices regarding how care is provided; description of how tasks are divided between staff and/or clinics including informal systems work systems designed to overcome other barriers, including mandated tasks and same day appointments
(C1) PC/MH boundaries	Perceived physical and/or psychological barriers between primary care and mental health clinics provide barriers to care.
(C2) Time pressure	Overworked staff, working through admin/lunch time
(C3) Staff participation	Staff "buy-in", perceptions of mutual PC and MH participation, comfort with PC/MH referrals. It includes the use of formal and informal meetings to increase participation.
(D) Referral systems	Processes used to coordinate care may include specific barriers to the referral process. It including the use of electronic medical record, paging systems, checklists.
(E) Communication	Interpersonal communication, communication between PC and MH.
Patient complexity	Challenges due to complicated mental health conditions and/or medical comorbidities; patients have many health needs, including noncompliance issues

links between concepts suggested by the data. The authors refined the model through an iterative process of reviewing the data and group discussion.

Triangulation is valued in qualitative research because parallel perspectives across key informants can increase the credibility of qualitative analyses [39, 40]. We expected variability in how the intervention was implemented across sites because the design of work is path dependent, that is, the way that structure is modified is influenced by history and prior structure [41], and so work practices are likely to vary greatly by site. We also expected variability in the barriers and facilitators to implementation across sites. Therefore, we compared responses across sites to enhance the credibility of results and we specifically noted where conclusions were based on the report of key informants at only one site.

3. Results

We have developed a theory to understand that the leadership and organizational factors create barriers and facilitators to a locally adapted intervention designed to provide mental health care in the primary care setting (Figure 1). Definitions of emergent codes are presented in Table 3. Our analyses focused on factors associated with leadership (Factor A), organization (Factor B), and provider experiences (Factor C) as they were reported to impact both referral systems (Factor D) and communication (Factor E). The role of referral systems and communication with coordinated mental health care (Factor F) was not measured, but informed our conceptual framework and study design, and were discussed as important by participants. Below, we begin by discussing the two modes of coordination in PC/MHI, interpersonal communication between providers, and standardized referral systems. We present evidence regarding the influence of provider experiences on communication (Path C → E), and how referral systems are affected by both organizational factors (Path B → D) and provider experiences (Path C → D). We then review the evidence regarding how provider experiences are affected by organizational factors (Path B → C), and discuss how leadership can affect both organizational factors (Path A → B) and provider experiences (Path A → C). Finally, we conceptually discuss the role of patient factors in our model, depicted as the surrounding environment in Figure 1.

3.1. Communication between Primary Care and Mental Health. Communication between providers was relational, starting at the front lines. Primary care providers reported interacting with mental health staff on a personal level, building relationships, in order to generate trust and effective communication. At some sites, where the mental health worker was a psychologist rather than a psychiatrist, primary care providers indicated that they would have preferred MD to MD relations with a psychiatrist. Yet reported communication patterns varied. The source of this variation was not

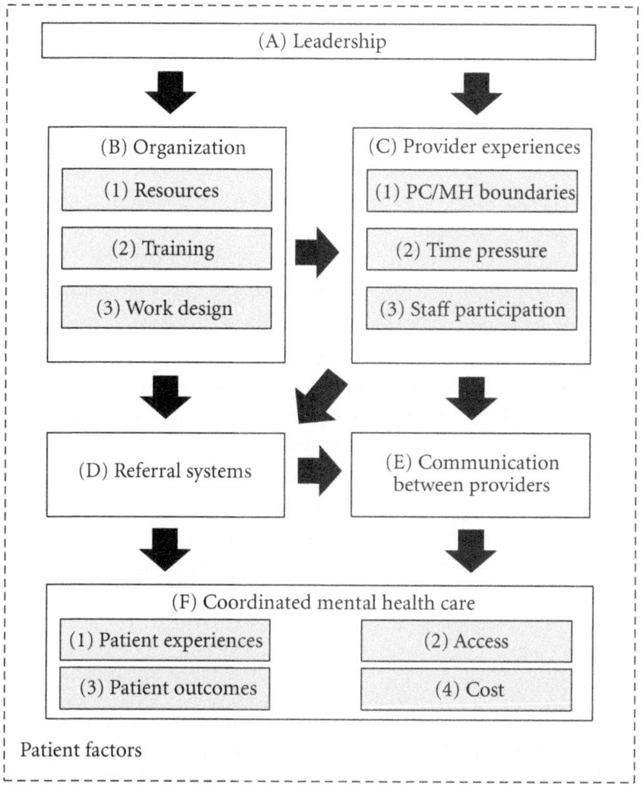

FIGURE 1: Theoretical framework of barriers and facilitators to locally-adapted PC/MHI implementation.

clear from the analyses, but may have been due to individual differences in preferences and attitudes.

Primary care providers who discussed communication barriers indicated that time pressures made it difficult to build relationships (Path C2 → E). Communication between PC and MH typically increased incrementally during the implementation of PC/MHI as the psychological boundaries between services decreased and staff increased their participation and involvement in integrated mental health care. As mental health staff started to work to address primary care needs, primary care began communicating more with mental health (Path C3 → E).

3.2. Referral Systems. The VA electronic medical record provides tools and templates so PC and MH providers can better communicate about patients and, when necessary, see patients sooner. Some examples included a consult screen being successful in increasing patient access and referrals; a triage checklist for PC to handle patients in crisis right away; and integrated medication lists to flag medication interactions. The electronic medical record provides information about how PC and MH are coordinating services for a patient through automated notification processes. This electronic communication appeared to facilitate interpersonal communication regarding patient care (Path D → E). Staff reported barriers due to inadequate information in the electronic medical record which included the quick consult screen not being detailed enough to provide needed information, follow-up appointments not being scheduled appropriately by specialists, and lack of certain fields which could provide increased coordination (e.g., the name of the primary mental health provider).

Appropriate staffing and funding to hire new employees were reported as important for referral system effectiveness (Path B1 → D). Some sites emphasized the need to hire more MH and PC providers. Staffing limitations were reported as barriers to implementing the desired work design for PC/MHI. For example, staffing limited colocation of psychologists that in turn limited the availability of same day access to mental health care or short-term therapies. Space resources were needed to allow staff to be colocated within the same space (Path B1 → B3) and to provide the staff needed to handle the additional mental health consults (Path B1 → D). Notably, leaders often reported that available space in primary care limited the amount of mental health staff that could be hired. Other staffing issues which may impact referral system effectiveness were staff turnover, inability to fill vacant positions, and Human Resources delays inhibiting timely hiring.

Referral systems were also reported to be affected by time pressure and training. Referrals through the electronic medical record were seen as more efficient when workload was high (Path C2 → E). Other sites reported that a lack of knowledge of the appropriate mental health referral processes limited the effectiveness of electronic referrals. Strategies for increasing referrals mentioned were training primary care staff (Path B2 → D) and developing referral templates (i.e., standardizing coordination) for the electronic medical record (Factor D). Primary care staff reported needing additional training for evidence-based mental health treatment. Staff from various sites reported receiving broad training regarding changes in work design (Path B2 → B3) and referral processes (Path B2 → D) but not necessarily in-depth training for how to handle specific problems (Path B2 → F). In one site, staff reported that training was needed for nurses (e.g., dealing with crisis patients during triage) and clerks (e.g., interacting with angry patients) in addition to primary care providers.

Unresolved conflicts between work design and patient mental health needs were identified as barriers to patient access that limited referral system effectiveness and efficiency. Primary care providers noted that formulary restrictions often made it difficult for them to adjust medications for mental health conditions (prescribing authority in VA is often limited by provider specialty) that increased the need for specialty care referrals (Path B3 → D). One mental health clinician reported that competing demands to focus improvement efforts on returning Veterans and traumatic brain injury led to a divided focus on primary care integration (Path B3 → D). Having an on-site mental health clinician was noted to help alleviate same day appointment concerns through warm hand-offs (Path B1 → B3 → D), where primary care providers would introduce patients to MH staff, who would then perform a short assessment. However, some primary care participants reported the use of beepers as an alternative method to manage scheduling and same day appointment access (Path B3 → D). Mental health at many sites responded to high demand for care by designing work (i.e., templates and protocols) to manage this demand (Path B3 → D). For example, at one site, mental health required a patient to be on the maximum medication dosage before being seen. Another site handled high demand for substance abuse care by mandating that mental health conditions be resolved before addressing substance abuse. In some sites, primary care staff reported ad-hoc workarounds to meet the criteria of the template to manage these access restrictions.

The intentional choices regarding how primary care and mental health work are organized (i.e., work design) created the potential for conflicts when coordination procedures were revised. Conflicts between intended improvements to work design with the broader patient care system created unintended consequences in referral systems (Path B3 → D). One type of conflict was observed between the design of routine and urgent mental health care. Some sites implemented an electronic scheduling system where open slots are available and patients in need of MH services can be given immediate access, but increasing the number of open appointment slots was reported to decrease access for regularly scheduled patients. A second type of conflict was observed in how referral systems were specified between services. Interservice referrals in VA were specified by formal or informal agreements, and these prior agreements set the context for unintended consequences when PC/MHI was implemented. In two sites, emergency room staff reacted to the addition of PC/MHI staff by attempting to shift responsibility for urgent mental health care to primary care. Other sites reported that specialty mental health staff began restricting access to only patients with the most severe conditions. Yet another site reported difficulties managing referrals to substance abuse for patients who also had mental health conditions.

3.3. Organizational Factors Influence Provider Experiences. The knowledge, skills, and abilities of staff were frequently mentioned as an important organizational resource for integrated care. Some examples of key relevant staff characteristics were motivation to work with and care for Veterans in particular, primary care providers who understand psychology, and competent mental health liaison nurses. Interviewees reinforced the need for collaboration among providers with differing levels and types of primary care and mental health skills. Interviews suggested that mutual awareness of collaboration opportunities was sufficient to create interactions. Persistence of colocated mental health staff in developing relationships and learning about how to address mental health needs in primary care was reported to slowly change primary care providers' participation (Path B1 → C3). At the point of the interviews, mental health staffing was not yet sufficient to handle the volume of work in many sites (B1 → C2). Time pressure was closely related to work design, where several sites reported efforts to redistribute workload across PC and MH (B3 → C2).

Mental health staff members were frequently colocated with primary care staff. Colocation was perceived as improving integration, referrals, and clinician accessibility in part because proximity increased familiarity between primary care and mental health staff (B3 → C3). Mental health providers reported that informal conversations with primary care providers, such as in hallways or over lunch, were particularly important in engaging primary care providers. Preexisting collaborative relationships between primary care and mental health were reported to facilitate the intervention (Path B3 → C3). In sites without these preexisting relationships, mental health providers reported actively seeking opportunities to demonstrate how mental health could help primary care. Mental health staff attendance at monthly primary care meetings was reported to increase primary care participation and engagement (Path B3 → C3). Employees noted that during these meetings, discussions about appropriate consults occurred, and leadership could provide a consistent message regarding the importance of coordinated mental health care.

Cultural norms and work patterns differ between PC and MH, so defining the boundaries of patient care responsibilities and dealing with preconceived notions of how patient mental health care should be coordinated are challenges that require on-going upkeep. Deterioration of interactions across PC and MH boundaries that arose over time was repeatedly described as turf wars and sometimes attributed to lack of resources (Path B1 → C1). For example, primary care providers were reported to be worried that PC/MHI would increase demand on their scarce resources, and at one site mental health providers were reported to redirect large numbers of patients to primary care for treatment who were previously treated in specialty mental health (e.g., personality disorders). Colocated mental health staff, who worked on the boundary between primary care and mental health, provided detailed information regarding these conflicts. The general theme is that boundary issues are not static but require continuing attention over time so as not to break down as staff and circumstances change.

3.4. The Role of Leadership in Integrated Care. PC/MHI implementation required collaboration between service leaders. At a minimum, engagement of both primary care and mental health leaders in a collaborative effort was needed to support the intervention. Clinic leaders indicated that the intervention benefitted from collaboration with leaders in administration, human resources, nursing service, and specialists in the needs of Veterans returning from Iraq and Afghanistan. Leadership was reported to be effective in bridging boundaries between services, resolving conflicts, requesting and allocating resources, and setting responsibilities for new staff.

PC/MHI is designed to act for multiple constituencies (e.g., PC, MH, and patients), and changes to work design and resources through the PC/MHI intervention affected how those constituencies perceived the intervention. In some cases, these issues were resolved by leader involvement and interservice negotiations. Leaders helped clinicians cross boundaries between PC and MH through formal and informal meetings (Path A → C1). In contrast, other leaders maintained or even strengthened these boundaries between PC and MH by acting as an intermediary between services rather than promoting direct interaction. Leaders were particularly important when conflicts arose across these PC/MH boundaries (i.e., turf wars) over responsibility for patients with urgent mental health needs.

Leadership was broadly identified as important in focusing available resources toward PC/MHI goals (Path A → B1). Sites that reported leaders to be supportive indicated that leadership was particularly valuable for staff recruitment and space allocation. Informants who reported poor leadership support reported long delays for necessary resources, such as changes in the referrals systems that would improve communication. Further, leaders at all levels (e.g., service chiefs, nurse managers) were reported to have an important role in developing training programs that provided mental health knowledge, skills, and abilities needed for the intervention (Path A → B2 → B1).

Informants also reported that leadership was an important factor in adjusting work design to improve patient access to mental health care (Path A → B3). Leadership was also reported to have some impact on staff participation (Path A → C3). Leaders were reported to have minimal direct influence in the intervention as changes in care required changes to provider behaviors, but active frontline leader engagement was reported as critical in supporting highly motivated providers (e.g., providing co-located space, supporting work redesign) thereby maintaining but not necessarily creating staff participation (Path A → B1 → C3).

3.5. Patient Factors. Data indicated that patient factors may affect the utilization and effectiveness of referral systems (Factor D), as well as the amount of communication needed between providers (Factor E). Informants reported the importance of differentiating patients with on-going chronic needs who need to see providers in a MH setting versus patients with short-term needs that can be handled in a PC setting. Providers would like to refer some of these complex patients to treatment programs or long-term care facilities but sometimes have difficulty finding the open slots. Regarding the effectiveness of referral systems, staff reported that patients were frequently noncompliant to prescribed treatment and missed appointments. In addition, complex patients require medication coordination that may increase the amount of communication needed between primary care and mental health.

4. Discussion

We developed a theory that posits leadership, provider experiences, and organizational factors as key influences on the successful implementation of new mental health coordination practices in real-world healthcare settings. Specifically, factors associated with leadership and organizational characteristics shaped provider experiences, all of which affected the degree to which mental health care was coordinated through referral mechanisms and communication among providers. Organizational factors and provider experiences were important because they set the structural and relational conditions that facilitated and hindered PC/MHI implementation. Though the relationships between individual provider attributes and intervention implementation are often meaningful, our findings suggest that the organizational processes supporting/constraining implementation are extremely important.

Leaders were able to affect provider experiences by providing opportunities for staff to work across professional boundaries, by resolving conflicts, and otherwise supporting staff who were working to implement the intervention. Leaders also were able to modify organizational factors by obtaining and allocating critical resources (e.g., personnel, space), developing training to close staff knowledge or skill shortages, and adjusting work responsibilities to address implementation challenges as they arose. Provider experiences and organizational factors directly impacted how referral systems and interprovider communication were implemented.

4.1. Practical Significance. This study is a first step toward an explanatory model of organizational coordination intervention implementation that could be applied to a wide range of mental health coordination problems. For example, in addition to outpatient coordination of depression care, transitions of mental health care between inpatient settings and primary care are important. A recent VA study suggests that transitions of mental health care after general medical hospitalizations are particularly important for patients with mental health conditions [42]. We propose that the implementation of coordination procedures between inpatient medicine and an outpatient mental health service is likely to be affected by the same set of factors (i.e., leadership, organization, and provider) as the PC/MHI intervention.

This study has direct, practical implications for mental health providers and managers who are considering implementing changes to how patient care is coordinated across multiple healthcare providers and especially when those providers operate across organizational boundaries (i.e., professional silos). In the context of local responses to a mandated intervention, both leadership and organizational factors (i.e., resources, training and work design) were identified as potential antecedents for the implementation of new referral systems and patterns of communication across providers. Provider factors (i.e., perceived PC/MHI boundaries, and staff participation in the intervention) were reported to be important but only indirectly affected by leaders. Sites in the current study either took advantage of preexisting collaborative relationships between primary care and mental health or utilized highly engaged key individuals to attenuate the boundaries between services and increase staff participation.

The PC/MHI intervention was designed to cross intraorganizational boundaries in that coordination procedures were implemented across PC and MH units within one healthcare facility. However, organizational boundaries can also be interorganizational. For example, coordination procedures could be implemented between independent fee-for-service PC and MH providers or provider groups. We propose that our model is also relevant for these types of interventions. That is, communication patterns between independent facilities such as these will likely depend on the strength of organizational boundaries, the time pressure experienced by staff, and the degree to which staff choose to participate in the intervention. Without a common health system as in VA, organizational boundaries may be stronger and participation may be more variable, but we suggest that the concepts will be similar. Accountable care organizations and medical homes being created in the private sector, for example, may have environments amenable to these types of interventions. Resources, training, and work design may also vary more across independent units and therefore implementing standardized referral procedures may be more challenging, but the key relationships between these concepts are likely to be the same. Because we expect increased variation in both organizational factors and provider experiences when implementing interventions across independent facilities, we expect that leadership will be even more important. Shared vision for the organizational change across independent facilities is likely to be particularly important when redesigning work, allocating resources, and bridging interorganizational boundaries.

4.2. Limitations and Future Research Directions. The dependent variable for our study was coordination, an operational dimension of integrated care, but we acknowledge that the clinical and financial dimensions of integration are important outcomes of PC/MHI. Patient experiences, patient access, patient outcomes, and cost data would be needed to judge whether the intervention was successful or not. Our study was only able to identify the factors that influenced the implementation process. That is, leadership, organization factors, and provider experiences may be important in changing coordination processes, but those processes may have negligible impact on outcomes. Thus, further research on the clinical, financial, and patient-centered impacts of the PC/MHI model in actual practice settings is recommended.

We did not design this study to measure the impact of patient factors on the intervention implementation. Healthcare integration is typically conceptualized as an organizational factor, but patient experiences of integrated care are an important dimension that is often overlooked in both theoretical and empirical work [26]. We acknowledge that patient preferences and mental health diagnoses vary in the types of referrals and amount of communication needed, and therefore patient factors may moderate the impact of leadership, organization factors, and provider experiences. For example, depression may be entirely managed within the primary care setting, particularly if colocated short-term therapy is available, whereas other mental health disorders, such as schizophrenia, may be managed in specialized clinics. Thus, the characteristics of the patient panel involved are likely to have considerable impact on leadership support, resources, and provider experiences. Our study was not designed to identify these links and thus our data is limited regarding how patient factors influence the delivery of mental health care in the primary care setting.

This study was limited in that sites were all sampled from VA, a healthcare network with unique organizational structures compared to other healthcare providers in the United States. Aspects such as its hierarchical structure and the influence it has on different medical centers, the degree to which it is a closed system, and its size, may limit the transferability of findings to other settings [41]. However, the purpose of the current study was theory building rather than theory testing and therefore purposeful sampling to identify the processes of interest was appropriate rather than random sampling to identify population parameters [43]. Our use of multiple sites strengthens the emergent theory because identified processes are not limited to a single group of healthcare providers. Theory building is an iterative process that involves analysis of multiple cases and additional research is needed to determine whether and how certain dimensions of the current theory are limited to VA. Some reported barriers (e.g., turf wars) may not be as relevant for coordination between fee-for-service facilities, but we propose that the concepts presented are likely to generalize across contexts. Because our theory is based on local responses to a national mandate to provide integrated mental health care, results may be most directly applicable to responses to national or state-level policy changes (e.g., licensure scope, mental health equity) but may also apply to any local organizational changes intended to improve coordination. Although the specific factors may vary, the concepts identified in the current study are common in studies of organizational intervention barriers and facilitators [32–34]. We propose that our framework of leadership, organization factors, and provider experiences is relevant to the implementation of any intervention designed to create coordination procedures.

We acknowledge that clearly specified interventions with stronger evidence may be more easily marketed to clinicians and may be viewed as easier to adopt by local leaders [18], but research has not focused adequately on understanding situations where "evidence-based" interventions are not available or do not fit with local conditions. Intervention implementation research in clinical settings tends to focus on either adoption [18, 19, 34] or spread [44–46] of evidence-based practices. This type of implementation research is designed to identify the factors that maximize implementation fidelity of a standardized intervention that is being promoted as a best practice. However, establishing fidelity to a standardized guideline may not be optimal for all sites [44]. Recent research suggests that interventions that are tailored to be consonant with local norms, resources, and patterns of practice may be more sustainable than standardized interventions [45]. Furthermore, healthcare settings face problems for which there may not be clear evidence-based solutions available [46, 47]. There are many studies of implementation barriers and facilitators but no general framework to explain how these barriers and facilitators affect organizational changes [32–34]. The current study provides a framework of barriers and facilitators that can be used to study local tailoring and adaption of planned organizational changes.

Future research on the implementation of interventions designed to improve coordination would benefit from careful initial measurement of the identified organizational, leadership and provider/cultural/social factors to assess baseline capacities relevant for implementation. Repeated measurements of these and related factors over time would allow for exploration of the extent to which they mediate/moderate key intervention outcomes. For example, organizational boundaries due to social and cognitive differences between professions may interfere with intervention implementation [48]. Leadership was the only factor that we identified as an exogenous variable; that is, our interviews did not indicate that leadership was influenced by organizational or provider factors, but rather that leadership influenced each of those factors. Repeated measurement of leadership behaviors and communication across these boundaries could provide evidence that leadership can improve implementation of a coordination intervention by interpersonal interactions between professions. Future research would benefit from exploring the qualities and practices of leaders who effectively support the boundary spanning activities of providers that are essential to providing coordinated mental health care.

5. Conclusions

We used grounded theory to develop a conceptual framework that identifies leadership, provider experiences, and organization factors as key antecedents to local changes when new coordination practices are implemented in healthcare settings. Our results suggest that current organizational resources, training, and work design along with psychological barriers between units, time pressure, and barriers to staff participation in the new coordination procedures at a site are each important factors to consider before implementing an organizational coordination intervention. Results may apply to any local changes intended to improve organizational coordination.

Acknowledgments

Financial support was provided in part from Department of Veterans Affairs, Veterans Health Administration, Office of Research and Development Grant (IIR no. 05-221) and three VA Office of Academic Affiliations HSR&D postdoctoral fellowships. The views expressed in this paper are those of the authors and do not necessarily reflect the position or policy of the Department of Veterans Affairs or the United States government.

References

[1] E. H. Wagner, B. T. Austin, C. Davis, M. Hindmarsh, J. Schaefer, and A. Bonomi, "Improving chronic illness care: translating evidence into action," *Health Affairs*, vol. 20, no. 6, pp. 64–78, 2001.

[2] M. Butler, R. L. Kane, D. McAlpine et al., "Integration of mental health/substance abuse and primary care," *Evidence Report/Technology Assessment*, no. 173, pp. 1–362, 2008.

[3] E. P. Post and W. W. Van Stone, "Veterans Health Administration primary care-mental health integration initiative," *North Carolina Medical Journal*, vol. 69, no. 1, pp. 49–52, 2008.

[4] A. S. Pomerantz and S. L. Sayers, "Primary care-mental health integration in healthcare in the Department of Veterans Affairs," *Families, Systems & Health*, vol. 28, no. 2, pp. 78–82, 2010.

[5] E. P. Post, M. Metzger, P. Dumas, and L. Lehmann, "Integrating mental health into primary care within the Veterans Health Administration," *Families, Systems & Health*, vol. 28, no. 2, pp. 83–90, 2010.

[6] P. A. Brawer, R. Martielli, P. L. Pye, J. Manwaring, and A. Tierney, "St. Louis Initiative for Integrated Care Excellence (SLI^{2}CE): integrated-collaborative care on a large scale model," *Families, Systems & Health*, vol. 28, no. 2, pp. 175–187, 2010.

[7] J. A. Barber, L. M. Frantsve, S. Capelli, and K. A. Sanders, "Implementation and evaluation of an integrated care program in a VA medical center," *Psychological Services*, vol. 8, pp. 282–293, 2011.

[8] J. S. Funderburk, D. E. Sugarman, S. A. Maisto et al., "The description and evaluation of the implementation of an integrated healthcare model," *Families, Systems & Health*, vol. 28, no. 2, pp. 146–160, 2010.

[9] M. Tai-Seale, M. E. Kunik, A. Shepherd, J. Kirchner, and A. Gottumukkala, "A case study of early experience with implementation of collaborative care in the veterans health administration," *Population Health Management*, vol. 13, no. 6, pp. 331–337, 2010.

[10] J. Kirchner, C. N. Edlund, K. Henderson, L. Daily, L. E. Parker, and J. C. Fortney, "Using a multi-level approach to implement a primary care mental health (PCMH) program," *Families, Systems & Health*, vol. 28, no. 2, pp. 161–174, 2010.

[11] W. J. Katon, E. H. Lin, M. Von Korff et al., "Collaborative care for patients with depression and chronic illnesses," *The New England Journal of Medicine*, vol. 363, no. 27, pp. 2611–2620, 2010.

[12] A. S. Pomerantz, B. Shiner, B. V. Watts et al., "The white river model of colocated collaborative care: a platform for mental and behavioral health care in the medical home," *Families, Systems & Health*, vol. 28, no. 2, pp. 114–129, 2010.

[13] L. V. Rubenstein, E. F. Chaney, S. Ober et al., "Using evidence-based quality improvement methods for translating depression collaborative care research into practice," *Families, Systems & Health*, vol. 28, no. 2, pp. 91–113, 2010.

[14] J. Tew, J. Klaus, and D. W. Oslin, "The behavioral health laboratory: building a stronger foundation for the patient-centered medical home," *Families, Systems & Health*, vol. 28, no. 2, pp. 130–145, 2010.

[15] P. Jivanjee and A. Robinson, "Studying family participation in system-of-care evaluations: using qualitative methods to examine a national mandate in local contexts," *Journal of Behavioral Health Services and Research*, vol. 34, no. 4, pp. 369–381, 2007.

[16] P. M. Schyve, "The evolution of external quality evaluation: observations from the Joint Commission on Accreditation of Healthcare Organizations," *International Journal for Quality in Health Care*, vol. 12, no. 3, pp. 255–258, 2000.

[17] M. Wensing, H. Wollersheim, and R. Grol, "Organizational interventions to implement improvements in patient care: a structured review of reviews," *Implementation Science*, vol. 1, article 2, 2006.

[18] C. B. Stetler, L. J. Damschroder, C. D. Helfrich, and H. J. Hagedorn, "A Guide for applying a revised version of the PARIHS framework for implementation," *Implementation Science*, vol. 6, article 99, 2011.

[19] L. J. Damschroder, D. C. Aron, R. E. Keith, S. R. Kirsh, J. A. Alexander, and J. C. Lowery, "Fostering implementation of health services research findings into practice: a consolidated framework for advancing implementation science," *Implementation Science*, vol. 4, article 50, 2009.

[20] G. Young, M. P. Charns, K. Desai et al., "Patterns of coordination and clinical outcomes: a study of surgical services," *Health Services Research*, vol. 33, no. 5, pp. 1211–1236, 1998.

[21] M. P. Charns and M. Schaefer, *Health Care Organization: A Model For Management*, Prentice Hall, Englewood Cliffs, NJ, USA, 1983.

[22] M. P. Charns, G. J. Young, J. Daley, S. Khuri, and W. Henderson, Eds., *Coordination and Patient Care Outcomes*, Imperial College, London, UK, 2000.

[23] C. J. Peek, "Planning care in the clinical, operational, and financial worlds," in *Collaborative Medicine Case Studies: Evidence in Practice*, R. Kessler and D. Stafford, Eds., pp. 25–38, Springer, New York, NY, USA, 2008.

[24] S. Thielke, S. Vannoy, and J. Unutzer, "Integrating mental health and primary care," *Primary Care*, vol. 34, no. 3, pp. 571–592, 2007.

[25] J. M. Pyne, J. C. Fortney, S. P. Tripathi, M. L. Maciejewski, M. J. Edlund, and D. K. Williams, "Cost-effectiveness analysis of a rural telemedicine collaborative care intervention for depression," *Archives of General Psychiatry*, vol. 67, no. 8, pp. 812–821, 2010.

[26] S. J. Singer, J. Burgers, M. Friedberg, M. B. Rosenthal, L. Leape, and E. Schneider, "Defining and measuring integrated patient care: promoting the next frontier in health care delivery," *Medical Care Research and Review*, vol. 68, no. 1, pp. 112–127, 2011.

[27] E. F. Harkness and P. J. Bower, "On-site mental health workers delivering psychological therapy and psychosocial interventions to patients in primary care: effects on the professional practice of primary care providers," *Cochrane Database of Systematic Reviews*. vol. 21, no. 1, DC000532, 2009.

[28] K. Charmaz, *Constructing Grounded Theory: A Practical Guide Through Qualitative Analysis*, Sage, Thousand Oaks, Calif, USA, 2006.

[29] J. P. Spradley, *The Ethnographic Interview*, Wadsworth, Belmont, California, USA, 1979.

[30] J. M. Johnson, "In-depth interviewing," in *Handbook of Qualitative Research*, J. F. Gubrium and J. A. Holstein, Eds., pp. 103–119, Sage, Thousand Oaks, Calif, USA, 2002.

[31] W. Miller and B. Crabtree, "Depth interviewing," in *Doing Qualitative Research*, W. Miller and B. Crabtree, Eds., pp. 89–107, Sage, Thousand Oaks, Calif, USA, 2nd edition, 1999.

[32] M. Johnson, R. Jackson, L. Guillaume, P. Meier, and E. Goyder, "Barriers and facilitators to implementing screening and brief intervention for alcohol misuse: a systematic review of qualitative evidence," *Journal of Public Health*, vol. 33, pp. 412–421, 2011.

[33] R. A. Price, J. Zapka, H. Edwards, and S. H. Taplin, "Organizational factors and the cancer screening process," *Journal of the National Cancer Institute Monographs*, vol. 2010, no. 40, pp. 38–57, 2010.

[34] D. M. Schalk, M. L. Bijl, R. J. Halfens, L. Hollands, and G. G. Cummings, "Interventions aimed at improving the nursing work environment: a systematic review," *Implementation Science*, vol. 5, article 34, 2010.

[35] C. Auerbach and L. Silverstein, *Qualitative Data: An Introduction to Coding and Analysis*, New York University, New York, NY, USA, 2003.

[36] "NVivo qualitative data analysis software," in *Book NVivo Qualitative Data Analysis Software, Version 2*, QSR International, Southport, UK, 2002.

[37] B. G. Glaser and A. L. Strauss, *The Discovery of Grounded Theory*, Transaction Publishers, Piscataway, NJ, USA, 1967.

[38] E. H. Bradley, L. A. Curry, and K. J. Devers, "Qualitative data analysis for health services research: developing taxonomy, themes, and theory," *Health Services Research*, vol. 42, no. 4, pp. 1758–1772, 2007.

[39] Y. S. Lincoln and E. G. Guba, *Naturalistic Inquiry*, Sage, Newbury Park, Calif, USA, 1985.

[40] C. Erzberger and G. Prein, "Triangulation: validity and empirically-based hypothesis construction," *Quality and Quantity*, vol. 31, no. 2, pp. 141–154, 1997.

[41] D. Wilsford, "Path dependency, or why history makes it difficult but not impossible to reform health care systems in a big way," *Journal of Public Policy*, vol. 14, no. 3, pp. 251–283, 1994.

[42] J. K. Benzer, J. L. Sullivan, S. Williams, and J. F. Burgess, "One-year cost implications of using mental health care after discharge from a general medical hospitalization," *Psychiatric Services*, vol. 63, pp. 672–678, 2012.

[43] K. M. Eisenhardt and M. E. Graebner, "Theory building from cases: opportunities and challenges," *Academy of Management Journal*, vol. 50, no. 1, pp. 25–32, 2007.

[44] R. Grol and J. Grimshaw, "From best evidence to best practice: effective implementation of change in patients' care," *The Lancet*, vol. 362, no. 9391, pp. 1225–1230, 2003.

[45] J. H. Ford II, D. Krahn, M. Wise, and K. A. Oliver, "Measuring sustainability within the veterans administration mental health system redesign initiative," *Quality Management in Health Care*, vol. 20, pp. 263–279, 2011.

[46] M. Magoni, P. Okong, L. Bassani, P. K. Namaganda, S. Onyango, and M. Giuliano, "Implementation of a programme for the prevention of mother-to-child transmission of HIV in a Ugandan hospital over five years: challenges, improvements and lessons learned," *International Journal of STD and AIDS*, vol. 18, no. 2, pp. 109–113, 2007.

[47] G. L. Jackson, A. A. Powell, D. L. Ordin et al., "Developing and sustaining quality improvement partnerships in the VA: the colorectal cancer care collaborative," *Journal of General Internal Medicine*, vol. 25, supplement 1, pp. 38–43, 2010.

[48] E. Ferlie, L. Fitzgerald, M. Wood, and C. Hawkins, "The non-spread of innovations: the mediating role of professionals," *Academy of Management Journal*, vol. 48, no. 1, pp. 117–134, 2005.

Prevalence and Severity of Depression and Its Association with Substance Use in Jimma Town, Southwest Ethiopia

Andualem Mossie,[1] Dagmawi Kindu,[2] and Alemayehu Negash[3]

[1]*Department of Biomedical Sciences, College of Health Sciences, Jimma University, Ethiopia*
[2]*College of Health Sciences, Debre Tabor University, Ethiopia*
[3]*Department of Psychiatry, College of Health Sciences, Jimma University, Ethiopia*

Correspondence should be addressed to Andualem Mossie; andualemm2000@gmail.com

Academic Editor: Martin Alda

Background. Depression is a significant contributor to the global burden of disease and affects 350 million people worldwide. Substance use could be the risk factor for depression. *Objective.* We aim to determine the prevalence and severity of depression and its association with substance use. *Methods.* A cross-sectional study was conducted on a sample of 650 respondents in Jimma town in March 2014. A multistage stratified sampling method was conducted. Structured questionnaire and Beck's Depression Inventory (BDI-II) scale were used for data collection. Data analysis was done using the SPSS Version 20.0 for Windows. *Results.* The participation rate of respondents was 590/650 (90.77%). The proportion of females was 300 (50.9%). The current prevalence of depression was 171 (29.0%). Based on the BDI-II grading of the severity of depression, 102 (59.6%) had mild, 56 (32.7%) had moderate, 13 (7.6%) had severe depression. In the present study, age of 55 years and above [OR = 5.94, CI: 2.26–15.58], being widowed [OR = 5.18, CI: 1.18–22.76], illiterates [OR = 9.06, CI: 2.96–27.75], khat chewing [OR = 10.07, CI: 5.57–18.25], cigarette smoking [OR = 3.15, CI: 1.51–6.58], and shisha usage [OR = 3.04, CI: 1.01–9.19] were significantly and independently associated with depression. *Conclusion.* The finding depicted that depression was a moderate public health problem. Advanced age, being widowed, illiterate, khat chewing, and cigarette and shisha smocking could be the potential risk factors for depression. Risk reduction is recommended.

1. Introduction

World Health Organization (WHO) has reported that about 450 million people worldwide suffer from mental illness and one in four people meets criteria of mental illness at some point in their life [1, 2]. Among the mental disorders, depression is a disease of the global burden affecting 350 million people worldwide [3]. A study conducted on adult populations of USA reported that lifetime prevalence of major depressive disorder was 16.2% and 12-month prevalence was 6.6% [4]. Surveys conducted in 16 European countries found that 27% of adult Europeans are affected by depression: at least one mental disorder in a 12-month period [5, 6]. The burden of the disease is higher by 50% in females than in males [7]. The prevalence of depression in low and middle income countries (LMIC) ranged from 11.1 to 53%. The burden is highest in Afghanistan, Middle East, and North and Sub-Saharan African countries [8]. It was reported that the prevalence of depression in Ethiopia is 9.1% [9].

Depression disorder presents with depressed mood, loss of interest or pleasure, decreased energy, feelings of guilt or low self-worth, disturbed sleep or appetite, poor concentration, problem of thinking and making decisions, and, in severe stages, recurring thoughts of death or suicide [10]. Depending on the number and severity of symptoms, a depressive episode can be categorized as mild, moderate, or severe. An individual with a mild depressive episode will have some difficulties in continuing with ordinary work and social activities but will probably not cease to function completely. On the other hand, it is very unlikely that the individual with severe depressive episode will be able to continue with social, work, or domestic activities, except to a very limited extent. As for moderate depression, the individual would normally have more than the five symptoms that are needed to make the diagnosis of depression. Moderate episodes have a severity that is intermediate between mild and severe depressions [11].

Depression has many possible causes, including mood disturbance, genetic vulnerability, chronic stressful life, use of psychoactive substances, and medical problems. It is believed that several of these forces interact to bring depression [10, 11].

Areas in the brain that are affected in cases of depression are the prefrontal cortex, cingulated gyrus, amygdala, hippocampus, thalamus, and hypothalamus. These brain regions are involved in the regulation of motivation, eating, sleeping, energy level, circadian rhythm, and responses to rewarding and aversive stimuli, which are all abnormal in depressed people [12].

Neurotransmitters that are depleted in patients with depression are serotonin that helps regulate sleep, appetite, and mood and inhibits pain. Reduced serotonin secretion is recorded in patients with depression [13]. Norepinephrine triggers anxiety and is involved in some types of depression. It determines motivation and reward. Norepinephrine and serotonin (5-HT) modulate subcortical and cortical functions that their shortage in states of depression and anxiety contributes to abnormalities in sleep, concentration, attention and memory, arousal states, appetite, and libido [14]. Furthermore, their modulation of the cortical-hippocampal-amygdala pathways regulates responses to aversive, stressful, and fearful experience along with modulation of the affective aspects of memory [15].

Several studies confirmed that major depression is associated with a state of reduced dopamine and treated with monoamine oxidase inhibitors [16]. Problems in dopamine secretion have been associated with psychosis, a severe form of distorted thinking, hallucinations, or delusions. Dopamine is thought to play a role during substance abuse [17].

Psychoactive substance use, such as khat (*Catha edulis*), alcohol, and tobacco have become the rising risk factors for major mental health problems worldwide [18]. Khat (*Catha edulis*), which is commonly used in the study area, contains a psychoactive substance, cathinone, which stimulates the central nervous system analogous to amphetamine. Its mechanism of action is believed to be mediated via its sympathetic like action in the body [19].

A common side effect of khat use is insomnia, a condition that the users sometimes try to overcome with intake of sedatives or alcohol. The withdrawal symptoms after prolonged khat use are lethargy, mild depression, slight trembling, and recurrent bad moods [20].

Although tobacco contains thousands of chemicals, the main active ingredient that acts in the brain and produces addiction is nicotine. Many of the effects of nicotine are produced through its action on both the central and peripheral nervous systems [21]. Alcohol, a brain depressant and intoxicant, is the most commonly used psychoactive substance by both mentally healthy people and mentally ill people [22].

Depression has severe consequences on the productive human force and social areas which calls the attention of care providers for early diagnosis, proper treatment, and intervention. Although the prevalence of khat use and its physiological and psychosocial effects were studied, there is still limited knowledge on the association between substance use and depression in Jimma town at community level. Therefore, the main aim of the present study is to determine the prevalence and severity of depression and its association with the risk factors such as substance use.

2. Research Methods

This cross-sectional, community based study was conducted from 15 February 2014 to 15 March 2014 in Jimma town. The town's total population was estimated to be 130,254. People of ≥18 years of age were included in the study.

Out of thirteen kebeles of Jimma town, six kebeles were selected using a lottery method and 650 households were selected using a systematic random sampling. Once the households were identified, one adult family member was selected randomly using the lottery method. The sample size was calculated using multistage sampling formula; the prevalence rate of depression (p) was taken to be 26.3% from the previous study [23], with the confidence level of 95% and margin of error of 5%. Contingency of 10% for the nonresponse rate was added and multiplied by 2 for the design effect assuming that the source population is heterogeneous and multistage sampling was taken.

Beck's Depression Inventory revision II (BDI-II) [24] screening questionnaire has been employed for screening depression and for grading its severity. BDI has a high degree of sensitivity and specificity for detecting depression. BDI scoring was conducted as follows: normal depression (0–13), mild depression (14–19), moderate depression (20–28), and severe depression (29–63). World Health Organization (WHO) drug addiction questionnaire [25] was adopted and modified to make it relevant to the objectives of the study. The magnitude of khat chewing, alcohol consumption, and cigarette smoking was evaluated using this questionnaire.

To improve the quality of the data, the questionnaire was pretested on 32 randomly selected subjects who were not included in the study samples. Questionnaires were translated from the English language into local language and back-translated to English language for the sake of consistency. A two-day training was given for 6 psychiatric nurses as data collectors. The questionnaires were checked for their completeness during data cleaning and the incomplete ones were discarded. Data analysis was carried out using SPSS Version 20.0 for Windows. Frequency tables were used to summarize categorical data. The associations between predictor and outcome variables were measured using Chi-square test. Multivariate logistic regression analysis was conducted to control confounders and to identify the independent contribution of each variable to the outcome variable.

Ethical clearance was obtained from Jimma University Ethical Review Board. Participants' consent was taken and confidentiality was maintained.

2.1. Operational Definitions. First, we define substances use: substances that are commonly used in the study site are alcohol, khat, cigarette, and shisha. Second, we define current chewers: they represent the proportion of respondents who were chewing khat within 30 days before the study. Third, we define nonchewers: they represent the proportion of respondents who were not chewing khat within 30 days before the study. Fourth, we define current smokers: They represent the proportion of respondents who were smoking cigarettes within 30 days before the study. Fifth, we define nonsmokers: they represent the proportion of respondents who were not smoking cigarettes within 30 days before the study. Sixth, we define current alcohol users: they represent the proportion of respondents who were drinking alcohol (beer, whisky, local araki, or gin) within 30 days before the study. Seventh, we define lifetime drinkers: they represent the proportion of respondents who had ever drunk alcohol in their lifetime. Eighth, we define non-alcohol users: they represent the proportion of respondents who were not drinking alcohol within 30 days before the study. Shisha is an oriental tobacco pipe with a long, flexible tube connected to a container, where the smoke is cooled by passing through water. Shisha smoking, also called hookah, water pipe, or hubble-bubble smoking, is a way of smoking tobacco, sometimes mixed with fruit or molasses sugar, through a bowl and hose or tube.

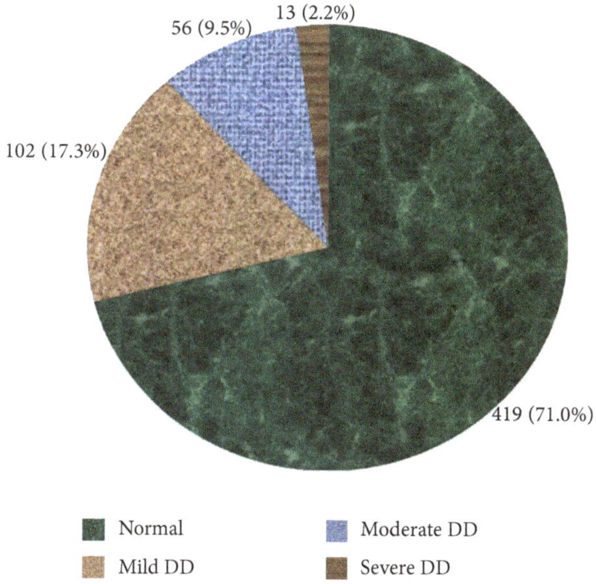

FIGURE 1: Severity of depression disorder in Jimma town, Southwest Ethiopia ($n = 590$). According to Beck's Depression Inventory, cutoff value ≤13 is normal; score of 14–19 is mild depression; score of 20–28 is moderate depression; score of 29–63 is severe depression. Four hundred nineteen participants were normal and 29% had depression, out of which 17.3% had mild depression, 9.5% had moderate depression, and 2.2% had severe depression.

3. Results

Among 650 respondents, the participation rate was 590 (90.8%). The current prevalence of depression was 171 (29.0%). According to BDI-II grading scale, 102 (17.3%) participants had mild depression, 56 (9.5%) participants had moderate depression, and 13 (2.2%) participants had severe depression, as presented in Figure 1. The magnitude of depression increases with age (Table 1). The prevalence of depression increases to 56.4% as the age advances above 55 years. Age above 55 years is 5.9 times more likely to have depression than lower age groups.

As per gender, in comparison with males, significantly larger proportion, 90 (52.6%), of females had depression (AOR = 2.43; 95% CI: 1.43, 4.13). The highest prevalence of depression was recorded among widows (85.0%) and illiterates (64.4%) as presented in Tables 1 and 3.

Out of the total respondents, 200 (33.9%) khat chewers, 203 (34.4%) alcohol users, 60 (10.2%) cigarette smokers, and 22 (3.7%) shisha users were recorded. One hundred four (52.0%) khat chewers, 38 (63.3%) cigarette smokers, 75 (36.9%) alcohol users, and 15 (68.2%) shisha smokers had depression episodes. There was a significant association between depression and substance use ($p < 0.05$) as shown in Tables 2 and 3.

Those sociodemographic and substance use related variables that have shown a significant association with depression episodes were tested by multivariate logistic regression analysis. Age, sex, marital status, educational status, khat chewing, cigarette smoking, and shisha usage were found to be the risk factors for depression as presented in Table 3. The logistic regression model revealed that the odds of developing depression for 55 years of age and above was as follows: AOR = 5.94; 95% CI: 2.26–15.58. Regarding marital status, widowed individuals were five times more likely to develop depression in comparison with the singles (AOR = 5.18; 95% CI: 1.18–22.76). Illiterate individuals were nine times more likely to develop depression as compared to educated people (AOR = 9.06; 95% CI: 2.96–27.75).

Similarly, khat chewers had tenfold risk of developing depression as compared to nonchewers (AOR = 10.07; 95% CI: 5.57–18.25). Cigarette smokers were approximately three times more likely to develop depression compared to nonsmokers (AOR = 3.15; 95% CI: 1.51–6.58) and shisha users had threefold higher risk for having depression compared to nonshisha users (AOR = 3.04; 95% CI: 1.01–9.19).

4. Discussion

Burden of depression poses a substantial public health challenge. In the present study, the current prevalence of depression in the community was 29%. This result is in agreement with the study done in Uganda which has reported prevalence of depression of 29.3% [26]. A slightly lower prevalence of depression compared to the current finding has been reported by studies conducted in Ethiopia and France: 26.3% [27] and 26.5% [28], respectively. A much lower prevalence of depression was reported in studies conducted in South Africa and Malaysia: 9.7% [29] and 6.3% [30], respectively. A much higher prevalence of depression, 54.5%, was reported in a study conducted in Nigeria [31]. The possible explanation for the higher prevalence of depression

Table 1: Association between depression and sociodemographic variables in Jimma town, Southwest Ethiopia ($n = 590$).

Variables		Total, $n = 590$ N (%)	Depression Yes, $n = 171$ n (%)	No, $n = 419$ n (%)	χ^2	p value
Sex	Male	290 (49.1)	81 (27.9)	209 (72.1)		
	Female	300 (50.9)	90 (30.0)	210 (70.0)	31.00	0.001
Age	18–24	183 (63.1)	33 (18.0)	150 (82.0)		
	25–34	188 (31.9)	48 (24.5)	140 (74.5)		
	35–44	102 (17.3)	33 (32.4)	69 (67.6)	36.46	0.000
	45–54	62 (10.5)	26 (41.9)	36 (58.1)		
	≥55	55 (9.3)	31 (56.4)	24 (43.6)		
Marital status	Single	242 (41.0)	61 (25.2)	181 (74.8)		
	Married	312 (52.9)	84 (23.9)	228 (73.1)	38.59	0.000
	Divorced	16 (2.7)	9 (56.2)	7 (43.8)		
	Widowed	20 (3.4)	17 (85.0)	3 (15.0)		
Occupation	Merchant	213 (36.1)	51 (23.9)	162 (76.1)		
	Employed	61 (10.3)	21 (34.4)	40 (65.6)		
	Unemployed	56 (9.5)	18 (32.1)	38 (67.9)	36.06	0.000
	Housewife	134 (22.7)	55 (41.0)	79 (59.0)		
	Students	102 (17.3)	15 (13.8)	94 (86.2)		
	Others*	24 (4.1)	11 (64.7)	6 (35.3)		
Educational status	Illiterate	45 (7.6)	29 (64.4)	16 (35.6)		
	1° School	140 (23.7)	49 (35.0)	91 (65.0)		
	2° School	207 (35.1)	50 (27.1)	151 (72.9)	29.47	0.000
	Certificate	38 (6.4)	11 (28.9)	27 (71.1)		
	Diploma	84 (14.2)	12 (14.3)	72 (85.7)		
	Degree plus	76 (12.9)	14 (18.4)	62 (81.6)		

*Farmers, pension.

Table 2: Association between depression and substance use in Jimma town, Southwest Ethiopia ($n = 590$).

Variables		Total, $n = 590$ N (%)	Depression Yes, $n = 171$ n (%)	No, $n = 419$ n (%)	χ^2	p value
Current khat chewing	Yes	200 (33.9)	104 (52.0)	96 (48.0)	77.88	0.000
	No	390 (66.1)	67 (17.2)	323 (82.8)		
Current cigarette smoking	Yes	60 (10.2)	38 (63.3)	22 (36.7)	38.29	0.000
	No	530 (89.8)	133 (25.1)	397 (74.9)		
Current alcohol intake	Yes	203 (34.4)	75 (36.9)	128 (63.1)	9.53	0.002
	No	387 (65.6)	96 (24.8)	291 (75.2)		
Current shisha use	Yes	22 (3.7)	15 (68.2)	7 (31.8)	17.06	0.000
	No	568 (96.3)	156 (27.5)	412 (72.5)		

disorder in the present study could be associated with the high production distribution and consumption of khat. Khat is grown abundantly in Jimma area. Many people chew khat in this place for different purposes. In most cases, khat chewing is accompanied by coffee drinking, cigarette smoking, and shisha usage and after these substances people used to drink alcohol to reduce the excitatory effect of khat and nicotine. Regular usage of all these substances could be the potential predisposing factors for depression.

In the current study, advanced age is strongly associated with the occurrence of depression and the result of this study is consistent with other previous findings conducted in USA [32] and Malaysia [30]. Age of 55 years and above was approximately six times more likely to develop depression as compared with age of 18–24 years. This could be due to disturbances of sleep, appetite, and sexual activities and due to an imbalance of neurotransmitters in the brain for nerve impulse transmission as age increases. Depressive

TABLE 3: Multivariate logistic regression analysis for the association of different variables with depression episode in Jimma town, Southwest Ethiopia ($n = 590$).

Variables	Categories	Total respondents n (%)	Depression episodes n (%)	AOR (95% CI)	p values
Age	18–24	183 (31.0)	131 (31.0)	1.00	
	25–34	188 (31.9)	188 (31.9)	0.89 (0.46–1.73)	0.732
	35–44	102 (17.3)	102 (17.3)	1.55 (0.70–3.41)	0.281
	45–54	62 (10.5)	62 (10.5)	3.04 (1.24–7.41)	0.015
	55+	55 (9.3)	55 (9.3)	5.94 (2.26–15.58)	0.000
Sex	Male	290 (49.2)	290 (49.2)	1.00	
	Female	300 (50.9)	300 (50.8)	2.43 (1.43–4.13)	0.001
Marital status	Single	242 (41.0)	242 (41.0)	1.00	
	Married	312 (52.9)	312 (52.9)	0.75 (0.42–1.35)	0.335
	Divorced	16 (2.7)	16 (2.7)	1.49 (0.41–5.48)	0.547
	Widowed	20 (3.4)	20 (3.4)	5.18 (1.18–22.77)	0.029
Education	Illiterate	45 (7.6)	45 (7.6)	9.06 (2.96–27.75)	0.000
	Primary	140 (23.7)	140 (23.7)	4.13 (1.70–10.08)	0.002
	Secondary	207 (35.1)	207 (35.1)	3.14 (1.38–7.12)	0.006
	Certificate	38 (6.4)	38 (6.4)	4.36 (1.41–13.43)	0.010
	Diploma	84 (14.2)	84 (14.2)	1.00 (0.37–2.74)	1.000
	Degree+	76 (12.9)	76 (12.9)	1.00	
Current khat chewing	Yes	200 (33.9)	104 (52%)	10.07 (5.57–18.25)	0.000
	No	390 (66.1)	67 (17.2%)	1.00	
Current cigarette smoking	Yes	60 (10.2)	38 (63.3%)	3.15 (1.51–6.58)	0.002
	No	530 (89.8)	133 (25.1%)	1.00	
Current alcohol intake	Yes	203 (34.4)	75 (36.9%)	1.05 (0.63–1.76)	0.856
	No	387 (65.6)	96 (24.8%)	1.00	
Current shisha use	Yes	22 (3.7)	15 (68.2%)	3.04 (1.01–9.19)	0.049
	No	568 (96.3)	156 (27.5%)	1.00	

1.00 = reference categories. All variables were adjusted to differentiate between predictors and confounders.

symptoms are significantly higher among elders above the age of 55 years. The possible explanation is that as the age advances, several problems related to aging come into picture including deterioration of body functions and hormonal secretions and metabolic activities, decreased quality of life, and higher mortality from comorbid medical conditions which contribute to the development of depression.

In the present study, females were found to be twice more vulnerable to depression than males. This report is consistent with a study conducted in Turkey [33]. This could be due to a low social and economic status, cultural discrimination, the affective nature of females response to stressful life, and hormonal changes during puberty; postpartum and post-menopausal periods and taking contraceptive pills have been incriminated as possible factors for the higher prevalence of depression among women.

According to the present findings, depression was significantly associated with educational status. The prevalence of depression was nine times higher among illiterates compared to educated samples. The result is in agreement with studies conducted in South Africa [29] and Turkey [33]. The possible explanation for this could be the fact that individuals with low socioeconomic and educational status were given less value to their self-esteem and live a stressful life as compared with educated individuals. In addition, educated people have better understanding of the risk factors of depression compared to illiterates.

In this study, depression has shown a significant association with marital status. Widowed individuals were five times more likely to develop depression as compared to single individuals. The result of this report was in line with the study conducted in Ethiopia [27, 34, 35]. This could be due to the fact that the loss of a spouse or lovers has been identified as one of the most stressful life events, requiring more psychological therapy compared to many others.

Depression was significantly associated with khat chewing. The probability of developing depression episodes among khat chewers is tenfold higher than that among nonchewers. This result is consistent with the study conducted in Jimma University [18, 23] and with WHO expert analysis [36]. Some authors propose that depression episodes disappeared during khat chewing sessions [22]. But these depressive symptoms crop up on cessation of khat use. This might be due to the fact that khat contains psychoactive chemicals cathinone and cathine that have amphetamine like action in the brain which activates the release of monoaminergic neurotransmitters such as dopamine [37] in the limbic system, resulting in reward sensations but after the cessation of khat, it leads to depression.

The result of the present study indicated that depression shows a significant association with current cigarette smoker. This result demonstrates that smokers have developed depression symptom three times greater than non-smokers. The present finding is in agreement with the study conducted by Pasco et al. [38]. However, other works in literature explained that depression and smoking show bidirectional relationship [39]. Substance use increases the risk of major depressive disorder [40]. Persons with major depression tend to abuse substances and have difficulties when they try to stop. There are thousands of chemicals other than nicotine present in cigarette smoke, of which one or several may affect mood in the same way as a group of antidepressant medications called monoamine oxidase inhibitors or (MAOIs) does [41]. These MAOIs effectively increase levels of specific neurotransmitters involved in the regulation of mood. Smoking, therefore, may be one way for depressed individuals to alleviate depressive symptoms.

5. Conclusion

To sum up, the magnitude of depression episodes recorded so far was found to be a moderate public health problem. The strongest association was recorded in the present study between depressive episodes and substance use. Chronic regular use of a psychoactive plant, khat, could be a potential risk factor. Khat chewing is accompanied by cigarette smoking and alcohol drinking. Avoidance of risk factors for depression is such a commendable preventive measure. Psychological and pharmacological therapies are equally important as well.

Conflict of Interests

The authors declare that they have no conflict of interests.

Authors' Contribution

All the authors contributed equally to the conception and design of the study, analysis and interpretation of the data, and drafting the paper. Finally, they all approved the final version.

Acknowledgments

The authors are grateful to Jimma University for its support. The authors also thank all the data collectors and the study participants who have kindly given them the necessary information.

References

[1] World Health Organization, *Promoting Mental Health: Concepts Emerging Evidence Practice*, Summary Report, World Health Organization, Geneva, Switzerland, 2004.

[2] World Health Organization, *The World Health Report: 2001: Mental Health: New Understanding, New Hope*, World Health Organization, Geneva, Switzerland, 2001.

[3] World Health Organization, *The World Health Report 2002-Reducing Risks, Promoting Healthy Life*, World Health Organization, Geneva, Switzerland, 2002.

[4] R. C. Kessler, P. Berglund, O. Demler et al., "The epidemiology of major depressive disorder: results from the national comorbidity survey replication (NCS-R)," *The Journal of the American Medical Association*, vol. 289, no. 23, pp. 3095–3105, 2003.

[5] T. Fryers, T. Brugha, Z. Morgan et al., "Prevalence of psychiatric disorder in Europe: the potential and reality of meta-analysis," *Social Psychiatry and Psychiatric Epidemiology*, vol. 39, no. 11, pp. 899–905, 2004.

[6] E. S. Paykel, T. Brugha, and T. Fryers, "Size and burden of depressive disorders in Europe," *European Neuropsychopharmacology*, vol. 15, no. 4, pp. 411–423, 2005.

[7] H.-U. Wittchen and F. Jacobi, "Size and burden of mental disorders in Europe—a critical review and appraisal of 27 studies," *European Neuropsychopharmacology*, vol. 15, no. 4, pp. 357–376, 2005.

[8] D. Akena, J. Joska, E. A. Obuku, T. Amos, S. Musisi, and D. J. Stein, "Comparing the accuracy of brief versus long depression screening instruments which have been validated in low and middle income countries: a systematic review," *BMC Psychiatry*, vol. 12, article 187, 2012.

[9] S. Hailemariam, F. Tessema, M. Asefa, H. Tadesse, and G. Tenkolu, "The prevalence of depression and associated factors in Ethiopia: findings from the National Health Survey," *BMC International Journal of Mental Health Systems*, vol. 6, article 3, 2012.

[10] M. Marcus, M. T. Yasamy, M. van Ommeren, D. Chisholm, and S. Saxena, "Depression: a global public health concern," in *Proceedings of the 65th World Health Assembly*, World Health Organization, Geneva, Switzerland, May 2012, http://www.who.int/mediacentre/events/2012/wha65/journal/.

[11] World Health Organization, *The Global Burden of Disease 2004 Update*, 2008, http://www.who.int/healthinfo/global_burden_disease/GBD_report_2004update_full.pdf.

[12] E. J. Nestler, M. Barrot, R. J. DiLeone, A. J. Eisch, S. J. Gold, and L. M. Monteggia, "The neurobiology of depression," *Neuron*, vol. 34, no. 1, pp. 13–25, 2002.

[13] M. J. Owens and C. B. Nemeroff, "Role of serotonin in the pathophysiology of depression," *Clinical Chemistry*, vol. 40, no. 2, pp. 288–295, 1994.

[14] D. S. Charney, "Monoamine dysfunction and the pathophysiology and treatment of depression," *Journal of Clinical Psychiatry*, vol. 59, supplement 14, pp. 11–14, 1998.

[15] K. J. Ressler and C. B. Nemeroff, "Role of serotonergic and noradrenergic systems in the pathophysiology of depression and anxiety disorders," *Depression and Anxiety*, vol. 12, supplement 1, pp. 2–19, 2000.

[16] B. W. Dunlop and C. B. Nemeroff, "The role of dopamine in the pathophysiology of depression," *Archives of General Psychiatry*, vol. 64, no. 3, pp. 327–337, 2007.

[17] A. S. Brown and S. Gershon, "Dopamine and depression," *Journal of Neural Transmission/General Section*, vol. 91, no. 2-3, pp. 75–109, 1993.

[18] Y. Gelaw and A. Haile-Amlak, "Khat chewing and its socio-demographic correlates among the staff of Jimma University," *Ethiopian Journal of Health Development*, vol. 18, no. 3, pp. 179–184, 2005.

[19] I. Dhaifalah and J. Šantavý, "Khat habit and its health effect: a natural amphetamine," *Biomedical Papers*, vol. 148, no. 1, pp. 11–15, 2004.

[20] E. B. Erica, G. Falkay, and A. Gabor, "Khat a controversial plant," *The Middle Europian Journal of Medicine*, vol. 121, pp. 604–614, 2009.

[21] R. Jain and K. Mukherjee, "Biological Basis of nicotine addiction," *Indian Journal of Pharmacology*, vol. 35, no. 5, pp. 281–289, 2003.

[22] K. Graham, A. Massak, A. Demers, and J. Rehm, "Does the association between alcohol consumption and depression depend on how they are measured?" *Alcoholism: Clinical and Experimental Research*, vol. 31, no. 1, pp. 78–88, 2007.

[23] D. Tekalign, M. Andualem, and T. Markos, "Khat chewing and mental distress: a community based study, Jimma Town, Southwest Ethiopia," *Ethiop Journal of Health Sciences*, vol. 21, no. 1, pp. 37–45, 2011.

[24] A. T. Beck, R. A. Steer, R. Ball, and W. Ranieri, "Comparison of beck depression inventories-IA and-II in psychiatric outpatients," *Journal of Personality Assessment*, vol. 67, no. 3, pp. 588–597, 1996.

[25] R. G. Smart, P. H. Hughes, L. D. Johnston et al., "A methodology for student drug-use surveys," World Health Organization Offset Publication 50, WHO, Geneva, Switzerland, 1983.

[26] E. Kinyanda, J. Tugumisirize, and S. Ndyanabangi, "Poverty, life events and the risk for depression in Uganda," *Society of Psychiatric Epidemiology*, vol. 46, no. 1, pp. 35–44, 2011.

[27] S. Mogga, M. Prince, A. Alem et al., "Outcome of major depression in Ethiopia," *British Journal of Psychiatry*, vol. 189, pp. 241–246, 2006.

[28] K. Ritchie, S. Artero, I. Beluche et al., "Prevalence of DSM—IV psychiatric disorder in the French elderly population," *The British Journal of Psychiatry*, vol. 184, no. 2, pp. 147–152, 2004.

[29] M. Tomlinson, A. T. Grimsrud, D. J. Stein, D. R. Williams, and L. Myer, "The epidemiology of major depression in South Africa: results from the South African Stress and Health study," *South African Medical Journal*, vol. 99, no. 5, pp. 368–373, 2009.

[30] M. Sherina, R. L. Sidik, M. Aini, and H. Norhidayati, "The prevalence of depression among elderly in an urban area of Selangor, Malaysia," *The International Medical Journal*, vol. 4, no. 2, pp. 57–67, 2005.

[31] O. M. Aiyelero, H. O. Kwanashie, T. L. Sheikh, and I. M. Hussaini, "Some socio-demographic features of mood disorders presented by patients attending a northern Nigerian tertiary health institution clinic," *Journal of Applied Pharmaceutical Science*, vol. 1, no. 6, pp. 92–95, 2011.

[32] A. Fiske, J. L. Wetherell, and M. Gatz, "Depression in older adults," *Annual Review of Clinical Psychology*, vol. 5, pp. 363–389, 2009.

[33] M. Topbafl, F. Yaris, G. Can, M. Kapuca, and K. Sayar, "The effect of sociodemographic factors and medical status on depressive symptoms of the inhabitants of nursing home and community-dwelling elders in Trabzon-Turkey," *Bulletin of Clinical Psychopharmacology*, vol. 14, pp. 57–60, 2012.

[34] N. Deyessa, Y. Berhane, A. Alem, U. Hogberg, and G. Kullgren, "Depression among women in rural Ethiopia as related to socioeconomic factors: a community-based study on women in reproductive age groups," *Scandinavian Journal of Public Health*, vol. 36, no. 6, pp. 589–597, 2008.

[35] P. J. Clayton, J. A. Halikas, and W. L. Maurice, "The depression of widowhood," *British Journal of Psychiatry*, vol. 120, no. 554, pp. 71–77, 1972.

[36] World Health Organization, *Promoting Mental Health: Concepts Emerging Evidence Practice*, Summary Report, Geneva, Switzerland, 2004.

[37] N. B. Patel, "Mechanism of action of cathinone: the active ingredient of khat (*Catha edulis*)," *East African Medical Journal*, vol. 77, no. 6, pp. 329–332, 2000.

[38] J. A. Pasco, L. J. Williams, F. N. Jacka et al., "Tobacco smoking as a risk factor for major depressive disorder: population-based study," *British Journal of Psychiatry*, vol. 193, no. 4, pp. 322–326, 2008.

[39] N. Breslau, S. P. Novak, and R. C. Kessler, "Psychiatric disorders and stages of smoking," *Biological Psychiatry*, vol. 55, no. 1, pp. 69–76, 2004.

[40] L. C. Dierker, S. Avenevoli, K. R. Merikangas, B. P. Flaherty, and M. Stolar, "Association between psychiatric disorders and the progression of tobacco use behaviors," *Journal of the American Academy of Child & Adolescent Psychiatry*, vol. 40, no. 10, pp. 1159–1167, 2001.

[41] L. S. Covey, A. H. Glassman, and F. Stetner, "Cigarette smoking and major depression," *Journal of Addictive Diseases*, vol. 17, no. 1, pp. 35–46, 1998.

19

Late-Life Depressive Symptoms, Religiousness, and Mood in the Last Week of Life

Arjan W. Braam,[1,2] Marianne Klinkenberg,[3] Henrike Galenkamp,[1] and Dorly J. H. Deeg[1]

[1] *Longitudinal Aging Study Amsterdam, Department of Epidemiology and Biostatistics, EMGO Institute for Health and Care Research, VU University Medical Center Amsterdam, Van der Boechorststraat 7, 1081 BT Amsterdam, The Netherlands*
[2] *Department of Emergency Psychiatry & Department of Specialist Training, Altrecht Geestelijke Gezondheidszorg, Utrecht, The Netherlands*
[3] *Integraal Kankercentrum Nederland, Amsterdam, The Netherlands*

Correspondence should be addressed to Arjan W. Braam, a.braam@vumc.nl

Academic Editor: Raphael M. Bonelli

Aim of the current study is to examine whether previous depressive symptoms modify possible effects of religiousness on mood in the last week of life. After-death interviews with proxy respondents of deceased sample members of the Longitudinal Aging Study Amsterdam provided information on depressed mood in the last week of life, as well as on the presence of a sense of peace with the approaching end of life. Other characteristics were derived from interviews with the sample members when still alive. Significant interactions were identified between measures of religiousness and previous depressive symptoms (CES-D scores) in their associations with mood in the last week of life. Among those with *previous* depressive symptoms, church-membership, church-attendance and salience of religion were associated with a greater likelihood of depressed mood in the last week of life. Among those *without* previous depressive symptoms, church-attendance and salience of religion were associated with a higher likelihood of a sense of peace. For older adults in the last phase of life, supportive effects of religiousness were more or less expected. Fore those with recent depressive symptoms, however, religiousness might involve a component of existential doubt.

1. Introduction

One important aspect of religion is how it may guide people through questions about the end of life. For some religious believers, it is clear that death only implies a transition. Others are less convinced, and may doubt about the existence of a transition, or about the conclusion of a judgement on their moral behaviour. In a previous study, we focused on the role of religiousness with respect to aspects of mood in the last week of life, as observed in a sample of older adults in The Netherlands [1]. Several aspects of religiousness were included, but none of them was associated with depressed mood in the last week of life, as reported by surviving relatives. Nonetheless, church attendance earlier in life predicted a "sense of peace" with the approaching end of life. Therefore, only modest support was found for the adaptive potential of religion in the last week of life. A possibly maladaptive aspect was not identified in this first report. Furthermore—although the analyses were adjusted for effects of previous depressive symptoms—the first study did not focus on those who were prone to depression during their lifetime.

The Netherlands represents a highly secularized country, but the older generation has still grown up in a society in which religious traditions had a prominent role, and many older people still endorse religious beliefs [2]. An ongoing debate in The Netherlands, especially among psychologists of religion and mental health professionals, is about the question whether religious beliefs, instead of giving support, may provoke depressive symptoms, such as feelings of guilt [3]. Indeed, for older people with a depressive syndrome, feelings of guilt were more often reported for the Calvinist Protestants and Roman Catholics, compared to nonchurch members [4]. The same was true for complaints of psychomotor inhibition, especially among depressed Protestants, but among the nondepressed, there were no denominational differences in guilt or psychomotor inhibition. Therefore, the relationship between facets of religiousness and mood seems to differ between the depressed and the nondepressed.

The last phase of life may follow different trajectories, such as with a gradual or rapid physical decline, and the mental demands will vary across the different types of illness. The last phase of life is characterized by inevitable adjustments for many older adults. There is a large need of informal and formal care, and many have to face a transfer to a different living environment [5]. In a recent study from the US, Hui and colleagues described fairly high levels of spiritual distress (such as feeling despair and brokenness, from an existential point of view) among patients with advanced cancer [6]. As expected, spiritual distress was associated with depression.

On the other hand, several studies among terminally ill patients showed associations between Spiritual Well-being Scale scores and lower levels of psychological distress [7, 8]. As some content overlap may occur between spiritual well-being and emotional well-being (or its reverse, psychological distress), these studies included statistical adjustment for depressive symptoms. Which aspects of religiousness and spirituality specifically determined the association with psychological distress in the terminally ill is difficult to say because the measure of spiritual well-being combines several aspects. One study included the belief in a hereafter as a distinct variable, and this was associated with lower levels of hopelessness, but not with feelings of anxiety or depression [9]. A complementary finding by Van Laarhoven and colleagues, in a small sample of advanced cancer patients, was the association of an explicit agnostic perspective on death and afterlife with higher levels of hopelessness [10]. The authors also described a negative association, but only at a nonsignificant level, between an explicit religious attitude and depression. In a palliative care study, a significant negative association with depression or anxiety disorder was found for church-attendance, but not for religious affiliation, prayer, or subjective religiousness [11].

With respect to the association between religiousness and the course of depression, several studies (from the US, Netherlands, and Australia), have shown that intrinsic religious motivation (or salience of religion) was associated with a quicker remission of the depression [12]. Findings in the literature about the association between church-attendance and the course of depression are however less consistent [13].

Clinical experience and epidemiological evidence have made clear that depression and depressive symptoms (or "subthreshold" depression) tend to recur, and for a minority, to persist, also in later life [14–16]. Therefore, the best predictor of depression is previous depression, and likewise, we expect that the vulnerability to depression will also predict depressed mood in terminal patients. With respect to the possible role of religiousness in this last phase of life, little is known about how an existing vulnerability to depression interferes with supportive or undermining effects of religiousness.

The current, population-based study focuses on relationships between aspects of religiousness and mood in the last week of life, as reported by surviving relatives of deceased sample members of the Longitudinal Aging Study Amsterdam (LASA) [17]. Information on religiousness was also obtained from the LASA respondents who were interviewed during lifetime about several aspects of religious life, as well as about depressive symptoms. In our previous study, we found that previous depressive symptoms predicted depressed mood, anxiety, and lack of sense of peace in the last week of life [1]. The current study aims to examine whether previous depressive symptoms modify associations between aspects of religiousness and mood in the last week of life, either giving way to a supportive potential of religiousness (e.g., for salience of religion), or to maladaptive effects (e.g., for certain convictions such as belief in hell).

2. Methods

2.1. Sample. The Longitudinal Aging Study Amsterdam (LASA) is an ongoing interdisciplinary study on predictors and consequences of changes in autonomy and well-being in the aging population. The LASA cohort is based on a nationwide random sample of older adults between the ages of 55 and 85, stratified for age, sex, and expected mortality five years into the study. Registries of 11 municipalities in areas in the West (mostly secularized, including Amsterdam), North-east (predominantly Protestant), and South (predominantly Roman Catholic) of The Netherlands provided the sampling frame [18, 19]. The realized number of respondents in the LASA baseline interview cycle in 1992/1993 amounted to 3,107. Respondents were interviewed in their homes by intensively supervised interviewers. Three years later, in 1995/1996, all respondents were approached for the T2 interview cycle. The participation rates and numbers of decedent respondents are shown in Figure 1. Between T2 and T3 (1998/1999), 342 respondents died. The database of LASA contains contact information about two persons close to the sample member, such as the partner, a child, sibling, or other person who had had close contact. Wherever possible, one proxy respondent was selected, who had been involved in the last three months of the sample member, and who was willing and able to participate. The proxy respondent was approached with a letter with information on the study, followed by a telephone call, to make an appointment for the interview, which was held in the home of the proxy respondent. This research method is known in the literature as "retrospective/after-death approach" or "proxy interview" [20]. The number of proxy respondents amounted to 270, mainly children (50%) and spouses (33%) of the sample members.

2.2. Measures

2.2.1. Mood in the Last Week of Life. The interview with the proxy respondent included a one-item question on whether the sample member showed feelings of depression in the last week of life. Scores were 0 (absence of depressed mood) or 1 (presence of depressed mood). Furthermore, the proxy respondents were asked to estimate whether the sample member experienced a sense of peace with the approaching

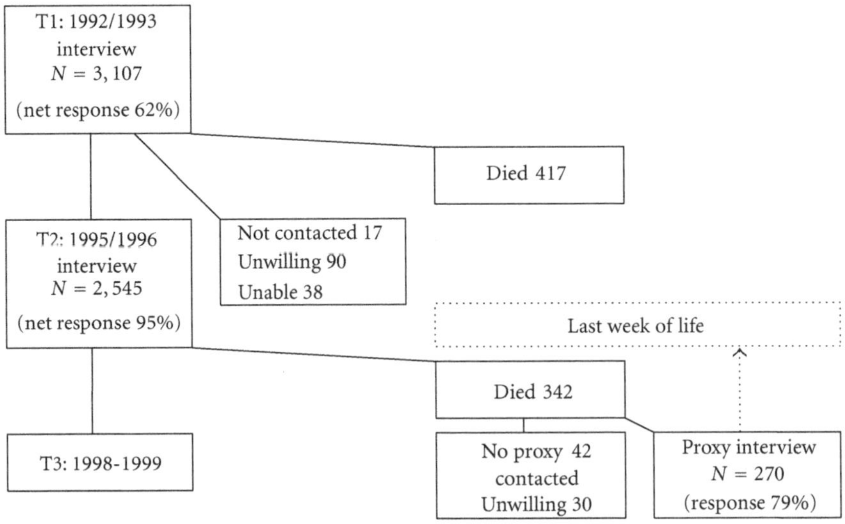

Figure 1: Flowchart of sampling times of the proxy interviews of deceased respondents of the Longitudinal Aging Study Amsterdam between T2-T3.

end of life. This was scored as 0 (sense of peace-absent) or 1 (sense of peace present).

2.2.2. Religiousness. Data on *religious affiliation* and *church attendance* were obtained during the first assessment cycle of LASA. Religious affiliation included: Protestant, Roman Catholic, and nonreligious affiliation. The Protestant group consisted of several denominations, but most with origins in the Reformed/Calvinist protestant tradition. The religious affiliation of the parents was also asked, and was coded as: (1) both parents and sample member affiliated; (2) parents affiliated, sample member not affiliated (first generation secularized); (3) neither parents nor sample member affiliated (second generation secularized). Church-attendance was assessed using five response categories, ranging from "once a year or less" (1) to "once a week or more" (5).

The second LASA assessment cycle contained questionnaires on orthodox religious beliefs and salience of religion. The level of adherence to traditional (Christian) religious beliefs was assessed at T2 by the Orthodoxy Scale, which has been regularly used in studies by the Dutch Social and Cultural Planning Office (SCP) [2]. Doctrines included are (asked as "Do you believe in"): life after death, heaven, purgatory, hell, the devil, the actual existence of Adam and Eve, and the Bible as God's word. Answer could be "yes" (score = 1) or "no" (score = 0), yielding a score range of 0–7 (Cronbach's alpha 0.86).

Salience of religion was assessed using two items of a religious salience scale [21]: "My religious faith/philosophy of life has a pronounced impact on my daily life" and "When I take important decisions, my religious faith/philosophy of life plays a considerable role." Response categories range between "totally disagree" (0) to "totally agree" (5). Salience of religion was also probed in the proxy interview, using the same items ("Salience-according-to-proxy").

2.2.3. Previous Depressive Symptoms Assessed in the LASA Respondent Interview. Depressive symptoms were measured using the Center for Epidemiologic Studies Depression Scale [22]. Subjects were asked how often they experienced each of 20 symptoms during the previous week. The response categories ranged from 0 ("rarely or none of the time") to 3 ("most of or all the time"), yielding a score range of 0 to 60 (Cronbach $\alpha = 0.83$). A CES-D score of 16 or higher has generally been used as indicative for clinically relevant depressive symptoms, including both minor or subthreshold depression and major depression [23, 24]. Therefore, in the stratified analyses, this cutoff was applied.

2.2.4. Covariates from the LASA Respondent Interview. Demographic characteristics of the sample member included age of death, sex, education in years, and marital status (married versus widowed, divorced, or never married).

The number of *major chronic diseases* was assessed at T2, by explicitly asking the respondents whether or not they had or had had any of the following seven conditions: chronic lung disease, cardiac disease, peripheral artery disease, stroke, diabetes mellitus, arthritis, and cancer [25].

2.2.5. Covariates from the Proxy Interview

Physical State. The proxy respondents were asked about the presence of serious physical symptoms in the last week of life of the sample member: fatigue, pain, shortness of breath, confusion, and nausea and/or vomiting. Responses (0 "no" and 1 "yes") were summed to obtain a symptom burden score (range 0–5).

Cognitive change between the measurement in 1995/1996 and 3 months before death was assessed using the six-item short form Informant Questionnaire on Cognitive Decline in the Elderly [26]. For every item, the proxy respondent answered on a five-point scale (range 1–5; Cronbach α = 0.93). Higher sum scores indicate cognitive decline.

Time Intervals. The duration of the periods between the T2 interview and death, and between death and the proxy interview were included to adjust for any influence of time on the outcomes.

Whether the sample members had *expected death* and had been *aware of the approaching end* was estimated by the proxy respondents, with "yes," "no," or "more or less" as response categories. When both questions were answered with "yes," it is assumed that the sample member clearly realized the approaching end.

2.3. Statistical Procedure. In the previous paper, associations with the two outcome variables on mood in the last week of life—feeling depressed and sense of peace—were analysed for each of the religious variables, using logistic regression analysis, computing odds ratios (OR) and 95% confidence intervals (95% CI) [1]. Adjustment was made for the covariates with significant associations with the dependent variables, as was evident from prior bivariate and multivariate analyses (also carried out in the stratified subgroups of interest with and without previous depressive symptoms). As there was variation in item nonresponse between the variables, the maximal number of sample members was included in each of the analyses.

Modification of the association with the outcome variables was examined by including the product term between previous depressive symptoms as assessed on T2 (79%) or on T1 (21%, with missing scores at T2) and each of the religion variables in the subsequent logistic regression models. To avoid multicollinearity between first-order terms and product terms, product terms were formed by multiplying the centered (deviation from the mean) scores of both components [27]. The level of statistical significance was set at $P < 0.05$ for main effects, and at $P < 0.10$ for interaction effects, as the power of statistical tests for higher order terms is generally lower than for first order terms [27, 28]. To facilitate interpretation of the interactions, the associations between the religion variables and the outcome variables were examined using logistic regression analyses, adjusted for relevant covariates and stratified for two contrasting subgroups: those who had low levels of depressive symptoms at a previous assessment (CES-D score < 16) and those who had high levels of depressive symptoms (CES-D ≥ 16).

3. Results

3.1. Characteristics of the Sample. The majority of the sample (Table 1) was male, which is in accordance with the higher expected mortality among males. Mean age of death amounted to 80 years. About one-third was Protestant, one-third Roman Catholic, and one-third nonaffiliated. One-third of the sample members used to attend church on a weekly basis. As examples of items of the orthodoxy, 57% of the sample members reported to believe in heaven, and 30% reported to believe in hell. Salience of religion received higher scores by the sample members at T2, compared to the report by the proxy respondents. The Cohen κ for inter-rater agreement was fair for both salience items (.27 and .25). Depressed mood in the last week of life was reported for 28% of the sample members and sense of peace for 76%.

Bivariate associations between covariates and mood in the past week of life have been reported in the previous publication [1]. Depressive symptoms, assessed in previous LASA interviews, significantly predicted the presence of depressed mood in the last week of life ($t = -2.9$, $P = .005$), as well as the absence of a sense of peace ($t = 4.3$, $P = .000$). Neither the duration of the period between the T2 interview and death, nor the duration between death and the proxy interview had significant associations with depressed mood ($t = 0.6$, $P = .573$; $t = -1.1$, $P = .263$) or with sense of peace ($t = -0.7$, $P = .459$; $t = 0.2$, $P = .869$). These time periods did not significantly interact with depressive symptoms assessed in the previous LASA interview and depressed mood or sense of peace in the last week of life (results on request). Similarly, the type of relationship between the respondent and the proxy (whether or not this was the partner or child) did not interact with the association between depressive symptoms and mood in the last week of life (results on request).

Serious physical symptoms and cognitive decline were significantly associated with depressed mood in the last week of life ($t = -4.2$, $P < .001$, and $t = -2.6$, $P = .009$, resp.). In contrast, cognitive decline and higher age were positively associated with a sense of peace ($t = 2.0$, $P = .043$; $t = 2.3$, $P = .024$).

3.2. Interactions with Previous Depressive Symptoms. The results of the tests for interactions are shown in Table 2. For depressed mood in the last week of life, previous depressive symptoms significantly interacted with religious affiliation, church-attendance, and orthodox beliefs. For sense of peace, previous depressive symptoms significantly interacted with religious affiliation, church-attendance, and salience according to proxy. The nature of the interactions is illustrated using stratified analyses. Table 3 summarizes the associations between the religious variables and the proxy's reports on depressed mood and sense of peace in the last week of life, both for those who had high and low CES-D scores at an earlier assessment. Two main patterns emerge.

First, among those with previous depressive symptoms (CES-D ≥ 16), there was a significantly higher risk of depressed mood in the last week of life for those who were affiliated with a church, for those who attended church on a more frequent basis, and for those for whom religion was salient according to the proxy respondent. Although only at the level of a statistical trend, the same was found for those with higher orthodoxy scores. No significant association was found between salience of religion and depressed mood in the last week of life.

The second pattern pertains to the other outcome, sense of peace in the last week of life. Here, for those *without* previous depressive symptoms (CES-D < 16), there was a higher chance on a sense of peace for those who used to go to church on a regular basis, and for those for whom religion was salient according to the proxy respondent.

TABLE 1: Characteristics of deceased sample members of the Longitudinal Aging Study Amsterdam (LASA) between 1995 and 1998.

	n	Range	Mean	(SD)	%
Sex (% female)	270				38.1
Age of death	270	59–91	80.4	(7.5)	
Time interval: last respondent interview–death (days)	269	8–1321	589	(330)	
Time interval: death proxy interview (days)	270	131–1479	789	(316)	
Last respondent interview					
Marital state (% married)	263				47.1
Education (years)	263	5–18	8.6	(3.4)	
Number of major chronic diseases	270	0–7	1.6	(1.2)	
Depressive symptoms (% ≥16) [$n = 56$ at T1, $n = 211$ at T2]	267	0–44	10.4	(8.6)	21.7
Religious affiliation	270				
Protestant					31.9
Roman Catholic					28.9
Other					1.5
Nonaffiliated(2)					37.8
Church attendance in 1992 (LASA baseline interview)	270	1–5	2.7	(1.8)	
Orthodoxy scale	203	0–6	2.9	(2.3)	
Salience of religion, last interview with sample member	203	0–8	5.1	(2.1)	
Interview with proxy respondent					
Cognitive decline *according to proxy respondent* (1)	238	1–5	3.8	(0.8)	
Serious physical symptoms in the last week of life(1)	259	0–5	2.2	(1.3)	
Mood in last week of life *according to proxy respondent*					
Depressed mood	233				28.2
Sense of peace—absent	204				23.5
Salience of religion *according to proxy respondent*	268	0–8	3.5	(3.1)	
Expected death/aware of approaching end (both "yes", %)	270				53.0

(1) High scores indicate more problems.
(2) Among the nonaffiliated: one or both parent(s) affiliated 61% ($n = 59$) and both parents nonaffiliated 39% ($n = 38$) (9 had missing value).

3.3. Denominational Background. Additional analyses (Table 4) revealed that among those with previous depressive symptoms, the risk of depressed mood was, at trend level, somewhat more evident for Roman Catholics, compared to the nonaffiliated. Among those without previous depressive symptoms, affiliation showed a gradual increase in the likelihood of experiencing a sense of peace in the last week of life; compared to second generation secularized, the difference for the first generation secularized was not significant (OR 2.46), reached trend-level for Roman Catholics (OR 3.15), and was significant for Protestants (OR 3.52). The confidence intervals showed, however, a considerable overlap, indicating that the differences between the three denominational groups do not differ significantly.

4. Discussion

The current contribution focused on the role of religiousness in the association between previous depressive symptoms and mood in the last week of life. Information was partly obtained from interviews, as the sample members participated in a prospective population-based study, and partly from after-death interviews with relatives of the deceased sample members.

The previous report on these data showed that there were no significant associations between aspects of religiousness and depressed mood in the last week of life in the full sample [1]. However, the current study shows that among those with *previous* depressive symptoms in the last interview cycle (on average about two years before death), several aspects of religiousness were associated with an increased likelihood of depressed mood in the last week of life: church-attendance, (Roman Catholic) church-membership, and salience of religion (salience-according-to-proxy).

In contrast, among those *without* previous depressive symptoms, church-attendance, church-membership, and salience of religion (salience-according-to-proxy) were associated with a higher likelihood of a sense of peace with the approaching end of life. This sense of peace had the lowest reports among the nonchurch members with nonaffiliated parents (second generation secularized).

The finding that religiousness is associated with depressed mood in the last week of life for those who had previous depressive symptoms, at least at the level of

Table 2: Interaction effects between previous depressive symptoms and aspects of religiousness for mood (depressed mood or sense of peace) in the last week of life, according to proxy respondents; results of logistic regression analyses; results printed in bold are statistically significant.

	Depressed mood in last week of life (according to proxy) interaction with previous depressive symptoms (CES-D)[a]				Sense of peace with approaching end of life (according to proxy) interaction with previous depressive symptoms (CES-D)[b]			
	N	B (SE)	Wald	*P*	*N*	B (SE)	Wald	*P*
Church members versus nonaffiliated	216	**0.08(0.04)**	**3.8**	**.050**	192	**−0.13 (0.05)**	**7.9**	**.005**
Church attendance	218	**0.02 (0.01)**	**3.6**	**.058**	194	**−0.03(0.01)**	**6.8**	**.009**
Orthodox beliefs	162	**0.03 (0.01)**	**5.6**	**.018**	156	−0.01 (0.01)	0.2	.644
Salience of religion	163	0.01 (0.01)	0.3	.615	154	−0.01 (0.02)	0.5	.482
Salience according to proxy	217	−0.01 (0.01)	0.2	.650	193	**−0.01 (0.01)**	**3.4**	**.067**

[a] Adjusted for effects by physical distress (according to proxy respondent) and cognitive decline (according to proxy respondent).

[b] Adjusted for effects by age of death, physical distress (according to proxy respondent), and expectance of death/awareness of the approaching end (according to proxy respondent).

TABLE 3: Mood in the last week of life, as reported by proxy respondents of deceased sample members of the Longitudinal Aging Study Amsterdam between 1995 and 1998: associations with aspects of religiousness, stratified for previous depressive symptoms.

		Depressed mood in last week of life (according to proxy)[a]					Sense of peace with approaching end of life (according to proxy)[b]				
		N	Wald	*P*	OR	95% CI	*N*	Wald	*P*	OR	95% CI
Previously nondepressed	Church members versus nonaffiliated	171	0.1	.739	0.88	0.42–1.86	151	2.3	.129	1.92	0.83–4.45
	Church attendance [1–5]	173	0.0	.942	1.01	0.83–1.23	153	**4.5**	**.034**	**1.31**	**1.02–1.68**
	Orthodox beliefs [0–6]	131	0.1	.770	0.97	0.81–1.17	123	0.6	.433	1.08	0.89–1.33
	Salience of religion [0–8]	131	0.8	.360	0.92	0.76–1.11	124	1.3	.250	1.14	0.91–1.41
	Salience according to proxy [0–8]	173	0.1	.707	1.02	0.91–1.15	152	**4.1**	**.042**	**1.15**	**1.00–1.32**
Previously depressed (CES-D ≥ 16)	Church members versus nonaffiliated	45	**4.9**	**.028**	**9.05**	**1.28–64.02**	41	0.7	.412	0.51	0.10–2.56
	Church attendance [1–5]	45	**6.4**	**.011**	**2.32**	**1.21–4.44**	41	1.1	.300	0.79	0.51–1.23
	Orthodox beliefs [0–6]	32	*3.5*	*.060*	*1.58*	*0.98–2.55*	30	1.1	.299	1.24	0.83–1.86
	Salience of religion [0–8]	32	1.6	.207	1.41	0.83–2.40	30	1.8	.174	0.68	0.39–1.18
	Salience according to proxy [0–8]	44	**4.0**	**.046**	**1.40**	**1.00–1.93**	41	0.4	.540	0.92	0.70–1.20

Results printed in **bold** are statistically significant (*italics*: trend).
[a]Adjusted for effects by physical distress (according to proxy respondent) and cognitive decline (according to proxy respondent).
[b]Adjusted for effects by age of death, physical distress (according to proxy respondent), and expectance of death/awareness of the approaching end (according to proxy).

TABLE 4: Religious affiliation and mood in the last week of life, as reported by proxy respondents of deceased sample members of the Longitudinal Aging Study Amsterdam between 1995 and 1998: stratified for previous depressive symptoms.

		Depressed mood in last week of life (according to proxy)[b]					Sense of peace with approaching end of life (according to proxy)[b]				
		N	Wald	*P*	OR	95% CI	*N*	Wald	*P*	OR	95% CI
Previously nondepressed	Protestant[a]	57	1.4	.245	0.52	0.17–1.57	47	**4.3**	**.039**	**3.52**	**1.07–11.58**
	Roman Catholic[a]	58	0.0	.885	0.93	0.32–2.65	49	*3.8*	*.053*	*3.15*	*0.99–10.08*
	First-generation secularized[a]	29	0.1	.774	1.17	0.40–3.48	35	2.1	.144	2.46	0.74–8.25
	Second-generation secularized	17			1		21			1	
Previously depressed (CES-D ≥ 16)	Protestant[a]	15	0.5	.502	1.78	0.33–9.55	14	0.1	.718	1.47	0.18–11.72
	Roman Catholic[a]	11	*2.8*	*.095*	*4.67*	*0.77–28.47*	12	1.5	.220	0.27	0.04–2.11
	First-generation secularized[a]	11	0.0	.999	1.00	0.15–6.53	9	0.4	.518	0.50	0.06–4.09
	Second-generation secularized	11			1		7			1	

Results printed in **bold** are statistically significant (*italics*: trend).
[a]Reference group is second generation secularized (nonaffiliated respondents with nonaffiliated parents).
[b]Nonadjusted because of too low number of respondents; when adjusted as in Table 3, the results are slightly stronger but with problematic wide 95% CI's.

subthreshold depression, is appealing and raises the question what mechanism is at work. In discussing theories on death anxiety, Kastenbaum considers that death concern belongs to the core Christian conceptions [29]. He states that it is possible that Christian doctrine may intensify both anxiety, living in dread of judgment, and serenity, even with longing and impatience. Kastenbaum calls for more elaborate empirical research to understand the psychological and social key factors through which individuals and families come to terms with both the "dread" and the "welcome" of Christian death. The current results seem to offer empirical support for the existence of both positions.

Church-attendance showed the greatest contrast between those with and without previous depressive episodes. The level of orthodoxy of Christian beliefs showed a contrast as well, but was significant only at the level of a statistical trend in those with previous depressive symptoms. Thus, the cognitive (doctrinal) aspects of religiousness do not seem to represent the main explanation, whereas behavioural and motivational aspects (as measured with church-attendance and salience of religion) do come to the fore. The emotional facet, the feeling of being accepted by the deity, or abandoned, could be even more central. Especially feelings of abandonment by God are known to have high correlations with depression, and, hypothetically, may result in a deeper crisis when the belief in sustainment by the deity seems to be out of grasp [30]. Future research should also address the emotional facet of religiousness in this context.

In the current sample of older adults, there was still considerable membership of religious denominations, but the nonaffiliated represented a sizable group. About one-third of this group had nonaffiliated parents as well. The main impression is that the nonaffiliated had the least disadvantages (least depressed mood in the last week of life) in case of previous depressive symptoms. On the other hand, for those without previous depressive symptoms, the non-affiliated who had nonaffiliated parents as well had the least advantages with respect to sense of peace. Perhaps, this group may no longer have access to the supportive aspects of religious faith, in contrast to the first generation secularised. It should however be noted that the denominational differences in the current study were statistically modest or even weak, because of small group numbers in the stratified analyses.

The contemporary society of The Netherlands should be characterized as highly secularized, and in younger samples, the first-generation secularized represents a large group. Some convictions and remnants of doctrines may persist, along with spiritual feelings, rituals, and new beliefs, such as feelings about reincarnation. With respect to the needs and strengths of secularized older adults when facing death, future research may include aspects of spirituality and other dimensions of meaning in life. For those who have been raised within a religious tradition, inclusion of measures of intrinsic and extrinsic religious motivation is warranted, as well as deeper inquiry into the contents of beliefs, to reveal which church doctrines and which motivations are more sustaining and supportive and which are more depressing.

Salience of religion as reported by the proxy respondent, but not salience as reported by the sample member, was associated with a sense of peace in the last week of life. One may therefore assume that the proxy respondents (especially the spouses) used to have similar religious beliefs and practices as the respondents had during their lives. On the one hand, the results from the current study might show how religiousness of the proxy respondent helped to cope with the loss of the relative. On the other had, the considerable degree of personal involvement of the proxy respondents may have influenced the results. The current study focuses, however, on effect modification by a variable that was assessed earlier in life: previous depressive symptoms. Apparently, the global assessment of mood in the last week of life by the proxy respondents did not prevent that more or less opposing results for the nondepressed and depressed still could be described.

One limitation of the current study is that mood in the last week of life was not directly observed in the respondents when they were terminally ill, but was assessed retrospectively. For the current sample, Klinkenberg and colleagues verified some information obtained from the proxy respondents with reports from physicians [31]. The proxy respondents seemed to provide accurate information with respect to chronic physical conditions. As Addington-Hall and McPherson (2001) point out in their review about the validity of after-death interviews, some studies provided evidence that there is little correspondence between the sample member and the proxy respondent about topics like depressed mood [32]. According to research on the concordance of patient and caregiver reports, both patient and caregiver depression were common predictors of disagreement [33]. Although the results of the current study closely examined for effects of previous depressive symptoms, further reasons for nonconcordance could not be ruled out. The same is true for recall bias by the proxy respondents, many of whom were interviewed after two years. An important concern regarding research about the end of life in the general population remains the difficulty of timely identification of respondents, and if they can be identified, few will be able or allowed to participate. Interviews with surviving relatives therefore will remain a source of knowledge about the last phase of life. Another limitation is that both outcomes consisted of one-item measures. One recommendation for future research is to examine the state of mood more fully. Meanwhile, psychometrically acceptable measures of the quality of the dying experience have become available, such as two versions of the quality of dying in long-term care instrument [34]. A related point is that the current study did not include measures on, partly overlapping, concepts such as spiritual distress, or death anxiety [6, 35]. Measures on emotional aspects of religiousness, spirituality, and secular sources of meaning in life may be included in further research.

The current results suggest that vulnerability to depression is an important aspect for the direction of the relationship between religiousness and mood in the last phase of life. It should be underlined that replication is desirable, both employing quantitative and qualitative research methods, before any recommendations can be done to professionals in the field of palliative care. Recent guidelines and recommendations for the quality of spiritual care—as a dimension of palliative care—provide suggestions for screening questions to assess spiritual life in patients in palliative care, to keep an eye on spiritual distress or religious struggle, and how to integrate spiritual issues into the treatment plan [36]. Verifying the recent history of depressive symptoms may provide a cue to detect any religious struggle or other severe existential doubts, which may possibly represent an additional burden for those in the last phase of life.

Conflict of Interests

No competing financial interests exist.

Acknowledgments

The data reported on were collected in the context of the Longitudinal Aging Study Amsterdam, which is financed primarily by The Netherlands Ministry of Welfare, Health, and Sports. The study of religious resources and common mental disorders was supported by a grant by The Netherlands Organisation for Health Research and Development (ZON-MW Grant 2003-05769). The results of the current study have been presented at the VIIth European Conference of the IAGG, Bologna, Italy, April 16, 2011.

References

[1] A. W. Braam, M. Klinkenberg, and D. J. H. Deeg, "Religiousness and mood in the last week of life: an explorative approach based on after-death proxy interviews," *Journal of Palliative Medicine*, vol. 14, no. 1, pp. 31–37, 2011.

[2] J. W. Becker and J. S. J. de Wit, *Secularisation in the Nineties; Churches as Institution, Tenets of Beliefs, and a Forecast*, Sociaal en Cultureel Planbureau, The Hague, The Netherlands, 2000.

[3] A. A. de Lely, W. W. van den Broek, P. G. H. Mulder, and T. K. Birkenhäger, "Symptoms of depression in strict Calvinist patients and in patients without religious affiliations: a comparison," *Tijdschrift voor Psychiatrie*, vol. 51, no. 5, pp. 279–289, 2009.

[4] A. W. Braam, C. M. Sonnenberg, A. T. F. Beekman, D. J. H. Deeg, and W. van Tilburg, "Religious denomination as a symptom-formation factor of depression in older Dutch citizens," *International Journal of Geriatric Psychiatry*, vol. 15, no. 5, pp. 458–466, 2000.

[5] M. Klinkenberg, G. Visser, M. I. Broese van Groenou, G. van der Wal, D. J. H. Deeg, and D. L. Willems, "The last 3 months of life: care, transitions and the place of death of older people," *Health and Social Care in the Community*, vol. 13, no. 5, pp. 420–430, 2005.

[6] D. Hui, M. de la Cruz, S. Thorney, H. A. Parsons, M. Delgado-Guay, and E. Bruera, "The frequency and correlates of spiritual distress among patients with advanced cancer admitted to an acute palliative care unit," *American Journal of Hospice and Palliative Medicine*, vol. 28, no. 4, pp. 264–270, 2011.

[7] J. T. Chibnall, S. D. Videen, P. N. Duckro, and D. K. Miller, "Psychosocial-spiritual correlates of death distress in patients with life-threatening medical conditions," *Palliative Medicine*, vol. 16, no. 4, pp. 331–338, 2002.

[8] C. S. McClain, B. Rosenfeld, and W. Breitbart, "Effect of spiritual well-being on end-of-life despair in terminally-ill cancer patients," *The Lancet*, vol. 361, no. 9369, pp. 1603–1607, 2003.

[9] C. McClain-Jacobson, B. Rosenfeld, A. Kosinski, H. Pessin, J. E. Cimino, and W. Breitbart, "Belief in an afterlife, spiritual well-being and end-of-life despair in patients with advanced cancer," *General Hospital Psychiatry*, vol. 26, no. 6, pp. 484–486, 2004.

[10] H. W. M. van Laarhoven, J. Schilderman, C. A. H. H. V. M. Verhagen, K. C. Vissers, and J. Prins, "Perspectives on death and an afterlife in relation to quality of life, depression, and hopelessness in cancer patients without evidence of disease and advanced cancer patients," *Journal of Pain and Symptom Management*, vol. 41, no. 6, pp. 1048–1059, 2011.

[11] K. G. Wilson, H. M. Chochinov, M. G. Skirko et al., "Depression and anxiety disorders in palliative cancer care," *Journal of Pain and Symptom Management*, vol. 33, no. 2, pp. 118–129, 2007.

[12] V. Payman and B. Ryburn, "Religiousness and recovery from inpatient geriatric depression: findings from the PEJAMA Study," *Australian and New Zealand Journal of Psychiatry*, vol. 44, no. 6, pp. 560–567, 2010.

[13] A. W. Braam, "Religion/spirituality and mood disorders," in *Religion/Spirituality and Psychiatry* , P. Huguelet and H. G. Koenig, Eds., pp. 97–113, Cambridge University Press, New York, NY, USA, 2009.

[14] L. L. Judd, H. S. Akiskal, J. D. Maser et al., "A prospective 12-year study of subsyndromal and syndromal depressive symptoms in unipolar major depressive disorders," *Archives of General Psychiatry*, vol. 55, no. 8, pp. 694–700, 1998.

[15] I. Colman, K. Naicker, Y. Zeng, A. Ataullahjan, A. Senthilselvan, and S. B. Patten, "Predictors of long-term prognosis of depression," *Canadian Medical Association Journal*, vol. 183, no. 17, pp. 1969–1976, 2011.

[16] A. T. F. Beekman, S. W. Geerlings, D. J. H. Deeg et al., "The natural history of late-life depression: a 6-year prospective study in the community," *Archives of General Psychiatry*, vol. 59, no. 7, pp. 605–611, 2002.

[17] M. Klinkenberg, D. L. Willems, G. van der Wal, and D. J. H. Deeg, "Symptom burden in the last week of life," *Journal of Pain and Symptom Management*, vol. 27, no. 1, pp. 5–13, 2004.

[18] M. I. Broese van Groenou, T. G. van Tilburg, E. D. de Leeuw, and A. C. Liefbroer, "Data collection," in *Living Arrangements and Social Networks of Older Adults*, C. P. M. Knipscheer, J. de Jong Gierveld, T. G. van Tilburg, and P. A. Dykstra, Eds., pp. 185–197, VU University Press, Amsterdam, The Netherlands, 1995.

[19] D. J. H. Deeg, T. van Tilburg, J. H. Smit, and E. D. de Leeuw, "Attrition in the longitudinal aging study Amsterdam: the effect of differential inclusion in side studies," *Journal of Clinical Epidemiology*, vol. 55, no. 4, pp. 319–328, 2002.

[20] C. J. McPherson and J. M. Addington-Hall, "Judging the quality of care at the end of life: can proxies provide reliable information?" *Social Science and Medicine*, vol. 56, no. 1, pp. 95–109, 2003.

[21] A. J. A. Felling, J. Peters, and O. Schreuder, *Believing and Living: A National Study Into Contents and Consequences of Religious Beliefs*, Kerkebosch, Zeist, The Netherlands, 1986.

[22] L. S. Radloff, "The CES-D scale: a self-report depression scale for research in the general population," *Applied Psychological Measurement*, vol. 1, no. 3, pp. 385–401, 1977.

[23] L. F. Berkman, C. S. Berkman, S. Kasl et al., "Depressive symptoms in relation to physical health and functioning in the elderly," *American Journal of Epidemiology*, vol. 124, no. 3, pp. 372–388, 1986.

[24] A. T. F. Beekman, D. J. H. Deeg, J. van Limbeek, A. W. Braam, M. Z. de Vries, and W. van Tilburg, "Criterion validity of the Center for Epidemiologic Studies Depression Scale (CES-D): results from a community-based sample of older subjects in the Netherlands," *Psychological Medicine*, vol. 27, no. 1, pp. 231–235, 1997.

[25] D. M. W. Kriegsman, B. W. J. H. Penninx, J. T. M. van Eijk, A. J. P. Boeke, and D. J. H. Deeg, "Self-reports and general practitioner information on the presence of chronic diseases in community dwelling elderly. A study on the accuracy of patients' self-reports and on determinants of inaccuracy," *Journal of Clinical Epidemiology*, vol. 49, no. 12, pp. 1407–1417, 1996.

[26] J. F. M. de Jonghe, B. Schmand, M. E. Ooms, and M. W. Ribbe, "The Dutch short form informant questionnaire on cognitive decline in the elderly (IQCODE-N)," *Tijdschrift voor Gerontologie en Geriatrie*, vol. 28, no. 5, pp. 224–229, 1997.

[27] L. S. Aiken and S. G. West, *Multiple Regression: Testing and Interpreting Interactions*, Sage, Newbury Park, Calif, USA, 1991.

[28] S. Greenland, "Interactions in epidemiology: relevance, identification, and estimation," *Epidemiology*, vol. 20, no. 1, pp. 14–17, 2009.

[29] R. Kastenbaum, *The Psychology of Death*, Free Association Books, London, UK, 3d edition, 2000.

[30] A. W. Braam, A. C. Schrier, W. C. Tuinebreijer, A. T. F. Beekman, J. J. M. Dekker, and M. A. S. De Wit, "Religious coping and depression in multicultural Amsterdam: a comparison between native Dutch citizens and Turkish, Moroccan and Surinamese/Antillean migrants," *Journal of Affective Disorders*, vol. 125, no. 1–3, pp. 269–278, 2010.

[31] M. Klinkenberg, J. H. Smit, D. J. H. Deeg, D. L. Willems, B. D. Onwuteaka-Philipsen, and G. van der Wal, "Proxy reporting in after-death interviews: the use of proxy respondents in retrospective assessment of chronic diseases and symptom burden in the terminal phase of life," *Palliative Medicine*, vol. 17, no. 2, pp. 191–201, 2003.

[32] J. Addington-Hall and C. McPherson, "After-death interviews with surrogates/bereaved family members: some issues of validity," *Journal of Pain and Symptom Management*, vol. 22, no. 3, pp. 784–790, 2001.

[33] J. M. Hauser, C. H. Chang, H. Alpert, D. Baldwin, E. J. Emanuel, and L. Emanuel, "Who's caring for whom? Differing perspectives between seriously ill patients and their family caregivers," *American Journal of Hospice and Palliative Medicine*, vol. 23, no. 2, pp. 105–112, 2006.

[34] J. C. Munn, S. Zimmerman, L. C. Hanson et al., "Measuring the quality of dying in long-term care," *Journal of the American Geriatrics Society*, vol. 55, no. 9, pp. 1371–1379, 2007.

[35] G. Gesser, P. T. P. Wong, and G. T. Reker, "Death attitudes across the life-span: the development and validation of the Death Attitude Profile (DAP)," *Omega*, vol. 18, no. 2, pp. 113–128, 1987.

[36] C. Puchalski, B. Ferrell, R. Virani et al., "Improving the quality of spiritual care as a dimension of palliative care: the report of the consensus conference," *Journal of Palliative Medicine*, vol. 12, no. 10, pp. 885–904, 2009.

Mental Health Services Required after Disasters: Learning from the Lasting Effects of Disasters

A. C. McFarlane[1] and Richard Williams[2]

[1] *Department of Psychiatry, Centre for Traumatic Stress Studies, The University of Adelaide, Adelaide SA 5000, Australia*
[2] *Mental Health Strategy, Welsh Institute for Health and Social Care, University of Glamorgan and Ty Bryn, St Cadoc's Hospital, Aneurin Bevan Health Board, NHS Wales, Lodge Road, Caerleon, Gwent NP 18 3XQ, UK*

Correspondence should be addressed to A. C. McFarlane, alexander.mcfarlane@adelaide.edu.au

Academic Editor: Rachel Yehuda

Disasters test civil administrations' and health services' capacity to act in a flexible but well-coordinated manner because each disaster is unique and poses unusual challenges. The health services required differ markedly according to the nature of the disaster and the geographical spread of those affected. Epidemiology has shown that services need to be equipped to deal with major depressive disorder and grief, not just posttraumatic stress disorder, and not only for victims of the disaster itself but also the emergency service workers. The challenge is for specialist advisers to respect and understand the existing health care and support networks of those affected while also recognizing their limitations. In the initial aftermath of these events, a great deal of effort goes into the development of early support systems but the longer term needs of these populations are often underestimated. These services need to be structured, taking into account the pre-existing psychiatric morbidity within the community. Disasters are an opportunity for improving services for patients with posttraumatic psychopathology in general but can later be utilized for improving services for victims of more common traumas in modern society, such as accidents and interpersonal violence.

1. Introduction

Disasters, by their nature, are events that are unanticipated when and where they occur and are situations in which the protective mechanisms of a civil society are particularly likely to fail. Globally, there is an average of at least one disaster every day, the frequency of disasters is rising with climate change, as are the numbers of people involved with increasing population densities but, overall, the proportionate mortality caused by natural disasters has fallen.

Conversely, the morbidity caused by people's exposure to trauma is rising and a substantial portion of the health effects lies in the psychosocial and mental ill health domains, and this is placing a rising burden on services that are often very stretched already [1].

In response, an approach is required that is built of public health interventions for groups of people. Practical and community support are critical in the immediate aftermath of events though rarely should mental health professionals provide that care. In addition a population-based approach enables primary and secondary preventative intervention to be offered and it facilitates evidence-based practice. This paper uses the term psychosocial care to describe these population-based interventions and to differentiate them from the mental healthcare that is provided by primary care and specialist mental health services, usually, later in the trajectory of events.

There is predictable psychiatric morbidity in populations who are exposed to disasters. The most common effects include distress and grief, and, less frequently, but nonetheless commonly, anxiety disorders and depression [2]. People's attempts at self-medication for the stress, often with alcohol, may lead them into harm and substance use disorders, which may also mask mood and anxiety disorders and postpone their recognition.

Tol and van Ommeren say [2] "*... mental health and psychosocial support programmes ... are increasingly a standard component of humanitarian response.*" Thus, this topic is of global concern. However, the capacities of mental health systems across the world vary widely. While the evidence on the effectiveness of interventions that is available now remains far from complete, it is sufficient to enable us to outline a generic model of care that can be adapted to particular circumstances [3].

This paper outlines how psychosocial and mental health resources should be developed in the setting of particular events that can then be mobilised at times of disaster to deal with an entire population. It provides a framework based on enabling nonmental health trained responders to provide psychosocial care and identifying people who have unmet needs arising from mental disorders on whom to focus the work of mental health services.

This paper reflects on the literature about disasters and the authors' personal experiences following a number of events in which they have been involved. They include the long-term effects of a major naval disaster that occurred in 1964, two major bushfire disasters in Australia, the Iraqi occupation in Kuwait in 1990, the bombings in London in 2005, and the compound disaster of 2011 in Fukushima, Japan. However, the lessons about people's need for psychosocial care and mental healthcare also apply to more common everyday traumas.

Disasters are collective events that evoke a great deal of public concern and distress. The normal methods and structures of civil administration are seriously challenged during and following major incidents [4]. In their wake, major resources are mobilized to assist the survivors. An irony is that smaller scale events occur every day within families and communities. They may be as traumatizing to particular people as are the larger scale events that evoke so much, usually short-term public engagement. But the common small-scale traumatic events, such as, domestic violence and abuse have similar adverse long-term consequences for people's psychological and social wellbeing [5–7]. They attract less concentrated public concern despite there being much to learn from disasters for day-to-day practice and vice versa.

2. The Societal Impacts of Disasters

The lessons learned from each disaster must inform governments' policies, strategic planning, design and operation of services, and clinical practice so that a cycle of learning and knowledge acquisition continues within all societies and communities. Thereby, people and communities can be assisted to become more resilient and services more appropriate to their needs. Many studies have focused on assessing the prevalence of PTSD among survivors of natural and technological disasters. However, Norris [7] has highlighted in a review of 225 studies that the quality of more recent research is, if anything, declining due to small samples and short followups. This is evidence that knowledge and practice in this field can be repetitive iterations with less than optimal learning from past lessons. Tol and van Ommeren [2] also call for more evidence for psychosocial care, in particular.

Each disaster is unique and poses unusual challenges. Therefore, it is not possible to prescribe in detail simple solutions to the requirements for providing psychosocial and mental health care following them. However, experience, from the 1993 World Trade Centre Bombing, has brought significant improvements in evacuation procedures, leading to the 9/11 evacuations being highly successful [8]. The corollary is that rapid evolution of strategic and operational plans must continue through all phases of each disaster in order to adapt the general plan that was formed beforehand to ensure that it fits the particular circumstances of the disaster with which the responsible authorities are dealing at the time. To this end, planners responsible for the emergency preparedness of many communities, regions, and nations are developing and testing template plans for responding to a range of disastrous situations. Various organizations have provided generic frameworks and/or standards that are capable of adaptation for different societies and which are able to recognise fully people's differing cultures [1, 9, 10].

Often, disasters include single or a small series of incidents that occur suddenly, such as, the bombings in London on 7 July 2005 [11]. Others are characterised by drawn out events, such as, flooding and fires that start suddenly, but may persist for weeks. These types of event cause enormous nondisordered distress, which is an anticipated response that affects a large proportion of the populations affected but also substantial rates of anxiety disorders and depression probably because the traumatic effects persist for many months [2, 12, 13]. Plans for both types of disaster must include plans for responding effectively to the psychosocial and mental health needs of the affected populations.

One of the major reasons for deaths in disaster is the failure of technology to control the natural environment. In the modern world, we see nature as being a containable and controllable dimension of our existence. Engineering design has done much to manage the forces of nature. People tend to take this for granted so that there is horror when these defenses are breached [14]. The impact of disasters tends to be much more destructive in Third World countries because of the fragility of their engineering infrastructure.

Often, disasters are major turning points or benchmarks in the history of communities. The Tangshan earthquake that occurred in the height of the Cultural Revolution in the China on 28 July 1976 demonstrates this. 242,000 people were killed and a further 164,000 were badly injured [15]. While the gang of four had a campaign in the media about concern for the victims, they used this as an environment to attack Deng Xiaoping, their political opponent. They were seen by their statements to be callous and indifferent to the suffering of so many bereaved and traumatised people [16]. Within four months, Madam Mao had been arrested and the tyranny of the gang of four had been ended. This was the beginning of the liberation of modern China.

Disasters are also the turning points in many of the safety measures that are used to protect and organize civilized society. After the sinking of the Titanic, for example, very strict rules were created for the number of lifeboats and buoyancy devices in relation to passengers [17, 18]. The changes in airport security following 11 September 2001 provide another example. This paper advises on certain lessons for mental healthcare that can be derived from past experience and research.

Disasters are also events in which the survivors are generally less stigmatised than when they are involved in singular events. This is partly because there is an acceptance of the general vulnerability of the community, rather than adverse outcomes being attributed to individual people's lack of resilience [19].

One of the greatest challenges is to create awareness among politicians and health agencies about the time course and the patterns of immediate, medium-term and longer term psychosocial and mental health needs of affected populations. In the initial aftermath, there is public outpouring of care and concern. However, communities recover, move on, and forget [20]. But, this is the very time at which the mental health needs of disaster-affected communities pose challenges because a relatively small proportion of survivors are most in need of services that address their longer term adverse outcomes. Their needs interact with the existing morbidity within affected communities, but reshape its presentation and understanding.

3. Types of Disasters

The type of event is important when considering the rates of morbidity following disasters and designing the types of health services that are required to deal effectively with affected populations. Furthermore, the impact of disasters is changing as our countries become more densely populated.

Some events are geographically circumscribed. They may have clear margins of demarcation between the people who are affected and those who are not, such as, in major fires. In other disasters, such as, earthquakes and storms, there is a gradient of destruction from the epicenter. The Enschede fireworks factory disaster affected people who came from a defined geographical region [21, 22]. In these circumstances, disaster services should be carefully integrated with the existing primary and secondary health care networks that particular people use at such times. Similarly, the flooding in England in 2007 affected populations in certain parts of the country by invading their homes and workplaces, and the impacts on the affected communities are likely to be long-term.

Travel accidents and terrorism pose a current challenge. They may affect commuter transport systems, which have localized effects on particular communities, but they may be remote from where the events take place. The Sarin attack in Tokyo and the terrorist bombings in Madrid of 2004 are examples. The significant majority of the people affected are from local communities. Another example is the Clapham rail disaster in London, in which many of the people affected lived in a more distant county that was not otherwise involved in the event [23]. In contrast, if major international transport systems, such as, trains or aircraft are targeted, the survivors come from widely distributed regions and nations. The Bali terrorist bombing is an example.

Hence, planning for the types of health services required should be cognizant of these substantial differences. After the bombing in Bali, for example, retrieving large numbers of seriously burnt people was an extreme challenge to health systems in Australia. There was no established plan for their retrieval from a place where the health care systems were inadequate.

Other disasters may affect people from widely distributed geographical regions. The immediate and short-term responses are required at the place at which the event occurs, but short-, medium-, and longer term services are required at a distance or on a distributed basis. In other words, the systems of mental healthcare that are required in the immediate aftermath of the event in which the survivors and the relatives of people who have died congregate are very different to those that are required in the medium and longer terms as people return to their regions of domicile. However, it is important to the continuity of care that the immediate responses and the longer term ones are well coordinated. Thus, unique, but different, outreach systems of care are required in these differing circumstances, and there are challenges to create effective communication systems to sustain individual care plans that may involve many service providers that are separated geographically.

The impact of a disaster is influenced substantially by the duration of the warning and impact phases. Evacuation systems can be put in place if there is a significant period of anticipation, such as, with storms.

The terrorist attacks on New York on September 11 were particularly challenging because they affected local communities, tourists, and international business people. However, at least one major company, which was based in one of the twin towers, had a major incident plan that was well planned and rehearsed regularly. While, there were other factors that affected their survival, the staff of that company suffered fewer fatalities; staff knowing what to do was an important factor.

The major events in Fukushima in Japan in 2011 illustrate another important feature of large-scale disasters, which is that, often, they transcend the traditional division categorization of natural and human-made disasters. The crisis began with an earthquake, which led to a tsunami, the inundation of a nuclear power plant, and radiation hazard. The traumatizing features were multiple, unfolded in full view of the world, and, together, affected directly a very large number of people and an even greater number in Japan and across the world through the economic consequences. The effects on people's mental health are still emerging and are likely to be long term.

4. Research into the Psychosocial and Mental Health Impacts of Disasters

4.1. Types of Disaster Studies. When considering the prevalence and types of reactions to disasters, it is important to understand the variety of methodologies that have been used. This is because there are so many different approaches that have been used and many have substantial weaknesses [12, 13]. Commonly, there are four sampling methodologies used in disaster research. Each has certain strengths but, importantly, weaknesses too.

4.1.1. Samples of Convenience. Frequently, researchers examine samples of convenience, given the chaos and confusion that occur in the aftermath of disasters. It is difficult to form broad generalizations from these studies. Nonetheless, samples of convenience play an important role in disaster research because, frequently, groups of survivors pose particular challenges with regards to their needs for health services. An example is of the studies conducted after the earthquake in Turkey, which examined various groups, such as, people in emergency housing [24, 25].

4.1.2. Treatment Seeking Samples. Clinicians working in disaster settings have often conducted specific examinations of the people who approach them to seek treatment [26]. These studies may assist clinicians to understand when people may present the nature of their complaints and the clinical needs of populations in similar circumstances.

4.1.3. Longitudinal Studies. Increasingly, longitudinal studies have been conducted, such as, those after the Enschede Fire Works disaster [27]. They demonstrate the patterns of longer term morbidity and are useful in modeling the aetiology of posttraumatic morbidity and how this can be best addressed by health services. They tend to be uncommon in disaster research [28].

4.1.4. Special Subpopulations. Emergency service personnel are an important group who are at particular risk in disasters. A number of studies have identified the impacts of major disasters against the background of the chronic strains of their roles. Children also evoke particular interest.

A core issue that complicates the interpretation of the data is that, often, the sampling is not representative. Also, there is a tendency to not include the people who are most severely affected because of the demands imposed by involving them in postdisaster studies.

However, some studies, which use stratified epidemiological samples, have looked at representative cohorts with comparison groups [6]. An example is the study of the Yun Nan Earthquake by Cao et al. [29], which examined the populations of three villages at increasing distances from the epicenter of an earthquake in China. The people in these villages were compared with those in a village unaffected by the earthquake that was demographically very similar. This approach addresses the issue of exposure as well as the background problem of the prevalence of morbidity in the community by presuming this to be the same for people who live in the unexposed village.

4.2. The Psychosocial and Mental Health Impacts of Disasters. Disasters and terrorism capture human attention and concern, but public interest tends to be relatively short lived [20, 30]. Often, their long-term morbidity is underestimated by planners and health and social welfare providers [31]. While concern for the survivors and the relatives of people who are killed, seriously injured or missing, is potent in the immediate aftermath of these events, it tends to be forgotten in the longer term. The impacts on the lives and mental health of the staff who care for people who suffer profound injuries in disasters and long-lasting impairments afterwards are also neglected. A meta-analysis documents population-level behavioral and psychological consequences of terrorist incidents [32].

The Inter-Agency Standing Committee (IASC) is formed by the heads of a broad range of UN and non-UN humanitarian organisations. In 2007, it published Guidelines on Mental Health and Psychosocial Support in Emergency Settings [9]. That document segments the psychosocial and psychiatric consequences into groups. Tol and van Ommeren [2] highlighted that there are a range of consequences of disasters. They remind us that "*... mental health practitioners in humanitarian settings frequently encounter people with severe pre-existing neuropsychiatric disorders ...*" and "*... disasters and armed conflicts ... impact the social conditions that shape mental health, through increased poverty, threats to human rights, domestic and community violence and changes social relations.*" In summary, these groups include people who have:

(1) pre-existing social problems (e.g., extreme poverty, belonging to a group that is discriminated against, marginalized, or politically oppressed);

(2) emergency-induced social problems (e.g., family separation; disruption of social networks; destruction of community structures, resources and trust; increased gender-based violence);

(3) emergency-induced distress (e.g., grief, anticipated or nonpathological distress and distress in which the symptoms may appear similar to those of acute distress disorder, posttraumatic stress disorder, and/or depression);

(4) emergency-induced mental disorders: depression and anxiety disorders, (including acute stress disorder and PTSD), substance misuse, and sustained personality changes;

(5) humanitarian aid-induced social problems (e.g., undermining of community structures or traditional support mechanisms);

(6) humanitarian aid-induced psychological problems (e.g., anxiety and depression due to lack of information about food distribution or due to poor management of the information that is provided);

(7) pre-existing mental health or psychiatric problems (e.g., severe mental disorder, alcohol abuse).

It is important to have an overview of the wider panoply of risks and effects that emergencies, major incidents, and disasters of all kinds may have because, very importantly for policy, service planning, and clinical practice, many people fall into more than a single group. Furthermore, the groups are by no means separate because the effects of one type of consequence may act as risk or exacerbating factors for others. Recent experience highlights the overlaps. Extensive flooding in parts of the UK in 2007 and Australia in 2011 rendered the homes of a large number of people uninhabitable. This posed immediate problems for their safety and domicile and many risks to the health and mental health of the public [12, 13, 33]. It also threatened essential local services (e.g., power supplies, sewerage, and availability of potable water) because they were engulfed or because staff of those services were affected.

Thus, many people who were not directly involved in the emergency also had the services on which they depend affected or put at risk. The risks to essential services include the preoccupation of staff with other matters, problems with transport and locating people. All of these effects become secondary stressor, which, when persistent, as in the case of flooding, are potent perpetuators of people's distress and provoke delayed mental disorders such as depression [12, 13, 33]. They pose threats to care, including mental healthcare, in affected communities. People who are not directly involved in disasters are also at risk, if they require continuity of mental health services.

A specific challenge in disasters is to assess the health and welfare needs of first responders and staff of the emergency services involved in rescuing survivors and retrieving the bodies or remains of the people who have been killed [34]. Emergency service personnel are trained to carry out this work and, but many fewer have effective support networks to assist them to deal with the adversity. Staff training should include structured systems to build and support the resilience of staff. Staff who care for people who have multiple or long-term injuries also require consideration. Often, the capacity for support structures to contain and deal with these circumstances is overwhelmed by events.

The effects of emergencies on the needs of people for psychosocial and mental health services require planners to consider the practical requirements of four main groups of people as indicated in Table 1.

All of these groups (see Table 1) acquire psychosocial needs and a smaller but substantial proportion may develop mental disorders. Planners must take account of each one. They must also be aware of the ripple effects whereby the pool of people involved tends to grow by association and of the needs to coordinate planning of immediate and medium and long-term responses sometimes over wide geographical areas depending on the nature of the events and the origins of the people involved. These challenges require appointment of knowledgeable and experienced specialist advisers who respect and understand the existing healthcare and support networks for the people who are exposed to disasters, as well as recognising the cultural preferences of people who are affected.

Positively, disasters can be used as circumstances for creating much greater awareness and skill about psychopathology in communities and as examples of the importance for all mental healthcare services providing planned and coordinated programmes of care. Training mental health professionals to provide responsive services at the time of a disaster can be utilized later to deal with the more ubiquitous and day-to-day trauma that exists with great prevalence in all countries. Presently, much of this morbidity is unrecognized and poorly treated.

Table 1: Groups with different mental health needs following disasters.

(i) People who are at risk of distress, mental health problems, and mental disorders, principally anxiety, depressive, and substance use disorders, consequent on their direct and indirect involvement in events and who present new and additional demands on mental health services.
(ii) People who have continuing needs for mental health services for preexisting conditions, but whose care is threatened by challenges to the "business continuity" of preexisting mental health services consequent on network and community dislocation.
(iii) People whose involvement in an emergency provokes or precipitates the relapse of a preexisting mental disorder.
(iv) People who are responders and whose mental health might be put at raised risk consequent on their work.

5. Lessons from Research

5.1. The Reactions of Survivors and Professionals. In the immediate aftermath of disasters, survivors tend to seek out their own networks of support, if they are available. This desire should be recognised and actively supported. The majority of people has a natural stoicism and tends to minimize their focus on the psychosocial impact and anticipate improvement in their distress. On the other hand, professionals usually feel an obligation to assist and often encourage people to seek counseling. However, they should focus more on individual person's distress and must guard against exaggerating the psychosocial and mental health risks or apprehension about survivors ability to cope. This conflict means that it is critical for survivors' perspectives to be respected and addressed.

On the other hand, tendencies to exaggerate personal hardiness and the stigma and shame of seeking help with social, psychological, and mental health needs must be carefully managed in any service intervention provided. People who are involved (staff as well as survivors) may use avoidance as a psychological strategy for dealing with their distress.

Critical consequences that must be planned for when delivering health services include the confusion that people may experience about the meaning of their experiences and the frequency with which people who are psychologically distressed present with physical symptoms. This occurs particularly often in war veterans but also after disasters. McFarlane and Papay et al. [35] studied the pattern of presentation of firefighters to their general practitioners and their histories of health complaints after the Ash Wednesday bushfires. Many of these men had attended their general practitioners to complain of a range of physical symptoms, which they experienced to a significantly greater degree than another group of fire officers who had similar rates of injury and exposure but did not have posttraumatic stress disorder [36]. Often, the general practitioners did not recognise the symptoms as being indicators of a possible psychiatric disorder.

The importance of this section is that it alerts planners to the importance of designing services, which take into account the integrated physical and psychological needs and preferences of affected people. It also reminds us that any services offered should be based on planners and practitioners sound understanding of the issues that arise from different cultural and societal preferences, expectations, and needs.

5.2. Resilience. While there is longstanding evidence that a substantial number of people who are exposed to disasters develop psychopathology for short, medium, or longer periods of time, there is growing international interest in how and why many and so more people who are involved in disasters do not develop mental disorders.

There is an increasing evidence that many people appear to be resilient to the deleterious sustained psychosocial impacts that are experienced by a most of the people who are involved [37]. In addition, there is also a small but slowly increasing number of studies showing that some people may suffer distress in the short-term but also derive certain psychosocial developmental advantages too. One of the intentions of this work is to learn lessons for how we might reduce the risk of mental disorder that is imposed by people's exposure to a wide variety of stressors, and it is leading to the development of public mental health services.

Sapienza and Masten [38] and Masten and Narayan [39] provide summaries of the development of the concept of resilience and research evidence in two recent papers that focus on children. Other recent work has researched the resilience of groups of people and communities. This is termed collective resilience as compared with personal resilience, which covers the resilience of particular people. It showed that strangers who are thrown together by circumstance to face disaster as a group often develop collective resilient patterns of behaviour very quickly in their immediate response to unfolding major incidents and that this phenomenon is not limited to communities or groups of people who are well-known to each other. These patterns of behaviour were found in the people caught in the underground rail carriages in the bombings in London on 7 July, 2005 [40].

Personal and collective resilience offers psychosocial advantages that buffer the ill effects of disasters on people's mental health. This prompts a question about whether it is possible to prepare people and communities for the possibility of disaster in ways that strengthen them and mitigate the risks of mental disorder without provoking widespread fear and anxiety. As yet, there is little research into the effectiveness of resilience building [33]. However, presently, programmes are in hand in a number of countries that are intended to promote the resilience of people and communities.

While promoting resilience is a broad societal matter and not a direct call upon health services, there is an increasingly popular argument for including it in the spectrum of psychosocial services that are required in mature cross-agency plans for responding to disasters [33].

5.3. Psychopathology. The most consistent finding from disaster studies is that intensity of people's exposure is the critical determinant of their risk of psychopathology [29, 41]. Exposure is defined by a combination of the threat to particular persons and groups of people and the losses that they sustain [42]. Measuring exposure is not a straightforward issue. Sometimes, it is defined by a group in terms of being a member of the community that has suffered greatly or according to personal loss.

A difficulty in interpreting findings from research is that exposure is affected by other factors that modify, intensify, or buffer its affects. Recently, for example, meta-research has shown that availability of psychosocial support or otherwise has a very substantial moderating effect on the risk generated by exposure [43]. This finding emphasises the importance of planning services in advance. However, it is difficult to directly compare many studies because of the different time intervals that have elapsed from the point of the disaster to the point of the investigation [12, 13]. In all populations exposed to major incidents, there is an expected process of natural remission and this impacts on the prevalence rates according to the time that has elapsed after an event.

Disaster is only one type of traumatic experience that can affect people's lives. One way of understanding the comparative effect of different categories of traumatic events is to look at general community stratified population samples and examine the prevalence of disaster exposure. The National Mental Health and Wellbeing Survey conducted in 2007 [44] in Australia looked at 10,600 people. PTSD (diagnosed using ICD-10 criteria) was found to be the most common anxiety disorder. One of the problems with the methodology in these studies is that they ask people about only one event. Among the Australian population, 20% of men and 13% of women had been exposed to disasters. Compared with the rates of PTSD following most of the other major stressors that were examined in this population, the rates were significantly less than those after events involving interpersonal violence. The 12-month prevalence among the disaster-exposed population using DSM-IV criteria was 2.3%. Although this is a small percentage, it reflects a long tail of effect because for many of the people the disaster may have occurred many years previously.

As set out above, there are a substantial percentage of people in any disaster-affected community who are already suffering from psychiatric disorders as well as those who become unwell due to the disaster. This frames an enduring challenge to disentangle the interaction between these two groups. In other words, the percentages of people who have never previously suffered from psychiatric disorder and who emerge with a diagnosis after trauma are of particular interest. The way in which the existing psychopathology is changed in terms of its phenomenology and longitudinal course is an equally critical question. Most disaster studies to date have not made this differentiation. This latter question is of particular importance in respect of the observations of Kessler et al. [45] in the National Comorbidity Study.

It demonstrated that PTSD could be a disorder that runs a significantly chronic course in approximately 40% of people who are so diagnosed. The positive perspective is that, in 60%, the disorder ameliorates by 72 months and community-based treatments appear to have beneficial effects. Long-term studies of disasters are few with the 33-year followup of the Aberfan mudslide disaster showing that 46% of the childhood survivors had had PTSD at some stage, and 29% had that diagnosis at followup [46]. The Piper Alpha oilrig disaster of 1988 ten years later found that, 21% of the survivors was found to have PTSD [47]. Studies, such as, these indicate that people who have had a high intensity exposure have a significant risk of prolonged and enduring morbidity. This is the challenge for health services namely, anticipating, identifying, and treating people in the long-term as well as the short-term need following these events.

While studies measure anxiety disorders, such as, PTSD, fewer measure the prevalence of mood disorders though the studies that do show that depression is commonly comorbid with PTSD or occurs in the absence of PTSD [12, 13, 48, 49]. While particular interest is focused on PTSD following disastrous events, there is, now, an increasingly substantial body of evidence demonstrating that the whole range of psychiatric disorders emerge with an increased risk following these events. Bonanno et al. [50] offer an authoritative review of the literature relating to the psychosocial and mental health costs of disasters. They say, "*People exposed to disaster show myriad psychological problems, including PTSD, grief, depression, anxiety, stress-related health costs, substance abuse, and suicidal ideation.*"

A study that one of us [51] conducted looking at 200 motor vehicle survivors, a substantial group developed major depression alone in the absence of PTSD [52]. Equally, many people with PTSD had significant degrees of comorbidity. Similarly, the growing volume of good quality research into mental health of the UK armed forces is beginning to reveal that the most common disorders among veterans who have served in Iraq are depression (53% of those with a mental disorder), anxiety disorders (18%) PTSD (16%), and substance misuse (12%) [53]. These findings emphasise the importance of research in future examining the broad pattern of morbidity [12, 13, 48].

6. Effective Interventions

6.1. An Evidence-Informed Model of Care. The interventions recommended by IASC and the Sphere Project's standards are intended for adoption in all parts of the world, societies, and cultures [9, 10]. They are based on the best available evidence. It is imperative that frameworks for disaster mental healthcare are adaptable. A recent paper states that "*Mental health care is desperately needed throughout the developing world*" and it reports that Aceh province in Indonesia is testing a novel approach, which minimizes reliance on psychiatrists [54]. The guidance from IASC, Sphere, and NATO is intended to be applicable in a wide range of differently resourced countries.

Tol and van Ommeren [2] draw attention to the four layered pyramid of intervention that these sources commend comprising of psychosocial care for most survivors and their relatives delivered by nonmental healthcare practitioners combined with mental healthcare that is targeted on people who have diagnosed disorders that is delivered by people who are trained to do so [55]. They draw attention to a recent review of the grey literature that has compared currently popular practices with the evidence for effective practices. They point out that the most rigorous evidence supports specialised practices for intervening with people who have PTSD and depression.

Other bodies have recommended similar approaches to intervention that are intended to be economical with precious trained mental health practitioners who are often of limited availability in many countries. One such approach is the strategic stepped model of care that has been adopted as nonbinding guidance by NATO [1]. It is also based on the best available evidence. Forbes et al. [55] have advocated a stratified approach to psychosocial and mental health care. In 2009, Williams and Bisson brought together work undertaken in Europe with the NATO Guidance to produce a set of principles that is informed by the best evidence available. Table 2 illustrates a stratified model of care [56].

6.2. Intervening in the Rescue and Immediate Recovery Phase. There is a growing professional consensus and slowing rising evidence that a series of psychosocial interventions should be applied immediately after disasters. This approach is based on the principles of psychological first aid. Recently, the WHO published its guide on PTSD for field workers [57].

The philosophy for the psychosocial and mental health interventions is the PIES model that has been developed from the military, namely that services provided should be based on their proximity, immediacy of response, expectancy of recovery, and simplicity.

It is critical is to make people feel safe and to assist in decreasing their anxiety immediately after a disaster impacts. It involves providing information and dealing with the immediate survival, welfare, and humanitarian needs, if requested. People should be provided with reassurance and physical comfort. Those in pain from injuries should be given good pain relief.

However, providing immediate counseling risks creating a false belief that there will be no long-term morbidity and, furthermore, counseling immediately after disasters has not been shown to be effective. So, it is important to manage carefully access of counselors to survivors. This involves vetting offers for help and credentialing service providers. It is important that there is active interaction between disaster services on-scene and the staff who provide inpatient care for injured persons at a distance because, otherwise, people who require psychosocial support may slip through the usual channels.

In this phase, some people may develop an acute stress reaction, which may be termed acute stress disorder (ASD) if the experiences are severe and cause dysfunction. On first examination, people who have this disorder may experience symptoms that are similar to those of distress, on one hand, and, on the other hand, those experienced by people who suffer PTSD later. Therefore, great care is required

Table 2: Interventions in the aftermath of disasters.

Level	Intervention	Target population	Examples of interventions	Interventions conducted by
1	Psychological first aid (PFA)	Most of the people who are affected	Restoring immediate safety Restoring contact with loved ones	All responders and aid workers
2	Community development	Communities after large-scale events	Schools, sports, meetings, newsletters to unite groups of people	All responders and aid workers
3	Skills for psychosocial recovery (SPR)	People whose distress is sustained by bereavement or secondary stressors	Brief needs assessment Problem-solving Social support	Healthcare practitioners and workers trained in the skills
4	Psychosocial interventions for medium- and long-term problems	People whose distress is sustained and associated with functional impairment	Trauma-focused cognitive behaviour therapy	Staff of mental healthcare facilities

in distinguishing people who are temporarily distressed from those who have ASD and, after a month, PTSD. The most reliable feature is how well people recover over time. Distressed but resilient people recover quickly but may experience quite debilitating experiences for a while. People with an ASD recover more slowly. Progressive mitigation or diminution of their intrusive recollections of the disaster differentiates people who develop PTSD from those who do not. The definition of PTSD precludes its diagnosis until a month after the event. These findings have led the National Institute for Health and Clinical Excellence in the UK (NICE) [58] to recommend that a stance of watchful waiting be adopted for around four weeks after the start of events before treatment for PTSD is initiated. During the interval, survivors should be offered support that is based on the principles of psychological first aid [59] and further assessment. Therefore, one of the primary aims in this phase is to screen the population and make some assessment of people who are at particular risk in the future. However, earlier treatment should be provided if people's distress is unusual or particularly intense.

In the rescue and early recovery phases, it is best to use local health providers, if possible, because they are embedded in the affected communities, trusted, and know the culture and local circumstances. During this phase, it is also critical to develop a training programme for general practitioners who are likely to be the contact points for people who require long-term services. Even if they are not particularly skilled in the mental health domain at this point, they are the people who tend to be consulted by survivors in the aftermath of the disaster. They are well placed to distinguish people who require psychosocial care from those who need specialist mental healthcare.

7. Developing Services

7.1. Policy Development. The services, including the mental health services, that are required following a disaster only work effectively if planners anticipate the need for them, understand the dynamic shifts in need that occur with the passage of time, and are clear about how these services are to work with other agencies that offer psychosocial responses.

Mental health services for moderate- and large- scale emergencies should be well integrated with humanitarian aid, welfare, and psychosocial care in disaster response plans. This requires that lessons learned through research and experience are translated in integrated ways into policy at four levels:

(1) government policies;

(2) strategic policies for service design;

(3) service delivery policies; and

(4) policies for good clinical practice.

Each of these four levels of policy should be influenced by the kinds of evidence that this paper summarises. Policy at each level should be ethical. There are important roles for practitioners who are skilled in mental healthcare and experienced and trained in disaster management to provide advice to the authorities as they develop each of these aspects of policy and conduct operations in the face of disaster. The principles developed by Williams et al. [56] cover all four policy levels. Cultural and ethical values should permeate each level of policy and planning.

Government policies are required to set the aims and objectives for psychosocial and mental healthcare responses. They should specify the requirement for services to be designed, developed, and delivered that offer mental healthcare that is integrated into all disaster response plans. The responsible authorities should bring together evidence from research with expert consensus, their knowledge of the country, its society and cultures, and the profile of risks to design services. They should plan programmes for managing the performance of the services in meeting the objectives that are identified for them.

Service delivery policies concern how particular services function and relate to their partner services and how affected populations are guided into and through them according to the evidence and awareness of the preferences and needs of people who are likely to use them. Therefore, service delivery policies include evidence- and values-based models of care, care pathways, and protocols and guidelines for care as well as processes for demand management, audit, and review. Policies for good clinical practice concern how clinical staff take account of the needs and personal and cultural preferences of patients, deploy their clinical skills, and work with patients to decide how guidelines, care pathways, and protocols are to be interpreted in individual cases.

Major incident mental health services should be built upon the existing clinical skills and preparedness within each community to deal with day-to-day disasters. Furthermore, the services that provide psychosocial support and those that provide mental healthcare should be an integral part of the major incident or disaster plans for every community. This challenges community leaders' planning and training and raises their needs for knowledge and skill. One way in which the latter task can be approached is by ensuring that the skills that are developed are made available within communities by, for example, the mental health services being available to the survivors of, for example, motor vehicle accidents, house fires, criminal assaults.

Additionally, there are phases and time windows that are critical to service planning, design and delivery as Williams et al. [56] concur.

Planning in advance of warning of possible disaster should be ubiquitous. It should cover five domains of service requirement:

(i) medical rescue and immediate intervention services;

(ii) continuing physical healthcare;

(iii) recovery and rehabilitation services;

(iv) business continuity for preexisting services for the general population (which may, otherwise, be depleted as a consequence of disasters with secondary consequential affects on communities);

(v) psychosocial and mental health services.

Demands vary significantly across the different time-scales and narratives of each disaster. Thought is required about the profile of services required as a disaster unfolds and in the rescue, recovery, and restoration phases. The need for medical services is greatest in the early phases. By contrast, the specialist mental health services are most required later. Psychosocial services are required in the immediate aftermath and recovery phases and have a continuing contribution into the restoration phase.

7.2. Time Windows for Service Planning

7.2.1. The Predisaster Phase. In the predisaster phase, it is critical to ensure that each community has a plan for providing psychosocial and mental healthcare after disasters and that the plan includes immediate and medium- and long-term components. This means that these plans should be flexible and responsive to differing types of disaster by, for example, including the means to alert distant communities to the requirement to plan medium- and long-term responses if the people involved come from wider rather than local geographical areas. The problem is that disaster plans are too often designed around the most recently impacting event, which, in probability, may not be the event that occurs next. It is a challenge to maintain a pool of disaster experience and of staff who are interested in the absence of a real threat.

It is a challenge to involve mental health services at this stage. Planners tend to see the critical issues as being emergency surgical services and hospital management plans. While those facilities are critical, mental health services should be given an enhanced priority because failure to include them in this stage of the planning means that it is harder to achieve their engagement later. This has implications for training. Decisions of this nature tend only to be made if the government policies include them, and mental healthcare is explicitly specified in strategic designs for services. Otherwise, the resources required, as predicted by appropriate appraisals of the risks, may not be forthcoming.

Practice in all phases must be ethical, and this calls for a framework of public health ethics (as compared with personal health care ethics) to be adopted during the predisaster planning phase. An example of such a successful framework is provided by the work on public health and policy ethics conducted by the UK government in its preparations for an influenza pandemic, which was tested in 2009-10. Additionally, the Madrid Framework can be used to test how well policies deal with the values and evidence that are inherent in designing and delivering services [56, 60].

7.2.2. The Disaster or Incident Warning Phase. Plans should be put into effect during the period when there is an increased risk of disaster, such as, the summer in bushfire prone zones or during the period when a weather system is emerging as a major threat. This requires acceptance of the heightened danger at all four levels of policymaking and practice. Otherwise, denial results in loss of time that is vital for detailed planning. This occurred in the cyclone that devastated Darwin on Christmas Day in 1975. The disaster warnings were largely ignored because, on 24 December, everybody was busy with their Christmas preparations [61]. Similar denial took place before the floods in the Netherlands of 1953.

Taking this advice means accepting that there are many instances in which a warning arises, but no disaster follows. it is critically important to be adaptive and for risk appraisal to be flexible during this period because each event poses new challenges.

7.2.3. The Phase of Disaster Occurrence. As disasters unfold, there is often little that can be done. There are many events, such as, the Kobe earthquake [62], which occurs in such a brief time frame that no action is possible. Other disasters, such as, fires and floods, have a more enduring course. It is critical to be tolerant of loss of control during this stage, and face the sense of helplessness and unpredictability of chance.

Often, the immediate impressions of a disaster scene for members of the public and staff of the rescue services who are first to arrive are one of such utter chaos and devastation that it is difficult to know where or how to begin work. That experience is immobilizing, and anticipation of what the scene may be like should be built into training along with sound leadership if rescue teams are to acclimatize and begin work rapidly. The terror impact of the attack on the

World Trade Centre Towers, for example, was dramatic and the survivors struggled to express their feelings in a way that was understood [63].

At these early times, it is not unreasonable for people who are in emergency service roles, such as, ambulance services staff and firefighters, to behave in self-protective ways, rather than taking needless risks. High levels of risk were run by fire officers who went into the World Trade Centre on September 11 because they failed to adequately assess the potential for the buildings to collapse. Survival demands flexibility of risk appraisal and the ability to switch into rescue mode when this becomes a viable proposition.

Paradoxically, one of the difficulties for staff who come to disasters later in the aftermath is that the awfulness and horror have abated. Often, there is a dreadful silence and stillness in the aftermath of destruction. The contrast between the aftermath and the event often makes it very difficult for those people who have not experienced a disaster to understand the horror and the awfulness of what has been experienced by survivors and the staff of the rescue services.

One of the predicaments of disaster survivors is that they have been through a time warp of horrors which people not present struggle to grasp. Thus, it is easy for the psychosocial and mental health issues to be ignored in this chaos.

7.2.4. The Rescue Phase. In the rescue phase, it is critical to assess the assets and resources that are available within the community to address the needs of the population. While the focus is on attending to the acute physical needs of affected people, it is also important to make a preliminary assessment of the survivors' potential long-term needs [64]. Often, new leadership structures emerge in communities as they deal with the unpredictability of the emergency. Acceptance of the fluidity of this situation is a critical part of the capacity of the responding services to face the threat and cope in the disorganisation that follows traumatic events. Sometimes, there is a conflict for staff of the health services between attending to the needs of their families and going to work as a rescuer or health provider. This dilemma is most acute for the emergency service workers, and they require continuing contact with their families, good leadership, support, regular rest, food and breaks, and engagement as members of teams if they are to give of their best.

Knowing about how people behave in the face of disaster and the longer-term potential for psychosocial effects is important not solely within the health services at this time, but when providing support for and understanding the behaviour of survivors. This frames another important item for training staff, including, particularly, major incident commanders (MICs), well before events occur.

As events unfold, identification of survivors and their needs for acute physical care is an immediate priority. Threat to life is the immediate priority and threat to limb and other morbidity follows. While the prospects for people having immediate needs for psychiatric care are small (estimated as 1 in 1,000 survivors), it is important to establish if any survivor is in immediate need of specialist mental health services. Similarly, few people's behaviour is grossly disorganized. Often, managing staff and volunteers who want to help is a more substantial challenge.

Well before events occur, planners should respond to their obligations to rescuers and relief workers by providing them with effective leadership, training, supervision, defined expectations, and support and these functions must be available to staff throughout their work in an emergency. It is important to assess if the size and impact of the disaster require reciprocal assistance from similar services from outside the immediate area to augment local capacity. Plans for reciprocal responses in major emergencies must be in existence prior to any disaster.

7.2.5. The Medium-Term Recovery Phase. The central role of primary healthcare services should be considered carefully in the recovery phase. Good quality care for physical injuries and adequate pain relief can do much to benefit people's psychosocial states. All psychosocial and mental health services should be integrated with the primary healthcare services and be placed in similar locations so they do not compete. Continuing professional support and education should be provided.

The mental health practitioners who deal with traumatized survivors and their relatives in the medium-term should be well trained in evidence-based assessment and treatment skills that are required for dealing with posttraumatic mental disorders of all types including depression and anxiety disorders. They should use a multidisciplinary approach and have strong links with the primary healthcare networks that recovering people continue to require. The staff who provide these services should be aware of the interaction between the emerging posttraumatic morbidity and existing psychiatric morbidity within the community. Consultants should be involved in monitoring the emerging morbidity and ensuring that groups of people who are at risk receive services. Planning for future service development should be continuous.

Experience shows that there is poor uptake of specialist services in the mediumterm after disasters. This requires plans for active outreach that is based on the screening that has been conducted in the previous phase to define the populations that are at risk. Addressing communities' mental health literacy is another critical challenge at this point because of the divergence of the beliefs. The population should be monitored for behaviors, such as, self-harm and patterns of substance use, that may indicate risk indirectly and depression and anxiety disorders. Also, this is the time when other events in civilian life may raise the risks of re-traumatisation for fire, ambulance, and police officers, for example.

7.2.6. The Long-Term Reestablishment Phase. Throughout all phases of recovery, practitioners should ensure that people who have been involved in disasters have optimal outcomes [65]. Although the number of people who develop persistent mental disorders is relatively small, their needs may be substantial and last for lengthy periods. Some people require maintenance treatment. However, there is a common tendency to withdraw services prematurely. Additionally, there may be an interval, sometimes an extended interval, before some people develop disorders, such as, depression and PTSD [66]. Thus, new cases tend to emerge for many years after disasters. This means that specialist services are likely to be required to address the needs of the survivors of the many lesser disastrous events as well as the major disasters that have befallen the population in the same geographical area.

After any disaster, there is always the requirement to identify what has worked and what has gone wrong. Reviews should be initiated during the earlier phases but become the focus of particular consideration during the long-term phase. There are lessons to be learned for policy, planning, organisations, leadership, and management of responses. The reestablishment phase provides opportunities to review and address the clinical skills of the professional staff of the mental health services with a view to ensuring that they are adequately trained, and that emerging professional lessons have been identified and learned.

7.2.7. The Chronic Posttraumatic Reestablishment Phase. General public interest in disaster-affected communities dies quickly. On the long term, the mental health services can play a critical role in maintaining recognition of the continuing additional needs of affected communities.

The staff of the mental health services who are involved in responding to disasters should also actively manage reintegration of the specialized services with the mainstream structures [67]. Often, additional funds that were made available to discharge disaster response services are withdrawn. This presents challenges because the people who have long-term mental health needs may still require active interventions [68, 69]. All-too-often, the prevalence and impacts of past and future disasters and other major incidents within affected communities are underestimated as is the role of the psychological trauma that stems from disasters in determining the patterns of background psychiatric morbidity in affected communities.

In some disasters, there is also the important challenge of dealing with coroners' courts, legal systems, and compensation claims. The cumbersome delays and the procedural slowness of legal processes can be a substantial cause of further psychosocial aggravation for survivors.

8. Conclusion

Looking back, there has been a striking, rapid, and dramatic change in scientific understanding of and public approaches to recognising and managing the psychosocial trauma that may occur as a consequence of disasters. The position taken in this paper is that psychosocial and mental healthcare services should be planned and actively integrated components of all disaster relief and broader healthcare responses.

This requires attention to learning the lessons from research and from survivors' stories about the requirements for psychosocial care of populations of people and mental health services for people who develop depression, anxiety, and/or substance use disorders. There is a strong consensus in the evidence about the types of disorders that people may suffer after disasters. The evidence of effectiveness is stronger for intervening with people who have disorders, though the rising interest in public mental health should propel more research into the needs for and effectiveness of psychosocial care.

The WHO has espoused the principals for immediate psychosocial care, and there is a strong expert consensus on basing this work on psychological first aid.

Critically, achieving what is required also requires continuing negotiation with policymakers, managers and clinical staff of all relevant disciplines and backgrounds. Often, emergency preparedness managers and emergency service leaders welcome greater knowledge of the psychosocial and mental health impacts of disasters and that evidence-informed expert consensus frameworks of response that have great similarity are now available.

The challenge of maintaining the skills developed in the aftermath of the disaster is only met if service delivery models and clinical skills are extended into other settings. The WHO Burden of Disease has emphasised the importance of motor vehicle accidents as a critical cause of morbidity. Furthermore, people who are chronically mentally ill are often the victims of trauma and violence. Thus, this paper could be considered as describing a microcosm of mental healthcare that should allow lessons to be learned for developing services for people who are exposed to less extreme events. The skills learnt by staff of the mental health services can then be effectively transmitted into their work with the survivors of small but no less painful day-to-day traumatic events. Reciprocally, that advance will provide critical skills among managers and practitioners to meet the needs of their community if it were to be affected by a disaster.

Governments should lead by actively engaging in continuing policy development to take account of our emerging knowledge. At the same time, people who are involved at each of the four levels of policy require active support and assistance. Practical steps that can assist in these regards include creating centres of excellence, such as, the WHO centre in Kobe. Also, developing collaborative associations with researchers and colleagues across the world is vital as is developing education in a variety of institutions and professions that build upon our accumulating knowledge. Only then will systems have been created that are based on cycles of improvement in which the lessons from disasters assist in better management of the survivors of the large, small, and personal disasters that occur daily in all societies.

References

[1] "Psychosocial Care for People Affected by Disasters and Major Incidents: A Model for Designing, Delivering and Managing Psychosocial Services for People Involved in Major Incidents, Conflict, Disasters and Terrorism," 2012, http://www.health-planning.co.uk/nato/.

[2] W. A. Tol and M. van Ommeren, "Evidence-based mental health and psychosocial support in humanitarian settings:

gaps and opportunities," *Evidence-Based Mental Health*, vol. 15, pp. 25–26, 2012.

[3] "Australian Guidelines for the Treatment of Adults with Acute Stress Disorder and Posttraumatic Stress Disorder," http://www.acpmh.unimelb.edu.au/resources/resource-asdptsd_guidelines.html.

[4] A. C. McFarlane and B. Raphael, "Ash Wednesday: the effects of a fire," *Australian and New Zealand Journal of Psychiatry*, vol. 18, no. 4, pp. 341–351, 1984.

[5] M. Creamer, P. Burgess, and A. C. Mcfarlane, "Post-traumatic stress disorder: findings from the Australian National Survey of Mental Health and well-being," *Psychological Medicine*, vol. 31, no. 7, pp. 1237–1247, 2001.

[6] A. C. McFarlane and M. Van Hooff, "Impact of childhood exposure to a natural disaster on adult mental health: 20-year longitudinal follow-up study," *British Journal of Psychiatry*, vol. 195, no. 2, pp. 142–148, 2009.

[7] F. H. Norris, "Epidemiology of trauma: frequency and impact of different potentially traumatic events on different demographic groups," *Journal of Consulting and Clinical Psychology*, vol. 60, no. 3, pp. 409–418, 1992.

[8] G. Proulx and R. F. Fahy, "Evacuation of the World Trade Center: what went right?" in *Proceedings of the CIB-CTBUH International Conference on Tall Buildings*, Malaysia, October 2003.

[9] Inter-Agency Standing Committee, IASC Guidelines on Mental Health and Psychosocial Support in Emergency Settings, Geneva, Switzerland, 2007.

[10] *The Sphere Project, Humanitarian Charter and Minimum Standards in Disaster Response*, Hobbs, Southampton, UK, 2011.

[11] C. R. Brewin, P. Scragg, M. Robertson, M. Thompson, P. D'Ardenne, and A. Ehlers, "Promoting mental health following the london bombings: a screen and treat approach," *Journal of Traumatic Stress*, vol. 21, no. 1, pp. 3–8, 2008.

[12] C. Stanke, V. Murray, R. Amlot et al., "The effects of flooding on mental health: findings and recommendations from a review of the literature," *Public Library of Science Currents: Disasters*. In press, http://currents.plos.org/disasters/article/the-effects-of-flooding-on-mental-health-outcomes-and-recommendations-from-a-review-of-the-literature/.

[13] V. Murray, H. Caldin, R. Amlot et al., *The Effects of Flooding on Mental Health*, Health Protection Agency, London, UK, 2011.

[14] L. Weisaeth and A. Tonnessen, "Responses of individuals and groups to consequences of technological disaster and radiation exposure," in *Terrorism and Disaster: Individual and Community Mental Health Interventions*, R. Ursano, C. Fullerton, and A. Norwood, Eds., Cambridge Universtity Press, Cambridge, UK, 2003.

[15] BBC, "1976: Chinese earthquake kills hundreds of thousands," in *On This Day*, British Broadcasting Corporation, 1976.

[16] J. Chang, *Wild Swans*, Simon and Schuster, London, UK, 1991.

[17] "Lifeboats for all not ordered by law (1912, April 17)," *New York Times*, 1912.

[18] D. A. Butler, *Unsinkable: The Full Story of the R.M.S. Titanic*, DaCapo Press, Cambridge, UK, 2002.

[19] A. C. McFarlane, "Attitudes to victims: issues for medicine, the law & society," in *Proceedings of the 8th International Symposium on Victimology*, M. Sumner, Ed., Australian Insitute of Criminology, Canberra, Australia, 1996.

[20] L. Weisaeth, "PTSD: vulnerability and protective factors," *Bailliere's Cinical Psychiatry, International Practice and Research*, vol. 2, pp. 217–228, 1996.

[21] P. G. V. D. Velden, L. Grievink, R. J. Kleber et al., "Post-disaster mental health problems and the utilization of mental health services: a four-year longitudinal comparative study," *Administration and Policy in Mental Health and Mental Health Services Research*, vol. 33, no. 3, pp. 279–288, 2006.

[22] L. Weisaeth, "A study of behavioural responses to an industrial disaster," *Acta Psychiatrica Scandinavica*, vol. 80, no. 355, supplement, pp. 13–24, 1989.

[23] C. Selly, E. King, R. Peveler, K. Osola, N. Martin, and C. Thompson, "Post-traumatic stress disorder symptoms and the Clapham rail accident," *British Journal of Psychiatry*, vol. 171, pp. 478–482, 1997.

[24] M. Başoğlu, E. Şalcıoğlu, and M. Livanou, "Traumatic stress responses in earthquake survivors in Turkey," *Journal of Traumatic Stress*, vol. 15, no. 4, pp. 269–276, 2002.

[25] E. Şalcioğlu, M. Başoğlu, and M. Livanou, "Long-term psychological outcome for non-treatment-seeking earthquake survivors in Turkey," *Journal of Nervous and Mental Disease*, vol. 191, no. 3, pp. 154–160, 2003.

[26] A. C. McFarlane, "Posttraumatic morbidity of a disaster. A study of cases presenting for psychiatric treatment," *Journal of Nervous and Mental Disease*, vol. 174, no. 1, pp. 4–14, 1986.

[27] E. O. Noorthoorn, J. M. Havenaar, H. A. De Haan, Y. R. Van Rood, and W. A. H. J. Van Stiphout, "Mental health service use and outcomes after the enschede fireworks disaster: a naturalistic follow-up study," *Psychiatric Services*, vol. 61, no. 11, pp. 1138–1143, 2010.

[28] J. Drury and R. Williams, "Children and young people who are refugees, internally displaced persons and victims and perpetrators of war and mass violence," *Current Opinion in Psychiatry*, vol. 25, no. 4, pp. 277–284, 2012.

[29] H. Cao, A. C. McFarlane, and S. Klimidis, "Prevalence of psychiatric disorder following the 1988 Yun Nan (China) earthquake—the first 5-month period," *Social Psychiatry and Psychiatric Epidemiology*, vol. 38, no. 4, pp. 204–212, 2003.

[30] A. Kardiner, *The Traumatic Neuroses of War*, Hoeber, New York, NY, USA, 1941.

[31] A. C. McFarlane and B. van der Kolk, "Trauma and its challenge to society," in *Traumatic Stress: The Effect of Overwhelming Experience on Mind, Body and Society*, B. van der Kolk, A. C. McFarlane, and L. Weisaeth, Eds., Guilford, New York, NY, USA, 1996.

[32] C. DiMaggio and S. Galea, "The behavioral consequences of terrorism: a meta-analysis," *Academic Emergency Medicine*, vol. 13, no. 5, pp. 559–566, 2006.

[33] R. Whittle, W. Medd, H. Deeming et al., *After the Rain—Learning the Lessons from Flood Recovery in Hull*, Lancaster University, Lancaster, UK, 2010.

[34] J. P. Wisnivesky, S. L. Teitelbaum, A. C. Todd et al., "Persistence of multiple illnesses in World Trade Center rescue and recovery workers: a cohort study," *The Lancet*, vol. 378, no. 9794, pp. 888–897, 2011.

[35] A. C. McFarlane and P. Papay, "Multiple diagnoses in posttraumatic stress disorder in the victims of a natural disaster," *Journal of Nervous and Mental Disease*, vol. 180, no. 8, pp. 498–504, 1992.

[36] A. L. Del Gaizo, J. D. Elhai, and T. L. Weaver, "Posttraumatic stress disorder, poor physical health and substance use behaviors in a national trauma-exposed sample," *Psychiatry Research*, vol. 188, no. 3, pp. 390–395, 2011.

[37] F. H. Norris, M. Tracy, and S. Galea, "Looking for resilience: understanding the longitudinal trajectories of responses to stress," *Social Science and Medicine*, vol. 68, no. 12, pp. 2190–2198, 2009.

[38] J. K. Sapienza and A. S. Masten, "Understanding and promoting resilience in children and youth," *Current Opinion in Psychiatry*, vol. 24, no. 4, pp. 267–273, 2011.

[39] A. S. Masten and A. J. Narayan, "Child development in the context of disaster, war, and terrorism: pathways of risk and resilience," *Annual Review of Psychology*, vol. 63, pp. 227–257, 2012.

[40] J. Drury, C. Cocking, and S. Reicher, "Everyone for themselves? A comparative study of crowd solidarity among emergency survivors," *British Journal of Social Psychology*, vol. 48, no. 3, pp. 487–506, 2009.

[41] I. V. E. Carlier and B. P. R. Gersons, "Stress reactions in disaster victims following the Bijlmermeer plane crash," *Journal of Traumatic Stress*, vol. 10, no. 2, pp. 329–335, 1997.

[42] A. C. McFarlane, "The aetiology of post-traumatic morbidity: predisposing, precipitating and perpetuating factors," *British Journal of Psychiatry*, vol. 154, pp. 221–228, 1989.

[43] F. H. Norris, M. J. Friedman, P. J. Watson, C. M. Byrne, E. Diaz, and K. Kaniasty, "60,000 disaster victims speak—part I. An empirical review of the empirical literature, 1981–2001," *Psychiatry*, vol. 65, no. 3, pp. 207–239, 2002.

[44] T. Slade, A. Johnston, M. Teesson et al., "The Mental Health of Australians 2. Report on the 2007 National Survey of Mental Health and Wellbeing," Canberra, Australia, 2009.

[45] R. C. Kessler, A. Sonnega, E. Bromet, M. Hughes, and C. B. Nelson, "Posttraumatic stress disorder in the national comorbidity survey," *Archives of General Psychiatry*, vol. 52, no. 12, pp. 1048–1060, 1995.

[46] L. Morgan, J. Scourfield, D. Williams, A. Jasper, and G. Lewis, "The Aberfan disaster: 33-year follow-up of survivors," *British Journal of Psychiatry*, vol. 182, pp. 532–536, 2003.

[47] A. M. Hull, D. A. Alexander, and S. Klein, "Survivors of the piper alpha oil platform disaster: long-term follow-up study," *British Journal of Psychiatry*, vol. 181, pp. 433–438, 2002.

[48] R. Williams and D. A. Alexander, "Conflict, terrorism and disasters: the psychosocial consequences for children," in *Conflict and Catastrophe Medicine: A Practical Guide*, A. Hopperus Buma, Ed., Springer, London, UK, 2nd edition, 2009.

[49] A. Shaw and S. Shaw, "The psychosocial effect of a community-wide disaster on children: planning for terrorism," in *Bioterrorism—Psychological and Public Health Interventions*, R. Ursano, A. Norwood, and C. Fullerton, Eds., Cambridge University Press, Cambridge, UK, 2004.

[50] G. A. Bonanno, C. R. Brewin, K. Kaniasty, and A. M. La Greca, "Weighing the costs of disaster: consequences, risks, and resilience in individuals, families, and communities," *Psychological Science in the Public Interest, Supplement*, vol. 11, no. 1, pp. 1–49, 2010.

[51] A. C. McFarlane, M. Atchison, and R. Yehuda, "The acute stress response following motor vehicle accidents and its relation to PTSD," *Annals of the New York Academy of Sciences*, vol. 821, pp. 437–441, 1997.

[52] M. Tracy, F. H. Norris, and S. Galea, "Differences in the determinants of posttraumatic stress disorder and depression after a mass traumatic event," *Depression and Anxiety*, vol. 28, no. 8, pp. 666–675, 2011.

[53] J. F. Ikin, M. R. Sim, M. C. Creamer et al., "War-related psychological stressors and risk of psychological disorders in Australian veterans of the 1991 Gulf War," *British Journal of Psychiatry*, vol. 185, pp. 116–126, 2004.

[54] G. Miller, "Who needs psychiatrists?" *Science*, vol. 335, no. 6074, pp. 1294–1298, 2012.

[55] D. F. Forbes, M. Creamer, and D. Wade, "Psychological support and recovery in the aftermath of natural disaster," *International Psychiatry*, vol. 9, no. 1, pp. 15–17, 2012.

[56] R. Williams, J. Bisson, D. Ajdukovic et al., "Guidance for Responding to the Psychsocial and Mental Health Needs of People Affected by Disasters or Major Incidents," http://www.healthplanning.co.uk/principles/.

[57] World Health Organization, "War Trauma Foundation, and World Vision International, Psychological first aid: Guide for field workers," WHO Geneva, Switzerland, 2011.

[58] "Post-Traumatic Stress Disorder (PTSD): The management of PTSD in adults and children in primary and secondary care," www.nice.org.uk/nicemedia/pdf/CG026NICEguideline.pdf.

[59] D. Forbes, V. Lewis, T. Varker et al., "Psychological first aid following Trauma: implementation and evaluation framework for high-risk organizations," *Psychiatry*, vol. 74, no. 3, pp. 224–239, 2011.

[60] M. Marinker, *Constructive Conversations in Health: About Policy and Values*, Radcliffe Publishing, Oxford, UK, 2006.

[61] G. Parker, "Psychological disturbance in Darwin evacuees following cyclone Tracy," *Medical Journal of Australia*, vol. 1, no. 21, pp. 650–652, 1975.

[62] K. J. Tierney and J. D. Goltz, "Emergency response: lessons learned from the Kobe earthquake," *Scientific Commons*, 1997.

[63] B. van der Kolk, "Trauma and memory," in *Traumatic Stress: The Effects of Overwhelming Experience on Mind, Body and Society*, B. van der Kolk, A. C. McFarlane, and L. Weisaeth, Eds., Guilford Press, New York, NY, USA, 1996.

[64] M. L. Meewisse, M. Olff, R. Kleber, N. J. Kitchiner, and B. P. R. Gersons, "The course of mental health disorders after a disaster: predictors and comorbidity," *Journal of Traumatic Stress*, vol. 24, no. 4, pp. 405–413, 2011.

[65] S. E. Perlman, S. Friedman, S. Galea et al., "Short-term and medium-term health effects of 9/11," *The Lancet*, vol. 378, no. 9794, pp. 925–934, 2011.

[66] K. H. Holgersen, C. A. Klöckner, H. Jakob Boe, L. Weisæth, and A. Holen, "Disaster survivors in their third decade: trajectories of initial stress responses and long-term course of mental health," *Journal of Traumatic Stress*, vol. 24, no. 3, pp. 334–341, 2011.

[67] L. I. Sederer, C. B. Lanzara, S. M. Essock, S. A. Donahue, J. L. Stone, and S. Galea, "Lessons learned from the New York State mental health response to the September 11, 2001, attacks," *Psychiatric Services*, vol. 62, no. 9, pp. 1085–1089, 2011.

[68] C. S. North, D. E. Pollio, R. P. Smith et al., "Original research: trauma exposure and posttraumatic stress disorder among employees of New York City companies affected by the september 11, 2001 attacks on the World Trade Center," *Disaster Medicine and Public Health Preparedness*, vol. 5, supplement 2, pp. S205–S213, 2011.

[69] L. E. Thorpe and S. Friedman, "Health consequences of the world trade center disaster: a 10th anniversary perspective," *Journal of the American Medical Association*, vol. 306, no. 10, pp. 1133–1134, 2011.

Symptom Endorsement and Sociodemographic Correlates of Postnatal Distress in Three Low Income Countries

Amanda J. Nguyen, Emily E. Haroz, Tamar Mendelson, and Judith Bass

Department of Mental Health, Johns Hopkins School of Public Health, 624 North Broadway, 8th Floor, Baltimore, MD 21205, USA

Correspondence should be addressed to Amanda J. Nguyen; aparke38@jhu.edu

Academic Editor: Axel Steiger

Background. Maternal mental illness has been implicated in adverse child development outcomes. Factors such as context and culture may influence experiences of maternal distress and explain differences in outcomes across settings. *Methods.* We analyzed baseline data from 5,647 mothers in Ethiopia, India (Andhra Pradesh), and Vietnam participating in an ongoing cohort study (Young Lives) to compare symptom endorsement and sociodemographic correlates of distress. Maternal distress was assessed using the Self-Reporting Questionnaire-20 Items (cutoff: ≥8). Logistic regressions were stratified by sample to identify correlates of distress. *Results.* Symptom endorsement was similar among distressed women, particularly with regard to feeling unhappy (76%, 80%, and 79%). Notable differences were observed in three items assessing Depressive Thoughts, which were most highly endorsed in Ethiopia (49%–56%). Having a child experiencing a life-threatening event was correlated with distress in all three samples. A variety of correlates were unique to only one sample. *Conclusions.* There were multiple similarities but also notable differences across sites in the expression and correlates of maternal distress. Feeling unhappy appears to be a hallmark feature of distress. Correlates highlight the relationship between distress and indicators of poverty, child wellbeing, and economic shocks. Differences demonstrate the value of further exploration of cross-cultural differences.

1. Background

Depressive and anxiety disorders are a leading contributor to global disability, accounting for more than half of the total neuropsychiatric burden of disease [1]. These disorders present a higher burden among women than men with particular implications for women of childbearing age, for whom depression is the number one cause of disease burden in both high and low resource settings [2]. A systematic review of studies from low and middle income countries (LMIC) reported a weighted mean depression prevalence of 19.8% in the postnatal period, indicating that the burden may be higher in low resource as compared with high-resource settings [3]. Additionally, studies suggest women may be at higher risk for anxiety disorders during the perinatal period [4]. Although less research has focused on perinatal anxiety or broader categories of distress, focusing on depression alone is problematic because symptoms of depression and anxiety often cooccur [5, 6]. Therefore, in the present study we examine a broader construct of maternal distress, defined as elevated depressive, anxious, and somatic symptoms within the perinatal period. These mental health problems cause significant role impairment and have been implicated in a range of negative child development outcomes [7–9] such as problems related to infant growth and cognitive development [10, 11], greater number of diarrheal episodes and poorer adherence with recommended immunization schedules [12], and heightened risk of insecure attachment and child behavioral problems [5, 13].

Culture can influence the expression of distress and other mental health problems and must be considered when studying mental health cross-culturally [14]. There is growing recognition that symptom presentation of common mental disorders may vary across individuals and groups, which results in diverse clinical presentations and potential for different risk factors and responses to treatment [15–19]. For example, findings that appetite changes are not reliably associated with perinatal depression [20] and that sadness presents as less of a core feature in late life depression [21] suggest improved accuracy of the identification of these types of problems among various subgroups. The prevalence of specific depressive and anxiety symptoms has also been shown to vary across cultures [16, 22, 23], and in certain populations standardized screening instruments have been found to be less informative than indigenous measures for capturing common mental health problems [24, 25]. Likewise, researchers have examined the impacts of potential cultural differences in somatization on depression case finding and outcomes [26–28]. However, exploration of culture's impact on more general maternal distress has been underexplored in the literature to date.

A number of social and demographic factors have also been found to vary by context in their association with increased risk for maternal common mental disorders (CMD) in LMIC [3, 7]. Fisher et al. [3] identified 47 studies across 17 countries on depression either during pregnancy or in the year following birth. Reported risk factors included social and economic circumstances (poverty, economic hardship, young age, being an ethnic minority, and being unmarried), family and relationship stressors (intimate partner problems, family conflict, low social support, and having many children), pregnancy factors (unwanted or unintended pregnancy, poor maternal health during pregnancy, pregnancy complications, and past abortion or stillbirth), and child factors (having an infant with health problems, prolonged infant crying, experiencing the death of a child, and having a female child in certain cultures). Higher education, having employment, being in the ethnic majority, and receiving postpartum care were identified as protective factors.

The current study explores the experience of clinically significant levels of maternal distress symptoms across three LMIC settings, Ethiopia, India (Andhra Pradesh), and Vietnam. These settings share challenges common to low income countries, such as high poverty and susceptibility to natural disasters, but also represent diverse cultural and sociodemographic perspectives. Ethiopia is an ethnically and linguistically diverse country where, in addition to the predominant Christian and Muslim religions, many people simultaneously adhere to indigenous belief systems [29, 30]. India, a majority Hindu country with Muslim and Christian minorities, has historically been characterized by a caste system that has influenced social norms and access to resources [31]. The people of Vietnam are predominantly Kinh ethnicity, with many small ethnic minority groups [29]. Family, education, and social structures in Vietnam have been influenced by the "three teachings" of Confucianism, Taoism, and Buddhism; a majority of the Vietnamese also report participating in ancestor worship [30]. With respect to sociodemographic indicators, in 2002 at the time of baseline data collection, the three countries differed in their levels of disadvantage, with Vietnam ranked highest in the United Nations Development Program (UNDP) Human Development Index (109) relative to India (124) and Ethiopia (168) [32]. Consistent with these rankings, Vietnam was characterized by longer life expectancy and higher rates of adult literacy and secondary school enrollment than the other two countries, with India ranking below Vietnam and Ethiopia reporting the poorest outcomes of the three countries in these domains [32]. The aims of this paper were to (1) compare endorsement of specific symptoms by mothers meeting criteria for maternal distress in these three settings and (2) evaluate the consistency of associations between maternal distress and recognized risk factors. These aims were exploratory, as the literature does not suggest clear predictions regarding how cultural and contextual differences across our samples will affect expression and correlates of maternal distress.

2. Methods

This cross-sectional, secondary analysis uses baseline data collected in Ethiopia, India (Andhra Pradesh), and Vietnam in 2002 as part of Young Lives (YL), an ongoing, longitudinal study of childhood poverty [33, 34]. Although YL is also following a Peruvian cohort, Peru was not included in this study as the mental health symptom-level data are not publicly available. The countries were selected for inclusion in the Young Lives study to reflect a diversity of experiences in LMIC [33]. At the time when baseline data were collected, Ethiopia was in the midst of a famine, was slipping back on progress made toward millennium development goals, and had high mortality, adult illiteracy, and child malnutrition. India was showing mixed progress toward development goals and also had high adult illiteracy and child malnutrition. By contrast, Vietnam had relatively lower levels of mortality, child malnutrition, and adult illiteracy [32]. This breadth of experience allows for an exploration of how context may affect experiences of maternal distress.

Data were collected in each country on approximately 2000 mothers of infant children using sentinel site surveillance. Detailed sampling methods and rationale have been described elsewhere [35]. Briefly, local experts identified 20 sites in each country to represent a range of geographic and socioeconomic environments, with oversampling of high poverty areas. For each site, lists of households with a child aged 6–18 months were compiled by observation and door-to-door surveys. One hundred index children and their caregivers were randomly sampled from each site to participate in the study.

The study team has published a detailed methods guide regarding research ethics and procedures [36]. Interviewers in all four sites were trained using a standard interviewer handbook (available at the UK Data Service [34]) that addressed ethics and consent, enrollment and interviewing procedures, and instructions for completion of each section of the common questionnaire. Training included role plays and practice sessions aimed at measuring the same items across the samples, while interviewer feedback during training was used to improve local translations [36]. Pilot studies were carried out in each country to evaluate the suitability of the questionnaire [37], and all interviews were completed in the local language of the primary caregiver. Informed consent was obtained for all adult participants, and the baseline survey obtained a response rate of over 90% in each of the three countries [37]. Ethical approval for the Young Lives study was granted by London School of Hygiene and Tropical Medicine [38]. While there were no exclusion criteria for the original data collection, this analysis excludes primary caregivers other than the biological mother ($n = 108$) and those missing mental health data (n = 255), resulting in 5647 cases: n = 1906, 1886, and 1855 in Ethiopia, Andhra Pradesh, and Vietnam, respectively.

2.1. Maternal Distress Caseness and Symptoms. A case of probable clinically relevant maternal distress was classified by the YL team using the Self-Reporting Questionnaire-20 Items (SRQ-20), a brief screening and case-finding (i.e., nondiagnostic) scale recommended by the World Health Organization for application in LMIC [39]. The SRQ-20 consists of 20 yes/no questions (no = 0; yes = 1) regarding somatic, depressive/anxious, and cognitive/energy symptoms experienced in the past 30 days (see Figure 1 x-axis for a list of all symptoms), summed to create a scale score ranging from 0 to 20 with higher scores indicating greater severity [40]. The scale has been translated and validated across several LMIC with sensitivity and specificity for psychiatric problems (as assessed in diagnostic interviews) ranging from 63 to 90% and 44 to 95%, respectively [39]. In India, cutoff scores of both 6 [41] and 8 or higher [42] have previously been used, although a more recent study reported an optimal cutoff of 12 or 13 among primary care attendees [43]. Early Ethiopian work identified optimal cutoffs of 8 or higher among clinic attendees and 5 or higher among nonclinic attendees [44], while a recent study using the SRQ specifically with perinatal women reported cutoffs of 3 or 7 and higher but noted study limitations in the ability to identify an optimal cutoff [45]. As the SRQ had not previously been validated in Vietnam, the English instrument was translated, back-translated, and validated with an optimal cutoff of 8 or higher [46]. Although the most efficient cutoff for determining caseness may vary by setting, a review of validation studies shows that a commonly used cut point is ≥ 8 for identifying a probable clinically significant case of maternal distress [40]. The YL dataset includes a binary case variable classifying women with probable distress by SRQ-20 scores below versus at or above 8 [37]. We also used the 20 symptom items to examine symptom endorsement among these samples.

2.2. Sociodemographic Correlates of Maternal Distress. Potential correlates of maternal distress were selected for analysis based on identification in prior research [3] and are listed in Table 1. Maternal factors include maternal age (in years), marital status, education level, and participation in livelihoods activities. Marital status was reported as married, single, divorced, or widowed but was recoded as binary (married/not married) for analysis due to low numbers of nonmarried women. Maternal education was defined on the basis of completion of primary school (yes/no). For livelihood, mothers reported the number of economic activities they participated in during the prior 12 months; this was coded as none (0), one (1), and two or more (2). Disability status was explored but excluded from the final analysis because the low number of disabled mothers precluded meaningful comparisons. Time lived in the community was also initially considered but excluded as it made no significant contribution to variance in the outcome across any of the three countries and was not supported by prior literature.

Table 1: Potential maternal distress correlates considered in analysis.

Maternal	Pregnancy/child	Household
Age	Unwanted pregnancy	Wealth index
Marital status	Antenatal care[2]	Urban/rural setting
Education	Child age	Economic shock
Disability status[1]	Child sex	More than 3 children
Livelihood activities	Long-term health problem	Death of a child
Cognitive social capital	Life-threatening incident	
Group membership	Birth weight[1]	
Social support[2]		
Citizenship activities[2]		
Years lived in community[2]		

[1]Excluded from initial multiple regression models.
[2]Excluded from final models after stepwise deletion.

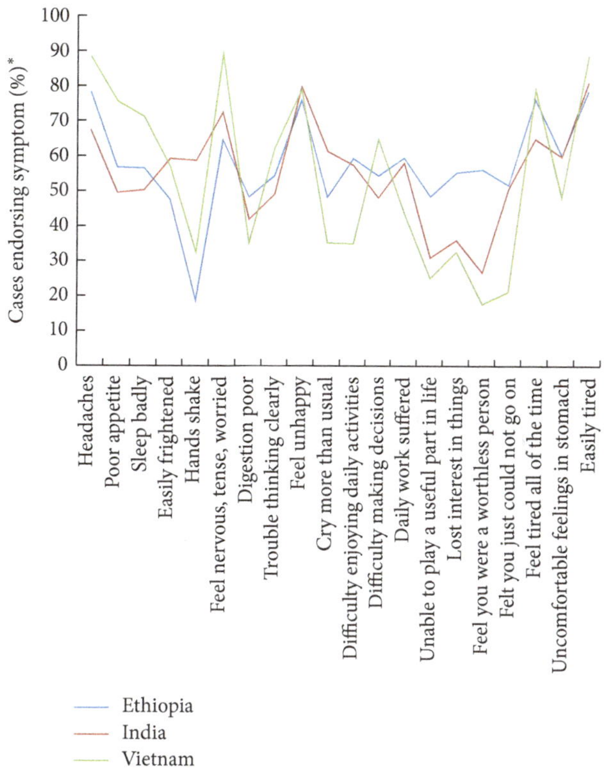

*Based on the number of respondents for each symptom, ranging from 93.8% (unable to play a useful part in life) to 99.4% (headaches)

Figure 1: Prevalence of SRQ-20 symptom endorsement* in those identified as probable maternal CMD cases, by country.

In addition to child age (months) and sex, pregnancy and child factors included whether or not the mother wanted the pregnancy (yes/no) and the child has a long-term health problem (recorded as the presence or absence of a long-term health problem) or has experienced a life-threatening event (recorded as whether or not the child had experienced a serious illness or injury where the mother believed the child might die). Birth weight was considered for inclusion but excluded due to missing data in approximately 50% of observations. Whether the mother had received antenatal care (none = 0; any = 1) was also explored but excluded from the final models due to lack of significant associations.

Household factors included community setting (urban/rural), number of children (dichotomized at 1–3 versus more than 3), having ever experienced the death of a child (yes/no), a household wealth index, and recent economic shocks. Household wealth index was a composite variable calculated by the YL team from a number of housing, consumption, and service factors, producing a continuous score ranging from 0 (lowest wealth) to 1 (highest wealth). Economic shocks were measured using a list of events the mother may have experienced since being pregnant with the index child, which negatively impacted household welfare (e.g., natural disaster, job loss, failed crops, severe illness or injury, migration, family death, and new educational expenses). These experiences were categorized as a binary variable indicating whether the household had experienced an economic shock (yes/no).

In light of previous research into the role of social capital in these same samples [47], a number of social capital variables (group membership, social support, citizenship, and cognitive social capital) were also considered. Group membership quantified the number of organizations the mother was a part of, analyzed as 0, 1-2, and 3 or more groups. Cognitive social capital (CSC) was a composite variable evaluating the mother's sense of community belonging, trust, and positive perception of others, analyzed as a low/medium (0) and high (1) CSC. Social support (the number of group, individual, and organizational sources from which the mother received social support in the past year, analyzed as 0, 1–4, and 5 or more sources) and citizenship activities (a binary none/some record of the mother's activities to join others in her community to enact change) were not included in the final models due to lack of significant contribution to variance.

2.3. Statistical Analysis. The analysis of individual symptom prevalence within the subset of those identified as probable cases (i.e., those with SRQ-20 scores at or above 8) was calculated by country using cross-tabulation. Chi-square analyses were used to evaluate differences in symptom prevalence across countries. Missing data were excluded for the symptom analysis, so that the proportion of endorsement for all symptoms was calculated based on the number of responses to each question rather than the total number of cases. The missingness of symptom responses ranged from 2.5% (unable to play a useful part in life) to 0% (sleep badly) in Ethiopia, 13.3% (unable to play a useful part in life) to 0.8% (headaches) in Andhra Pradesh, and 6.6% (lost interest in things) to 0.3% (uncomfortable feelings in stomach) in Vietnam.

Analyses of potential correlates of distress caseness were conducted separately for each of the three countries. Univariate associations were explored using simple logistic regression. With the exception of birth weight and maternal disability, all variables were entered into a multiple linear regression model to test for collinearity using variable inflation factors (VIFs), which produced mean VIFs of 1.44, 1.26, and 1.34 for Ethiopia, Andhra Pradesh, and Vietnam, respectively, with no VIF greater than 3 indicating minimal collinearity. The multiple logistic regression models were further evaluated by stepwise removal of nonsignificant variables including years lived in the community, antenatal care, citizenship activities, and social support. All variables retained after stepwise removal for any of the three countries were included in the final multiple logistic regression models for all three countries to enable cross-country comparisons. Maternal age, child age, and child sex were included regardless of their level of association with the outcome because of their recognized relevance to maternal mental distress. Population average estimates were derived using generalized estimating equations (GEE) with robust standard errors to account for clustered sampling, which explained 3%, 22%, and 10% of the variance in Ethiopia, Andhra Pradesh, and Vietnam, respectively. The amount of correlate missing data was limited. With the exception of the social support variable, which was missing 18% total (52% in Ethiopia), all included variables had missingness of less than 5%. Multiple imputation using chained equations [48] was used to provide appropriate standard errors to account for missing data.

3. Results

Demographic characteristics of each of the three study populations are presented in Table 2. All three samples represent women with average age in the mid-20s (mean ranging from 24 to 27 by country) approximately 1 year since childbirth, reporting low to moderate household wealth (mean wealth index 0.21–0.44), with a considerable length of time lived (means of 9–17 years) in predominantly rural (66–80%) communities. There were statistically significant differences in proportion of the Ethiopian, Indian, and Vietnamese samples, respectively, in terms of completing primary education (21, 40, and 73%), participating in multiple economic activities (13, 19, and 71%), and experiencing economic shocks (70, 44, and 42%). There were also significant differences in proportion of unwanted pregnancies (37, 8, and 17%), lack of antenatal care (52, 11, and 24%), and death of a child (26, 11, and 6%). Based on the cutoff score on the SRQ-20 of at least 8 symptoms, prevalence of probable clinically significant maternal distress was 33% in Ethiopia, 30% in Andhra Pradesh, and 21% in Vietnam, as previously reported in Harpham et al. [37].

3.1. Symptom Endorsement. Mothers identified as probable cases endorsed an average of 11.4 (SD = 2.8) symptoms in Ethiopia, which was slightly higher than the 10.7 (SD = 2.3) in Andhra Pradesh and 10.6 (SD = 2.6) in Vietnam ($p < 0.001$). Mothers who were identified as *not* probable cases endorsed an average of 3.1 (SD = 2.2) symptoms in Ethiopia and 3.2 (SD = 2.1) in Andhra Pradesh, slightly higher than the 2.6 (SD = 2.2) in Vietnam ($p < 0.001$).

Figure 1 displays the prevalence for endorsing each symptom among probable cases by country. In Ethiopia, over three-quarters of cases reported being easily tired, having

TABLE 2: Sample demographics by country.

	Ethiopia (n = 1906)	India (n = 1886)	Vietnam (n = 1855)	p value*
Household wealth index (mean, SD)	0.21 (.17)	0.41 (.20)	0.44 (2.23)	<0.001
Maternal age in years (mean, SD)	27.4 (6.3)	23.7 (4.3)	27.2 (5.8)	<0.001
Years lived in community (mean, SD)	15.5 (10.6)	9.1 (7.7)	17.4 (11.2)	<0.001
Age of child in months (mean, SD)	11.6 (3.6)	11.7 (3.5)	11.6 (3.2)	0.122
Number of children (mean, SD)	3.6 (2.4)	2.0 (1.2)	1.9 (1.2)	<0.001
Index child is female (%)	47.01	45.92	48.41	0.310
Marital status (%)				<0.001
Married	86.62	99.42	97.68	
Divorced	7.92	0.32	1.08	
Single	3.52	0.11	1.02	
Widowed	1.94	0.16	0.22	
Urban setting (%)	33.95	25.5	19.95	<0.001
Education level (%)				<0.001
Completed primary	21.14	40.40	72.83	
Did not complete primary	73.19	59.49	27.17	
Livelihood activities in past year (%)				<0.001
None	42.81	50.37	6.74	
One	43.70	30.65	22.16	
Two or more	13.48	18.98	71.11	
Unwanted pregnancy (%)	37.15	8.01	17.20	<0.001
Experienced economic shock (%)	70.41	43.80	42.37	<0.001
Child life-threatening incident (%)	30.43	22.59	12.88	<0.001
Child long-term health problem (%)	10.02	4.40	4.26	<0.001
Death of a child (%)	26.50	11.13	5.82	<0.001
Group membership (%)				<0.001
Low (0)	23.03	70.78	73.26	
Medium (1-2)	55.93	28.58	24.69	
High (3 or more)	12.01	0.32	2.05	
Cognitive social capital (%)				<0.001
Low/medium	11.23	5.14	9.38	
High	87.46	92.52	90.40	
% meeting distress criteria (i.e., ≥8 symptoms)	33.0	30.1	21.2	<0.001

*Comparisons using chi-square for categorical variables, ANOVA for continuous variables.

headaches, feeling tired all the time, and feeling unhappy (78.6, 78.3, 76.3, and 76%, resp.), while shaking hand was the least reported symptom (18.7%). In Andhra Pradesh, the most common symptoms were being easily tired and feeling unhappy (81.2 and 79.9%), whereas only a quarter of cases reported feeling like they were a worthless person (26.8%). In Vietnam, six symptoms were reported by over three-quarters of cases, feeling nervous, being easily tired, headaches, being tired all the time, being unhappy, and poor appetite (89.2, 88.9, 88.5, 79.2, 79.1, and 75.5%), while a quarter or less reported feeling worthless, feeling you just could not go on, and being unable to play a useful part in life (17.8, 21.2, and 25.1%).

Chi-square tests indicated statistically significant differences between endorsement prevalence among probable cases by country for 19 of the 20 questions at $p \leq 0.001$; variation in a subset of symptoms appeared to be particularly visible. On three items, Vietnam differed markedly from Ethiopia and Andhra Pradesh, respectively; these included higher reporting of poor appetite (75.5%, compared to 56.8% and 49.6%), lower endorsement of feeling one could not go on (21.2%, compared to 51.8% and 50.7%), and less difficulty enjoying daily activities (35%, compared to 59.4% and 57.5%). There were also three symptoms in which the symptom prevalence in Ethiopia was notably higher relative to Andhra Pradesh and Vietnam, respectively. These included feeling unable to play a useful part in life (48.6%, compared to 31% and 25%), loss of interest in things (55.3% compared to 36.1% or 32.6%), and feeling worthless (56.2% relative to 26.8% and 17.8%). Shaking hands also appeared to be relatively uncommon in Ethiopia (18.7%) compared to Andhra Pradesh (58.8%). One item, "Do you feel unhappy?," produced similar endorsement levels (76–80%, X^2 = 2.87, p = 0.238) in all three countries.

Table 3: Correlates of maternal distress.

	Ethiopia		Andhra Pradesh		Vietnam	
	OR	95% CI	OR	95% CI	OR	95% CI
Maternal age (years)	1.01	[0.99, 1.03]	1.03*	[1.00, 1.06]	1.00	[0.97, 1.03]
Child age (months)	1.00	[0.97, 1.04]	1.01	[0.98, 1.04]	1.01	[0.98, 1.05]
Female (versus male) child	0.94	[0.77, 1.15]	0.83	[0.70, 1.00]	0.96	[0.82, 1.13]
Household wealth index	0.47	[0.10, 2.11]	0.15**	[0.07, 0.34]	0.12**	[0.06, 0.23]
Urban (versus rural) setting	1.73*	[1.00, 2.98]	1.56	[0.50, 4.89]	2.82**	[1.71, 4.64]
No partner (versus having partner)	1.32	[0.99, 1.74]	2.29	[0.90, 5.79]	3.52**	[1.98, 6.24]
Low (versus more than primary) education	1.15	[0.79, 1.69]	1.23	[1.00, 1.51]	1.04	[0.82, 1.33]
Unwanted (versus wanted) pregnancy	1.92**	[1.62, 2.27]	1.07	[0.61, 1.88]	0.81	[0.55, 1.20]
Having > 3 (versus 1–3) children	1.40*	[1.08, 1.81]	1.06	[0.60, 1.89]	1.18	[0.82, 1.69]
Experiencing an economic shock (versus not)	1.96**	[1.43, 2.69]	1.29	[0.97, 1.73]	2.34**	[1.73, 3.16]
Child life-threatening incident (versus not)	1.86**	[1.51, 2.28]	1.43**	[1.16, 1.77]	1.60**	[1.17, 2.19]
Child long-term health problem (versus not)	1.46	[0.99, 2.16]	2.15**	[1.50, 3.09]	3.72**	[2.31, 6.01]
Death of a child (versus not)	1.12	[0.87, 1.43]	1.11	[0.82, 1.51]	1.73**	[1.16, 2.57]
Maternal livelihood activities (ref: none)						
One	1.02	[0.77, 1.35]	1.11	[0.83, 1.50]	0.65**	[0.48, 0.86]
Two or more	1.37	[0.94, 1.98]	1.17	[0.80, 1.70]	0.58**	[0.42, 0.79]
Maternal group membership (ref: low)						
Med	0.94	[0.70, 1.24]	1.16	[0.95, 1.42]	1.32*	[1.00, 1.74]
High	1.72*	[1.11, 2.68]	0.61	[0.11, 3.40]	1.18	[0.59, 2.38]
High (versus low/medium) CSC	0.57*	[0.37, 0.89]	0.67	[0.42, 1.07]	0.48**	[0.36, 0.64]

*$p < 0.05$.
**$p < 0.01$.
Population averages from multiple logistic regression using GEE estimation with robust standard errors.

3.2. Sociodemographic Correlates. Table 3 presents the relative odds of maternal distress with 95% confidence intervals for each of the correlates of interest. In Ethiopia, having an unwanted pregnancy (OR = 1.92, $p < 0.001$), having more than three children (OR = 1.40, $p = 0.010$), experiencing an economic shock (OR = 1.96, $p < 0.001$), the index child having a life-threatening health event (OR = 1.86, $p < 0.001$), and having high (relative to low) group membership (OR = 1.72, $p = 0.015$) were all associated with increased odds of poor mental health. However, having high (relative to low/medium) cognitive social capital (OR = 0.57, $p = 0.013$) was associated with decreased odds of poor mental health. Marginally significant results included living in urban settings (OR = 1.73, $p = 0.049$), having no partner (1.32, $p = 0.054$), and having a child with a long-term health problem (OR = 1.46, $p = 0.054$).

In Andhra Pradesh, increasing maternal age (OR = 1.03, $p = 0.034$) and the index child experiencing a life-threatening event (OR = 1.43, $p = 0.001$) or having a long-term health problem (OR = 2.15, $p < 0.001$) were all associated with increased odds of poor mental health. However, higher household wealth (OR = 0.15, $p < 0.001$) was associated with decreased odds of poor mental health. Marginally significant findings were found for low maternal education (OR = 1.23, $p = 0.050$) and having a female index child (OR = 0.83, $p = 0.052$).

In Vietnam, being unmarried (OR = 3.52, $p < 0.001$), living in an urban setting (OR = 2.82, $p < 0.001$), experiencing an economic shock (OR = 2.34, $p < 0.001$), the index child having a life-threatening event (OR = 1.60, $p = 0.003$) or long-term health condition (OR = 3.72, $p < 0.001$), and having experienced the death of a child (OR = 1.72, $p = 0.007$) were associated with higher odds of maternal distress. However, higher household wealth (OR = 0.12, $p < 0.001$), participating in *any* livelihood activities (one: OR = 0.65, $p = 0.003$; two or more: OR = 0.58, $p = 0.001$), and having high cognitive social capital (OR = 0.48, $p < 0.001$) were all associated with lower odds of maternal distress. Marginally significant findings were found for being involved in a medium (relative to low) number of groups (OR = 1.32, $p = 0.048$).

4. Discussion

The current study assessed symptom endorsement by mothers meeting criteria for maternal distress and evaluated the consistency of associations between maternal distress and recognized risk factors across three LMIC settings. We identified similar patterns of symptom prevalence across the three countries. In particular, there was high and consistent reporting of feeling unhappy among probable cases of maternal distress across all three samples. While the overall similarity between countries was striking, noteworthy exceptions regarding symptom endorsement, including higher reporting of cognitive symptoms in Ethiopia and higher reporting of low energy and somatic complaints in Vietnam, were also observed.

With regard to associated risk factors, negative life events and the index child experiencing either a life-threatening event or long-term health problem were consistently associated with increased odds of distress across all three samples. The reporting of unhappiness, a hallmark feature of depression, across the three settings is consistent with major cross-national studies reporting that as many as three-quarters of respondents report sadness as a symptom of depression [49–51]. Clinically, sadness in people not currently meeting criteria for depression has been shown in the US to be an important predictor of depressive disorder onset within the following year and is critical for preventive screening [52]. The stability of this symptom in the study samples suggests the potential for similar predictive utility in these settings, although with only cross-sectional data the relative risk of onset in these samples could not be assessed.

Variation in symptom prevalence rates was identified for the items assessing the mother's feelings of utility, interest in things, and feelings of worthlessness—three items which have previously been found to load onto a single "Depressive Thoughts" factor [53]. The Ethiopian sample endorsed all three of these symptoms at higher rates than the samples from Andhra Pradesh and Vietnam. Previous qualitative research among Ethiopians has suggested that cognitive features may be viewed as *causes* of distress, with symptoms manifesting as physical complaints in the head, heart, and stomach [54]. Vietnamese women were less likely to endorse these cognitive symptoms but reported high rates for being easily tired and tired all the time, as well as having headaches and poor appetites, which have previously been shown to load on "Decreased Energy" and "Somatic" factors [53]. This conforms with clinical suggestions that low energy and sleep problems can highlight depressive moods among southeast Asian women [55]. These differences may illustrate ways in which culture influences the local expression of maternal distress and presents potential areas for further research in treatment adaptations and developing better screening tools that identify women for services as well as providing an avenue for further exploration as to how these may interact with child health outcomes. For example, perhaps mental distress expressed in terms of low energy and health complaints may involve more functional impairment than cognitive expressions, which may in turn have more adverse effects on children's healthy development.

We identified both common and distinct correlates of maternal distress across the three study samples. As previously mentioned, the most consistent findings related to negative life events and the index child experiencing a life-threatening event or long-term health problem. These factors were associated with increased odds of distress in all three settings. Higher levels of group membership also displayed a trend toward increased odds of distress across samples, which replicates a previous finding in this same sample [47] and has also been observed elsewhere [56]. As these data are cross-sectional, the causal relationship between group membership and maternal distress is unclear. Noting that support from groups was measured separately from group membership, however, one could potentially conclude that group membership itself does not offer support and may present an additional stressor for mothers. It is also noteworthy that social support itself did not explain additional variance in outcomes and was excluded from the final adjusted models; this may have been due to the higher percentage of missing data in this variable, rather than a true lack of association.

Higher wealth and cognitive social capital were generally associated with lower odds of maternal distress, consistent with prior literature [57, 58]. The higher odds of distress associated with maternal age in Andhra Pradesh were somewhat unexpected, as the women represented a rather homogenously aged group of women averaging in the mid-20s; the increased odds were minimal and may have been found by chance. Maternal distress was not associated with child age (within the range of 6–18 months), consistent with prior findings that maternal depression stabilizes after the first six months after childbirth [59]. Failure to replicate prior research findings of associations for marital status and cognitive social capital in the Indian sample is likely due to the minimal variation across these characteristics in that sample. This raises some question as to whether these factors are truly less prevalent in the population of poor mothers in Andhra Pradesh or whether the process of sentinel site surveillance does not fully represent the source population of poor mothers in that region. Likewise, the lack of association between maternal distress and wealth in Ethiopia may reflect the higher poverty level in this group as a whole rather than a true absence of impact.

A number of associations also emerged that were unique to each setting. Exclusive to Ethiopia, both having an unwanted pregnancy and having more than three children elevated risk for maternal mental distress. Unique to Andhra Pradesh, child sex (female) was marginally protective, although this runs counter to prior findings of increased risk of maternal distress associated with female children in the Indian context [60]. Vietnam was the only setting in which experiencing the death of a child remained significantly associated with mental distress after adjusting for all other factors, and having a child with a long-term health problem—while trending toward higher odds in all countries—was the strongest predictor of increased odds of mental distress in Vietnam. Lastly, participation in livelihood activities appeared to be differentially associated depending on context: in both Andhra Pradesh and Ethiopia, two or more livelihood activities in the past year trended toward increased odds of distress, whereas *any* livelihood activities in Vietnam were associated with significantly *decreased* odds of distress.

These unique results support the hypothesis that it is not absolute poverty but relative deprivation and its associated adversities within a context that may take the greatest toll on maternal mental health [58, 61]. The distressed women in Ethiopia appear to live in an environment in which poor women with low education are disempowered to make decisions about reproductive health and healthcare for themselves and their families; the result may be that large families place particular strain maternal resources. The context in India, with the lowest proportion of unplanned pregnancies, highest utilization of antenatal care, and over 99% of women in the sample married, suggests that when women have greater control over their reproductive health, economic factors such as wealth, livelihoods, and economic shocks may be more dominant influences on their wellbeing. And in Vietnam, where more women were completing basic education and participating in livelihoods, child wellbeing appears to be the domain most associated with maternal mental health. The direction of causality is unclear, but as prior literature has also documented high levels of distress among Vietnamese mothers of children with disabilities [62], it is possible that this finding reflects an impact of poor child health on maternal distress. These are all hypotheses as to the different mechanisms influencing maternal distress across these contexts, which deserve further empirical evaluation. The findings on the correlates of maternal distress should be interpreted within the historical context. As YL baseline data were collected in 2002, the relevance of identified correlates may be different for women today based on recent social and cultural developments.

One promising direction for future research involves evaluation of potential associations of maternal distress expression and correlates with child health outcomes and, in particular, how these associations may vary across settings. For example, in a four-country analysis of the YL data, Harpham et al. [37] report associations between maternal common mental disorders (CMD) and child nutritional status in India and Vietnam, but not in Peru and Ethiopia. Medhin et al. [63] also reported no significant associations between common mental disorders and child health in Ethiopia, whereas Hadley et al. [64] found strong associations in the same country. Data are still being collected on women in the YL study; thus, future studies can build on the current analysis to examine how variation in symptom prevalence and correlates may be predictive of longitudinal health and wellbeing outcomes for both the mother and child.

4.1. Limitations. Although the procedures of the Young Lives data collection included translation and pilot testing, the standardized YL instrument did not include potentially relevant local idioms of distress; as a result, we may have missed capturing culturally specific symptoms of distress in the three settings. Also, for these specific populations of postpartum women, the cut point of 8 or more symptoms was only explicitly validated in the Vietnam sample [46]. It is probable that some misclassification of maternal distress cases occurred, which is likely to have attenuated the strength of the observed associations.

Additionally, oversampling for women living in poverty may have produced homogenous samples not reflective of the wider experience of mothers in these three countries, such that findings are likely not generalizable to the populations of postnatal women in each country, particularly in India, where the sample was drawn from only one region of the country. It was also difficult to explore certain correlates due to small sample sizes; for example, evaluating the experiences of widowed, divorced, or never married women separately was not possible given the infrequency with which these categories were reported. The cross-sectional nature of this study also precludes inference regarding cause and effect; future studies should examine these associations across time. The analysis also did not include factors such as disability status, paternal characteristics, and intimate partner relationship stressors, which have previously been shown to be associated with maternal distress [3] and which, if included, may have impacted the adjusted estimates. Finally, due to multiple testing some observed associations may have been found by chance; given the exploratory nature of the analysis, future research to replicate these findings is warranted.

5. Conclusions

A strength of this study is identification of common and distinct mental health experiences of poor mothers across three diverse settings in which postnatal distress is common and has been differentially associated with negative early child health indicators. This study supports the recognized association between poverty and maternal mental distress in LMIC settings. This cycle is particularly concerning due to the potential long-term negative impact on child health of psychologically distressed mothers. Distressed mothers are less able to care for themselves and their children or to leverage social supports to do so. At the same time, the stress of mothering a child with poor health can also increase the risk of maternal distress. A 15-year longitudinal study of childhood poverty in Ethiopia, Andhra Pradesh, Peru, and Vietnam is exploring questions of this nature. Baseline data indicated the association between these factors may be mediated by the culture in which the women live [37]. The current analysis supports this conclusion.

This study identified country-specific and unique patterns of symptom prevalence and sociodemographic correlates in the Ethiopia, Andhra Pradesh, and Vietnam samples. These results contribute to the literature on maternal mental health by identifying similarities and differences in symptom presentation with implications for clinical practice, as well as potential areas of divergence in the experience of maternal distress across LMIC contexts. Findings suggest that "feeling unhappy" is a consistent experience of maternal distress across cultures and may be leveraged for early screening and prevention. However, variation in symptom prevalence rates between settings was also notable. These findings highlight the value of further exploration of potential cross-cultural differences in experiences of maternal mental distress.

Abbreviations

YLD: Years lost due to disability
LMIC: Low and middle income country
UNDP: United Nations Development Program
CMD: Common mental disorders
SRQ-20: Self-Reporting Questionnaire-20 Items.

Disclaimer

The views expressed here are those of the authors. They are not necessarily those of Young Lives, the University of Oxford, DFID, or other funders.

Conflict of Interests

The authors declare they have no conflict of interests.

Authors' Contribution

Amanda J. Nguyen obtained the data, developed the study concept and design, performed the analysis, and drafted the paper. Emily E. Haroz helped to draft the paper and consulted on study design and analysis. Tamar Mendelson helped draft the paper. Judith Bass oversaw the conception and design of the study, consulted on the analysis, and helped to draft the paper. All authors read and approved the final paper.

Acknowledgments

Amanda J. Nguyen was supported by training Grant T32MH019545 from the National Institute of Mental Health. Emily E. Haroz was supported by training Grant T32MH103210 from the National Institute of Mental Health. Tamar Mendelson and Judith Bass are funded through a variety of grants and contracts. The data used in this paper come from Young Lives, a 15-year study of the changing nature of childhood poverty in Ethiopia, India (Andhra Pradesh), Peru, and Vietnam (http://www.younglives.org.uk/). Young Lives is funded by UK aid from the Department for International Development (DFID) and cofunded from 2010 to 2014 by the Netherlands Ministry of Foreign Affairs.

References

[1] H. A. Whiteford, L. Degenhardt, J. Rehm et al., "Global burden of disease attributable to mental and substance use disorders: findings from the Global Burden of Disease Study 2010," *The Lancet*, vol. 382, no. 9904, pp. 1575–1586, 2013.

[2] WHO, *The Global Burden of Disease: 2004 Update*, World Health Organization, Geneva, Switzerland, 2008.

[3] J. Fisher, M. C. de Mello, V. Patel et al., "Prevalence and determinants of common perinatal mental disorders in women in low- and lower-middle-income countries: a systematic review," *Bulletin of the World Health Organization*, vol. 90, no. 2, pp. 139G–149G, 2012.

[4] L. E. Ross and L. M. McLean, "Anxiety disorders during pregnancy and the postpartum period: a systematic review," *Journal of Clinical Psychiatry*, vol. 67, no. 8, pp. 1285–1298, 2006.

[5] C. Glasheen, G. A. Richardson, and A. Fabio, "A systematic review of the effects of postnatal maternal anxiety on children," *Archives of Women's Mental Health*, vol. 13, no. 1, pp. 61–74, 2010.

[6] F. Lamers, P. van Oppen, H. C. Comijs et al., "Comorbidity patterns of anxiety and depressive disorders in a large cohort study: the Netherlands Study of Depression and Anxiety (NESDA)," *Journal of Clinical Psychiatry*, vol. 72, no. 3, pp. 342–348, 2011.

[7] T. D. Wachs, M. M. Black, and P. L. Engle, "Maternal depression: a global threat to children's health, development, and behavior and to human rights," *Child Development Perspectives*, vol. 3, no. 1, pp. 51–59, 2009.

[8] N. M. Talge, C. Neal, and V. Glover, "Antenatal maternal stress and long-term effects on child neurodevelopment: how and why?" *Journal of Child Psychology and Psychiatry*, vol. 48, no. 3-4, pp. 245–261, 2007.

[9] B. R. H. Van den Bergh, E. J. H. Mulder, M. Mennes, and V. Glover, "Antenatal maternal anxiety and stress and the neurobehavioural development of the fetus and child: links and possible mechanisms. A review," *Neuroscience and Biobehavioral Reviews*, vol. 29, no. 2, pp. 237–258, 2005.

[10] J. Petzoldt, H.-U. Wittchen, F. Einsle, and J. Martini, "Maternal anxiety versus depressive disorders: specific relations to infants' crying, feeding and sleeping problems," *Child: Care, Health and Development*, 2015.

[11] V. Patel, N. DeSouza, and M. Rodrigues, "Postnatal depression and infant growth and development in low income countries: a cohort study from Goa, India," *Archives of Disease in Childhood*, vol. 88, no. 1, pp. 34–37, 2003.

[12] A. Rahman, Z. Iqbal, J. Bunn, H. Lovel, and R. Harrington, "Impact of maternal depression on infant nutritional status and illness: a cohort study," *Archives of General Psychiatry*, vol. 61, no. 9, pp. 946–952, 2004.

[13] P. J. Cooper and L. Murray, "Fortnightly review. Postnatal depression," *The British Medical Journal*, vol. 316, no. 7148, pp. 1884–1886, 1998.

[14] J. K. Bass, P. A. Bolton, and L. K. Murray, "Do not forget culture when studying mental health," *The Lancet*, vol. 370, no. 9591, pp. 918–919, 2007.

[15] L. J. Kirmayer, "Cultural variations in the clinical presentation of depression and anxiety: implications for diagnosis and treatment," *Journal of Clinical Psychiatry*, vol. 62, supplement 1, pp. 22–30, 2001.

[16] L. Marques, D. J. Robinaugh, N. J. LeBlanc, and D. Hinton, "Cross-cultural variations in the prevalence and presentation of anxiety disorders," *Expert Review of Neurotherapeutics*, vol. 11, no. 2, pp. 313–322, 2011.

[17] B. Harald and P. Gordon, "Meta-review of depressive subtyping models," *Journal of Affective Disorders*, vol. 139, no. 2, pp. 126–140, 2012.

[18] H. M. van Loo, P. de Jonge, J.-W. Romeijn, R. C. Kessler, and R. A. Schoevers, "Data-driven subtypes of major depressive disorder: a systematic review," *BMC Medicine*, vol. 10, article 156, 2012.

[19] J. Bühler, F. Seemüller, and D. Läge, "The predictive power of subgroups: an empirical approach to identify depressive symptom patterns that predict response to treatment," *Journal of Affective Disorders*, vol. 163, pp. 81–87, 2014.

[20] M. Kammerer, M. N. Marks, C. Pinard et al., "Symptoms associated with the DSM IV diagnosis of depression in pregnancy and post partum," *Archives of Women's Mental Health*, vol. 12, no. 3, pp. 135–141, 2009.

[21] J. J. Gallo and P. V. Rabins, "Depression without sadness: alternative presentations of depression in late life," *American Family Physician*, vol. 60, no. 3, pp. 820–826, 1999.

[22] R. Small, J. Lumley, and J. Yelland, "Cross-cultural experiences of maternal depression: associations and contributing factors for Vietnamese, Turkish and Filipino immigrant women in Victoria, Australia," *Ethnicity & Health*, vol. 8, no. 3, pp. 189–206, 2003.

[23] D. Saint Arnault and O. Kim, "Is there an Asian idiom of distress? Somatic symptoms in female Japanese and Korean students," *Archives of Psychiatric Nursing*, vol. 22, no. 1, pp. 27–38, 2008.

[24] Z. Steel, D. Silove, N. M. Giao et al., "International and indigenous diagnoses of mental disorder among Vietnamese living in Vietnam and Australia," *British Journal of Psychiatry*, vol. 194, no. 4, pp. 326–333, 2009.

[25] R. Youngmann, N. Zilber, F. Workneh, and R. Giel, "Adapting the SRQ for Ethiopian populations: a culturally-sensitive psychiatric screening instrument," *Transcultural Psychiatry*, vol. 45, no. 4, pp. 566–589, 2008.

[26] Z. Kalibatseva, F. T. L. Leong, and E. H. Ham, "A symptom profile of depression among Asian Americans: is there evidence for differential item functioning of depressive symptoms?" *Psychological Medicine*, vol. 44, no. 12, pp. 2567–2578, 2014.

[27] L. A. Uebelacker, D. Strong, L. M. Weinstock, and I. W. Miller, "Use of item response theory to understand differential functioning of DSM-IV major depression symptoms by race, ethnicity and gender," *Psychological Medicine*, vol. 39, no. 4, pp. 591–601, 2009.

[28] Y.-H. Um, H.-J. Huh, S.-Y. Kim, and J.-H. Chae, "Possible cultural effects on the increments of somatic symptoms in subjectively resilient depressed patients," *Asia-Pacific Psychiatry*, vol. 6, no. 3, pp. 259–266, 2014.

[29] The World Factbook, https://www.cia.gov/library/publications/the-world-factbook/.

[30] M. Juergensmeyer and W. C. Roof, Eds., *Encyclopedia of Global Religion*, SAGE Publications, Thousand Oaks, Calif, USA, 2011.

[31] International Institute for Population Sciences (IIPS), *Macro International: National Family Health Survey (NFHS-3), 2005-2006: India: Volume 1*, IIPS, Mumbai, India, 2007.

[32] United Nations Development Programme (UNDP), *Human Development Report 2002*, Oxford University Press, New York, NY, USA, 2002.

[33] Young Lives: An International Study of Childhood Poverty, http://www.younglives.org.uk/.

[34] S. Huttly and N. Jones, *Young Lives: an International Study of Childhood Poverty: Round 1, 2002*, SN: 5307, UK Data Service, Colchester, UK, 5th edition, 2014.

[35] I. Wilson, S. R. A. Huttly, and B. Fenn, "A case study of sample design for longitudinal research: young lives," *International Journal of Social Research Methodology*, vol. 9, no. 5, pp. 351–365, 2006.

[36] K. Brock and C. Knowles, *Young Lives Methods Guide*, Young Lives, Oxford, UK, 2011.

[37] T. Harpham, S. Huttly, M. J. De Silva, and T. Abramsky, "Maternal mental health and child nutritional status in four developing countries," *Journal of Epidemiology and Community Health*, vol. 59, no. 12, pp. 1060–1064, 2005.

[38] V. Morrow, "Practical ethics in social research with children and families in young lives: a longitudinal study of childhood poverty in Ethiopia, Andhra Pradesh (India), Peru and Vietnam," *Methodological Innovations Online*, vol. 8, pp. 21–35, 2013.

[39] M. Beusenberg and J. H. Orley, *A User's Guide to the Self Reporting Questionnaire (SRQ 20)*, World Health Organization, Geneva, Switzerland, 1994.

[40] T. Harpham, M. Reichenheim, R. Oser et al., "Measuring mental health in a cost-effective manner," *Health Policy and Planning*, vol. 18, no. 3, pp. 344–349, 2003.

[41] T. W. Harding, M. V. de Arango, J. Baltazar et al., "Mental disorders in primary health care: a study of their frequency and diagnosis in four developing countries," *Psychological Medicine*, vol. 10, no. 2, pp. 231–241, 1980.

[42] B. Sen, "An analysis of the nature of depressive phenomena in primary health care utilising multivariate statistical techniques," *Acta Psychiatrica Scandinavica*, vol. 76, no. 1, pp. 28–32, 1987.

[43] V. Patel, R. Araya, N. Chowdhary et al., "Detecting common mental disorders in primary care in India: a comparison of five screening questionnaires," *Psychological Medicine*, vol. 38, no. 2, pp. 221–228, 2008.

[44] F. Kortmann, "Psychiatric case finding in Ethiopia: shortcomings of the self reporting questionnaire," *Culture, Medicine and Psychiatry*, vol. 14, no. 3, pp. 381–391, 1990.

[45] C. Hanlon, G. Medhin, A. Alem et al., "Detecting perinatal common mental disorders in Ethiopia: validation of the self-reporting questionnaire and Edinburgh Postnatal Depression Scale," *Journal of Affective Disorders*, vol. 108, no. 3, pp. 251–262, 2008.

[46] T. Tuan, T. Harpham, and N. T. Huong, "Validity and reliability of the self-reporting questionnaire 20 items in Vietnam," *Hong Kong Journal of Psychiatry*, vol. 14, no. 3, pp. 15–18, 2004.

[47] M. J. De Silva, S. R. Huttly, T. Harpham, and M. G. Kenward, "Social capital and mental health: a comparative analysis of four low income countries," *Social Science and Medicine*, vol. 64, no. 1, pp. 5–20, 2007.

[48] M. J. Azur, E. A. Stuart, C. Frangakis, and P. J. Leaf, "Multiple imputation by chained equations: what is it and how does it work?" *International Journal of Methods in Psychiatric Research*, vol. 20, no. 1, pp. 40–49, 2011.

[49] N. Sartorius and WHO Collaborative Study on Standardized Assessment of Depressive Disorders, *Depressive Disorders in Different Cultures: Report on the WHO Collaborative Study on Standardized Assessment of Depressive Disorders/N. Sartorius ... [et al.]*, World Health Organization, Geneva, Switzerland, 1983.

[50] S. Bernert, H. Matschinger, J. Alonso, J. M. Haro, T. S. Brugha, and M. C. Angermeyer, "Is it always the same? Variability of depressive symptoms across six European countries," *Psychiatry Research*, vol. 168, no. 2, pp. 137–144, 2009.

[51] M. M. Weissman, "Cross-national epidemiology of major depression and bipolar disorder," *The Journal of the American Medical Association*, vol. 276, no. 4, pp. 293–299, 1996.

[52] W. W. Eaton, M. Badawi, and B. Melton, "Prodromes and precursors: epidemiologic data for primary prevention of disorders with slow onset," *The American Journal of Psychiatry*, vol. 152, no. 7, pp. 967–972, 1995.

[53] E. Iacoponi and J. D. J. Mari, "Reliability and factor structure of the Portuguese version of Self-Reporting Questionnaire," *International Journal of Social Psychiatry*, vol. 35, no. 3, pp. 213–222, 1989.

[54] R. Youngmann, S. Minuchin-Itzigsohn, and M. Barasch, "Manifestations of emotional distress among Ethiopian immigrants in Israel: patient and clinician perspectives," *Transcultural Psychiatry*, vol. 36, no. 1, pp. 45–63, 1999.

[55] A. Haque, "Mental health concepts in Southeast Asia: diagnostic considerations and treatment implications," *Psychology, Health & Medicine*, vol. 15, no. 2, pp. 127–134, 2010.

[56] C. U. Mitchell and M. LaGory, "Social capital and mental distress in an impoverished community," *City and Community*, vol. 1, no. 2, pp. 199–222, 2002.

[57] M. J. De Silva, K. McKenzie, T. Harpham, and S. R. A. Huttly, "Social capital and mental illness: a systematic review," *Journal of Epidemiology and Community Health*, vol. 59, no. 8, pp. 619–627, 2005.

[58] C. Lund, A. Breen, A. J. Flisher et al., "Poverty and common mental disorders in low and middle income countries: a systematic review," *Social Science and Medicine*, vol. 71, no. 3, pp. 517–528, 2010.

[59] L. Wang, T. Wu, J. L. Anderson, and J. E. Florence, "Prevalence and risk factors of maternal depression during the first three

years of child rearing," *Journal of Women's Health*, vol. 20, no. 5, pp. 711–718, 2011.

[60] V. Patel, M. Rodrigues, and N. DeSouza, "Gender, poverty, and postnatal depression: a study of mothers in Goa, India," *The American Journal of Psychiatry*, vol. 159, no. 1, pp. 43–47, 2002.

[61] V. Patel and A. Kleinman, "Poverty and common mental disorders in developing countries," *Bulletin of the World Health Organization*, vol. 81, no. 8, pp. 609–615, 2003.

[62] N. T. M. Thuy and H. L. Berry, "Social capital and mental health among mothers in Vietnam who have children with disabilities," *Global Health Action*, vol. 6, 2013.

[63] G. Medhin, C. Hanlon, M. Dewey et al., "The effect of maternal common mental disorders on infant undernutrition in Butajira, Ethiopia: the P-MaMiE study," *BMC Psychiatry*, vol. 10, article 32, 2010.

[64] C. Hadley, A. Tegegn, F. Tessema, M. Asefa, and S. Galea, "Parental symptoms of common mental disorders and children's social, motor, and language development in sub-Saharan Africa," *Annals of Human Biology*, vol. 35, no. 3, pp. 259–275, 2008.

22

Depression Treatment Patterns among Elderly with Cancer

Patricia A. Findley,[1] Chan Shen,[2] and Usha Sambamoorthi[3,4]

[1] *School of Social Work, Rutgers University, New Brunswick, NJ 08901, USA*
[2] *Department of Biostatistics, MD Anderson Cancer Center, The University of Texas, Houston, TX 77030, USA*
[3] *Department of Pharmaceutical Systems and Policy, School of Pharmacy, West Virginia University, Morgantown, WV 26506, USA*
[4] *Department of Community Health and Preventive Medicine, Morehouse School of Medicine, Atlanta, GA 30310, USA*

Correspondence should be addressed to Patricia A. Findley, pfindley@ssw.rutgers.edu

Academic Editor: Harm W. J. van Marwijk

Little is known about cancer treatment patterns among the elderly as depression and cancer in this older population have not been well explored. This study seeks to fill a gap in the literature by using data from the Medicare Current Beneficiary Survey from years 2000–2005 to examine depression treatment patterns among elderly diagnosed with both cancer and depression. Depression treatments examined include antidepressants with and without psychotherapy. We found that of those with both cancer and depression, 57.7% reported antidepressant use only, 19.7% received psychotherapy with or without antidepressants, and 22.6% had no depression treatment. We found those with greater comorbidity, of a minority race, with lower levels of education, and living in rural areas were less likely to receive treatment for depression. These findings highlight the need to address disparities in the treatment of depression in the elderly population with cancer.

1. Introduction

Cancer among the elderly has grown in prevalence, in 2007, 70% of those diagnosed with cancer in the United States were over 65 years of age, with 44% over the age of 75 [1]. Currently, among the US population there are 7 million people over the age of 65 living with cancer [2]. Projections from 2010 to 2030 estimate a 67% increase in cancer incidence among the US population that is 65 years and older, compared to an increase of only 11% in younger age groups [3]. Given the rapid increases in the number of elderly diagnosed with cancer, greater awareness, identification, evaluation, and treatment of depression this group has gained attention [4]. However, the elderly are not been specifically studied in current cancer studies. For example, in a metareview of 100 studies, the prevalence of depression among individuals of all ages with cancer was reported to have reached as high as 38%–58%, but these studies did not include the elderly [5].

Although depression has been recognized as detrimental to cancer prognosis, treatment, and related quality of life, not much is known about the treatment of depression among elderly with cancer. In one study that included both elderly and nonelderly, using data from community oncology practices in the US, individuals over age 60 were less likely to receive antidepressants compared to younger individuals [6]. Furthermore, it has been reported that the elderly with cancer are at risk of developing subthreshold forms of depression, meaning depression may go unrecognized and untreated [7]. In fact, it has been reported that overall, the elderly as a subgroup are vulnerable to the undertreatment of depression [7]. Treating depression in elderly with cancer may help to prevent the adverse changes associated with depression such as decreases in quality of sleep, relationships, and quality of life, as well as increases in pain and other symptoms of cancer [4]. Such treatment of depression may support better treatment outcomes for elderly diagnosed with cancer.

The examination of existing data on elderly patients with cancer could lead to better treatment of depression in this growing population of elderly with cancer. Therefore, the primary objective of the present study is to estimate the rates of depression treatment and to identify subgroup differences in treatment (or lack of treatment) for depression among the elderly who are diagnosed with cancer and depression. This study uses cross-sectional data from multiple years of the Medicare Current Beneficiary Survey (MCBS), a nationally representative survey of Medicare beneficiaries.

This study was approved by the Institutional Review Board of Rutgers University.

2. Methods

2.1. Study Design. This is a retrospective, cross-sectional study using data on the elderly derived from a nationally representative survey of Medicare beneficiaries. This is a descriptive study.

2.2. Data. Data for our study were obtained from the MCBS from 2000 to 2005. The MCBS is a rotating panel survey of a nationally representative sample of Medicare beneficiaries [8]. Survey data are collected by using in-depth computer-assisted personal interviews (CAPI) and are conducted every four months to capture healthcare utilization (including prescriptions filled) and non-Medicare payment sources reported by respondents. The MCBS provides both cross-sectional and longitudinal data on the health status, treatment, Medicare and non-Medicare utilization, prescription drug use, and expenditures of Medicare beneficiaries. These data also provide socioeconomic and demographic characteristics of the beneficiaries. The current study used the annual data from the calendar year 2000–2005 "Cost and Use" files.

2.3. Identification of Cancer. We identified individuals with cancer based on their responses to two survey questions in the MCBS. Survey respondents were asked whether "a doctor (ever) told (you) that (you) had any (other) kind of cancer, malignancy, or tumor other than skin cancer?" A similar question was asked about any diagnosis of skin cancer. We defined individuals with cancer based on an affirmative response to one or both of the questions. We included all cancers as the emotional response to a cancer diagnosis can vary by individual despite the type of cancer.

2.4. Identification of Diagnosed Depression. Diagnosed depression was identified using fee-for-service claims of the Medicare beneficiaries and based on the *International Classification of Diseases, 9th Edition, Clinical Modification* (ICD-9-CM) codes [9]. The ICD-9-CM codes we used were 296.2 (major depressive disorder, single episode), 296.3 (major depressive disorder, recurrent episode), 300.4 (neurotic depression), 309.1 (prolonged depressive reaction), and 311 (depression, not elsewhere classified). These codes were used to identify diagnosed depression in a prior published study [10].

2.5. Analytical Sample. Among the elderly with cancer and depression, we excluded beneficiaries who were not enrolled in Medicare throughout the entire calendar year to ensure we had complete annual data. We excluded those who were institutionalized (i.e., in a nursing home), who were enrolled in Medicare managed care, and who died during the observation years. We used only fully enrolled beneficiaries to ensure a uniform observation period. Since we derived psychotherapy use from claims, Medicare-managed enrollees were excluded because claims were not available for those individuals. Thus, the final sample for analysis consisted of data for 865 elderly Medicare beneficiaries who had both cancer and depression in the years from 2000 to 2005.

3. Measures

3.1. Dependent Variable

3.1.1. Depression Treatment: Antidepressant Use. We derived antidepressant use from self-reported prescription drug data. We could not use pharmacy claims because Medicare Part D was not enacted until 2006. For the MCBS, to minimize recall errors in medication use, a number of steps had been taken, including holding interviews at 4-month intervals, asking the survey respondents to bring prescription drug bottles to the interview, and providing the respondents with calendars on which to record their use of prescription drugs. We used drug names to identify antidepressants. Drugs included in the class of antidepressants were selective serotonin reuptake inhibitors (SSRI), serotonin/norepinephrine reuptake inhibitors (SNRI), tricyclics (TCA), tetracyclics, and monoamine oxidase inhibitors (MAOI) [11].

3.1.2. Treatment of Depression: Psychotherapy. We identified psychotherapy treatment from Medicare claims based on current procedural terminology (CPT) codes used in previous published analyses [12]. We categorized depression treatment patterns into three groups based on the use of antidepressants and receipt of psychotherapy: (1) no depression treatment; (2) antidepressant use only; (3) psychotherapy use with or without antidepressants. We did not distinguish psychotherapy with and without antidepressants because most of the people who received psychotherapy also reported antidepressant use, with less than 5% ($n = 46$) receiving psychotherapy only.

3.2. Independent Variables. Independent variables consisted of demographic characteristics: gender (male, female), race (white, minority), age (65–74 years, 75 and older), marital status (married, widowed, and other), and geographic region (urban/rural). Socioeconomic status consisted of education (less than high school, completed high school, some college, completed college, and above), poverty status (<200% of the poverty level, ≥200%), and access to care, which was measured with an indicator variable (yes, no) for prescription drug coverage. As noted previously, because Medicare Part D did not start until January 2006, we constructed a variable on the use of prescription drugs using the same method reported in published studies [13, 14]. We measured health status with a number of variables: general health perception (excellent/very good, good, and fair/poor); number of chronic medical conditions, which included arthritis, diabetes, heart disease, hypertension, stroke, respiratory conditions, and/or osteoporosis; difficulty with activities of daily living (ADLs) based on the number of ADL categories that were considered difficult (none, 1-2, and 3–6). We assessed lifestyle risk factors in two areas: body mass index (BMI) and smoking status. A BMI of less than 25 kg/m^2 indicates the individual is underweight or normal; a BMI in the range from 25 to 29.9 kg/m^2 indicates the individual is overweight; a BMI greater than 30 kg/m^2 indicates the individual is obese or morbidly obese [15]. We used three categories for smoking status (current smoker, past smoker, and never smoked). In multinomial logistic regressions, we combined the categories of current smoker and past smoker.

3.3. Statistical Techniques. We conducted both bivariate and multivariate analyses, and tested the group differences in depression treatment using chi-squared statistics. We employed multinomial logistic regression on the depression treatment categories to examine treatment patterns. From multinomial logistic regression, we transformed the parameter estimates to odds ratios and reported their corresponding 95% confidence intervals. In the multinomial regression, for the dependent variable, the reference group was "no depression treatment." We accounted for the complex design of the MCBS by conducting all these analyses with survey procedures in SAS 9.2 [16].

4. Findings

We found that 5% of the elderly with cancer were diagnosed with depression. This percentage remained consistent for all the years studied (data not shown but available upon request). A description of this study sample of 865 elderly Medicare beneficiaries with depression and cancer is provided in Table 1. The majority of beneficiaries in our sample were white women who lived in urban areas. About half (48%) of them had low income as measured by an annual income of less than 200% of the poverty threshold. Thirty-six percent had completed a high school education. Common physical conditions (not presented in tabular form) included arthritis (77%), hypertension (66%), and heart disease (47%). Forty-four percent had difficulty with at least one ADL.

In our sample, of those who reported depression, 57.7% were prescribed antidepressants *only*, 19.7% had psychotherapy with or without antidepressants, and 22.6% had no depression treatment (Table 2). Among the significant findings ($.01 < P < .05$), we found that a greater proportion of the elderly living in rural areas had no depression treatment compared to those living in urban areas (29.2% versus 20.6%). Compared to the elderly with less formal education, a higher proportion of the elderly with a college education received psychotherapy treatment of depression and a lower proportion had no treatment. For example, 13.5% of those with less than a high school education received psychotherapy compared with 28.2% of those who completed college; 25.6% of the elderly who did not complete high school had no depression treatment versus 17.2% in the group who completed college.

Table 1: Description of study sample with reported cancer and diagnosed depression. Medicare Current Beneficiary Survey, 2000–2005.

	N	Weighted %
Year		
2000	125	13.1
2001	127	14.3
2002	170	18.7
2003	158	18.9
2004	147	18.2
2005	138	16.8
Gender		
Female	593	69.5
Male	272	30.5
Race/ethnicity		
White	783	90.5
African American	27	3.0
Latino	32	4.1
Other	23	2.4
Age in years		
65–69	113	14.2
70–74	183	25.0
75–79	202	26.9
80+	367	33.9
Marital status		
Married	382	45.5
Widowed	370	41.5
Divorced/separated	87	10.6
Other	26	2.5
Community status		
Urban	635	76.7
Rural	230	23.3
Education		
Less than high school	221	25.6
High school	308	36.1
Some college	146	16.9
College	186	21.4
Poverty status		
LT 200%	427	47.8
≥200%	438	52.2
Prescription drug coverage		
Yes	683	80.1
No	182	19.9
Health status		
Excellent/very good	64	7.0
Good	191	22.6
Fair/poor	107	12.5
Functional status (ADL)		
No difficulties with ADLs	478	55.9
1-2	236	27.0
3–6	149	17.1
Smoking status		
Current smoker	73	9.0
Past smoker	452	52.7

Table 1: Continued.

	N	Weighted %
Never smoked	340	38.2
Body mass index		
Underweight/normal	383	42.1
Overweight	308	35.9
Obese	168	22.0

Note: Based on 865 person—years of elderly Medicare beneficiaries with reported cancer and diagnosed depression.
ADL: activity of daily living.

Table 3 summarizes findings from the multinomial logistic regression on depression treatment. In this analysis "no treatment" served as the reference group for the dependent variable, depression treatment. We assessed the fit of our model by evaluating the overall model and statistically testing the contribution of each of the independent variables. In terms of overall model evaluation, we tested the fit of the final model against a null or intercept-only model. We found that all tests (likelihood ratio, score, and Wald) were statistically significant at $P < .0001$ suggesting that at least one of the independent variables was associated with depression treatment categories. We also tested parameter estimates of each independent variable using Wald chi-square tests. Based on these tests, we observed that gender, female, and community status were significantly associated with depression treatment categories. None of the other variables were statistically significant. In terms of individual categories, nonwhites were less likely to receive antidepressants only compared to no treatment at all (adjusted odds ratio [AOR] 0.54; 95% confidence interval [CI] = 0.30–0.95). Those living in urban areas were more likely to receive antidepressants rather than no treatment (AOR 1.52; 95% CI = 1.04–2.23) and those with less than a high school education or at most a high school education were less likely to receive psychotherapy ([AOR 0.36; 95% CI = 0.15–0.83] and [AOR 0.43; 95% CI = 0.20–0.93], resp.). The elderly who had more chronic conditions were more likely to receive antidepressants only compared to no treatment (AOR 1.17; 95% CI = 1.00–1.36). Conversely, the elderly with one to two areas of impairment in activities of daily living were less likely to receive antidepressants (AOR 0.65; 95% CI = 0.43–0.99). All of these findings were statistically significant at the $.01 < P < .05$ level.

5. Discussion

To examine patterns of depression treatment among elderly Medicare beneficiaries with a diagnosis for both cancer and depression, we used data from the MCBS, a nationally representative survey of individuals enrolled in Medicare in years from 2000 to 2005. We found that 24% of our study sample received no treatment of their depression, whereas an overwhelming majority (76%) reported using antidepressants and/or psychotherapy. Unfortunately, there are no published studies with which to compare the findings of the current study. For the purpose of discussion, we compare our findings to studies conducted in the general population (i.e., included nonelderly).

When examining the type of treatment, only a minority (19.7%) of the elderly received psychotherapy with or without antidepressant medications. Fifty-seven percent of our sample reported using antidepressant medications *only*. This result is similar to what Akincigil et al. reported in their study using MCBS data from 2005 where 67.3% of the general elderly population was using antidepressants and 14.3% used psychotherapy [17]. These findings were not surprising given the current trends in the treatment for depression across the nation overall where there has been a shift toward an increased reliance on medications over psychotherapy in all age groups. This is evidenced in a longitudinal study of the general population using Medical Expenditure Panel Survey (MEPS) data from 1996 to 2005. In this study, Mackenzic et al. [18] found that among elderly with depression, rates of antidepressant use increased between 1996 and 2005, whereas the rates of psychotherapy decreased. Wei et al. also found the use of psychotherapy to be uncommon among the elderly diagnosed with depression, despite its acknowledged efficacy [12]. We suggest that the limited use of psychotherapy may be attributed to several factors, including help-seeking behavior among the elderly [18], racial or ethnic disparities in health care [19, 20], restricted access to specialty mental health providers [21], low cultural acceptance of psychotherapy as a treatment [22], and the high cost of psychotherapy [23].

We found a lack of depression treatment for some of the elderly in our study. The lack of treatment for depression in individuals with cancer might be related to the competing demands of healthcare management and the prioritization of treatment of cancer with other chronic physical conditions the individual may be experiencing [24]. It is important to note that we did not know the date of diagnosis. Therefore, we could not distinguish between the elderly who had completed cancer treatment and those who were actively receiving cancer treatment. Active cancer treatment would likely supersede treatment for depression, in particular because these patients would likely be seen by oncologists rather than primary care physicians who might provide more inclusive care [25]. Furthermore, although cancer treatment itself is known to induce depression, efforts to manage pain and fatigue might play a more prominent role over the treatment for depression [26]. It has been reported that prevalence of fatigue is greater than 50–70% in advanced cancer patients and the prevalence of pain is 80% in elderly patients with advanced cancer [27]. Therefore, the complexities of treating a serious chronic disease and the coordination of the medical care required to address the comorbid conditions may lead to a lower priority for the treatment for depression [28]. Additionally, detecting depression in an elderly cancer patient may require special consideration to address agedrelated issues such a memory loss. Traeger and Pirl recommend adapting standard depression assessments by adding additional questions that characterize functioning (e.g., tell me about a typical day) rather than relying on specific recall [29]. These adaptations allow the physician to gather pieces of necessary information

TABLE 2: Number and weighted percent of study sample by depression treatment. Medicare Current Beneficiary Survey, 2000–2005.

	AD only		Psyc w/o AD		No treatment		
ALL	*N*	Wt%	*N*	Wt%	*N*	Wt%	Sig.
	493	57.7	168	19.7	204	22.6	
Year							
2000	75	58.9	21	18.5	29	22.6	
2001	75	58.6	23	20.1	29	21.3	
2002	81	46.5	39	23.8	50	29.7	
2003	100	63.7	31	19.4	27	16.9	
2004	89	63.7	24	15.7	34	20.6	
2005	73	55.0	30	20.7	35	24.3	
Gender							
Female	329	56.3	130	22.4	134	21.3	
Male	164	60.7	38	13.8	70	25.5	
Race							
White	453	58.2	151	19.9	179	22.0	
Minorities	40	53.0	17	18.6	25	28.4	
Age in years							
65–74	171	58.9	65	21.7	60	19.4	
75 and older	322	56.9	103	18.5	144	24.6	
Marital status							
Married	221	57.6	61	16.8	100	25.6	
Widowed	210	58.3	77	21.0	83	20.7	
Other	62	55.7	30	26.2	21	18.1	
Community status							*
Urban	366	58.5	132	20.9	137	20.6	
Rural	127	54.8	36	16.0	67	29.2	
Education							*
LT HS	130	60.9	32	13.5	59	25.6	
HS	185	60.5	52	17.0	71	22.5	
Some college	73	50.8	35	24.7	38	24.5	
College	104	54.7	49	28.2	33	17.2	
Poverty status							
LT 200%	254	61.2	68	16.0	105	22.8	
≥200%	239	54.4	100	23.2	99	22.4	
Prescription drug coverage							
Yes	393	58.2	133	19.7	157	22.1	
No	100	55.3	35	20.1	47	24.6	
Health status							
Excellent/very good	141	55.4	49	20.0	65	24.7	
Good	154	59.7	50	19.6	59	20.8	
Fair/poor	195	57.5	69	19.9	80	22.6	
Functional status (ADL)							
No difficulties	275	57.5	94	20.5	109	22.0	
1-2 ADLs	125	53.4	49	21.0	62	25.6	
3–6 ADLs	91	63.5	25	15.9	33	20.5	
Smoking status							
Current smoker	43	59.6	12	16.7	18	23.7	
Past smoker	253	56.8	88	20.9	111	22.3	
Never smoked	197	58.4	68	18.9	75	22.7	
Body mass index							
Und/normal	202	52.5	79	22.2	102	25.3	
Overweight	177	58.6	60	18.7	71	22.7	

Table 2: Continued.

ALL	AD only		Psyc w/o AD		No treatment		Sig.
	N	Wt%	N	Wt%	N	Wt%	
	493	57.7	168	19.7	204	22.6	
Obese	109	64.3	28	17.3	31	18.5	
Number of chronic conditions							
0–2	201	54.9	67	18.7	101	26.4	
Three or more	292	59.7	101	20.5	103	19.8	

Note: Based on 865 person—years of elderly Medicare beneficiaries with cancer and depression using Medicare Current Beneficiary Survey 2000–2005. Asterisks represent significant group differences by depression treatment based on chi-squared tests.
AD: antidepressants; Psyc w/o: psychotherapy use with or without antidepressants; Sig: significance; Wt: weighted; ADL: activity of daily living; Und: underweight; HS: high school; LT: less than.
*$.01 \le P < .05$ [Note: only a single asterisk appears in the table].

to see if the patient meets the criteria for depression as defined by the Diagnostic and Statistical Manual of Mental Disorders-IV-TR [30].

Our findings with regard to racial differences in depression treatment are consistent with the national treatment patterns for the general population. Another study has reported increased depression among the minority elderly with chronic illnesses [31]. However, when analyzing the trends in antidepressant use among individuals, regardless of a diagnosis for depression, and based on national data comparing the trends in 1996 to those in 2005, Olfson and Marcus [32] found that increases in antidepressant use were evident across all racial groups examined, except for among African Americans, who had comparatively low rates of use in both years (1996, 3.61%; 2005, 4.51%). Akincigil et al. [17] found an uneven trend in racial differences in antidepressant use from 1992 to 2005 for the elderly in their study. Their study showed that all minorities received less antidepressant treatment compared to whites in 2002–2005, which is similar to our findings in our study period of 2000–2005.

With respect to geographic area, we found the rates of psychotherapy use were different between urban and rural areas, with those in urban areas receiving more treatment. This is inconsistent with a recent prospective study on a small sample that found no widespread differences between cancer survivors living in rural versus nonrural areas with respect to mental health resource use [22]. These authors suggested that some of the decreased use of mental health resources in rural areas may be due to poorer accessibility and availability of mental health professionals in those communities. It has also been reported that the elderly living in rural areas may rely on their religion more than formal mental health services to support them when depressed [33].

We found that education level also influenced the likelihood of receiving psychotherapy. Individuals who had attained a higher level of education (i.e., college) were more likely to receive psychotherapy compared to those who had attained only a high school education or less. This was not surprising. Other researchers have found that higher levels of education influence more positive attitudes toward the acceptance of mental health services, particularly for men [18].

This study has several strengths worth noting. We used a nationally representative data set on a large number of Medicare beneficiaries with cancer that includes comprehensive information obtained from the survey and Medicare claims. We included a number of relevant covariates and use of a case-finding algorithm for quality measures to identify depression [34]. We included the use of psychotherapy, a variable that is not usually analyzed in studies of the elderly with cancer.

Despite the noted strengths, our study findings need to be interpreted in the context of their limitations. With respect to selection bias, by focusing on diagnosed depression, we may have excluded individuals who were not diagnosed but were given treatment; thus, our treatment rates may be underestimated. We also identify those individuals who were first diagnosed for depression then subsequently treated for depression. Medicare-managed care enrollees were excluded; thus, generalizability is limited. Although we pooled multiple years, the sample size was too small to allow us to separately analyze psychotherapy without antidepressants, which may have implications for individuals with cancer who are undergoing treatment.

We did have a limitation with prescription benefit coverage. As prescription benefits under Medicare Part *D* were not implemented until 2006, the year after our study period; prescription drug use was self-reported. Self-reporting has been shown to be susceptible to underreporting [35]. Although efforts were taken to minimize bias in the self-reported pharmacy data, preliminary results from a validation study conducted by the Centers for Medicare and Medicaid Services (CMS) suggest that there is an underreporting rate of approximately 15–18% in the MCBS [35]. However, these data are heavily used in published studies of depression among many different types of populations [14, 36].

We could not control for clinical factors such as the specific type of cancer or duration and stage of cancer, which may be associated with the likelihood for depression treatment. However, by excluding individuals who died during the same calendar year for which they were included in the data set, we were able to control for end-stage cancer. By focusing on diagnosed depression, we may have excluded individuals who were not diagnosed but were given treatment; thus, our treatment rates may be underestimated.

TABLE 3: Adjusted odds ratios and 95% confidence intervals from multinomial logistic regression on depression treatment. Medicare Current Beneficiary Survey, 2000–2005.

	Antidepressant only			Psychotherapy with or without antidepressants		
	AOR	95% CI	Sig.	AOR	95% CI	Sig.
Year						
2000						
2001	1.01	[0.55, 1.85]		1.05	[0.48, 2.30]	
2002	0.56	[0.30, 1.04]		0.87	[0.42, 1.80]	
2003	1.38	[0.74, 2.57]		1.38	[0.60, 3.17]	
2004	1.14	[0.61, 2.15]		0.92	[0.40, 2.13]	
2005	0.79	[0.46, 1.35]		0.95	[0.44, 2.08]	
Gender						
Female	0.99	[0.58, 1.68]		1.95	[0.99, 3.84]	
Male						
Race						
White						
Minorities	0.54	[0.30, 0.95]	*	0.67	[0.26, 1.69]	
Age in years						
65–74						
75,+	0.83	[0.49, 1.41]		0.65	[0.35, 1.23]	
Marital status						
Married						
Widowed	1.39	[0.84, 2.28]		1.69	[0.85, 3.37]	
Other	1.20	[0.58, 2.49]		1.86	[0.74, 4.70]	
Community status						
Urban	1.52	[1.04, 2.23]	*	1.80	[0.98, 3.33]	
Rural						
Education						
LT HS	0.69	[0.35, 1.34]		0.36	[0.15, 0.83]	*
HS	0.78	[0.40, 1.51]		0.43	[0.20, 0.93]	*
Some college	0.70	[0.37, 1.34]		0.63	[0.31, 1.30]	
College						
Poverty status						
LT 200%	1.12	[0.74, 1.70]		0.73	[0.41, 1.30]	
≥200%						
Prescription drug coverage						
Yes						
No	0.94	[0.60, 1.46]		1.16	[0.63, 2.15]	
Health status						
Excellent/very good						
Good	1.27	[0.78, 2.07]		1.25	[0.74, 2.10]	
Fair/Poor	1.06	[0.65, 1.72]		1.37	[0.70, 2.65]	
Number of chronic conditions						
	1.17	[1.00, 1.36]	*	1.16	[0.94, 1.41]	
Functional status (ADL)						
No difficulties						
1-2 ADLs	0.65	[0.43, 0.99]	*	0.72	[0.40, 1.30]	
3–6 ADLs	0.95	[0.52, 1.72]		0.67	[0.34, 1.33]	
Smoking status						
Current smoker	1.00	[0.63, 1.60]		1.13	[0.64, 2.01]	
Other						
Body mass index						
Under/normal						

Table 3: Continued.

	Antidepressant only			Psychotherapy with or without antidepressants		
	AOR	95% CI	Sig.	AOR	95% CI	Sig.
			Overall model evaluation			
Test		Chi-square	DF	P-value		
Overweight	1.26	[0.81, 1.95]		1.10	[0.65, 1.87]	
Obese	1.63	[0.90, 2.95]		1.02	[0.45, 2.32]	
Likelihood ratio		291214.347	48	<.0001		
Score		283025.448	48	<.0001		
Wald		138.4648	48	<.001		

Note: Based on 865 person—years of elderly Medicare beneficiaries with cancer and depression using Medicare Current Beneficiary Survey 2000–2005. The regression also included intercepts. The reference group for the dependent variable was "No depression treatment." Asterisks represent significant differences in likelihood of depression treatment compared to the reference group based on multinomial logistic regression.
AOR: adjusted odds ratio; CI: confidence interval; Sig: significance; LT: less than; HS: high school; high school; ADL: activity of daily living.
*$.01 \le P < .05$.

Medicare-managed care enrollees were excluded; thus, generalizability is limited. Although we pooled multiple years, the sample size was too small to allow us to separately analyze psychotherapy without antidepressants, which may have implications for individuals with cancer who are undergoing treatment.

Another area of limitation that is not restricted to our study alone is the identification of depression by ICD-9-CM codes. Although this is an accepted method in numerous publications [37–40], relying on these codes results in a very heterogeneous population since the codes were creating for billing purposes and not for treatment purposes. Future research on smaller populations using prospective studies and/or chart reviews might gather qualitative data more representative of individuals with depression and demonstrate the nuances of treatment decision making.

Despite these limitations, our study adds to the nascent literature on cancer and depression treatment in the elderly. The treatment for depression remains a concern because of the impact of depression on the success of cancer treatment [4] and the individual's overall prognosis. As proposed by the Institute of Medicine, survivorship care plans for cancer survivors include treatment for depression [41]. Our findings suggest that providers and policy makers need to address the barriers to psychotherapy use for the elderly, particularly in rural areas. Furthermore, interventions should be developed to educate individuals with cancer on the role of depression in their overall health care needs. Such interventions should target minority racial groups and cancer survivors living outside of urban areas to promote the identification and evaluation of depression and the appropriate treatment of depression among the elderly with cancer.

Acknowledgment

The project was conducted under the auspices of West Virginia University CoHORTS (Collaborative Health Outcomes Research of Therapies and Services) Center funded by AHRQ (1R24HS018622-03) in which Dr. U. Sambamoorthi is a data repository core director and coinvestigator.

References

[1] National Cancer Policy Forum/Institute of Medicine, *Cancer in Elderly People: Workshop Proceedings*, National Academies Press, Washington, DC, USA, 2007.

[2] Center for Disease Control, "Cancer survivors in the United States, 2007," *Morbidity and Mortality Weekly Report*, vol. 60, no. 9, pp. 269–296, 2011.

[3] B. D. Smith, G. L. Smith, A. Hurria, G. N. Hortobagyi, and T. A. Buchholz, "Future of cancer incidence in the United States: burdens upon an aging, changing nation," *Journal of Clinical Oncology*, vol. 27, no. 17, pp. 2758–2765, 2009.

[4] M. I. Weinberger, A. J. Roth, and C. J. Nelson, "Untangling the complexities of depression diagnosis in older cancer patients," *Oncologist*, vol. 14, no. 1, pp. 60–66, 2009.

[5] M. J. Massie, "Prevalence of depression in patients with cancer," *Journal of the National Cancer Institute. Monographs*, no. 32, pp. 57–71, 2004.

[6] F. D. Ashbury, L. Madlensky, P. Raich et al., "Antidepressant prescribing in community cancer care," *Supportive Care in Cancer*, vol. 11, no. 5, pp. 278–285, 2003.

[7] A. S. Young, R. Klap, C. D. Sherbourne, and K. B. Wells, "The quality of care for depressive and anxiety disorders in the United States," *Archives of General Psychiatry*, vol. 58, no. 1, pp. 55–61, 2001.

[8] http://www.cms.hhs.gov/MCBS/.

[9] C. Buck, *2010 ICD-9-CM For Hospitals*, vol. 1–3, Saunders, Maryland Heights, Mo, USA, 2010.

[10] U. Sambamoorthi, B. Bean-Mayberry, P. A. Findley, E. M. Yano, and R. Banerjea, "Organization of care and diagnosed depression among women veterans," *American Journal of Managed Care*, vol. 16, no. 9, pp. 657–665, 2010.

[11] AHFS Drug Information 2009, micromedex online, facts and comparisons, 2011, http://www.ahfsdruginformation.com/.

[12] W. Wei, U. Sambamoorthi, M. Olfson, J. T. Walkup, and S. Crystal, "Use of psychotherapy for depression in older adults," *American Journal of Psychiatry*, vol. 162, no. 4, pp. 711–717, 2005.

[13] U. Sambamoorthi, M. Olfson, J. T. Walkup, and S. Crystal, "Diffusion of new generation antidepressant treatment among elderly diagnosed with depression," *Medical Care*, vol. 41, no. 1, pp. 180–194, 2003.

[14] S. Crystal, U. Sambamoorthi, J. T. Walkup, and A. Akincigil, "Diagnosis and treatment of depression in the elderly medicare population: predictors, disparities, and trends," *Journal of the American Geriatrics Society*, vol. 51, no. 12, pp. 1718–1728, 2003.

[15] BMI Classification [Internet], 2011, http://www.cdc.gov/healthyweight/assessing/bmi/adult_bmi/index.html.

[16] SAS Institute Inc., SAS 9. 2, 2009.

[17] A. Akincigil, M. Olfson, J. T. Walkup et al., "Diagnosis and treatment of depression in older community-dwelling adults: 1992–2005," *Journal of the American Geriatrics Society*, vol. 59, no. 6, pp. 1042–1051, 2011.

[18] C. S. Mackenzie, W. L. Gekoski, and V. J. Knox, "Age, gender, and the underutilization of mental health services: the influence of help-seeking attitudes," *Aging and Mental Health*, vol. 10, no. 6, pp. 574–582, 2006.

[19] R. G. Hood, "Confronting racial and ethnic disparities in health care," *Academic Medicine*, vol. 76, no. 6, pp. 584–585, 2001.

[20] A. Nelson, "Unequal treatment: confronting racial and ethnic disparities in health care," *Journal of the National Medical Association*, vol. 94, no. 8, pp. 666–668, 2002.

[21] T. D. Sequist, "Ensuring equal access to specialty care," *The New England Journal of Medicine*, vol. 364, no. 23, pp. 2258–2259, 2011.

[22] M. A. Andrykowski and J. L. Burris, "Use of formal and informal mental health resources by cancer survivors: differences between rural and nonrural survivors and a preliminary test of the theory of planned behavior," *Psycho-Oncology*, vol. 19, no. 11, pp. 1148–1155, 2010.

[23] S. C. Marcus and M. Olfson, "National trends in the treatment for depression from 1998 to 2007," *Archives of General Psychiatry*, vol. 67, no. 12, pp. 1265–1273, 2010.

[24] M. S. Klinkman, "Competing demands in psychosocial care: a model for the identification and treatment of depressive disorders in primary care," *General Hospital Psychiatry*, vol. 19, no. 2, pp. 98–111, 1997.

[25] L. E. Jones and C. C. Doebbeling, "Suboptimal depression screening following cancer diagnosis," *General Hospital Psychiatry*, vol. 29, no. 6, pp. 547–554, 2007.

[26] M. Extermann and A. Hurria, "Comprehensive geriatric assessment for older patients with cancer," *Journal of Clinical Oncology*, vol. 25, no. 14, pp. 1824–1831, 2007.

[27] A. Rao and H. J. Cohen, "Symptom management in the elderly cancer patient: fatigue, pain, and depression," *Journal of the National Cancer Institute. Monographs*, no. 32, pp. 150–157, 2004.

[28] B. Starfield, L. Shi, and J. Macinko, "Contribution of primary care to health systems and health," *Milbank Quarterly*, vol. 83, no. 3, pp. 457–502, 2005.

[29] L. Traeger and W. F. Pirl, "Approaching the treatment of depression in elderly cancer patients," *Aging Health*, vol. 6, no. 3, pp. 393–403, 2010.

[30] American Psychiatric Association, *Diagnostic and Statistical Manual of Mental Health Disorders*, American Psychiatric Association, Washington, DC, USA, 4th edition, 2000.

[31] M. Bazargan and V. P. Hamm-Baugh, "The relationship between chronic illness and depression in a community of urban black elderly persons," *Journals of Gerontology B*, vol. 50, no. 2, pp. S119–S127, 1995.

[32] M. Olfson and S. C. Marcus, "National patterns in antidepressant medication treatment," *Archives of General Psychiatry*, vol. 66, no. 8, pp. 848–856, 2009.

[33] J. Mitchell and D. Weatherey, "Beyond church attendance: religiosity and mental health among rural older adults," *Journal of Cross-Cultural Gerontology*, vol. 15, no. 1, pp. 37–54, 2000.

[34] National Quality Measures Clearinghouse [Internet], http://www.qualitymeasures.ahrq.gov/summary/summary.aspx?ss=-1&doc_id=11488.

[35] J. A. Poisal, "Reporting of drug expenditures in the MCBS," *Health Care Financing Review*, vol. 25, no. 2, pp. 23–36, 2003.

[36] C. M. Blanchette, L. Simoni-Wastila, F. Shaya, D. Orwig, J. Noel, and B. Stuart, "Health care use in depressed, elderly, cardiac patients and the effect of antidepressant use," *American Journal of Health-System Pharmacy*, vol. 66, no. 4, pp. 366–372, 2009.

[37] L. E. Egede, C. Ellis, and A. L. Grubaugh, "The effect of depression on self-care behaviors and quality of care in a national sample of adults with diabetes," *General Hospital Psychiatry*, vol. 31, no. 5, pp. 422–427, 2009.

[38] P. Findley, C. Shen, and U. Sambamoorthi, "Multimorbidity and persistent depression among veterans with diabetes, heart disease, and hypertension," *Health & Social Work*, vol. 36, no. 2, pp. 109–119, 2011.

[39] J. M. Gill, M. S. Klinkman, and Y. X. Chen, "Antidepressant medication use for primary care patients with and without medical comorbidities: a national electronic health record (EHR) network study," *Journal of the American Board of Family Medicine*, vol. 23, no. 4, pp. 499–508, 2010.

[40] K. M. Schneider, B. E. O'Donnell, and D. Dean, "Prevalence of multiple chronic conditions in the United States' Medicare population," *Health and Quality of Life Outcomes*, vol. 7, article 82, 2009.

[41] C. C. Earle, "Failing to plan is planning to fail: improving the quality of care with survivorship care plans," *Journal of Clinical Oncology*, vol. 24, no. 32, pp. 5112–5116, 2006.

Breastfeeding and Postpartum Depression: An Overview and Methodological Recommendations for Future Research

Carley J. Pope and Dwight Mazmanian

Department of Psychology, Lakehead University, 955 Oliver Road, Thunder Bay, ON, Canada P7B 5E1

Correspondence should be addressed to Carley J. Pope; cpope@lakeheadu.ca

Academic Editor: Janusz K. Rybakowski

Emerging research suggests that a relationship exists between breastfeeding and postpartum depression; however, the direction and precise nature of this relationship are not yet clear. The purpose of this paper is to provide an overview of the relationship between breastfeeding and postpartum depression as it has been examined in the empirical literature. Also, the potential mechanisms of action that have been implicated in this relationship are also explored. PubMed and PsycINFO were searched using the keywords: *breastfeeding* with *postpartum depression, perinatal depression, postnatal depression*. Results of this search showed that researchers have examined this relationship in diverse ways using diverse methodology. In particular, researchers have examined the relationships between postpartum depression and breastfeeding intention, initiation, duration, and dose. Due to a number of methodological differences among past studies we make some recommendations for future research that will better facilitate an integration of findings. Future research should (1) use standardized assessment protocols; (2) confirm diagnosis through established clinical interview when possible; (3) provide a clear operationalized definition for breastfeeding variables; (4) clearly define the postpartum period interval assessed and time frame for onset of symptoms; (5) be prospective or longitudinal in nature; and (6) take into consideration other potential risk factors identified in the empirical literature.

1. Introduction

Postpartum depression is a serious mental health condition that affects an estimated 13% to 19% of women who have recently given birth [1]. Postpartum depression is characterized as a persistent low mood in new mothers, which is often accompanied by feelings of sadness, worthlessness, and/or hopelessness. Postpartum depression differs from the "baby blues," as the "baby blues" is a briefer period of emotional disturbance (including dysphoria, tearfulness, mood lability, trouble sleeping, irritability, and anxiety) that is experienced by up to 4 in 5 women within the first few days following childbirth and usually remits within 10 days [1, 2].

Currently, the Diagnostic and Statistical Manual for Mental Disorders-Fifth Edition (DSM-5) classifies depression with peripartum onset as beginning during pregnancy or within the first four weeks postpartum [3]. The International Classification of Diseases (ICD) classifies postpartum depression as occurring within the first six weeks postpartum [4]. In contrast to the current criteria, some researchers recommend that this time frame be extended in future revisions of these guides to account for episode onset within the first six months postpartum [5]. Further, in spite of the current ICD and DSM-5 guidelines, many researchers use a time frame that ranges up to one year postpartum for onset of postpartum depression [1].

While the clinical profile of postpartum depression is similar to depression occurring at other times in a woman's life, it may differ in some respects due to the profound physiological changes occurring during pregnancy and the postpartum period [1, 6]. In fact, it is estimated that as many as 80% of postpartum women experience symptoms of mood disturbance within the first few days following childbirth [7]. Moreover, many postpartum women experience symptoms following pregnancy that are characteristic of depression, such as disturbances in appetite, energy, and sleep [8]. These factors make it difficult to differentiate onset of a clinically significant depressive disorder from common symptoms experienced as a result of childbirth and caring for a new infant.

While postpartum depression can be brief and remit unexpectedly, approximately 30% of women in community samples who experience postpartum depression continue to be depressed up to two years postpartum [9], and 50% of women from clinical samples continue to have major depression throughout, and in some cases beyond, the first year postpartum [10]. Furthermore, the illness course can vary and chronic depression for these women may consist of stable mild depression, stable major depression, or recurrent episodes of major depression without full remission between episodes [10].

2. Consequences of Postpartum Depression

Compared to depression occurring at other time points in a woman's life, there is some evidence to suggest that women experiencing postpartum depression are at an increased risk for comorbid obsessive compulsive disorder [11, 12] and anxiety [11, 13, 14]. For example, one study reported that 19.9% of women screening positive for postpartum depression at 2 weeks postpartum also screened positive for anxiety (compared to 1.3% of women who did not screen positive for postpartum depression; $p < 0.001$). In this same study, 25.7% of women screening positive for postpartum depression at 2 weeks postpartum also screened positive for obsessive compulsive symptoms (compared to 8.4% of women who did not screen positive for postpartum depression; $p < 0.001$). Suicidal ideation and thoughts of self-harm or thoughts of harming the infant are also reported to be more common in women with postpartum depression [15–18]. For instance, one study found that 30% of women who screened positive for postpartum depression endorsed at least some experience of thoughts of self-harm [17]. In another study, 41% of depressed mothers reported at least some thoughts regarding harming their infant compared to 7% of control mothers [15].

In addition to being at increased risk for comorbid disorders, postpartum depression is associated with numerous consequences in other domains [19]. Negative long-term consequences to the infant's social, emotional, cognitive, and physical development have been reported [20]. Children of mothers with a history of postpartum depression may also be at increased risk of developing psychosocial and emotional or behavioural disturbances [21], as well as intellectual disabilities [22]. Additionally, postpartum depression is associated with disturbance in mother-infant interactions and bonding, as well as deficient parenting and parental safety practices [20, 23]. Spinelli [24] has reported that infanticide is rare in women who are experiencing nonpsychotic postpartum depression, but infanticide is a possible serious and tragic consequence when postpartum depression is accompanied by psychosis. Although postpartum psychosis only occurs following one to two out of 1000 births [3], it can result in other serious and devastating consequences for the mother and the infant, as well as the rest of the family [25]. Often postpartum psychosis leads to hospitalization and considerable functional impairment [26]. There is, however, some debate concerning the degree to which psychosis is related to the unipolar variation of postpartum depression [24]. Emerging evidence suggests that postpartum psychosis is more likely a variant of bipolar disorder [27].

Due to the potential devastating consequences of postpartum depression for the mother, the infant, and their family, it is necessary that research clearly delineate the potential risk and protective factors for postpartum depression. Emerging research suggests that breastfeeding may offer protective benefits against postpartum depression [28]; however, the exact nature of the association between breastfeeding and postpartum depression remains unclear [29]. The purpose of this paper is to provide an overview of the association between breastfeeding and postpartum depression as it has been examined in the empirical literature. To conduct this review we searched PubMed and PsycINFO using the keywords: *breastfeeding* with *postpartum depression, perinatal depression, postnatal depression*. All original studies located through this search and reported in English examining the relationship between postpartum depression and breastfeeding were included.

3. Breastfeeding and Postpartum Depression

Initially the relationship between breastfeeding and postpartum depression was conceptualized to be unidirectional, with postpartum depression resulting in lower rates of breastfeeding initiation and early cessation [30]. More recently however, reports indicate that the relationship may be bidirectional in nature, suggesting that while postpartum depression may reduce rates of breastfeeding, not engaging in breastfeeding may increase the risk of postpartum depression. Additionally, there is some evidence that breastfeeding may protect against postpartum depression or assist in a swifter recovery from symptoms [28].

The association between breastfeeding and postpartum depression has been studied by a number of investigators, but the direction of this relationship and the question of whether it is a direct relationship still eludes us. Numerous studies on the topic of breastfeeding and postpartum depression have come to contrasting conclusions, likely a result of the interaction between the numerous and complex physiological, psychological, and sociocultural mechanisms potentially responsible for the relationship [31], as well as the use of varying methods for studying the association. Specifically, a number of researchers have reported no relationship between breastfeeding and postpartum depression (e.g., see [32]) and two early reports suggested that breastfeeding mothers have a higher risk of depression [33, 34]. In contrast, a number of more recent studies have revealed that women who formula feed have higher rates of depression than women who breastfeed (e.g., see [35]), while other researchers have shown that mothers who experience postpartum depression are at greater risk of early breastfeeding cessation (e.g., see [36]).

4. Breastfeeding Intention and Initiation

Intention to breastfeed refers to the perinatal decision to breastfeed an infant following childbirth, but the prenatal time frame may differ between studies depending on when this information was obtained (i.e., prospectively or retrospectively). Breastfeeding initiation refers broadly to the act of breastfeeding. Unfortunately, breastfeeding initiation is operationalized differently between investigations and may include women who attempt to breastfeed but discontinue shortly thereafter, women who exclusively breastfeed for long periods, women who used expressed breast milk, and women who supplement their infant with formula in addition to breastfeeding. These discrepancies can complicate our interpretation of the research. With that being said, a number of investigators have examined the relationship between breastfeeding intention or initiation and postpartum depression.

Some researchers have found no association between prenatal depressive symptoms and intention to breastfeed [37–40]. In contrast, Insaf and colleagues [41] did find that women with prenatal depressive symptoms were less likely to intend to breastfeed, though this study did not follow the women through to childbirth to determine initiation rates. Similarly, Fairlie and colleagues [42] also found that prenatal depressive symptoms were associated with a reduced intention to breastfeed (reported in the second trimester). However, follow-up in the postpartum period revealed that depressive symptoms during pregnancy were not associated with the actual initiation of breastfeeding, indicating that some of the women who initially reported that they did not intend to breastfeed changed their minds and attempted to breastfeed. Furthermore, Pippins and colleagues [43] found, in their longitudinal study following a large sample of pregnant women, that women with prenatal depressive symptoms were not less likely to initiate breastfeeding. Thus, it appears that women's prenatal intention to breastfeed may fluctuate, perhaps due to breastfeeding encouragement or education in the third trimester.

The potential relationship between breastfeeding intention and initiation and postpartum depression was further explored by Borra et al. [44]. In this large longitudinal study the investigators found that, in women who were not depressed before delivery, the risk of postpartum depression was decreased if they had intended to breastfeed and initiated breastfeeding. In contrast, women were at an increased risk for postpartum depression if they had not intended to breastfeed and initiated breastfeeding. Interestingly, Davey and colleagues [45] found that failure to breastfeed (when attempted) is associated with postpartum depressive symptoms. Also, women who never established breastfeeding were reported to have a 2.4-fold chance of developing depressive symptoms at 16 weeks postpartum compared to breastfeeding women [46].

5. Breastfeeding and Maternal Mood

A number of studies report that women who are not breastfeeding are more likely to have higher levels of depressive symptoms than women who are breastfeeding [35, 47–61]. For example, a recent longitudinal study by Nishioka and colleagues [57] found that at 5 months postpartum the proportion of mothers with an Edinburgh Postnatal Depression Scale [62] score of ≥9 (suggesting risk of postpartum depression) was significantly lower for women who were breastfeeding compared to women who were formula feeding ($p = 0.04$). Moreover, the inverse relationship between breastfeeding and postpartum depressive symptoms was found to persist even once age and education were controlled (OR = 0.28, $p = 0.007$) [63] and when income, race, previous history of depression, or current psychoactive medication use was controlled ($p < 0.001$) [64]. Interestingly, one study found that depression severity was not related to breastfeeding status in a group of women diagnosed with postpartum depression [65]. Thus, while breastfeeding may be associated with depressive symptoms, it may not influence the severity of the symptoms.

Although postpartum depression has been identified as a risk factor for early breastfeeding cessation [56], early negative breastfeeding experiences may be a risk factor for postpartum depression [66]. Further, it has also been suggested that breastfeeding may offer protective benefits against postpartum depression [28]. One study to report on the protective benefits of breastfeeding found that lower levels of depressive symptoms in the prenatal but not postnatal period predicted exclusive breastfeeding. Furthermore, breastfeeding duration was associated with a significant decrease in depressive symptom scores from childbirth to 3 months postpartum for women who initiated breastfeeding. These investigators also found that women who did not initiate breastfeeding did not experience changes in depressive symptoms over the first three postpartum months. After considering the findings collectively, the investigators postulated that breastfeeding alleviates depressive symptomology over time [28].

Additionally, results from a study by Mezzacappa and Katkin [67] lend further support to the premise that breastfeeding offers ameliorating effects on postpartum depressive mood symptoms. These investigators looked at the acute effects of breastfeeding on maternal mood and found that breastfeeding mothers experienced a decrease in negative mood from prefeeding to postfeeding. Moreover, bottle-feeding mothers experienced a decrease in positive mood from prefeeding to postfeeding. Thus, breastfeeding may offer both acute and long-term ameliorating effects on postpartum depression; however, further research is required to substantiate these initial findings.

6. Breastfeeding Duration

Breastfeeding duration has been found to be inversely related to postpartum depressive symptoms. A relationship has been found to persist even after controlling for socioeconomic status, age, and education level [68], as well as for past history of depression, increased life stress, and psychoactive medication use [64]. In particular, a number of studies have reported an association between postpartum depressive symptoms and early weaning [30, 69–75]. In fact, McLearn et al. [56] reported that mothers with depressive symptoms were less likely to continue breastfeeding through to two to four months postpartum compared to mothers without depressive symptoms (AOR = 0.73, $p < 0.001$).

A number of studies note that postpartum depressive symptoms preceded breastfeeding cessation [68, 76]. In a large prospective study of postpartum women, Taveras and colleagues [77] found that having higher depressive symptoms at two weeks postpartum was associated with discontinuation of breastfeeding at 12 weeks postpartum. Dennis and McQueen [36] reported similar findings. Specifically, depressive symptomology in the early postpartum period predicted early cessation of breastfeeding at eight weeks postpartum. Also, in a smaller prospective study, Galler et al. [78] found that depressive symptoms at seven weeks postpartum inversely predicted breastfeeding practices at seven weeks, three months, and six months postpartum, even after controlling for disadvantaged environmental conditions. Interestingly, these investigators did not find an association between depressive symptoms at six months postpartum and breastfeeding practices at the same time point.

More recently, Dennis and McQueen [36] found that after controlling for baseline depressive symptoms there was no relationship between infant feeding outcome (feeding method used, satisfaction with method, breastfeeding difficulties, and breastfeeding self-efficacy) at one week postpartum and the development of postpartum depressive symptoms (measured one and two months postpartum). However, the women in this study who reported high levels of postpartum depressive symptoms were significantly more likely to discontinue breastfeeding. These women were also more likely to report being unsatisfied with their infant-feeding method, experience breastfeeding difficulties, and report lower breastfeeding self-efficacy. Taken together, these findings suggested that over time depressive symptoms may influence breastfeeding outcomes to a point of discontinuation.

7. Breastfeeding Dose-Response Effect

A dose-response effect of breastfeeding on postpartum depression has been proposed. In a large study of women evaluated between 8 and 12 weeks postpartum, Thome et al. [79] found that exclusively breastfeeding mothers had lower mean depressive symptom scores compared to partial breastfeeding mothers. Relatedly, Ystrom [80] found that, at six months postpartum, both partially breastfeeding and exclusively bottle-feeding were significantly related to higher levels of depressive symptoms in postpartum women compared to those who exclusively breastfed. Furthermore, bottle-feeding was related to postpartum depression to a greater degree than partial breastfeeding. Also, when the investigator adjusted for baseline prenatal anxiety and depression (measured at 30 weeks of gestation) the relationship persisted, indicating that breastfeeding may reduce depressive symptoms or depressive symptoms may result in breastfeeding titration.

One other study compared exclusive breastfeeding to exclusive bottle-feeding [81]. These investigators found an inverse association between postpartum depression and exclusive breastfeeding continuation. Also, it has been found that as early as one week postpartum levels of depressive symptoms are inversely related to exclusive breastfeeding [82]. Moreover, Kendall-Tackett et al. [83] investigated the effects of breastfeeding on women at high risk for postpartum depression and sleep difficulties due to a history of being victims of sexual assault. These investigators reported a relationship between exclusive breastfeeding and fewer reported sleep difficulties and depressive symptoms compared to women who partially breastfed or bottle-fed their infant. Unfortunately these results are based on analyses of cross-sectional data, making the direction of the relationship in each case unclear.

8. Reciprocal Relational Findings

In light of conflicting reports that postpartum depression leads to early breastfeeding cessation (e.g., see [56]) and that breastfeeding leads to a reduction in postpartum depressive symptoms (e.g., see [67]), recent investigations have examined the possible reciprocal relationship. Specifically, it has been proposed that postpartum depression can lead to early breastfeeding cessation but breastfeeding continuation may also reduce levels of postpartum depressive symptoms [28]. For example, results of a study by Hamdan and Tamim [31] support the reciprocal relationship hypothesis. These investigators found that women who were breastfeeding at two months postpartum had a lower risk of postpartum depression at four months postpartum. On the other hand, women who had postpartum depression at two months postpartum were less likely to be breastfeeding at four months postpartum. Also, Hahn-Holbrook et al. [84] found that prenatal depressive symptoms predicted a reduced frequency of breastfeeding and earlier cessation within the first three months postpartum. These researchers also found that more frequent breastfeeding at three months postpartum was associated with greater subsequent declines in depressive symptom levels up to two years postpartum.

9. No Association or Nonsignificant Trends

A number of studies have reported no significant relationship between postpartum depression and breastfeeding status [32, 39, 85–91]. However, two of these studies did report finding a nonsignificant trend suggestive of an inverse association [86, 89]. In any case, most of these findings were incidental; the primary purpose of those investigations was not to evaluate the association between breastfeeding and postpartum depression. However, recent data analyzed in our lab also failed to find support for a relationship between breastfeeding intention and initiation when controlling for other risk factors for postpartum depression.

10. Conflicting Research Findings

A majority of studies do report some association between breastfeeding and postpartum depression; however the direction of the relationship is unclear and some of the findings conflict with one another. This is likely a reflection of both the complex processes responsible for the association between breastfeeding and postpartum depression and the differences between the study designs and the samples used. Dennis and McQueen [92] suggested that the contrasting findings may be due to differences in research methodology or study limitations. Some of the limitations include differences in definition and criteria for assessing breastfeeding. That is, a number of studies only classified breastfeeding as a "yes" or "no" dichotomy, failing to take into account partial breastfeeding (e.g., see [32, 39, 87, 88, 90]). Also, one of the methodological differences that makes integration and comparison of studies difficult pertains to various discrepancies in how postpartum depression is operationalized between studies. For instance, some studies used assessment instruments that were not specific to depression (e.g., see [87]) or used lower cut-off scores (e.g., see [88, 89]) compared to most investigations. Furthermore, some studies used samples with higher than normal rates of women reporting postpartum depression. For instance, Lau and Chan [89] found the rate of postpartum depression in their sample to be 34%, which is about double the estimated prevalence [1], likely a result of the low cut-off score they used. Also, some studies used women at high risk for postpartum depression. For instance, Kendall-Tackett et al.'s [83] investigation used women who reported a history of sexual assault, a proposed risk factor for postpartum depression [10]. Furthermore, for many of the studies, the primary focus was not to delineate the relationship between breastfeeding and depression [92], which likely explains many of the methodological or interpretive shortfalls noted.

11. Mechanism of Action

The mechanisms by which breastfeeding is affected by or affects postpartum depression have been assessed in a number of studies. Breastfeeding self-efficacy and negative breastfeeding perceptions have been implicated as playing a primary role in the relationship. Specifically, during the first week postpartum, depressed mothers have been found to be at increased risk for feeling unsatisfied with breastfeeding and were experiencing significant breastfeeding problems. They are also at risk for experiencing lower levels of breastfeeding self-efficacy compared to nondepressed mothers [36].

Furthermore, mothers' postpartum depressive symptoms were found in one study to be inversely related to the belief that breastfeeding is the best option for infant feeding and positively related to the beliefs that breastfeeding is private and breastfeeding is restrictive [93]. Additionally, in a study that did not find a relationship between breastfeeding and depressive symptoms, women who worried about breastfeeding were significantly more likely to develop depression than women who did not worry [32]. Similarly, Tamminen [94] found that women with more depressive symptoms also reported more breastfeeding difficulties, and Dennis [95] noted that level of depressive symptoms at one, four, and eight weeks postpartum was inversely related to breastfeeding self-efficacy at the corresponding time periods. This is a similar finding to that recorded by Dai and Dennis [96]. Collectively, this research suggests that it is not necessarily the postpartum depression per se that leads to reduced breastfeeding; it might be the mothers' negative perceptions of their breastfeeding experiences that are responsible.

Alternatively, complications with the mother-infant interaction may also play a role. One study reported that breastfeeding led to less burping, less intrusive stimulation (e.g., mother poking the infant or moving) during nipple-in and nipple-out periods, and more stroking (by the mother to the infant) as well as superior mother-infant interaction rating scores as rated by an observer. Further, these benefits were found to extend to both the depressed and nondepressed breastfeeding women [97]. Thus, breastfeeding may enhance the mother-child interaction, which may lead to improved maternal mental health.

Breastfeeding difficulties and lack of breastfeeding confidence are reported as common concerns for mothers with postpartum depressive symptoms [98]. Dennis and McQueen [36] suggested that the factors underlying the relationship between breastfeeding duration and postpartum depression are multifactorial. In other words, it is likely that the interplay between the mothers' negative cognitions and impaired mother-infant interaction, in addition to other factors, such as underlying physiological processes, are responsible for the emergence of postpartum depression. Moreover, depressive symptoms in the early postpartum period resulted in the mother being more vulnerable to feelings of low self-esteem and self-efficacy. As a consequence, the depressive symptoms and accompanying negative cognitions may reinforce perceived breastfeeding difficulties or may reduce the mothers' ability to accurately interpret infant cues, further perpetuating actual breastfeeding difficulties [36].

Also, breastfeeding is suggested to attenuate neuroendocrine responses to stress and may act to enhance maternal mood. Specifically, oxytocin and prolactin, hormones responsible for lactation, are suggested to have mood-ameliorating effects. Oxytocin in particular is a hormone that promotes feelings of nurturance and relaxation during nursing [99–101]. Also, lactation is suggested to attenuate cortisol stress responses [102] by decreasing stress hormone levels (especially cortisol) and enhancing sleep [103]. In addition to enhancing mood, a number of neuroendocrine mechanisms have been implicated in both breastfeeding failure and postpartum depression including gonadal/placental steroids and lactogenic hormones, as well as neuroendocrine pathways related to stress reactivity [104]. Moreover, it is also possible that only a subset of women who have a hormonal sensitivity are at risk for depressive symptoms in relation to breastfeeding cessation. Thus, future research aimed at assessing the specific circumstances whereby breastfeeding may offer protective or ameliorating benefits against postpartum depression is warranted and needed in order to make informed recommendations tailored to each new mothers' unique circumstance.

12. Future Research

Future researchers examining the relationship between breastfeeding and postpartum depression should consider the following methodological recommendations. These recommendations are made in an effort to make results of this research more comparable and to allow for an integration of findings to aid in conclusions and clinical recommendations. Future researchers should use standardized assessment protocols and cut-off values established by psychometric evaluations of the measures. Currently the Edinburgh Postnatal Depression Scale (EPDS) is among the most widely used empirically validated self-report screening measures for postpartum depression. Using a cut-off value of 13 or greater, this measure is reported to have a sensitivity of 68–86%, specificity of 78–96%, and positive predictive value of 67–73%

[62, 105]. When possible, diagnostic clarification through the use of established structured clinical interviews is ideal as this process is currently the gold standard for psychiatric diagnosis. Use of both the EPDS and diagnostic interviews can be valuable as each provides a different approach to examining the relationship between breastfeeding and postpartum depression. That is, information from the EPDS allows researchers to evaluate depressive symptoms on a continuum to examine whether breastfeeding status might be associated with more transient symptoms or subclinical levels of depression. The addition of a diagnostic interview allows researchers to evaluate whether breastfeeding is involved in clinically confirmed postpartum depression.

Future researchers should also specify and clearly define breastfeeding variables as well as the time intervals assessed for postpartum depression. Investigators should also make efforts to determine the time frame for onset of symptoms. Currently there is debate over the time frame at which a woman is considered to have onset of a postpartum depressive episode [1]. Diagnostic guidelines dictate time frames ranging from anytime during pregnancy to the first six weeks postpartum [3, 4]. However, many researchers and clinicians consider onset within the first year postpartum to be considered a postpartum depressive episode [1, 5]. Due to the lack of consensus regarding what constitutes postpartum onset and variation in the postpartum intervals investigated by researchers it is important that investigators are very clear about the interval addressed in their research. This is especially pertinent as various biological, environmental, and psychosocial factors that may influence the relationship between breastfeeding and postpartum depression can vary depending on the postpartum time period being assessed.

Research that is prospective or longitudinal in nature will also be helpful in evaluating the direction of the proposed relationship between breastfeeding and postpartum depression. This will facilitate inferences regarding the temporal relationship. Such designs should take into consideration other potential factors suggested to influence postpartum depression. Considering the role of other potential postpartum depression risk factors within the breastfeeding and postpartum depression dynamic will better facilitate interpretation of results. Some of the risk factors more commonly identified in research include low socioeconomic status [1, 31], poor social support [46], and history of depression [31, 43, 45, 53].

13. Conclusions

The primary purpose of this paper was to provide an overview of the potential relationships between breastfeeding and postpartum depression that have been suggested by research and to provide recommendations to facilitate comparisons between investigations. Due to numerous methodological discrepancies between studies it is difficult to draw conclusions at this time. Also, interpretations of research are impeded by many of the same conundrums that exist when attempting to empirically understand postpartum depression in general. For instance, much of the research is naturalistic in nature, restricting the ability to make causal inferences. Also, the physiological changes that occur over the course of pregnancy and the postpartum period are not completely understood and hormonal shifts during the postpartum period may influence women's mental health and well-being in different ways depending on the time period referenced. Improved standardization between future research investigations will promote comparison between studies. To facilitate comparison and integration of study findings in this area we recommend that future research protocols (1) use standardized assessment protocols; (2) confirm diagnosis through established clinical interview when possible; (3) provide a clear operationalized definition for breastfeeding variables; (4) clearly define the postpartum period interval assessed and time frame for onset of symptoms; (5) be prospective or longitudinal in nature; and (6) take into consideration other potential risk factors identified in the empirical literature.

Competing Interests

The authors declare that there are no competing interests regarding the publication of this paper.

Acknowledgments

C. J. Pope gratefully acknowledges financial support from the Canadian Institutes of Health Research.

References

[1] M. W. O'Hara and J. E. McCabe, "Postpartum depression: current status and future directions," *Annual Review of Clinical Psychology*, vol. 9, pp. 379–407, 2013.

[2] J. Heron, S. Haque, F. Oyebode, N. Craddock, and I. Jones, "A longitudinal study of hypomania and depression symptoms in pregnancy and the postpartum period," *Bipolar Disorders*, vol. 11, no. 4, pp. 410–417, 2009.

[3] American Psychiatric Association, *Diagnostic and Statistical Manual of Mental Disorders*, American Psychiatric Association, Washington, DC, USA, 5th edition, 2013.

[4] World Health Organization, *The ICD-10 Classification of Mental and Behavioural Disorders*, World Health Organization, 2010, http://www.who.int/classifications/icd/en/.

[5] V. Sharma and D. Mazmanian, "The DSM-5 peripartum specifier: prospects and pitfalls," *Archives of Women's Mental Health*, vol. 17, no. 2, pp. 171–173, 2014.

[6] M. Bloch, P. J. Schmidt, M. Danaceau, J. Murphy, L. Nieman, and D. R. Rubinow, "Effects of gonadal steroids in women with a history of postpartum depression," *The American Journal of Psychiatry*, vol. 157, no. 6, pp. 924–930, 2000.

[7] M. M. Buttner, M. W. O'Hara, and D. Watson, "The structure of women's mood in the early postpartum," *Assessment*, vol. 19, no. 2, pp. 247–256, 2012.

[8] M. W. O'Hara, J. A. Schlechte, D. A. Lewis, and E. J. Wright, "Prospective study of postpartum blues: biologic and psychosocial factors," *Archives of General Psychiatry*, vol. 48, no. 9, pp. 801–806, 1991.

[9] J. A. Horowitz and J. Goodman, "A longitudinal study of maternal postpartum depression symptoms," *Research and Theory for Nursing Practice*, vol. 18, no. 2-3, pp. 149–163, 2004.

[10] N. Vliegen, S. Casalin, and P. Luyten, "The course of postpartum depression: a review of longitudinal studies," *Harvard Review of Psychiatry*, vol. 22, no. 1, pp. 1–22, 2014.

[11] E. S. Miller, D. Hoxha, K. L. Wisner, and D. R. Gossett, "The impact of perinatal depression on the evolution of anxiety and obsessive-compulsive symptoms," *Archives of Women's Mental Health*, vol. 18, no. 3, pp. 457–461, 2014.

[12] E. J. Russell, J. M. Fawcett, and D. Mazmanian, "Risk of obsessive-compulsive disorder in pregnant and postpartum women: a meta-analysis," *Journal of Clinical Psychiatry*, vol. 74, no. 4, pp. 377–385, 2013.

[13] V. Hendrick, L. Altshuler, T. Strouse, and S. Grosser, "Postpartum and nonpostpartum depression: differences in presentation and response to pharmacologic treatment," *Depression and Anxiety*, vol. 11, no. 2, pp. 66–72, 2000.

[14] M. O'Brien, E. Buikstra, and D. Hegney, "The influence of psychological factors on breastfeeding duration," *Journal of Advanced Nursing*, vol. 63, no. 4, pp. 397–408, 2008.

[15] K. D. Jennings, S. Ross, S. Popper, and M. Elmore, "Thoughts of harming infants in depressed and nondepressed mothers," *Journal of Affective Disorders*, vol. 54, no. 1-2, pp. 21–28, 1999.

[16] C. J. Pope, B. Xie, V. Sharma, and M. K. Campbell, "A prospective study of thoughts of self-harm and suicidal ideation during the postpartum period in women with mood disorders," *Archives of Women's Mental Health*, vol. 16, no. 6, pp. 483–488, 2013.

[17] K. L. Wisner, D. K. Y. Sit, M. C. McShea et al., "Onset timing, thoughts of self-harm, and diagnoses in postpartum women with screen-positive depression findings," *JAMA Psychiatry*, vol. 70, no. 5, pp. 490–498, 2013.

[18] V. Lindahl, J. L. Pearson, and L. Colpe, "Prevalence of suicidality during pregnancy and the postpartum," *Archives of Women's Mental Health*, vol. 8, no. 2, pp. 77–87, 2005.

[19] C. J. Pope, V. Sharma, and D. Mazmanian, "Recognition, diagnosis and treatment of postpartum bipolar depression," *Expert Review of Neurotherapeutics*, vol. 14, no. 1, pp. 19–28, 2014.

[20] T. Field, "Postpartum depression effects on early interactions, parenting, and safety practices: a review," *Infant Behavior & Development*, vol. 33, no. 1, pp. 1–6, 2010.

[21] M. Korhonen, I. Luoma, R. Salmelin, and T. Tamminen, "A longitudinal study of maternal prenatal, postnatal and concurrent depressive symptoms and adolescent well-being," *Journal of Affective Disorders*, vol. 136, no. 3, pp. 680–692, 2012.

[22] V. A. Morgan, M. L. Croft, G. M. Valuri et al., "Intellectual disability and other neuropsychiatric outcomes in high-risk children of mothers with schizophrenia, bipolar disorder and unipolar major depression," *The British Journal of Psychiatry*, vol. 200, no. 4, pp. 282–289, 2012.

[23] E. Moehler, R. Brunner, A. Wiebel, C. Reck, and F. Resch, "Maternal depressive symptoms in the postnatal period are associated with long-term impairment of mother-child bonding," *Archives of Women's Mental Health*, vol. 9, no. 5, pp. 273–278, 2006.

[24] M. G. Spinelli, "Maternal infanticide associated with mental illness: prevention and the promise of saved lives," *The American Journal of Psychiatry*, vol. 161, no. 9, pp. 1548–1557, 2004.

[25] S. Ganjekar, G. Desai, and P. S. Chandra, "A comparative study of psychopathology, symptom severity, and short-term outcome of postpartum and nonpostpartum mania," *Bipolar Disorders*, vol. 15, no. 6, pp. 713–718, 2013.

[26] E. Robertson, I. Jones, S. Haque, R. Holder, and N. Craddock, "Risk of puerperal and non-puerperal recurrence of illness following bipolar affective puerperal (post-partum) psychosis," *The British Journal of Psychiatry*, vol. 186, no. 3, pp. 258–259, 2005.

[27] I. Brockington, "Postpartum psychiatric disorders," *The Lancet*, vol. 363, no. 9405, pp. 303–310, 2004.

[28] B. Figueiredo, C. Canário, and T. Field, "Breastfeeding is negatively affected by prenatal depression and reduces postpartum depression," *Psychological Medicine*, vol. 44, no. 5, pp. 927–936, 2014.

[29] C. C. Dias and B. Figueiredo, "Breastfeeding and depression: a systematic review of the literature," *Journal of Affective Disorders*, vol. 171, pp. 142–154, 2015.

[30] L. Seimyr, M. Edhborg, W. Lundh, and B. Sjögren, "In the shadow of maternal depressed mood: experiences of parenthood during the first year after childbirth," *Journal of Psychosomatic Obstetrics and Gynecology*, vol. 25, no. 1, pp. 23–34, 2004.

[31] A. Hamdan and H. Tamim, "The relationship between postpartum depression and breastfeeding," *International Journal of Psychiatry in Medicine*, vol. 43, no. 3, pp. 243–259, 2012.

[32] L. H. Chaudron, M. H. Klein, P. Remington, M. Palta, C. Allen, and M. J. Essex, "Predictors, prodromes and incidence of postpartum depression," *Journal of Psychosomatic Obstetrics & Gynecology*, vol. 22, no. 2, pp. 103–112, 2001.

[33] E. M. Alder and J. L. Cox, "Breast feeding and post-natal depression," *Journal of Psychosomatic Research*, vol. 27, no. 2, pp. 139–144, 1983.

[34] E. Alder and J. Bancroft, "The relationship between breast feeding persistence, sexuality and mood in postpartum women," *Psychological Medicine*, vol. 18, no. 2, pp. 389–396, 1988.

[35] M. W. Groër, "Differences between exclusive breastfeeders, formula-feeders, and controls: a study of stress, mood, and endocrine variables," *Biological Research for Nursing*, vol. 7, no. 2, pp. 106–117, 2005.

[36] C.-L. Dennis and K. McQueen, "Does maternal postpartum depressive symptomatology influence infant feeding outcomes?" *Acta Paediatrica*, vol. 96, no. 4, pp. 590–594, 2007.

[37] J. Barnes, A. Stein, T. Smith, and J. I. Pollock, "Extreme attitudes to body shape, social and psychological factors and a reluctance to breast feed. ALSPAC Study Team. Avon Longitudinal Study of Pregnancy and Childhood," *Journal of the Royal Society of Medicine*, vol. 90, no. 10, pp. 551–559, 1997.

[38] S. W. Jacobson, J. L. Jacobson, and K. F. Frye, "Incidence and correlates of breast-feeding in socioeconomically disadvantaged women," *Pediatrics*, vol. 88, no. 4, pp. 728–736, 1991.

[39] M. D. McKee, L. H. Zayas, and K. R. B. Jankowski, "Breastfeeding intention and practice in an urban minority population: relationship to maternal depressive symptoms and mother-infant closeness," *Journal of Reproductive and Infant Psychology*, vol. 22, no. 3, pp. 167–181, 2004.

[40] H. J. Lee, M. R. Rubio, I. T. Elo, K. F. McCollum, E. K. Chung, and J. F. Culhane, "Factors associated with intention to breastfeed among low-income, inner-city pregnant women," *Maternal and Child Health Journal*, vol. 9, no. 3, pp. 253–261, 2005.

[41] T. Z. Insaf, R. T. Fortner, P. Pekow, N. Dole, G. Markenson, and L. Chasan-Taber, "Prenatal stress, anxiety, and depressive symptoms as predictors of intention to breastfeed among Hispanic women," *Journal of Women's Health*, vol. 20, no. 8, pp. 1183–1192, 2011.

[42] T. G. Fairlie, M. W. Gillman, and J. Rich-Edwards, "High pregnancy-related anxiety and prenatal depressive symptoms as predictors of intention to breastfeed and breastfeeding initiation," *Journal of Women's Health*, vol. 18, no. 7, pp. 945–953, 2009.

[43] J. R. Pippins, P. Brawarsky, R. A. Jackson, E. Fuentes-Afflick, and J. S. Haas, "Association of breastfeeding with maternal depressive symptoms," *Journal of Women's Health*, vol. 15, no. 6, pp. 754–762, 2006.

[44] C. Borra, M. Iacovou, and A. Sevilla, "New evidence on breastfeeding and postpartum depression: the importance of understanding women's intentions," *Maternal and Child Health Journal*, vol. 19, no. 4, pp. 897–907, 2015.

[45] H. L. Davey, S. C. Tough, C. E. Adair, and K. M. Benzies, "Risk factors for sub-clinical and major postpartum depression among a community cohort of canadian women," *Maternal and Child Health Journal*, vol. 15, no. 7, pp. 866–875, 2011.

[46] D. Nielsen Forman, P. Videbech, M. Hedegaard, J. D. Salvig, and N. J. Secher, "Postpartum depression: identification of women at risk," *BJOG: An International Journal of Obstetrics & Gynaecology*, vol. 107, no. 10, pp. 1210–1217, 2000.

[47] M. Abou-Saleh, R. Ghubash, L. Karim, M. Krymski, and I. Bhai, "Hormonal aspects of postpartum depression," *Psychoneuroendocrinology*, vol. 23, no. 5, pp. 465–475, 1998.

[48] J. Astbury, S. Brown, J. Lumley, and R. Small, "Birth events, birth experiences and social differences in postnatal depression," *Australian Journal of Public Health*, vol. 18, no. 2, pp. 176–184, 1994.

[49] K. Green, H. Broome, and J. Mirabella, "Postnatal depression among mothers in the United Arab Emirates: socio-cultural and physical factors," *Psychology, Health and Medicine*, vol. 11, no. 4, pp. 425–431, 2006.

[50] M. W. Groer and K. Morgan, "Immune, health and endocrine characteristics of depressed postpartum mothers," *Psychoneuroendocrinology*, vol. 32, no. 2, pp. 133–139, 2007.

[51] K. H. Gross, C. S. Wells, A. Radigan-Garcia, and P. M. Dietz, "Correlates of self-reports of being very depressed in the months after delivery: results from the pregnancy risk assessment monitoring system," *Maternal and child health journal*, vol. 6, no. 4, pp. 247–253, 2002.

[52] P. Hannah, D. Adams, A. Lee, V. Glover, and M. Sandler, "Links between early post-partum mood and post-natal depression," *The British Journal of Psychiatry*, vol. 160, pp. 777–780, 1992.

[53] R. Jardri, J. Pelta, M. Maron et al., "Predictive validation study of the Edinburgh postnatal depression scale in the first week after delivery and risk analysis for postnatal depression," *Journal of Affective Disørders*, vol. 93, no. 1–3, pp. 169–176, 2006.

[54] A. Lane, R. Keville, M. Morris, A. Kinsella, M. Turner, and S. Barry, "Postnatal depression and elation among mothers and their partners: prevalence and predictors," *The British Journal of Psychiatry*, vol. 171, pp. 550–555, 1997.

[55] F. Mancini, C. Carlson, and L. Albers, "Use of the postpartum depression screening scale in a collaborative obstetric practice," *Journal of Midwifery and Women's Health*, vol. 52, no. 5, pp. 429–434, 2007.

[56] K. T. McLearn, C. S. Minkovitz, D. M. Strobino, E. Marks, and W. Hou, "Maternal depressive symptoms at 2 to 4 months post partum and early parenting practices," *Archives of Pediatrics and Adolescent Medicine*, vol. 160, no. 3, pp. 279–284, 2006.

[57] E. Nishioka, M. Haruna, E. Ota et al., "A prospective study of the relationship between breastfeeding and postpartum depressive symptoms appearing at 1-5 months after delivery," *Journal of Affective Disorders*, vol. 133, no. 3, pp. 553–559, 2011.

[58] T. Tammentie, M.-T. Tarkka, P. Åstedt-Kurk, and E. Paavilainen, "Sociodemographic factors of families related to postnatal depressive symptoms of mothers," *International Journal of Nursing Practice*, vol. 8, no. 5, pp. 240–256, 2002.

[59] A. Tashakori, A. Z. Behbahani, and R. D. Irani, "Comparison of prevalence of postpartum depression symptoms between breastfeeding mothers an non-breastfeeding mothers," *Iranian Journal of Psychiatry*, vol. 7, no. 2, pp. 61–65, 2012.

[60] R. Warner, L. Appleby, A. Whitton, and B. Faragher, "Demographic and obstetric risk factors for postnatal psychiatric morbidity," *The British Journal of Psychiatry*, vol. 168, no. 5, pp. 607–611, 1996.

[61] K. A. Yonkers, S. M. Ramin, A. J. Rush et al., "Onset and persistence of postpartum depression in an inner-city maternal health clinic system," *The American Journal of Psychiatry*, vol. 158, no. 11, pp. 1856–1863, 2001.

[62] J. L. Cox, J. M. Holden, and R. Sagovsky, "Detection of postnatal depression: development of the 10-item edinburgh postnatal depression scale," *British Journal of Psychiatry*, vol. 150, pp. 782–786, 1987.

[63] S. Dunn, B. Davies, L. McCleary, N. Edwards, and I. Gaboury, "The relationship between vulnerability factors and breastfeeding outcome," *Journal of Obstetric, Gynecologic, & Neonatal Nursing*, vol. 35, no. 1, pp. 87–97, 2006.

[64] D. C. Hatton, J. Harrison-Hohner, S. Coste, V. Dorato, L. B. Curet, and D. A. McCarron, "Symptoms of postpartum depression and breastfeeding," *Journal of Human Lactation*, vol. 21, no. 4, pp. 444–449, 2005.

[65] D. McCarter-Spaulding and J. A. Horowitz, "How does postpartum depression affect breastfeeding?" *MCN The American Journal of Maternal/Child Nursing*, vol. 32, no. 1, pp. 10–17, 2007.

[66] S. Watkins, S. Meltzer-Brody, D. Zolnoun, and A. Stuebe, "Early breastfeeding experiences and postpartum depression," *Obstetrics & Gynecology*, vol. 118, no. 2, part 1, pp. 214–221, 2011.

[67] E. S. Mezzacappa and E. S. Katkin, "Breast-feeding is associated with reduced perceived stress and negative mood in mothers," *Health Psychology*, vol. 21, no. 2, pp. 187–193, 2002.

[68] J. J. Henderson, S. F. Evans, J. A. Y. Straton, S. R. Priest, and R. Hagan, "Impact of postnatal depression on breastfeeding duration," *Birth*, vol. 30, no. 3, pp. 175–180, 2003.

[69] I. Akman, M. K. Kuscu, Z. Yurdakul et al., "Breastfeeding duration and postpartum psychological adjustment: role of maternal attachment styles," *Journal of Paediatrics and Child Health*, vol. 44, no. 6, pp. 369–373, 2008.

[70] D. E. Bick, C. MacArthur, and R. J. Lancashire, "What influences the uptake and early cessation of breast feeding?" *Midwifery*, vol. 14, no. 4, pp. 242–247, 1998.

[71] P. J. Cooper, L. Murray, and A. Stein, "Psychosocial factors associated with the early termination of breast-feeding," *Journal of Psychosomatic Research*, vol. 37, no. 2, pp. 171–176, 1993.

[72] O. G. Falceto, E. R. J. Giugliani, and C. L. C. Fernandes, "Influence of parental mental health on early termination of breastfeeding: a case-control study," *Journal of the American Board of Family Practice*, vol. 17, no. 3, pp. 173–183, 2004.

[73] S. S. Fergerson, D. J. Jamieson, and M. Lindsay, "Diagnosing postpartum depression: can we do better?" *American Journal of Obstetrics & Gynecology*, vol. 186, no. 5, pp. 899–902, 2002.

[74] T. A. Papinczak and C. T. Turner, "An analysis of personal and social factors influencing initiation and duration of breastfeeding in a large Queensland maternity hospital," *Breastfeeding Review*, vol. 8, no. 1, pp. 25–33, 2000.

[75] T. Pearlstein, M. Howard, A. Salisbury, and C. Zlotnick, "Postpartum depression," *American Journal of Obstetrics & Gynecology*, vol. 200, no. 4, pp. 357–364, 2009.

[76] S. Misri, D. A. Sinclair, and A. J. Kuan, "Breast-feeding and postpartum depression: is there a relationship?" *The Canadian Journal of Psychiatry*, vol. 42, no. 10, pp. 1061–1065, 1997.

[77] E. M. Taveras, A. M. Capra, P. A. Braveman, N. G. Jensvold, G. J. Escobar, and T. A. Lieu, "Clinician support and psychosocial risk factors associated with breastfeeding discontinuation," *Pediatrics*, vol. 112, no. 1, part 1, pp. 108–115, 2003.

[78] J. R. Galler, R. H. Harrison, M. A. Biggs, F. Ramsey, and V. Forde, "Maternal moods predict breastfeeding in Barbados," *Journal of Developmental and Behavioral Pediatrics*, vol. 20, no. 2, pp. 80–87, 1999.

[79] M. Thome, E. M. Alder, and A. Ramel, "A population-based study of exclusive breastfeeding in Icelandic women: is there a relationship with depressive symptoms and parenting stress?" *International Journal of Nursing Studies*, vol. 43, no. 1, pp. 11–20, 2006.

[80] E. Ystrom, "Breastfeeding cessation and symptoms of anxiety and depression: a longitudinal cohort study," *BMC Pregnancy and Childbirth*, vol. 12, article 36, 2012.

[81] M. E. Flores-Quijano, A. Córdova, V. Contreras-Ramírez, L. Farias-Hernández, M. Cruz Tolentino, and E. Casanueva, "Risk for postpartum depression, breastfeeding practices, and mammary gland permeability," *Journal of Human Lactation*, vol. 24, no. 1, pp. 50–57, 2008.

[82] T. J. Clifford, K. M. Campbell, K. N. Speechley, and F. Gorodzinsky, "Factors influencing full breastfeeding in a Southwestern Ontario community: assessments at 1 week and at 6 months postpartum," *Journal of Human Lactation*, vol. 22, no. 3, pp. 292–304, 2006.

[83] K. Kendall-Tackett, Z. Cong, and T. W. Hale, "Depression, sleep quality, and maternal well-being in postpartum women with a history of sexual assault: a comparison of breastfeeding, mixed-feeding, and formula-feeding mothers," *Breastfeeding Medicine*, vol. 8, no. 1, pp. 16–22, 2013.

[84] J. Hahn-Holbrook, M. G. Haselton, C. Dunkel Schetter, and L. M. Glynn, "Does breastfeeding offer protection against maternal depressive symptomatology?: a prospective study from pregnancy to 2 years after birth," *Archives of Women's Mental Health*, vol. 16, no. 5, pp. 411–422, 2013.

[85] D. L. Bogen, B. H. Hanusa, E. Moses-Kolko, and K. L. Wisner, "Are maternal depression or symptom severity associated with breastfeeding intention or outcomes?" *Journal of Clinical Psychiatry*, vol. 71, no. 8, pp. 1069–1078, 2010.

[86] E. K. Chung, K. F. McCollum, I. T. Elo, H. J. Lee, and J. F. Culhane, "Maternal depressive symptoms and infant health practices among low-income women," *Pediatrics*, vol. 113, no. 6, pp. e523–e529, 2004.

[87] J. L. Cox, Y. Connor, and R. E. Kendell, "Prospective study of the psychiatric disorders of childbirth," *British Journal of Psychiatry*, vol. 140, no. 2, pp. 111–117, 1982.

[88] A. Josefsson, L. Angelsiöö, G. Berg et al., "Obstetric, somatic, and demographic risk factors for postpartum depressive symptoms," *Obstetrics and Gynecology*, vol. 99, no. 2, pp. 223–228, 2002.

[89] Y. Lau and K. S. Chan, "Influence of intimate partner violence during pregnancy and early postpartum depressive symptoms on breastfeeding among chinese women in Hong Kong," *Journal of Midwifery and Women's Health*, vol. 52, no. 2, pp. e15–e20, 2007.

[90] T. O'Neill, P. Murphy, and V. T. Greene, "Postnatal depression—aetiological factors," *Irish Medical Journal*, vol. 83, no. 1, pp. 17–18, 1990.

[91] M. Ramsay, E. G. Gisel, J. McCusker, F. Bellavance, and R. Platt, "Infant sucking ability, non-organic failure to thrive, maternal characteristics, and feeding practices: a prospective cohort study," *Developmental Medicine & Child Neurology*, vol. 44, no. 6, pp. 405–414, 2002.

[92] C.-L. Dennis and K. McQueen, "The relationship between infant-feeding outcomes and postpartum depression: a qualitative systematic review," *Pediatrics*, vol. 123, no. 4, pp. e736–e751, 2009.

[93] J. R. Galler, R. H. Harrison, F. Ramsey, S. Chawla, and J. Taylor, "Postpartum feeding attitudes, maternal depression, and breastfeeding in Barbados," *Infant Behavior and Development*, vol. 29, no. 2, pp. 189–203, 2006.

[94] T. Tamminen, "The impact of mother's depression on her nursing experiences and attitudes during breastfeeding," *Acta Paediatrica Scandinavica. Supplement*, vol. 344, pp. 87–94, 1988.

[95] C. L. Dennis, "The breastfeeding self-efficacy scale: psychometric assessment of the short form," *Journal of Obstetric, Gynecologic, & Neonatal Nursing*, vol. 32, no. 6, pp. 734–744, 2003.

[96] X. Dai and C.-L. Dennis, "Translation and validation of the breastfeeding self-efficacy scale into Chinese," *Journal of Midwifery and Women's Health*, vol. 48, no. 5, pp. 350–356, 2003.

[97] T. Field, M. Diego, M. Hernandez-Reif, B. Figueiredo, S. Ezell, and V. Siblalingappa, "Depressed mothers and infants are more relaxed during breastfeeding versus bottlefeeding interactions: brief report," *Infant Behavior and Development*, vol. 33, no. 2, pp. 241–244, 2010.

[98] M. Edhborg, A.-S. Matthiesen, W. Lundh, and A.-M. Widström, "Some early indicators for depressive symptoms and bonding 2 months postpartum—a study of new mothers and fathers," *Archives of Women's Mental Health*, vol. 8, no. 4, pp. 221–231, 2005.

[99] A.-S. Matthiesen, A.-B. Ransjö-Arvidson, E. Nissen, and K. Uvnäs-Moberg, "Postpartum maternal oxytocin release by newborns: effects of infant hand massage and sucking," *Birth*, vol. 28, no. 1, pp. 13–19, 2001.

[100] A. Skalkidou, C. Hellgren, E. Comasco, S. Sylvén, and I. Sundström Poromaa, "Biological aspects of postpartum depression," *Women's Health*, vol. 8, no. 6, pp. 659–672, 2012.

[101] C. Viero, I. Shibuya, N. Kitamura et al., "Oxytocin: crossing the bridge between basic science and pharmacotherapy," *CNS Neuroscience & Therapeutics*, vol. 16, no. 5, pp. e138–e156, 2010.

[102] B. Figueiredo, C. C. Dias, S. Brandão, C. Canário, and R. Nunes-Costa, "Breastfeeding and postpartum depression: state of the art review," *Jornal de Pediatria*, vol. 89, no. 4, pp. 332–338, 2013.

[103] M. T. Tu, S. J. Lupien, and C.-D. Walker, "Diurnal salivary cortisol levels in postpartum mothers as a function of infant feeding choice and parity," *Psychoneuroendocrinology*, vol. 31, no. 7, pp. 812–824, 2006.

[104] A. M. Stuebe, K. Grewen, C. A. Pedersen, C. Propper, and S. Meltzer-Brody, "Failed lactation and perinatal depression: common problems with shared neuroendocrine mechanisms?" *Journal of Women's Health*, vol. 21, no. 3, pp. 264–272, 2012.

[105] L. Murray and A. D. Carothers, "The validation of the Edinburgh Post-natal depression scale on a community sample," *The British Journal of Psychiatry*, vol. 157, no. 2, pp. 288–290, 1990.

A Possible Role of Anhedonia as Common Substrate for Depression and Anxiety

Luigi Grillo

Via Ragazzi del 99, No. 45, 20010 San Giorgio su Legnano, Italy

Correspondence should be addressed to Luigi Grillo; luigi.grillo01@libero.it

Academic Editor: Wai-Kwong Tang

Depression and anxiety are often comorbid, in up to 70% of cases, and the level of one or the other may fluctuate, leading now to a diagnosis of depression, now to a diagnosis of anxiety. For these reasons, and for the presence of many other common factors, it has been suggested that both are part of the same continuum of problems and that they have a common substrate. This paper proposes the possibility that anhedonia may be an important component of this possible common substrate, and it tries to identify the mechanism with which anhedonia could contribute to causing both depression and anxiety. It also proposes an explanation why an intense pleasure could improve both depression and anxiety.

1. Introduction

Depression and anxiety are often comorbid, in up to 70% of cases [1], and the level of one or the other may fluctuate, leading now to a diagnosis of depression, now to a diagnosis of anxiety [2, 3]. Both are preceded and facilitated by stress, either recent [4–9] or dating back to childhood [10–12], they are often accompanied by the search for drugs [13–15], they are part of the symptoms of withdrawal from drugs [15], and they are associated with rumination (i.e., with lingering over the same gloomy thoughts) [16]. They are also characterized by anhedonia [17–22], a reduction of the ability to feel pleasures.

According to Cohen et al., "despite increased attention over the past 25 years on the comorbidity between depression and anxiety, there is still a great deal of uncertainty over why these two disorders are so highly comorbid" [23]. And according to Starr and Davila, "although several comorbidity theories exist, the most prominent ones attribute anxiety-depression comorbidity to shared structural components. For example, Clark and Watson's (1991) tripartite model hypothesizes that anxiety is uniquely defined by physiological hyperarousal and depression by anhedonia but that both disorders share the common thread of elevated negative affectivity. Other researchers have presented similar structural models, in which shared underlying factors account for depression-anxiety cooccurrence. The tripartite model and other structural models have greatly expanded our understanding of anxiety-depression comorbidity, providing a nuanced view of which aspects of anxiety and depressive symptoms are most likely to cooccur. However, these models do not sufficiently explain depression-anxiety cooccurrence, for several reasons. First, although a number of studies have supported the tripartite model's three factors, others have not. Second, studies have shown both that physiological hyperactivity is correlated with depression and that anhedonia is correlated with anxiety, contradicting the specificity hypothesis of the tripartite model and suggesting that cooccurrence is not entirely accounted for by the hypothesized shared substrates" [24].

Starr and Davila also propose a model of their own, in which "anxiety symptoms lead to depressive symptoms via maladaptive anxiety response styles," bearing in mind that "many anxious people may develop hopeless thoughts about their anxiety" and that "in turn, several researchers have identified hopelessness and related attributions as a key risk factor for depressive symptoms" [24]. The "hopeless thoughts" of many anxious people seem to reveal that they live in a situation of continuous severe stress.

For their intermingling, and for the presence of many common factors, the possibility has been proposed that depression and anxiety are both part of the same continuum of problems [25, 26] and that they have a common substrate [27–29] that some authors suggest might be anhedonia [22].

The presence of anhedonia both in anxiety and in depression could be explained by the fact that both conditions are induced by stress [6, 30], and stress—acute or chronic—is regularly accompanied and followed by anhedonia in humans [9, 17, 31, 32] and in animals [33, 34].

The reduction of the ability to feel pleasure caused by stressful events tends to be long-lasting. For instance, traumatic experiences in infancy may cause anhedonia in adult life in man [35] and in animals [36]. Naturally, we are talking about significant anhedonia: low-grade anhedonia is normally present even in healthy people [37] who have not suffered severe stress, as everyday adversities are more or less stressful, and in some cases humiliation or feeling subordinate [38] or a low income [39] is enough to reduce a person's capacity for pleasure.

2. Anhedonia and Depression

Anhedonia is a key symptom of major depression [31, 40, 41] and it can influence many of its symptoms. Let us consider, for example, apathy in depressed people. Each action normally tends to provide pleasure [42]. Even freeing oneself from an unpleasant or painful situation is a pleasure [43], and this pleasure is at the basis of the attempts to escape from difficult situations [44, 45]. If we are unable to feel pleasures, as in the case of anhedonia, the desire to perform the actions necessary to achieve them is reduced or disappears [46] and may result in various levels of apathy [47].

Even difficulty in concentrating and keeping up attention, present in depression, could depend on anhedonia. In fact, the ability to feel pleasures seems to influence the ability to perceive and connect sensory information and the ability to learn. For example, in animals, when two separate stimuli, which individually do not provoke pleasure, are mentally connected to each other, the formation of this new bond causes pleasure, and this is considered important for learning in general [48, 49]. In man, satisfying a curiosity is pleasant [50], just as it is pleasant to grasp an inner meaning [51], and the pleasure connected to awaiting a novelty (novelties are pleasant [52]) facilitates learning [53]. So, at least in part, the reduced capacity to apply oneself encountered in depressed people could depend on the scarcity or lack of their ability to feel these pleasures. Moreover, a reduced hedonic tone is associated with a reduction of the cognitive processes both in the first automatic phase and in the subsequent phases of processing sensations [41].

Even rumination, which is frequent in depression [54], could derive from anhedonia: the ability to feel pleasures, in fact, allows an extension of both verbal [55–57] and visual [56, 57] associations and improves rumination [58]. Also the gloomy mood of depressed persons could be partially explained by the fact that they have to lead a life without everyday pleasures and they are unable to be active in a satisfactory way.

3. Pleasures and Depression

Various pleasant sensations can improve both anhedonia and depression, and this fact seems to be a further suggestion that anhedonia can influence many of the symptoms of depression. In man, drugs are used by anhedonic persons, with or without psychiatric disturbances, to try to reduce their reward deficit [59], and opioids have had an important role in the treatment of depression [60]. Depressed persons sometimes use sweet or fatty foods as self-medication, according to some authors to compensate the loss of the ability to feel normal pleasures [59, 61]. In rats, an enriched environment improves depression [62, 63] and so do sweet or fatty foods [64].

All these pleasures that are able to have a positive influence on anhedonia and depression have one particular feature: they give a pleasure more intense than ordinary everyday pleasures. The intensity of the pleasure produced by opioids and other drugs is well known, and also sweet or fatty foods are very strong pleasures for both men and animals [65–67]. Besides the possibility of physical exercise (which is an important pleasure if voluntary [68, 69]), an enriched environment also implies continuous novelties [63], and novelties provide strong pleasure [70, 71].

Since depression is characterized by anhedonia, perhaps these pleasures must be particularly intense to be able to overcome the high threshold for pleasure that characterizes anhedonia: in this way, a certain number of depressed people could feel them even when normal pleasures are no longer felt.

The mechanism with which a strong pleasure seems able to have a positive influence on depression is still not clear. An improvement of depression should mean regaining the ability to enjoy the ordinary pleasures of life, an ability that had been lost or very much reduced because of anhedonia. But how could a single pleasure, however intense it may be, for example, a dose of drugs, allow the recovery of sensitivity of many other different, less intense pleasures, much more normal and everyday, the loss of which is the central factor of depression?

An answer might be suggested by a particular aspect of the pleasant stimuli: besides giving pleasure, they also allow simultaneous or subsequent pleasures to be felt more intensely for a certain period. For example, a single dose of drugs causes an increase of sensitivity to subsequent pleasures, both to drugs [72, 73] and to normal pleasures such as food and social play [72, 74–78]. Normal pleasures in turn increase the pleasure given both by drugs [77, 79, 80] and by other normal pleasures [81], so that, in conclusion, "the perceived value of present reward is built upon past reward exposure" [81]. The high threshold for pleasure due to anhedonia prevents depressed persons from enjoying normal everyday pleasures, but some sufficiently intense pleasures could overcome this threshold, still be perceived, and be able to increase and recover other pleasures previously faded or lost. In this way, anhedonic persons could recover the possibility of enjoying ordinary everyday pleasures and leading a more pleasant life for some time. This could explain the fact why only particularly intense pleasures seem to be able to improve anhedonia and depression.

4. Stress, Dynorphin, and Anhedonia

Many of the pleasures that are able to improve depression also improve anxiety. For example, in man, opioids can relieve both depression and anxiety [60, 82], and alcohol is sought to cope with both conditions [83–89]. In animals, an enriched environment [63, 90–93] and agreeable foods [94–96] can improve depression and anxiety. This could suggest that anhedonia might contribute to causing, in addition to depression, even anxiety. But if it is fairly understandable that anhedonia could cause many of the symptoms of depression [97], it is difficult to imagine how anhedonia could cause anxiety.

At this point, it could be useful to recall the mechanism with which stress can provoke anhedonia. Some hormones are released during intense or repeated stress: adrenalin and noradrenaline which help to combat stress by increasing the flow of blood and glucose to the muscles and the brain, and corticotropin-releasing hormone (CRH) which in turn provokes the release of cortisone, the action of which accompanies and reinforces that of adrenalin and noradrenaline. The CRH also releases another hormone, dynorphin [97–99], which reduces the release of dopamine in the nucleus accumbens [100, 101]. The dopamine released in the nucleus accumbens produces pleasure [44, 102], so that stress can reduce the ability to perceive pleasure by reducing dopamine through the action of dynorphin. (As well as dopamine, opioids too are involved in feeling pleasure [103], and it has been proposed that dopamine is more involved in the search for pleasure, while opioids are involved in its enjoyment [104]. However, the action of dopamine and that of opioids are closely interwoven and overlapped, since dopamine releases endogenous opioids [105–108], while the opioids in turn release dopamine in the nucleus accumbens [105]. In this chain of interconnections between dopamine and endogenous opioids, some authors believe that dopamine could be the "basic link" [109].) On account of its ability to cause anhedonia, dynorphin is considered to be responsible for depression due to stress [14].

Dynorphin is released not only in the case of stress, but also in the case of an excessive release of dopamine, for example, when taking drugs. All drugs cause a marked increase of dopamine in the nucleus accumbens [100, 102, 107], and the intense pleasure that they procure is in most cases the reason why they are initially sought [110, 111]. However, if the use of drugs continues, the pleasure is reduced more and more. This reduction seems to be a consequence of the excessive pleasure of the drugs: to counterbalance the excessive dopamine stimulus, which can be harmful, dynorphin is released [100, 112, 113], which reduces the dopamine with consequent anhedonia. The effect of dynorphin is long-lasting [100, 113], and it is considered responsible, not only for anhedonia, but also for withdrawal symptoms (anxiety, agitation, depression, etc.) which are perceived when the effect of the drug ceases [113]. To rid oneself of withdrawal symptoms it is necessary to take the drug again, even though the pleasure that it procures is very much reduced because of anhedonia. At this point the search for drugs becomes more and more compulsive and, from an optional way of behaviour, aimed at obtaining pleasure, it is transformed into a forced behaviour aimed at ridding the user of the painful states of distress and suffering that accompany withdrawal [110, 114, 115]. This is how addiction begins [116].

Among the negative states that are reported as hard to bear in the withdrawal syndrome, anxiety is particularly stressed and is considered a consequence of dynorphin. In fact, dynorphin provokes both anhedonia and anxiety. Its anxiogenic effect has not been considered in relation to anhedonia but has been considered a consequence of a direct action of dynorphin on the anxiogenic centres (in particular on the amygdala, through dynorphinic receptors—KOR, κ-opioid receptors—present in the amygdala) [97].

However, this possible direct action of dynorphin does not explain the fact that many substances or situations that provoke intense pleasures possess an anxiolytic effect: as we have seen, opioids and alcohol can improve anxiety in man, while in animals pleasant foods, an enriched environment, and alcohol have the same positive effect on anxiety. It is perhaps worth considering the possibility that a possible direct action of dynorphin on the anxiogenic centres may be accompanied by an indirect anxiogenic action mediated by the anhedonic effect of dynorphin. Some authors leave this possibility open: "Given the high comorbidity of depressive and anxiety disorders, KOR signalling and control of DA function may underlie the pathogenesis of both" [6]. A possible anxiogenic action through a reduction of DA (dopamine) function and consequent anhedonia would allow the unification of the action mechanism of dynorphin on both anxiety and depression and could help explain why an intense pleasure is able to improve both depression and anxiety. But how could anhedonia arouse anxiety, that is, arouse an inexplicable fear of a grave imminent and unknown danger?

5. Anhedonia and Anxiety

The image of the world we receive through what we see and hear has to be continuously reassembled and reorganized; otherwise it could become distorted and fragmented and could change so much that we hardly recognize it. As regards the visual aspect, "our perceptual impressions of an object and its context are in permanent flux as we move or as the object moves or transforms itself: the (perceived) world is not static but permanently physically changing" [117]. We must immediately realize that a foreshortening is not a real deformation, that an object that is partially hidden is not cut off but extends under the cover, that a cloud seen through the branches of a tree is not part of the tree, and so on. For example, every time we look at a three-dimensional object from a different angle "the observer should be expected to see an object of changing shape. The cube should undergo constant amoebic transformations… Fortunately, but surprisingly enough, this does not happen" [118, p. 71]. But perhaps this might happen if something interferes with the mechanism of the indispensable continuous reorganization and interpretation of an "amoebic" reality. In this case, the alterations might become evident, objects might seem deformed and frightening, sky and clouds might seem head-spinningly close to the observer, making the surrounding world flat and oppressive, and so on.

One of the possible factors that might interfere with the indispensable and continuous reconstruction of the world could be anhedonia. We have seen how, according to many researchers, our ability to feel pleasure can influence our ability to perceive and connect sensory information. As regards the visual aspect in particular, recognizing an expected image gives pleasure, and if the image is unexpected the pleasure is even greater [119]. Recognizing a shape in an ambiguous context gives pleasure [51] and this stimulates us to look for other ambiguous shapes to discover their correct shape [117]. Getting rid of visual ambiguity gives pleasure in the same way as escaping a danger, on condition that we feel sufficiently protected in the moments of uncertainty that accompany the attempt to understand [120]. Visual learning is also facilitated by a simultaneous pleasure, even if this pleasure is completely extraneous to vision [121].

If we do not feel these pleasures, as may happen in some cases of marked anhedonia, our ability continuously to correct and interpret the variable aspect of our surroundings might be reduced and various degrees of frightening alteration of the aspect of the environment might result. Even in a person without psychiatric pathologies, the sudden awareness of a deformation of the appearance of the environment, deformation that had always been present but had previously been ignored, may give rise to intense anxiety. An example of this can be found in "art and visual perception," a book by Rudolf Arnheim, former president of the Division on Psychology and the Arts of the American Psychological Association, where the author describes the distressed reaction of a student when, following a suggestion by the teacher, she became aware of the deformations assumed by the appearance of an object according to the viewpoint from which it was observed, deformations which she had always corrected automatically without realizing it. "It is very difficult for many persons to visualize the working of perspective, even when it is demonstrated to them with a yardstick. Recently an intelligent and sensitive young college student, to whom I tried to show the oblique shape of a box on the table, finally hid her face in sudden terror and exclaimed: 'It is true - how horrible!'" [118, p. 160]. And in the case reported by Arnheim it was only a completely explainable alteration of the appearance of a single small object.

Perhaps even just a very brief, but unexpected and inexplicable deformation of some aspect of the environment caused by anhedonia might give in some cases the sensation that the apparent normality of the objects is only a fragile veil, which could be torn and reveal inexplicable and frightening deformities. Even only the vague feeling that this might happen might induce indefinable, inexpressible fear of imminent catastrophe, generating a state of anxiety, the cause of which cannot be explained to other people because the sufferers cannot explain it to themselves.

In any case, the hypothesis that a reduction of the pleasures connected with vision, or with other sensory information, could create difficulties in the indispensable, unceasing reconstruction of an environment that is continuously "physically changing" [117], and that this could contribute to the onset of anxiety might perhaps help us explain why an intense pleasure is able to relieve temporarily not only depression but also anxiety.

6. How a Pleasure, Sufficiently Intense to Be Felt, Could Improve Not Only Depression but Also Anxiety?

If we accept that anhedonia can contribute, through sensory alterations and consequent alterations of the environment, to the onset of the anxiety that accompanies depression, it becomes possible to propose an explanation of the reason why some intense pleasures improve anxiety as well as depression: their antianxiety action could depend, like the antidepressive action, on their ability to make lost or faded pleasures be perceived again. In fact, if the recovered pleasures also included those felt when perceiving and correctly connecting sensory information, these pleasures might help to recover the normal, indispensable ability to reconstruct the continuously variable aspect of the environment, which would thus be safe and familiar again. In this way, a sufficiently intense pleasure could reduce, with anhedonia, both depression and anxiety and help to lead a normal life again, at least for a certain time.

Conflict of Interests

The author declares that there is no conflict of interests regarding the publication of this paper.

References

[1] Z. Wu and Y. Fang, "Comorbidity of depressive and anxiety disorders: challenges in diagnosis and assessment," *Shanghai Archives of Psychiatry*, vol. 26, no. 4, pp. 227–231, 2010.

[2] D. A. Katerndahl, A. C. Larme, R. F. Palmer, and N. Amodei, "Reflections on DSM classification and its utility in primary care: case studies in 'mental disorders,'" *The Primary Care Companion to the Journal of Clinical Psychiatry*, vol. 7, no. 3, pp. 91–99, 2005.

[3] D. E. Nease Jr., J. E. Aikens, and T. L. Schwenk, "Mental health disorders and their descriptive criteria in primary care: clarifying or confounding?" *Primary Care Companion to the Journal of Clinical Psychiatry*, vol. 7, no. 3, pp. 89–90, 2005.

[4] R. C. Brown, E. C. Berenz, S. H. Aggen et al., "Trauma exposure and Axis I psychopathology: a cotwin control analysis in Norwegian young adults," *Psychological Trauma*, vol. 6, no. 6, pp. 652–660, 2014.

[5] T. Ayazi, L. Lien, A. Eide, L. Swartz, and E. Hauff, "Association between exposure to traumatic events and anxiety disorders in a post-conflict setting: a cross-sectional community study in South Sudan," *BMC Psychiatry*, vol. 14, article 6, 2014.

[6] A. Van't Veer and W. A. Carlezon Jr., "Role of kappa-opioid receptors in stress and anxiety-related behavior," *Psychopharmacology*, vol. 229, no. 3, pp. 435–452, 2013.

[7] L. Gottlieb, H. Waitzkin, and J. Miranda, "Depressive symptoms and their social contexts: a qualitative systematic literature review of contextual interventions," *International Journal of Social Psychiatry*, vol. 57, no. 4, pp. 402–417, 2011.

[8] C. Person, M. Tracy, and S. Galea, "Risk factors for depression after a disaster," *Journal of Nervous and Mental Disease*, vol. 194, no. 9, pp. 659–666, 2006.

[9] D. A. Pizzagalli, R. Bogdan, K. G. Ratner, and A. L. Jahn, "Increased perceived stress is associated with blunted hedonic capacity: potential implications for depression research," *Behaviour Research and Therapy*, vol. 45, no. 11, pp. 2742–2753, 2007.

[10] E. L. Weiss, J. G. Longhurst, and C. M. Mazure, "Childhood sexual abuse as a risk factor for depression in women: psychosocial and neurobiological correlates," *American Journal of Psychiatry*, vol. 156, no. 6, pp. 816–828, 1999.

[11] J. L. Hamilton, B. G. Shapero, J. P. Stange, E. J. Hamlat, L. Y. Abramson, and L. B. Alloy, "Emotional maltreatment, peer victimization, and depressive versus anxiety symptoms during adolescence: hopelessness as a mediator," *Journal of Clinical Child and Adolescent Psychology*, vol. 42, no. 3, pp. 332–347, 2013.

[12] C. Heim and C. B. Nemeroff, "The role of childhood trauma in the neurobiology of mood and anxiety disorders: preclinical and clinical studies," *Biological Psychiatry*, vol. 49, no. 12, pp. 1023–1039, 2001.

[13] V. Jaquier, J. C. Flanagan, and T. P. Sullivan, "Anxiety and posttraumatic stress symptom pathways to substance use problems among community women experiencing intimate partner violence," *Anxiety, Stress and Coping*, vol. 28, no. 4, pp. 445–55, 2015.

[14] L. Lalanne, G. Ayranci, B. L. Kieffer, and P. E. Lutz, "The kappa opioid receptor: from addiction to depression, and back," *Frontiers in Psychiatry*, vol. 5, article 170, 2014.

[15] K. J. Hartwell, B. K. Tolliver, and K. T. Brady, "Biologic commonalities between mental illness and addiction," *Primary Psychiatry*, vol. 16, no. 8, pp. 33–39, 2009.

[16] S. Nolen-Hoeksema, B. E. Wisco, and S. Lyubomirsky, "Rethinking rumination," *Perspectives on Psychological Science*, vol. 3, no. 5, pp. 400–424, 2008.

[17] T. B. Kashdan, J. D. Elhai, and B. C. Frueh, "Anhedonia and emotional numbing in combat veterans with PTSD," *Behaviour Research and Therapy*, vol. 44, no. 3, pp. 457–467, 2006.

[18] L. K. Tremblay, C. A. Naranjo, S. J. Graham et al., "Functional neuroanatomical substrates of altered reward processing in major depressive disorder revealed by a dopaminergic probe," *Archives of General Psychiatry*, vol. 62, no. 11, pp. 1228–1236, 2005.

[19] C. Martin-Soelch, "Is depression associated with dysfunction of the central reward system?" *Biochemical Society Transactions*, vol. 37, no. 1, pp. 313–317, 2009.

[20] A. S. Farmer and T. B. Kashdan, "Affective and self-esteem instability in the daily lives of people with generalize social anxiety disorder," *Clinical Psychological Science*, vol. 2, no. 2, pp. 187–201, 2014.

[21] P. A. Frewen, D. J. Dozois, and R. A. Lanius, "Assessment of anhedonia in psychological trauma: psychometric and neuroimaging perspectives," *European Journal of Psychotraumatology*, vol. 3, article 8587, 2012.

[22] R. Admon, G. Lubin, J. D. Rosenblatt et al., "Imbalanced neural responsivity to risk and reward indicates stress vulnerability in humans," *Cerebral Cortex*, vol. 23, no. 1, pp. 28–35, 2013.

[23] J. R. Cohen, J. F. Young, B. E. Gibb, B. L. Hankin, and J. R. Z. Abela, "Why are anxiety and depressive symptoms comorbid in youth? A multi-wave, longitudinal examination of competing etiological models," *Journal of Affective Disorders*, vol. 161, pp. 21–29, 2014.

[24] L. R. Starr and J. Davila, "Responding to anxiety with rumination and hopelessness: mechanism of anxiety-depression symptom co-occurrence?" *Cognitive Therapy and Research*, vol. 36, no. 4, pp. 321–337, 2012.

[25] D. S. Baldwin, D. L. Evans, R. M. A. Hirschfeld, and S. Kasper, "Can we distinguish anxiety from depression?" *Psychopharmacology Bulletin*, vol. 36, supplement 2, pp. 158–165, 2002.

[26] M. E. Wadsworth, J. J. Hudziak, A. C. Heath, and T. M. Achenbach, "Latent class analysis of child behavior checklist anxiety/depression in children and adolescents," *Journal of the American Academy of Child and Adolescent Psychiatry*, vol. 40, no. 1, pp. 106–114, 2001.

[27] S. M. Paul, "Anxiety and depression: a common neurobiological substrate?" *Journal of Clinical Psychiatry*, vol. 49, Supplement, pp. 13–16, 1988.

[28] K. R. Merikangas, H. Zhang, S. Avenevoli, S. Acharyya, M. Neuenschwander, and J. Angst, "Longitudinal trajectories of depression and anxiety in a prospective community study: the Zurich Cohort Study," *Archives of General Psychiatry*, vol. 60, no. 10, pp. 993–1000, 2003.

[29] C. J. M. Colletti, R. Forehand, E. Garai et al., "Parent depression and child anxiety: an overview of the literature with clinical implications," *Child and Youth Care Forum*, vol. 38, no. 3, pp. 151–160, 2009.

[30] A. J. Grippo, K. D. Wu, I. Hassan, and C. S. Carter, "Social isolation in prairie voles induces behaviors relevant to negative affect: toward the development of a rodent model focused on co-occurring depression and anxiety," *Depression and anxiety*, vol. 25, no. 6, pp. E17–E26, 2008.

[31] R. Bogdan and D. A. Pizzagalli, "Acute stress reduces reward responsiveness: implications for depression," *Biological Psychiatry*, vol. 60, no. 10, pp. 1147–1154, 2006.

[32] J. W. Hopper, R. K. Pitman, Z. Su et al., "Probing reward function in posttraumatic stress disorder: expectancy and satisfaction with monetary gains and losses," *Journal of Psychiatric Research*, vol. 42, no. 10, pp. 802–807, 2008.

[33] P. Willner, R. Muscat, and M. Papp, "Cronic mild stress-induced anhedhonia: a realistic animal model of depression," *Neuroscience and Biobehavioral Reviews*, vol. 16, no. 4, pp. 525–534, 1992.

[34] A. Zurita, I. Martijena, G. Cuadra, M. L. Brandão, and V. Molina, "Early exposure to chronic variable stress facilitates the occurrence of anhedonia and enhanced emotional reactions to novel stressors: reversal by naltrexone pretreatment," *Behavioural Brain Research*, vol. 117, no. 1-2, pp. 163–171, 2000.

[35] D. G. Dillon, A. J. Holmes, J. L. Birk, N. Brooks, K. Lyons-Ruth, and D. A. Pizzagalli, "Childhood adversity is associated with left basal ganglia dysfunction during reward anticipation in adulthood," *Biological Psychiatry*, vol. 66, no. 3, pp. 206–213, 2009.

[36] M. Leventopoulos, H. Russig, J. Feldon, C. R. Pryce, and J. Opacka-Juffry, "Early deprivation leads to long-term reductions in motivation for reward and 5-HT1A binding and both effects are reversed by fluoxetine," *Neuropharmacology*, vol. 56, no. 3, pp. 692–701, 2009.

[37] J. Keller, C. B. Young, E. Kelley, K. Prater, D. J. Levitin, and V. Menon, "Trait anhedonia is associated with reduced reactivity and connectivity of mesolimbic and paralimbic reward pathways," *Journal of Psychiatric Research*, vol. 47, no. 10, pp. 1319–1328, 2013.

[38] P. Gilbert, S. Allan, S. Brough, S. Melley, and J. N. V. Miles, "Relationship of anhedonia and anxiety to social rank, defeat

and entrapment," *Journal of Affective Disorders*, vol. 71, no. 1–3, pp. 141–151, 2002.

[39] M. E. Silverman, P. Muennig, X. Liu, Z. Rosen, and M. A. Goldstein, "The Impact of socioeconomic status on the neural substrates associated with pleasure," *The Open Neuroimaging Journal*, vol. 3, pp. 58–63, 2009.

[40] S. Edwards and G. F. Koob, "Experimental psychiatric illness and drug abuse models: from human to animal, an overview," *Methods in Molecular Biology*, vol. 829, pp. 31–48, 2012.

[41] I. H. A. Franken, J. W. Van Strien, and I. M. T. Nijs, "Effect of hedonic tone on event-related potential measures of cognitive processing," *Psychiatry Research*, vol. 142, no. 2-3, pp. 233–239, 2006.

[42] J. W. Muschamp and W. A. Carlezon Jr., "Roles of nucleus accumbens CREB and dynorphin in dysregulation of motivation," *Cold Spring Harbor Perspectives in Medicine*, vol. 3, no. 2, Article ID a012005, 2013.

[43] M. Andreatta, A. Mühlberger, A. Yarali, B. Gerber, and P. Pauli, "A rift between implicit and explicit conditioned valence in human pain relief learning," *Proceedings of the Royal Society B: Biological Sciences*, vol. 277, no. 1692, pp. 2411–2416, 2010.

[44] S. Ikemoto and J. Panksepp, "The role of nucleus accumbens dopamine in motivated behavior: a unifying interpretation with special reference to reward-seeking," *Brain Research Reviews*, vol. 31, no. 1, pp. 6–41, 1999.

[45] G. Kohls, M. T. Perino, J. M. Taylor et al., "The nucleus accumbens is involved in both the pursuit of social reward and the avoidance of social punishment," *Neuropsychologia*, vol. 51, no. 11, pp. 2062–2069, 2013.

[46] M.-L. Cléry-Melin, L. Schmidt, G. Lafargue, N. Baup, P. Fossati, and M. Pessiglione, "Why don't you try harder? An investigation of effort production in major depression," *PLoS ONE*, vol. 6, no. 8, Article ID e23178, 2011.

[47] D. A. Pizzagalli, D. Iosifescu, L. A. Hallett, K. G. Ratner, and M. Fava, "Reduced hedonic capacity in major depressive disorder: evidence from a probabilistic reward task," *Journal of Psychiatric Research*, vol. 43, no. 1, pp. 76–87, 2008.

[48] A. M. J. Young, R. G. Ahier, R. L. Upton, M. H. Joseph, and J. A. Gray, "Increased extracellular dopamine in the nucleus accumbens of the rat during associative learning of neutral stimuli," *Neuroscience*, vol. 83, no. 4, pp. 1175–1183, 1998.

[49] M. H. Joseph, K. Datla, and A. M. J. Young, "The interpretation of the measurement of nucleus accumbens dopamine by in vivo dialysis: the kick, the craving or the cognition?" *Neuroscience and Biobehavioral Reviews*, vol. 27, no. 6, pp. 527–541, 2003.

[50] M. Jepma, R. G. Verdonschot, H. van Steenbergen, S. A. R. B. Rombouts, and S. Nieuwenhuis, "Neural mechanisms underlying the induction and relief of perceptual curiosity," *Frontiers in Behavioral Neuroscience*, vol. 6, article 5, 2012.

[51] C. Muth and C. C. Carbon, "The Aesthetic Aha. About the pleasure of having insights into Gestalt," *Acta Psychologica*, vol. 144, no. 1, pp. 25–30, 2013.

[52] B. C. Wittmann, N. Bunzeck, R. J. Dolan, and E. Düzel, "Anticipation of novelty recruits reward system and hippocampus while promoting recollection," *NeuroImage*, vol. 38, no. 1, pp. 194–202, 2007.

[53] N. Bunzeck and E. Düzel, "Absolute coding of stimulus novelty in the human substantia nigra/VTA," *Neuron*, vol. 51, no. 3, pp. 369–379, 2006.

[54] E. Watkins and R. G. Brown, "Rumination and executive function in depression: an experimental study," *Journal of Neurology Neurosurgery and Psychiatry*, vol. 72, no. 3, pp. 400–402, 2002.

[55] M. F. Mason and M. Bar, "The effect of mental progression on mood," *Journal of Experimental Psychology: General*, vol. 141, no. 2, pp. 217–221, 2012.

[56] G. Rowe, J. B. Hirsh, and A. K. Anderson, "Positive affect increases the breadth of attentional selection," *Proceedings of the National Academy of Sciences of the United States of America*, vol. 104, no. 1, pp. 383–388, 2007.

[57] M. Grol and R. D. Raedt, "Effects of positive mood on attentional breadth for emotional stimuli," *Frontiers in Psychology*, vol. 5, article 1277, 2014.

[58] F. Bahrami, R. Kasaei, and A. Zamani, "Preventing worry and rumination by induced positive emotion," *International Journal of Preventive Medicine*, vol. 3, no. 2, pp. 102–109, 2012.

[59] G. Martinotti, C. R. Cloninger, and L. Janiri, "Temperament and character inventory dimensions and anhedonia in detoxified substance-dependent subjects," *American Journal of Drug and Alcohol Abuse*, vol. 34, no. 2, pp. 177–183, 2008.

[60] P. L. Tenore, "Psychotherapeutic benefits of opioid agonist therapy," *Journal of Addictive Diseases*, vol. 27, no. 3, pp. 49–65, 2008.

[61] A. M. Leventhal, M. Brightman, K. J. Ameringer et al., "Anhedonia associated with stimulant use and dependence in a population-based sample of American adults," *Experimental and Clinical Psychopharmacology*, vol. 18, no. 6, pp. 562–569, 2010.

[62] M. L. Lehmann and M. Herkenham, "Environmental enrichment confers stress resiliency to social defeat through an infralimbic cortex-dependent neuroanatomical pathway," *Journal of Neuroscience*, vol. 31, no. 16, pp. 6159–6173, 2011.

[63] J. C. Brenes Sáenz, O. R. Villagra, and J. Fornaguera Trías, "Factor analysis of forced swimming test, sucrose preference test and Open Field test on enriched, social and isolated reared rats," *Behavioural Brain Research*, vol. 169, no. 1, pp. 57–65, 2006.

[64] J. Maniam and M. J. Morris, "Voluntary exercise and palatable high-fat diet both improve behavioural profile and stress responses in male rats exposed to early life stress: role of hippocampus," *Psychoneuroendocrinology*, vol. 35, no. 10, pp. 1553–1564, 2010.

[65] N. D. Volkow, G.-J. Wang, and R. D. Baler, "Reward, dopamine and the control of food intake: implications for obesity," *Trends in Cognitive Sciences*, vol. 15, no. 1, pp. 37–46, 2011.

[66] N. M. Avena, P. Rada, and B. G. Hoebel, "Evidence for sugar addiction: behavioral and neurochemical effects of intermittent, excessive sugar intake," *Neuroscience and Biobehavioral Reviews*, vol. 32, no. 1, pp. 20–39, 2008.

[67] T. Agurs-Collins and B. F. Fuemmeler, "Dopamine polymorphisms and depressive symptoms predict foods intake. Results from a nationally representative sample," *Appetite*, vol. 57, no. 2, pp. 339–348, 2011.

[68] W. J. Lynch, A. B. Peterson, V. Sanchez, J. Abel, and M. A. Smith, "Exercise as a novel treatment for drug addiction: a neurobiological and stage-dependent hypothesis," *Neuroscience and Biobehavioral Reviews*, vol. 37, no. 8, pp. 1622–1644, 2013.

[69] M. J. Morris, E. S. Na, and A. K. Johnson, "Voluntary running-wheel exercise decreases the threshold for rewarding intracranial self-stimulation," *Behavioral Neuroscience*, vol. 126, no. 4, pp. 582–587, 2012.

[70] C. M. Reichel and R. A. Bevins, "Competition between novelty and cocaine conditioned reward is sensitive to drug dose and

retention interval," *Behavioral Neuroscience*, vol. 124, no. 1, pp. 141–151, 2010.

[71] D. H. Zald, R. L. Cowan, P. Riccardi et al., "Midbrain dopamine receptor availability is inversely associated with novelty-seeking traits in humans," *Journal of Neuroscience*, vol. 28, no. 53, pp. 14372–14378, 2008.

[72] J. A. Kim, K. A. Pollak, G. O. Hjelmstad, and H. L. Fields, "A single cocaine exposure enhances both opioid reward and aversion through a ventral tegmental area-dependent mechanism," *Proceedings of the National Academy of Sciences of the United States of America*, vol. 101, no. 15, pp. 5664–5669, 2004.

[73] S. H. Criner, J. Liu, and G. Schulteis, "Rapid neuroadaptation in the nucleus accumbens and bed nucleus of the stria terminalis mediates suppression of operant responding during withdrawal from acute opioid dependence," *Neuroscience*, vol. 144, no. 4, pp. 1436–1446, 2007.

[74] V. Trezza, P. J. J. Baarendse, and L. J. M. J. Vanderschuren, "Prosocial effects of nicotine and ethanol in adolescents rats through partially dissociable neurobehavioral mechanisms," *Neuropsychopharmacology*, vol. 34, no. 12, pp. 2560–2573, 2009.

[75] V. Trezza and L. J. M. J. Vanderschuren, "Cannabinoid and opioid modulation of social play behavior in adolescent rats: differential behavioral mechanisms," *European Neuropsychopharmacology*, vol. 18, no. 7, pp. 519–530, 2008.

[76] M. Zhang and A. E. Kelley, "Opiate agonists microinjected into the nucleus accumbens enhance sucrose drinking in rats," *Psychopharmacology*, vol. 132, no. 4, pp. 350–360, 1997.

[77] K. J. Thiel, A. C. Okun, and J. L. Neisewander, "Social reward-conditioned place preference: a model revealing an interaction between cocaine and social context rewards in rats," *Drug and Alcohol Dependence*, vol. 96, no. 3, pp. 202–212, 2008.

[78] P. K. Olszewski, J. Alsiö, H. B. Schiöth, and A. S. Levine, "Opioids as facilitators of feeding: can any food be rewarding?" *Physiology & Behavior*, vol. 104, no. 1, pp. 105–110, 2011.

[79] K. K. Pitchers, V. Vialou, E. J. Nestler, S. R. Laviolette, M. N. Lehman, and L. M. Coolen, "Natural and drug rewards act on common neural plasticity mechanisms with ΔFosB as a key mediator," *The Journal of Neuroscience*, vol. 33, no. 8, pp. 3434–3442, 2013.

[80] S. Logue, J. Chein, T. Gould, E. Holliday, and L. Steinberg, "Adolescent mice, unlike adults, consume more alcohol in the presence of peers than alone," *Developmental Science*, vol. 17, no. 1, pp. 79–85, 2014.

[81] D. L. Wallace, V. Vialou, L. Rios et al., "The influence of DeltaFosB in the nucleus accumbens on natural reward-related behavior," *The Journal of Neuroscience*, vol. 28, no. 41, pp. 10272–10277, 2008.

[82] A. Colasanti, E. A. Rabiner, A. Lingford-Hughes, and D. J. Nutt, "Opioids and anxiety," *Journal of Psychopharmacology*, vol. 25, no. 11, pp. 1415–1433, 2011.

[83] V. V. Grant, S. H. Stewart, and C. D. Mohr, "Coping-anxiety and coping-depression motives predict different daily mood-drinking relationships," *Psychology of Addictive Behaviors*, vol. 23, no. 2, pp. 226–237, 2009.

[84] J. G. Murphy, A. M. Yurasek, A. A. Dennhardt et al., "Symptoms of depression and PTSD are associated with elevated alcohol demand," *Drug and Alcohol Dependence*, vol. 127, no. 1–3, pp. 129–136, 2013.

[85] R. M. Crum, L. La Flair, C. L. Storr et al., "Reports of drinking to self-medicate anxiety symptoms: longitudinal assessment for subgroups of individuals with alcohol dependence," *Depression and Anxiety*, vol. 30, no. 2, pp. 174–183, 2013.

[86] T. L. Simpson, C. A. Stappenbeck, J. A. Luterek, K. Lehavot, and D. L. Kaysen, "Drinking motives moderate daily relationships between PTSD symptoms and alcohol use," *Journal of Abnormal Psychology*, vol. 123, no. 1, pp. 237–247, 2014.

[87] R. S. Miranda-Morales, M. E. Nizhnikov, D. H. Waters, and N. E. Spear, "New evidence of ethanol's anxiolytic properties in the infant rat," *Alcohol*, vol. 48, no. 4, pp. 367–374, 2014.

[88] K. C. Young-Wolff, K. S. Kendler, N. D. Sintov, and C. A. Prescott, "Mood-related drinking motives mediate the familial association between major depression and alcohol dependence," *Alcoholism: Clinical and Experimental Research*, vol. 33, no. 8, pp. 1476–1486, 2009.

[89] P.-H. Kuo, C. O. Gardner Jr., K. S. Kendler, and C. A. Prescott, "The temporal relationship of the onsets of alcohol dependence and major depression: using a genetically informative study design," *Psychological Medicine*, vol. 36, no. 8, pp. 1153–1162, 2006.

[90] T. C. Goes, F. D. Antunes, and F. Teixeira-Silva, "Environmental enrichment for adult rats: effects on trait and state anxiety," *Neuroscience Letters*, vol. 584, pp. 93–96, 2015.

[91] R. Ravenelle, H. B. Santolucito, E. M. Byrnes, J. J. Byrnes, and S. T. Donaldson, "Housing environment modulates physiological and behavioral responses to anxiogenic stimuli in trait anxiety male rats," *Neuroscience*, vol. 270, pp. 76–87, 2014.

[92] N. Benaroya-Milshtein, N. Hollander, A. Apter et al., "Environmental enrichment in mice decreases anxiety, attenuates stress responses and enhances natural killer cell activity," *European Journal of Neuroscience*, vol. 20, no. 5, pp. 1341–1347, 2004.

[93] A. J. Grippo, E. Ihm, J. Wardwell et al., "The effects of environmental enrichment on depressive and anxiety-relevant behaviors in socially isolated prairie voles," *Psychosomatic Medicine*, vol. 76, no. 4, pp. 277–284, 2014.

[94] J. Maniam and M. J. Morris, "Long-term postpartum anxiety and depression-like behavior in mother rats subjected to maternal separation are ameliorated by palatable high fat diet," *Behavioural Brain Research*, vol. 208, no. 1, pp. 72–79, 2010.

[95] J. Maniam and M. J. Morris, "Palatable cafeteria diet ameliorates anxiety and depression-like symptoms following an adverse early environment," *Psychoneuroendocrinology*, vol. 35, no. 5, pp. 717–728, 2010.

[96] Y. M. Ulrich-Lai, A. M. Christiansen, M. M. Ostrander et al., "Pleasurable behaviors reduce stress via brain reward pathways," *Proceedings of the National Academy of Sciences of the United States of America*, vol. 107, no. 47, pp. 20529–20534, 2011.

[97] A. T. Knoll and W. A. Carlezon Jr., "Dynorphin, stress, and depression," *Brain Research*, vol. 1314, pp. 56–73, 2010.

[98] B. B. Land, M. R. Bruchas, J. C. Lemos, M. Xu, E. J. Melief, and C. Chavkin, "The dysphoric component of stress is encoded by activation of the dynorphin κ-opioid system," *The Journal of Neuroscience*, vol. 28, no. 2, pp. 407–414, 2008.

[99] M. R. Bruchas, B. B. Land, J. C. Lemos, and C. Chavkin, "CRF1-R activation of the dynorphin/kappa opioid system in the mouse basolateral amygdala mediates anxiety-like behavior," *PLoS ONE*, vol. 4, no. 12, Article ID e8528, 2009.

[100] A. W. Bruijnzeel, "Kappa-opioid receptor signaling and brain reward function," *Brain Research Reviews*, vol. 62, no. 1, pp. 127–146, 2009.

[101] V. I. Chefer, T. Czyzyk, E. A. Bolan, J. Moron, J. E. Pintar, and T. S. Shippenberg, "Endogenous κ-opioid receptor systems regulate mesoaccumbal dopamine dynamics and vulnerability to cocaine," *Journal of Neuroscience*, vol. 25, no. 20, pp. 5029–5037, 2005.

[102] N. D. Volkow, G.-J. Wang, J. S. Fowler, D. Tomasi, F. Telang, and R. Baler, "Addiction: decreased reward sensitivity and increased expectation sensitivity conspire to overwhelm the brain's control circuit," *BioEssays*, vol. 32, no. 9, pp. 748–755, 2010.

[103] M. F. Barbano and M. Cador, "Differential regulation of the consummatory, motivational and anticipatory aspects of feeding behavior by dopaminergic and opioidergic drugs," *Neuropsychopharmacology*, vol. 31, no. 7, pp. 1371–1381, 2006.

[104] K. C. Berridge, "Food reward: brain substrates of wanting and liking," *Neuroscience and Biobehavioral Reviews*, vol. 20, no. 1, pp. 1–25, 1995.

[105] R. Doron, L. Fridman, and G. Yadid, "Dopamine-2 receptors in the arcuate nucleus modulate cocaine-seeking behavior," *NeuroReport*, vol. 17, no. 15, pp. 1633–1636, 2006.

[106] A. R. Soderman and E. M. Unterwald, "Cocaine-induced mu opioid receptor occupancy within the striatum is mediated by dopamine D2 receptors," *Brain Research*, vol. 1296, pp. 63–71, 2009.

[107] G. F. Koob, "Dynamics of neuronal circuits in addiction: reward, antireward, and emotional memory," *Pharmacopsychiatry*, vol. 42, no. 1, pp. S32–S41, 2009.

[108] C. A. Schad, J. B. Justice Jr., and S. G. Holtzman, "Endogenous opioids in dopaminergic cell body regions modulate amphetamine-induced increases in extracellular dopamine levels in the terminal regions," *Journal of Pharmacology and Experimental Therapeutics*, vol. 300, no. 3, pp. 932–938, 2002.

[109] G. B. Stefano, E. Bianchi, M. Guarna et al., "Nicotine, alcohol and cocaine coupling to reward processes via endogenous morphine signaling: the dopamine-morphine hypothesis," *Medical Science Monitor*, vol. 13, no. 6, pp. RA91–RA102, 2007.

[110] S. L. Parylak, G. F. Koob, and E. P. Zorrilla, "The dark side of food addiction," *Physiology and Behavior*, vol. 104, no. 1, pp. 149–156, 2011.

[111] G. F. Koob and N. D. Volkow, "Neurocircuitry of addiction," *Neuropsychopharmacology*, vol. 35, no. 1, pp. 217–238, 2010.

[112] G. F. Koob, "Addiction is a reward deficit and stress surfeit disorder," *Frontiers in Psychiatry*, vol. 4, article 72, 2013.

[113] S. R. Ebner, M. F. Roitman, D. N. Potter, A. B. Rachlin, and E. H. Chartoff, "Depressive-like effects of the κ opioid receptor agonist salvinorin A are associated with decreased phasic dopamine release in the nucleus accumbens," *Psychopharmacology*, vol. 209, no. 2, pp. 241–252, 2010.

[114] G. F. Koob, "The role of CRF and CRF-related peptides in the dark side of addiction," *Brain Research*, vol. 1314, pp. 3–14, 2010.

[115] E. J. Khantzian, "The self-medication hypothesis of substance use disorders: a reconsideration and recent applications," *Harvard Review of Psychiatry*, vol. 4, no. 5, pp. 231–244, 1997.

[116] S. Edwards and G. F. Koob, "Neurobiology of dysregulated motivational systems in drug addiction," *Future Neurology*, vol. 5, no. 3, pp. 393–410, 2010.

[117] C. Muth, M. H. Raab, and C. C. Carbon, "The stream of experience when watching artistic movies. Dynamic aesthetic effects revealed by the Continuous Evaluation Procedure (CEP)," *Frontiers in Psychology*, vol. 6, article 365, 2015.

[118] R. Arnheim, *Art and Visual Perception: A Psychology of the Creative Eye*, University of California Press, Berkeley, Calif, USA, 1954.

[119] S. Van de Cruys and J. Wagemans, "Putting reward in art: a tentative prediction error account of visual art," *i-Perception*, vol. 2, no. 9, pp. 1035–1062, 2011.

[120] M. Jakesch, H. Leder, and M. Forster, "Image ambiguity and fluency," *PLoS ONE*, vol. 8, no. 9, Article ID e74084, 2013.

[121] A. R. Seitz, D. Kim, and T. Watanabe, "Rewards evoke learning of unconsciously processed visual stimuli in adult humans," *Neuron*, vol. 61, no. 5, pp. 700–707, 2009.

25

Influence of Spirituality on Depression, Posttraumatic Stress Disorder, and Suicidality in Active Duty Military Personnel

Laurel L. Hourani, Jason Williams, Valerie Forman-Hoffman, Marian E. Lane, Belinda Weimer, and Robert M. Bray

Behavioral Health and Criminal Justice Division, RTI International, 3040 Cornwallis Road, P.O. Box 12194, Research Triangle Park, NC 27709, USA

Correspondence should be addressed to Laurel L. Hourani, hourani@rti.org

Academic Editor: Harold G. Koenig

Understanding the role of spirituality as a potential coping mechanism for military personnel is important given growing concern about the mental health issues of personnel returning from war. This study seeks to determine the extent to which spirituality is associated with selected mental health problems among active duty military personnel and whether it moderates the relationship between combat exposure/deployment and (a) depression, (b) posttraumatic stress disorder (PTSD), and (c) suicidality in active duty military personnel. Data were drawn from the 2008 Department of Defense Survey of Health Related Behaviors Among Active Duty Military Personnel. Over 24,000 randomly selected active duty personnel worldwide completed an anonymous self-report questionnaire. High spirituality had a significant protective effect only for depression symptoms. Medium, as opposed to high or low, levels of spirituality buffered each of the mental health outcomes to some degree. Medium and low spirituality levels predicted depression symptoms but only among those with moderate combat exposure. Medium spirituality levels also predicted PTSD symptoms among those with moderate levels of combat exposure and predicted self-reported suicidal ideation/attempt among those never deployed. These results point to the complex relationship between spirituality and mental health, particularly among military personnel and the need for further research.

1. Introduction

A sizable amount of literature has focused on the influence of religiosity and spirituality on health outcomes. Many of these studies are summarized in the 2001 book: *Handbook of Religion and Health* [1] and in Koenig et al. [2]. Research has shown associations between both concepts of spirituality and religiosity and mental health. For example, studies have indicated a significant relationship between higher levels of religiosity and lower levels of depression [3, 4], particularly among those at high risk for depression [5]. The association between higher levels of spirituality and lower levels of depressive symptoms has been demonstrated in several different subpopulations, including adolescent girls [6], patients in an urban clinic [7], and terminally ill patients with cancer and AIDS [8]. In addition, findings from the Baltimore Epidemiologic Catchment Area Study indicated that individuals who reported ever seeking spiritual comfort at Wave 3 assessment had decreased odds of suicidal ideation at Wave 4 as compared to those who reported never seeking spiritual comfort at Wave 3 [9]. The literature examining the relationship between spirituality, religion, and anxiety disorders and suicide is less robust [10]. However, greater levels of spirituality have been associated with fewer anxiety symptoms among patients with advanced illness [11] and with lower posttraumatic symptom severity among survivors of violent trauma [12]. Krejci et al. [13] found that although sexual abuse victims and controls did not differ in terms of spiritual well-being, lower psychopathology including PTSD symptom scores, were associated with increased spiritual well-being in both groups.

Several hypotheses have emerged that explain spirituality's link with mental disorders. Dating back to the end of the 19th century, Durkheim's study of religiosity/spirituality and suicidal behaviors suggested that those with increased spirituality also had greater levels of social support, which effectively buffered against psychopathology and suicidal behaviors [14]. More recent studies have come to similar conclusions [2, 3]. Another mechanism may be that greater spirituality protects against mental disorders and/or suicide by increasing the ability to cope with stressors [15], deepening one's sense of purpose or meaning [16], and/or reducing feelings of hopelessness, which have been indicated as a predictor of suicide [17]. In contrast, it has been suggested that religious beliefs may exert a negative influence on mental health especially in the emotionally vulnerable by increasing fears or guilt, reinforcing neurotic tendencies [2].

There have been a few published studies investigating the relationship between spirituality/religiosity and mental disorders and suicide in veteran samples. In a recently published study by Berg [18], spiritual distress was related to both combat-related posttraumatic stress disorder (PTSD) and depression in a sample of Vietnam veterans. Subjective religiosity (the extent religious beliefs are a source of comfort/strength) was shown to be associated with both women veterans [19] and male veterans [20] with sexual assault experience. Spiritual well-being was also found to be a mediator of the effect of a mantra (a sacred word or phrase repeated over and over) intervention to decrease PTSD symptoms in veterans with military trauma [21]. Other studies have examined interventions that include a spirituality component to help promote resilience (Pargament and Sweeney [22]), reduce health risks (Niederhauser et al. [23]), integrate health promotion and wellness (Parker et al. [24]), and reduce PTSD symptoms in veterans exposed to trauma (Harris et al. [25]), though all indicate that further, more robust research is warranted in these areas.

Additional investigations in military populations are needed given the potential importance of spirituality in helping active duty service members cope with deployment as well as transition from deployed to nondeployed status during wartime. Although programs such as the Warrior Transition Units have been created, they are not currently able to fully meet the needs of all returning service members [26]. Thus, the role of spirituality as a coping mechanism in the transition from deployed to nondeployed status and various associated stressors from recent combat experience may be important [27]. Spiritual fitness was named as one of the eight domains comprising a new framework of Total Force Fitness, an initiative from the Chairman of the Joint Chiefs of Staff for maintaining the health, readiness, and performance of Department of Defense (DoD) service members [28]. As part of the Army's Comprehensive Soldier Program which is comprised of a spiritual fitness tracker that requires soldiers to respond to statements such as, "I am a spiritual person, my life has lasting meaning, I believe that in some way my life is closely connected to all humanity and all the world," this program has come under recent controversy [29, 30]. The recommendations call for the development of evidence-based spiritual support policies and programs and integrating chaplains as primary providers of such services [31]. In 2010, DoD and the Department of Veterans Affairs (VA) launched a joint strategic action implementation plan under the DoD/VA Integrated Mental Health Strategy to increase understanding of chaplains' roles in primary care within the military treatment system and VA; to support continuity in the role of chaplains between the services and VA; to identify ways to facilitate access to mental health care through collaboration with community clergy and faith communities. Investigation of the relationship between spirituality and mental health problems is particularly important given that active duty members have particularly high rates of suicidal ideation and extreme anxiety as compared to reports from general population samples [32–34].

The present study seeks to address two research aims. The first aim is to determine the extent to which spirituality is associated with selected mental health problems (i.e., depression, PTSD, and suicidality) among active duty military personnel controlling for potential demographic, coping, and service-related variables. We hypothesize that high spirituality, defined as the self-reported importance of religious/spiritual beliefs in life and decision making, is protective against depression, PTSD, and suicidality. Although the measure used in this study combines both concepts of religiosity and spirituality, we refer to the broader concept of spirituality to encompass the combination of the concepts in this measure throughout this paper.

The second aim is to determine whether spirituality moderates the relationship between combat exposure/deployment and these mental health problems. We hypothesize that high levels of spirituality will buffer the association between combat exposure/deployment and depression, PTSD, and suicidality.

2. Materials and Methods

2.1. Subjects. Data were drawn from the 2008 DoD Survey of Health Related Behaviors Among Active Duty Military Personnel (2008 HRB Survey) [29]. The survey consists of a randomly selected representative sample of active duty military personnel from the Army, Navy, Marine Corps, Air Force, and Coast Guard. A two-stage replacement cluster sample proportional to size was employed in which geographic areas were clustered and randomly selected in the first stage, and individuals within the clusters were randomly selected in the second stage. All active duty members were eligible except for recruits, academy cadets, and persons who were absent without leave or incarcerated. The final sample of participants consisted of 28,546 military personnel (5,927 Army, 6,637 Navy, 5,117 Marine Corps, 7,009 Air Force, and 3,856 Coast Guard), who completed self-administered questionnaires anonymously. The overall response rate was 70.6%. Although the number of missing items tended to increase with the length of the questionnaire, the response rate was high relative to most military surveys, and most items showed less than a 5% missing rate. Data were weighted to represent all active duty personnel, meaning that the results of the survey represent population estimates of the entire active force. The current study included only the DoD services (Army, Navy, Air Force, and Marine Corps) for a study total of 24,690.

2.2. Survey Procedures. The majority (97%) of the 32-page anonymous self-report questionnaires were obtained during onsite visits to 64 military installations worldwide by the study team. The rest were obtained from questionnaires mailed to respondents who were unable to attend group sessions. At the group sessions, survey data collection field teams described the purpose of the study, assured participants of anonymity, informed participants of the voluntary nature of the survey, distributed introductory handouts, ensured that an ombudsperson was present for each group administration to attest that teams explained the voluntary nature of participation, and showed personnel the correct procedures for marking the questionnaire. Team members then distributed the optical-mark questionnaires to participants, who completed and returned them. On average, the questionnaire required about an hour to complete. Institutional Review Board approval was obtained from RTI International and DoD. Additional sampling and methodological details have been reported and published elsewhere [35].

2.3. Key Measures

2.3.1. Demographics. Demographics included gender (male and female) race/ethnicity (white non-Hispanic, black non-Hispanic, Hispanic, and other), highest level of education (high school diploma or less, some college, and college degree or more) age group (17–20, 21–25, 26–34, and 35 or older), and military pay grade (E1–E3 junior enlisted, E4–E6 middle enlisted, E7–E9 senior enlisted, W1–W5 warrant officer, O1–O3 junior commissioned officers, and O4–O10 middle and senior officers).

2.3.2. Spirituality. Respondents were asked to what extent they agreed with two questions regarding the importance of religious/spiritual beliefs and the degree to which religious/spiritual beliefs influenced their decision making. Items were "My religious/spiritual beliefs are a very important part of my life" and "My religious/spiritual beliefs influence how I make decisions in my life," each rated on a 4-point scale from strongly agree to strongly disagree. Respondents' spirituality was categorized as high if they reported "strongly agree" to both questions, moderate if they reported either "strongly agree" or "agree" to at least one of the questions, and low if they reported either "disagree" or "strongly disagree" to both questions. These items were adapted from those used in the National Survey on Drug Use and Health [36].

2.3.3. Combat Exposure. Exposure to combat and related circumstances was measured using a modified version of the 17-item Combat Experiences Scale of the Deployment Risk and Resilience Inventory [37]. These items assess exposure to incoming fire, mines, improvised explosive devices, firing on the enemy, viewing dead bodies or human remains, interaction with enemy prisoners of war, and similar circumstances that may be relevant. Each item asked how many times the respondent was exposed, and response options were 0 (0 times), 1 (1 to 3 times), 2 (4 to 12 times), 3 (13 to 50 times), and 4 (51 or more times). All items were summed, and the sum score was used to create a categorical combat exposure item where a score equal to zero was considered "deployed but no exposure to combat," a score from 1 to 9 was classified as "low/moderate combat exposure," and a score of 10 or greater was considered as "moderate/high combat exposure." A fourth category was added to capture personnel who had not been deployed. These cutoffs were subsequently examined with factor analysis and item scoring methods suggesting that these categories captured meaningful distinctions between groups of scores.

2.3.4. Coping. Respondents were asked to identify the types of strategies that they use to cope when they "feel pressured, stressed, depressed, or anxious." The list of strategies included items that assess both approach-oriented and problem-solving strategies ("Think of a plan to solve the problem," "Talk to a friend or family member," and "Exercise or play sports") and avoidant coping ("Have a drink," "Light up a cigarette," and "Get something to eat").

2.3.5. Depression. Depression was assessed using the 10-item short version of the Center for Epidemiologic Studies Depression Scale (CESD-10). Cutoff scores for depressive symptoms were greater than or equal to 10. Andresen and colleagues [38] found good predictive accuracy when they compared the CESD-10 to the full-length 20-item version of the CES-D.

2.3.6. PTSD. PTSD symptom severity was assessed using the PTSD Checklist, Civilian Version (PCLC) [39], a 17-item self-report instrument that asks respondents to rate the extent to which they have been bothered by PTSD symptoms during the previous 30 days using a 5-point scale (1: not at all and 5: extremely). PCLC items parallel DSM-IV PTSD symptom criteria B, C, and D, and a variety of studies support the use of the PCLC as a valid and reliable screening instrument [40–42]. The HRB Survey, and other DoD studies, prefer the PCLC over the military version of the PCL because the military version ignores symptoms from nonmilitary experiences and can miss common causes of deployment or war-related PTSD in women (e.g., sexual assault rather than combat) as well as deployment-related exacerbations of PTSD symptoms if the original inciting trauma is not military related [35]. The standard cutoff was used such that if the sum was greater than or equal to 50, the participant was classified as positive for PTSD; those with scores less than 50 were considered not to have PTSD [39].

2.3.7. Suicidal Ideation and Attempt. Suicidal ideation was assessed by asking respondents about the occurrence of suicidal thoughts within the past year. A dichotomous item indicated any thoughts of suicide versus no thoughts of suicide. This particular item has also been used as a first-level screen for suicidal ideation in previous studies of military personnel [35]. Suicide attempts were assessed by asking respondents whether they had attempted suicide within the past year. A dichotomous item indicated any suicide attempt versus no suicide attempt. Individuals responded based on

TABLE 1: Prevalence of mental health outcomes by spirituality level*.

	Overall prevalence (%) $N = 24{,}690$	Prevalence among spirituality levels		
		High $N = 5{,}692$	Medium $N = 11{,}639$	Low $N = 6{,}102$
Depression	30.6	24.9[a]	32.2[b]	32.1[b]
PTSD	10.7	8.8[a]	10.9[b]	11.6[b]
Suicide attempt, past year	2.2	1.8	2.4	2.0
Suicide contemplation, past year	4.6	4.2[a]	4.3[a,b]	5.3[b]
Suicide (attempt or contemplation), past year	6.0	5.5	5.9	6.5

*Excludes missing responses; Ns are unweighted.
[a,b]Estimates for spirituality column differences for depression, PTSD, and suicide contemplation not sharing a common superscript are significantly different at $P < 0.05$.

their own definitions of what it meant to them as having seriously considered or attempted suicide. A third item was created that indicated past year suicide contemplation or attempt versus no suicide contemplation or attempt.

2.4. Statistical Analyses. Analyses were conducted using SUDAAN [43] to account for the complex sampling design. Aim 1, the determination of basic prevalence of mental health problems across levels of spirituality and the associations of spirituality with these outcomes, was examined using simple frequencies and crosstabs. Multiple predictor logistic regression models were used to assess the prevalence of mental health outcomes by levels of the key independent variables of spirituality and combat exposure. Aim 2, examination of the moderation or hypothesized buffering effect of greater spirituality on the negative mental health impacts of combat exposure, was addressed with logistic regression models, which included spirituality by combat exposure interaction terms. Significant interaction parameters indicated that the effect of different levels of spirituality was not consistent across levels of combat exposure. For example, although high versus low spirituality may provide modest protection against depression for those not deployed, in the high deployment group the impact could be much greater, with high spirituality personnel showing less combat exposure-related depression relative to their lower spirituality peers. The reference category for spirituality was changed to "high" for models involving interactions because this category was the most dissimilar from the other two and would better highlight differential effects of combat exposure on the mental health outcomes. All regression models included gender, age, race/ethnicity, pay grade, and education as control measures.

3. Results

An estimated 30.6% of active duty personnel met screening criteria for depression on the CES-D, 10.7% met screening criteria for PTSD on the PCLC, and 6.0% reported either seriously considering or attempting suicide in the past year (Table 1). As shown in Table 1, 23.1% fell into the high spirituality category, 48.7% fell into the medium spirituality level, and 28.2% fell into the low spirituality level. Lowest rates of all mental health outcomes (except suicide attempts) were observed in the highest spirituality level.

To address the first aim, Table 2 presents the influence of spirituality on mental health outcomes and controlling for demographic and service-related variables. Moderate spirituality had a significant protective effect only for depression. Risk factors for both depression and PTSD were being female, being in younger age groups, non-Hispanic ethnicity, junior-enlisted pay grades, avoidant coping behaviors, and those with moderate or high combat exposure. Results were similar for suicidality with the exception that age and gender effects were not significant. Active coping behaviors were protective for each outcome.

To address the second aim, Table 3 displays the odds ratios and confidence intervals for the logistic models that included combat exposure by spirituality interactions to test the buffering effect of greater spirituality. Four interactions were significant, indicating that the magnitude of the odds ratio for one or more comparisons of spirituality's impact on mental health were conditional on level of combat exposure. To illustrate these differences in patterns, Table 4 shows the adjusted marginal estimates for the mental health outcomes for spirituality levels crossed with the four combat exposure categories. The logistic regression models with interactions effects for combat exposure and spirituality revealed several instances where the impact of combat exposure on mental health was conditional on level of spirituality. Two interactions were significant for spirituality and combat exposure with depression as the dependent variable. Within the low-to-moderate combat exposure group, high spirituality showed a significantly more pronounced buffering effect of exposure on depression. As indicated in Table 4, rates of depression for the high spirituality group within low-moderate combat exposure (21.3%) was considerably lower than the rate in the medium and low spirituality groups (31.1% and 27.3%, resp.). High spirituality was also associated with a more pronounced protective influence against PTSD compared to those with medium spirituality in the low-moderate combat exposure group. (4.4% versus 6.4%). Finally, and counter to expectations, for those in the nondeployed group, medium spirituality was associated with significantly lower likelihood of suicidality relative to those

Table 2: Logistic regression model parameters, interactions not included.

Independent variables	DV Depression OR (95% CI)	PTSD OR (95% CI)	Suicidality OR (95% CI)
Intercept	0.19 (0.14–0.25)*	0.02 (0.01–0.03)*	0.02 (0.02–0.04)*
High spirituality	0.99 (0.90–1.10)	1.16 (0.99–1.37)	1.11 (0.90–1.36)
Moderate spirituality	1.12 (1.01–1.25)*	1.08 (0.91–1.27)	0.96 (0.78–1.17)
Low spirituality	ref	ref	ref
Male	ref	ref	ref
Female	1.64 (1.49–1.79)*	1.63 (1.39–1.91)*	1.24 (1.04–1.47)*
17–20	1.32 (1.10–1.58)*	1.25 (0.94–1.66)	0.98 (0.69–1.39)
21–25	0.96 (0.83–1.12)	0.97 (0.82–1.14)	0.86 (0.67–1.12)
26–34	0.85 (0.74–0.98)*	0.93 (0.76–1.15)	0.79 (0.63–0.99)*
35 or older	ref	ref	ref
Non-Hispanic white	ref	ref	ref
Non-Hispanic black	1.08 (0.98–1.19)	1.01 (0.82–1.24)	1.45 (1.12–1.87)*
Hispanic	1.10 (1.00–1.21)	1.10 (0.90–1.34)	1.46 (1.16–1.83)*
Non-Hispanic other	1.26 (1.10–1.46)*	1.45 (1.21–1.74)*	1.97 (1.56–2.49)*
High school or less	ref	ref	ref
Some college	1.10 (1.00–1.20)*	1.08 (0.93–1.26)	0.96 (0.82–1.12)
College degree or more	1.10 (0.94–1.28)	0.95 (0.76–1.18)	0.98 (0.80–1.21)
E1–E3	1.79 (1.34–2.39)*	3.97 (2.12–7.45)*	2.37 (1.27–4.43)*
E4–E6	1.57 (1.23–2.00)*	2.96 (1.62–5.41)*	2.15 (1.23–3.74)*
E7–E9	1.15 (0.85–1.54)	1.89 (0.97–3.68)	1.68 (0.99–2.84)
W1–W5	0.88 (0.73–1.07)	0.76 (0.17–3.51)	1.71 (0.90–3.24)
O1–O3	1.13 (0.89–1.42)	1.88 (0.89–3.97)	1.69 (0.96–2.98)
O4–O10	ref	ref	ref
Not deployed	0.99 (0.87–1.13)	1.12 (0.91–1.38)	1.08 (0.89–1.31)
No combat exposure	ref	ref	ref
Moderate combat exposure	1.14 (1.04–1.26)*	1.11 (0.88–1.39)	0.84 (0.74–0.96)*
High combat exposure	1.52 (1.35–1.72)*	3.57 (3.00–4.26)*	1.28 (1.06–1.56)*
Active coping	0.68 (0.65–0.72)*	0.67 (0.62–0.73)*	0.65 (0.58–0.73)*
Avoidant coping	3.21 (3.02–3.41)*	3.10 (2.80–3.43)*	1.90 (1.70–2.12)*

with high spirituality (4.6% versus 6.4%) compared to this relationship in other combat exposure categories.

4. Discussion

This study examined the relationship between spirituality, combat exposure, and mental health among a large, population-based sample of active duty military personnel. Overall, spirituality had a positive influence on depression but not on suicidality. This relationship held while controlling for demographic variables, coping behaviors, and combat exposure; however, there was only limited support for the hypothesis that high spirituality would moderate the relationship between combat exposure and mental health outcomes. Findings showed that spirituality did buffer depression and PTSD symptoms but only among those with low-moderate combat exposure. On the other hand, a medium level of spirituality, relative to a high level, was protective of self-reported suicidal ideation/attempt only among those never deployed. This suggests that high levels of spirituality may be associated with greater suicidal ideation or attempt in this nondeployed subgroup of military personnel. It is certainly possible that this subgroup of nondeployed personnel had admitted to suicidal ideation during predeployment screening accounting for their nondeployment. Further research on this group may help elucidate whether this nondeployed group is coming into the service with higher levels of suicidal ideation or whether they are being screened out on mandatory predeployment health assessment forms. This also has implications for chaplains, social workers, and other service providers. Although wounded warriors have captured the attention of the media and have become a priority for service provisions and policy making in the military, these findings suggest that this should not be at the exclusion of those military personnel who have not been deployed.

These results point to the complex relationship between spirituality and mental health, particularly among military personnel. Although consistent with studies that found a relationship between depression and spirituality in various

TABLE 3: Logistic regression model parameters, interactions included.

Independent variables	DV Depression OR (95% CI)	PTSD OR (95% CI)	Suicidality OR (95% CI)
High spirituality	ref	ref	ref
Moderate spirituality	1.07 (0.91–1.27)	0.73 (0.51–1.02)	1.27 (0.85–1.89)
Low spirituality	0.98 (0.85–1.13)	0.81 (0.52–1.27)	1.06 (0.68–1.65)
Male	ref	ref	ref
Female	1.63 (1.49–1.79)*	1.63 (1.40–1.90)*	1.24 (1.04–1.47)*
17–20	1.33 (1.11–1.60)*	1.25 (0.94–1.67)	0.98 (0.69–1.40)
21–25	0.96 (0.83–1.11)	0.97 (0.82–1.14)	0.87 (0.67–1.12)
26–34	0.85 (0.74–0.97)*	0.93 (0.76–1.15)	0.79 (0.63–0.99)*
35 or older	ref	ref	ref
Non-Hispanic white	ref	ref	ref
Non-Hispanic black	1.08 (0.98–1.19)	1.01 (0.82–1.24)	1.44 (1.12–1.86)*
Hispanic	1.10 (0.99–1.21)	1.10 (0.90–1.33)	1.46 (1.17–1.83)*
Non-Hispanic other	1.27 (1.10–1.46)*	1.46 (1.22–1.75)*	1.97 (1.57–2.49)*
High school or less	ref	ref	ref
Some college	1.10 (1.00–1.20)*	1.08 (0.93–1.26)	0.96 (0.82–1.12)
College degree or more	1.10 (0.95–1.28)	0.95 (0.76–1.18)	0.99 (0.80–1.21)
E1–E3	1.79 (1.33–2.40)*	3.95 (2.10–7.42)*	2.39 (1.28–4.47)*
E4–E6	1.55 (1.21–1.99)*	2.92 (1.59–5.37)*	2.16 (1.24–3.74)*
E7–E9	1.14 (0.84–1.54)	1.87 (0.95–3.66)	1.68 (1.00–2.84)
W1–W5	0.87 (0.71–1.06)	0.75 (0.16–3.50)	1.70 (0.89–3.23)
O1–O3	1.11 (0.88–1.40)	1.85 (0.88–3.93)	1.69 (0.96–2.97)
O4–O10	ref	ref	ref
Not deployed	1.18 (0.97–1.42)	1.14 (0.76–1.69)	1.56 (1.08–2.26)*
No combat exposure	ref	ref	ref
Moderate combat exposure	0.83 (0.65–1.05)	0.69 (0.44–1.07)	1.08 (0.66–1.75)
High combat exposure	1.42 (1.14–1.77)*	2.97 (1.94–4.56)*	1.64 (0.97–2.80)
Active coping	0.68 (0.65–0.72)*	0.67 (0.62–0.73)*	0.65 (0.58–0.73)*
Avoidant coping	3.21 (3.02–3.41)*	3.10 (2.80–3.43)*	1.89 (1.70–2.11)*
High spirituality, nondeployed	NA	NA	NA
High spirituality, no exposure	NA	NA	NA
High spirituality, moderate exposure	NA	NA	NA
High spirituality, high exposure	NA	NA	NA
Medium spirituality, nondeployed	0.81 (0.65–1.01)	1.01 (0.65–1.58)	0.55 (0.35–0.87)*
Medium spirituality, no exposure	NA	NA	NA
Medium spirituality, moderate exposure	1.55 (1.20–2.01)*	2.05 (1.22–3.43)*	0.70 (0.37–1.30)
Medium spirituality, high exposure	1.09 (0.84–1.41)	1.41 (0.86–2.31)	0.65 (0.34–1.24)
Low spirituality, nondeployed	0.80 (0.63–1.01)	0.93 (0.54–1.61)	0.77 (0.48–1.24)
Low spirituality, no exposure	NA	NA	NA
Low spirituality, moderate exposure	1.42 (1.07–1.88)*	1.46 (0.81–2.65)	0.81 (0.46–1.43)
Low spirituality, high exposure	1.10 (0.78–1.56)	1.06 (0.57–2.00)	0.89 (0.42–1.89)

Note: NA indicates interaction term included reference level of one or more predictors and was not estimable.

TABLE 4: Adjusted estimates of spirituality by combat exposure.

Combat exposure	Not deployed			No exposure			Low-moderate exposure			High exposure		
Spirituality	High	Med	Low	High	Med	Low	High	Med	Low	High	Med	Low
Depression	27.8	25.1	23.1	24.7	26.0	24.2	21.3	31.1	27.3	31.7	35.2	33.3
PTSD	7.1	5.3	5.5	6.3	4.7	5.2	4.4	6.4	5.2	16.7	17.0	14.8
Suicidality	6.4	4.6	5.3	4.2	5.3	4.5	4.5	4.0	3.9	6.8	6.7	6.4

civilian populations, they are not consistent with the Berg [18] study that related spiritual distress with combat-related PTSD among Vietnam veterans, although that study used a different measure of spirituality than the present study. Further, these findings suggest that the buffering role of spirituality in mental health is limited, dependent on type of mental health problem investigated, and may be potentially overwhelmed by great stress, such as high levels of combat exposure. That is, the buffering effect of spirituality may operate within a limited window of stress (e.g., it may not make a difference for those with low amounts of stress or challenges but may be overwhelmed by greater stressors). This effect may also account for studies that have identified negative consequences of high spirituality. That is it may be suggested that high combat exposure may increase emotional vulnerability leading to poorer mental health among highly spiritual personnel. It is clear that spirituality/religiosity plays an important but complex role in the mental health of military personnel and must be investigated within the context of both a wide range of potential covariates and individual mental health indicators or diagnoses. Findings also suggest that it may be beneficial to enhance chaplain involvement across the entire deployment cycle (before, during, and after), ensuring that service members are encouraged to attend to their spiritual needs in whatever manner makes sense to them, and to integrate spiritual assessment into physical and mental health care to improve care of the whole individual. These findings extend those by Edlund et al. [44] using a similar measure who found a strong negative relationship between religiosity and substance abuse in the US population. Given the strong comorbidity of our mental health outcomes with substance abuse, future research should examine the effect of spirituality on mental health controlling for those who abstain from alcohol and other substances on religious grounds.

Among the limitations of this research is the self-report and cross-sectional nature of the data, which limits the ability to make casual inferences. The use of mental health screening measures does not imply clinical diagnoses. Due to the length of the questionnaire, the number of missing items tended to increase slightly with its length. However, the overall response rate was high relative to other military surveys, and most missing items showed less than a 5% missing rate. Although there is limited or a lack of psychometric data on some scales (e.g., coping behaviors scale) used in the survey, all have been utilized successfully in previous military surveys. It should be noted that the definition of spirituality used in this study is an operational one reflecting the specific language of the questionnaire items used to measure what may be thought of as a combination of conceptual definitions. Although religiosity and spirituality are intimately linked, it is widely acknowledged that the two should be studied as distinct concepts in research studies [45]. A large portion of prior research has focused on religiosity (generally used to refer to affiliation with organized and institutional religion) [46], but in recent years there has been an increasing focus on studying the impact of spirituality (generally more personal [2] or broadly defined as an individual's existential relationship with God [47, 48]) on mental health outcomes, specifically depression, anxiety, and suicide. Operational definitions of both constructs have varied widely and often overlap in their assessment [48, 49] as was done in the current study to be consistent with educational materials used in military settings [29]. Unfortunately this combined measure, based on the SAMHSA items, lacks psychometric information. Further studies would benefit from more comprehensive and rigorous measures of spirituality that specified the components of spirituality, such as forgiveness of self and others, and included religion measures, such as religious commitment. Investigating characteristics that differentiate between high, medium, and low levels of spirituality may be particularly informative. Further research into the theory and mechanism by which spirituality is associated with mental health is also warranted.

5. Conclusions

In conclusion, the most important finding of this study is that high spirituality appears to have some protective effect for depression and PTSD, but only for those in the low-moderate combat exposure group. This extends and qualifies previous findings of both positive and negative associations between religiosity and mental health outcomes in this and other populations. A number of additional topics for further investigation are identified emphasizing the need for evaluation of potential interventions including spiritual resilience programs implemented by the military.

Acknowledgments

The authors wish to thank Mr. Justin Faerber for his editorial assistance. This study was funded by Contract GS-10F-00971, Task Order W81XWH-07-F-0538 from the Department of Defense to RTI International. The views, opinions, and findings contained in this paper are those of the authors and should not be construed as an official Department of Defense position, policy, or decision, unless so designated by other official documentation.

References

[1] H. G. Koenig, M. E. McCullough, and D. B. Larson, *Handbook of Religion and Health*, Oxford University Press, New York, NY, USA, 2nd edition, 2001.

[2] H. G. Koenig, "Research on religion, spirituality, and mental health: a review," *Canadian Journal of Psychiatry*, vol. 54, no. 5, pp. 283–291, 2009.

[3] J. Maselko, S. E. Gilman, and S. Buka, "Religious service attendance and spiritual well-being are differentially associated with risk of major depression," *Psychological Medicine*, vol. 39, no. 6, pp. 1009–1017, 2009.

[4] L. Miller, V. Warner, P. Wickramaratne, and M. Weissman, "Religiosity and depression: ten-year follow-up of depressed mothers and offspring," *Journal of the American Academy of Child and Adolescent Psychiatry*, vol. 36, no. 10, pp. 1416–1425, 1997.

[5] L. Miller, P. Wickramaratne, M. J. Gameroff, M. Sage, C. E. Tenke, and M. M. Weissman, "Religiosity and major

depression in adults at high risk: a ten-year prospective study," *American Journal of Psychiatry*, vol. 169, no. 1, pp. 89–94, 2012.
[6] A. Desrosiers and L. Miller, "Relational spirituality and depression in adolescent girls," *Journal of Clinical Psychology*, vol. 63, no. 10, pp. 1021–1037, 2007.
[7] B. R. Doolittle and M. Farrell, "The association between spirituality and depression in an Urban clinic," *Primary Care Companion to the Journal of Clinical Psychiatry*, vol. 6, no. 3, pp. 114–118, 2004.
[8] C. J. Nelson, B. Rosenfeld, W. Breitbart, and M. Galietta, "Spirituality, religion, and depression in the terminally ill," *Psychosomatics*, vol. 43, no. 3, pp. 213–220, 2002.
[9] D. Rasic, J. A. Robinson, J. Bolton, O. J. Bienvenu, and J. Sareen, "Longitudinal relationships of religious worship attendance and spirituality with major depression, anxiety disorders, and suicidal ideation and attempts: findings from the Baltimore epidemiologic catchment area study," *Journal of Psychiatric Research*, vol. 45, no. 6, pp. 848–854, 2011.
[10] G. Glas, "Anxiety, anxiety disorders, religion and spirituality," *Southern Medical Journal*, vol. 100, no. 6, pp. 621–625, 2007.
[11] K. S. Johnson, J. A. Tulsky, J. C. Hays et al., "Which domains of spirituality are associated with anxiety and depression in patients with advanced illness?" *Journal of General Internal Medicine*, vol. 26, no. 7, pp. 751–758, 2011.
[12] K. M. Connor, J. R. T. Davidson, and L. C. Lee, "Spirituality, resilience, and anger in survivors of violent trauma: a community survey," *Journal of Traumatic Stress*, vol. 16, no. 5, pp. 487–494, 2003.
[13] M. J. Krejci, K. M. Thompson, H. Simonich et al., "Sexual trauma, spirituality, and psychopathology," *Journal of Child Sexual Abuse*, vol. 13, no. 2, pp. 85–103, 2004.
[14] E. Durkeim, *Suicide: A Study in Sociology*, Free Press, New York, NY, USA, 1951, Translated by J. A. Spaulding & G. Simpson.
[15] H. G. Koenig, L. K. George, and P. Titus, "Religion, spirituality, and health in medically ill hospitalized older patients," *Journal of the American Geriatrics Society*, vol. 52, no. 4, pp. 554–562, 2004.
[16] D. R. Williams and M. J. Sternthal, "Spirituality, religion and health: evidence and research directions," *The Medical Journal of Australia*, vol. 186, no. 10, supplement, pp. S47–S50, 2007.
[17] A. T. Beck, R. A. Steer, M. Kovacs, and B. Garrison, "Hopelessness and eventual suicide: a 10-year prospective study of patients hospitalized with suicidal ideation," *American Journal of Psychiatry*, vol. 142, no. 5, pp. 559–563, 1985.
[18] G. Berg, "The relationship between spiritual distress, PTSD and depression in Vietnam combat veterans," *The Journal of Pastoral Care & Counseling*, vol. 65, no. 1-2, pp. 6:1–6:11, 2011.
[19] B. H. Chang, K. M. Skinner, and U. Boehmer, "Religion and mental health among women veterans with sexual assault experience," *International Journal of Psychiatry in Medicine*, vol. 31, no. 1, pp. 77–95, 2001.
[20] B. H. Chang, K. M. Skinner, C. Zhou, and L. E. Kazis, "The relationship between sexual assault, religiosity, and mental health among male veterans," *International Journal of Psychiatry in Medicine*, vol. 33, no. 3, pp. 223–239, 2003.
[21] J. E. Bormann, L. Liu, S. R. Thorp, and A. J. Lang, "Spiritual wellbeing mediates PTSD change in veteranswith military-related PTSD," *International Journal of Behavioral Medicine*. In press.
[22] K. I. Pargament and P. J. Sweeney, "Building spiritual fitness in the army: an innovative approach to a vital aspect of human development," *American Psychologist*, vol. 66, no. 1, pp. 58–64, 2011.
[23] V. P. Niederhauser, J. Maddock, F. LeDoux, and M. Arnold, "Building strong and ready army families: a multirisk reduction health promotion pilot study," *Military Medicine*, vol. 170, no. 3, pp. 227–233, 2005.
[24] M. W. Parker, G. F. Fuller, H. G. Koenig et al., "Soldier and family wellness across the life course: a developmental model of successful aging, spirituality, and health promotion, part II," *Military Medicine*, vol. 166, no. 7, pp. 561–570, 2001.
[25] J. I. Harris, C. R. Erbes, B. E. Engdahl et al., "The effectiveness of a trauma focused spiritually integrated intervention for veterans exposed to trauma," *Journal of Clinical Psychology*, vol. 67, no. 4, pp. 425–438, 2011.
[26] K. D. Drescher, M. Burgoyne, E. Curran et al., "Issues of grief, loss, honor and remembrance: spirituality and work with military personnel and their families," in *Living and Surviving in Harm's Way*, S. M. Freeman, B. A. Moore, and A. Freeman, Eds., pp. 437–465, Routledge, New York, NY, USA, 2009.
[27] A. Fontana and R. Rosenheck, "Trauma, change in strength of religious faith, and mental health service use among veterans treated for PTSD," *Journal of Nervous and Mental Disease*, vol. 192, no. 9, pp. 579–584, 2004.
[28] D. J. Hufford, M. J. Fritts, and J. E. Rhodes, "Spiritual fitness," *Military Medicine*, vol. 175, no. 8, pp. 73–87, 2010.
[29] B. Hagerty, Army's "Spiritual Fitness" Test Angers Some Sodiers, 2011, http://www.npr.org/2011/01/13/132904866/armys-spiritual-fitness-test-angers-some-soldiers.
[30] J. Leopold, Army's "Spiritual Fitness" Test Comes Under Fire, 2011, http://truth-out.org/index.php?option=com_k2&view=item&id=268:army's-"spiritual-fitness"-test-comes-under-fire.
[31] R. L. Seddon, E. Jones, and N. Greenberg, "The role of chaplains in maintaining the psychological health of military personnel: an historical and contemporary perspective," *Military Medicine*, vol. 176, no. 12, pp. 1357–1361, 2011.
[32] P. A. F. McNulty, "Reported stressors and health care needs of active duty navy personnel during three phases of deployment in support of the war in Iraq," *Military Medicine*, vol. 170, no. 6, pp. 530–535, 2005.
[33] J. D. Snarr, R. E. Heyman, and A. M. S. Slep, "Recent suicidal ideation and suicide attempts in a large-scale survey of the U.S. air force: prevalences and demographic risk factors," *Suicide and Life-Threatening Behavior*, vol. 40, no. 6, pp. 544–552, 2010.
[34] Department of the Army, *The Army Health Promotion, Risk Reduction, and Suicide Prevention Report 2010 (the Red Book)*, Department of the Army, Washington, DC, USA, 2010.
[35] R. M. Bray, M. R. Pemberton, M. E. Lane, L. L. Hourani, M. J. Mattiko, and L. A. Babeu, "Substance use and mental health trends among U.S. military active duty personnel: key findings from the 2008 DoD health behavior survey," *Military Medicine*, vol. 175, no. 6, pp. 390–399, 2010.
[36] Substance Abuse and Mental Health Services Administration, "*Results from the 2010 National Survey on Drug Use and Health: summary of national findings*," NSDUH Series H-41, HHS Publication no. (SMA) 11-4658, Substance Abuse and Mental Health Services Administration, Rockville, Md, USA, 2011.
[37] D. W. King, L. A. King, and D. S. Vogt, *Manual for the Deployment Risk and Resilience Inventory (DRRI): A Collection of Measures for Studying Deployment Related Experiences of Military Veterans*, Nation Center for PTSD, Boston, Mass, USA, 2003.
[38] E. M. Andresen, J. A. Malmgren, W. B. Carter, and D. L. Patrick, "Screening for depression in well older adults: evaluation of a short form of the CES-D," *American Journal of Preventive Medicine*, vol. 10, no. 2, pp. 77–84, 1994.

[39] F. W. Weathers, B. T. Litz, J. A. Huska, and T. M. Keane, *The PTSD Checklist—Civilian Version (PCL-C)*, National Center for PTSD, Boston, Mass, USA, 1994.

[40] S. M. Keen, C. J. Kutter, B. L. Niles, and K. E. Krinsley, "Psychometric properties of PTSD checklist in sample of male veterans," *Journal of Rehabilitation Research and Development*, vol. 45, no. 3, pp. 465–474, 2008.

[41] K. J. Ruggiero, K. Del Ben, J. R. Scotti, and A. E. Rabalais, "Psychometric properties of the PTSD checklist—civilian version," *Journal of Traumatic Stress*, vol. 16, no. 5, pp. 495–502, 2003.

[42] A. J. Lang and M. B. Stein, "An abbreviated PTSD checklist for use as a screening instrument in primary care," *Behaviour Research and Therapy*, vol. 43, no. 5, pp. 585–594, 2005.

[43] Research Triangle Institute, *SUDAAN Language Manual, Release 10.0*, Research Triangle Institute, Triangle Park, NC, USA, 2008.

[44] M. J. Edlund, K. M. Harris, H. G. Koenig et al., "Religiosity and decreased risk of substance use disorders: is the effect mediated by social support or mental health status?" *Social Psychiatry and Psychiatric Epidemiology*, vol. 45, no. 8, pp. 827–836, 2010.

[45] D. B. Larson and J. P. Swyers, *Scientific Research on Spirituality and Health: A Consensus Report* , National Institute for Healthcare Research, Rockville, Md, USA, 1998.

[46] A. B. Cohen and H. G. Koenig, "Religion, religiosity and spirituality in the biopsychosocial model of health and ageing," *Ageing International*, vol. 28, no. 3, pp. 215–241, 2003.

[47] C. Puchalski and A. L. Romer, "Taking a spiritual history allows clinicians to understand patients more fully," *Journal of Palliative Medicine*, vol. 3, no. 1, pp. 129–137, 2000.

[48] D. R. Hodge, "Developing a spiritual assessment toolbox: a discussion of the strengths and limitations of five different assessment methods," *Health and Social Work*, vol. 30, no. 4, pp. 314–323, 2005.

[49] D. R. Hodge, "Spiritual assessment: a review of major qualitative methods and a new framework for assessing spirituality," *Social Work*, vol. 46, no. 3, pp. 203–214, 2001.

26

Symptom Profile and Severity in a Sample of Nigerians with Psychotic versus Nonpsychotic Major Depression

Increase Ibukun Adeosun and Oyetayo Jeje

Federal Neuropsychiatric Hospital, Yaba, 8 Harvey Road, PMB 2008, Lagos, Nigeria

Correspondence should be addressed to Increase Ibukun Adeosun; dr.increase.adeosun@gmail.com

Academic Editor: Martin Alda

The therapeutic strategies in managing patients with psychotic major depression (PMD) differ from those with non-psychotic major depression (NMD), because of differences in clinical profile and outcome. However, there is underrecognition of psychotic symptoms in depressed patients. Previous studies in Western population suggest that certain symptom patterns, apart from psychosis which may be concealed, can facilitate the discrimination of PMD from NMD. These studies may have limited applicability to sub-Saharan Africa due to cross-cultural differences in the phenomenology of depression. This study compared the rates and severity of depressive symptoms in outpatients with PMD ($n = 129$) and NMD ($n = 117$) using the Structured Clinical Interview for Depression (SCID) and Hamilton Depression Rating Scale (HAM-D). Patients with PMD had statistically significantly higher rates of suicidal ideation, suicidal attempt, psychomotor agitation, insomnia, and reduced appetite. Patients with NMD were more likely to manifest psychomotor retardation and somatic symptoms. PMD was associated with greater symptom severity. On logistic regression analysis, suicidal ideation, psychomotor disturbances, insomnia, and somatic symptoms were predictive of diagnostic status. The presence of these symptoms clusters may increase the suspicion of occult psychosis in patients with depression, thereby informing appropriate intervention strategies.

1. Introduction

Depression is a common psychiatric disorder estimated to affect about 1 out of 5 people in their lifetime [1]. It is a leading cause of disability, projected to become the second leading contributor to the global burden of disease by the year 2020 [2]. Clinically, a major depressive episode or disorder is characterised by the presence of depressed mood, loss of interest, low energy, and significant changes in sleep, appetite, weight, and psychomotor activity. Other symptoms include indecisiveness, feelings of worthlessness, guilt, and suicidality [3, 4].

Epidemiological evidence indicates that about 19 to 25% of patients with major depression have psychotic symptoms, typically delusions and hallucinations [5]. In comparison to Nonpsychotic major depression (NMD), patients with psychotic major depression (PMD) have a worse clinical course characterised by higher rates of recurrence,treatment resistance, suicidality, psychosocial impairment, overall symptom severity, and comorbidity [6–9].

Research has shown that there is underdetection of psychotic symptoms in depressed patients because psychotic symptoms may be subtle, intermittent, underreported, or deliberately concealed due to fear of embarrassment or stigma [10]. Considering the worse outcome in PMD, it is critical to identify features that could facilitate the clinical discrimination of PMD from NMD in addition to the presence or absence of psychotic symptoms.

Furthermore, the common notion that the severity of symptoms is an index of the presence of psychosis in depressed patients has been challenged by recent research findings indicating that psychosis is not inextricably linked to a higher severity of depressive symptoms [5, 7].

The majority of previous studies comparing the pattern and severity of symptoms in PMD versus NMD found that depressed patients with psychosis were more likely to manifest insomnia, psychomotor agitation, guilt, cognitive impairment, suicidal ideation, and suicidal attempt [10–14]. PMD was also associated with greater severity of depressive symptoms. Findings regarding differences in the prevalence and severity of anxiety, diurnal variation, hypochondriasis, and depressed mood are less consistent [15]. Forty et al. [11] found wide variations in severity in both patients with PMD and NMD, and showed that severity alone is not the determinant of psychosis in patients with depression. Rates of up to 15% of psychosis have been reported in patients with mild to moderate level of severity of depressive symptoms [5].

Previous authors have reported the phenomenology and correlates of depression in Africans, as well as certain differences between unipolar and bipolar depression [16–24]. However, there is limited information on the symptom and severity profile of patients with PMD in comparison to NMD using standardised instruments. Cross-cultural differences in the phenomenology of depression may limit the applicability of findings from Western countries to a sub-Saharan African population [25]. For instance, depression is more likely to be manifestd with somatic symptoms in Africans, whereas symptoms such as guilt, worthlessness, and suicidality common in Caucasians may occur with less frequency [5, 16–25]. Furthermore, ethnocultural differences are known to exist in the prevalence and manifestation of psychotic symptoms [26]. On account of these, previous authors have highlighted the need to examine the presentation of PMD and NMD from diverse ethnic and socio-cultural settings [12, 27].

This study therefore aimed to compare the rates and severity of symptoms of depression between patients with PMD and those with NMD among out-patients attending a major psychiatric care facility in Nigeria. Elucidations of these differences have implications for accurate diagnosis, timely intervention, and treatment planning. Based on the extant literature, we hypothesised that there are significant differences between PMD and NMD in frequency and severity of depressive symptoms.

2. Materials and Methods

2.1. Subjects. Consecutively presenting out-patients (n = 246) with PMD and NMD attending the largest mental health care facility in Nigeria, Federal Neuro-Psychiatric Hospital Yaba, were recruited into the sample over a period of four months (from January to April 2012). Exclusion criteria were subjects below the age of 18 years, the presence of comorbid medical/neurological disorders, mood/psychotic disorders due to a general medical condition, and other comorbid psychiatric disorders.

2.2. Procedure. Ethical approval was obtained from the institution's research and ethical committee. Consecutively presenting patients were invited to participate in the study and subjects were recruited following the provision of informed consent. There were only seven refusals and these did not differ significantly from the recruited sample in terms of demographic characteristics. Patients were recruited at the study setting following comprehensive psychiatric and medical assessment by consultant psychiatrists and senior residents in psychiatry. They were recruited at first contact with the facility prior to commencement of treatment. The researchers had access to patients clinical records (case notes) and in most cases collateral information by accompanying family members. Clinical diagnoses of depression were ascertained with the Structured Clinical Interview for DSM-1V Axis I Disorder (SCID) [28]. Comparisons were made between patients with PMD and NMD regarding the prevalence and severity of symptoms of depression using the SCID and the Hamilton Depression Rating Scale (HAM-D) [29], respectively. Interviewer-based instruments were completed by trained researchers with a minimum of 2-year postgraduate residency training in psychiatry. Interrater assessments from 10 joint interviews during a pretest yielded reliability coefficients, K = 0.90 for depression (SCID), K = 0.88 for "other somatic symptoms," and r = 0.89 for HAM-D.

2.3. Measures

2.3.1. Sociodemographic Questionnaire. The questionnaire was designed by the authors to elicit information about the age, gender, marital status, highest level of education and employment status of the participants. The literate participants completed the questionnaire by themselves. The researchers read out the questions and response options to those who were not literate and recorded the responses they volunteered.

2.3.2. SCID. The Structured Clinical Interview for DSM-1V Axis I Disorder (SCID) was administered to ascertain the diagnosis of depressive disorder (PMD and MD) in the participants. It also provided rating of symptoms of depression ranging from 1 (none), 2 (subthreshold), to 3 (threshold). Depressive symptoms were regarded as present (positive) only if the response items were rated as 3. In addition to the symptom profile elicited with the SCID, we also included the item "other somatic symptoms" in order to capture certain somatic symptoms (such as heat or peppery sensations in the head or body; heaviness or tension in the head; emptiness or feelings of fluid in the head; and crawling sensations) which have been shown by previous authors to be common or uniquely expressed among Africans [20–24]. In view of the fact that the expression of these symptoms may be related to the cultural idioms of distress or the use of somatic metaphors [25], "other somatic symptoms" were painstakingly probed clinically to ascertain their nature, quality, and frequency. For instance, patients were asked to describe these symptoms in detail including the use of local language in order to clarify if symptoms such as heat/pepper/crawling sensation were merely somatic metaphors or met the definition of tactile hallucinations or somatic delusions. When the symptoms are accompanied by delusional interpretation/explanations or the patients have clear somatic delusions or tactile hallucination (not merely a somatic metaphor) on further probing, these are regarded as psychotic symptoms. On the other hand if they were only idiomatic expressions or pseudo-hallucination occurring exclusively during mood episodes, they were regarded as nonpsychotic symptoms.

Table 1: Socio-demographic characteristics of the participants.

Variables	PMD (n = 129) n (%)	NMD (n = 117) n (%)	Total	χ^2	P
Gender					
Male	38 (29.5)	46 (39.3)	84	2.652	0.103
Female	91 (70.5)	71 (60.7)	162		
Marital status					
Married	83 (64.3)	62 (53.0)	145	3.266	0.071
Not married	46 (35.7)	55 (47.0)	101		
Employment status					
Employed	56 (43.4)	44 (37.6)	100	0.857	0.355
Unemployed	73 (56.6)	73 (62.4)	146		
Level of education					
Primary/none	38 (29.5)	22 (18.8)	60	4.066	0.131
Secondary	53 (41.1)	59 (50.4)	112		
Tertiary	38 (29.5)	36 (30.8)	74		
	Mean (SD)	Mean (SD)		t	
Age	39.94 (13.47)	39.85 (13.22)		0.051	0.960

2.3.3. Hamilton Depression Rating Scale (HAM-D). It was administered by the researcher to rate the severity of depressive symptoms in the participants. It is a 21-item interviewer based instrument, but only the first 17 items responses were summed up to determine the severity of depressive symptoms.

2.4. Statistical Analyses. Data was analysed with the SPSS version 16. The sociodemographic and clinic characteristics were compared using chi-square for categorical variables and t-test for continuous variables. The primary outcome of interest was the presence or absence of symptoms of depression in patients with PMD versus NMD. This was compared using chi-square. Group comparison of symptom severity (mean total HAM-D) score was conducted with the independent Student's t-tests. To test for independent significant relationships, significant variables on bivariate analysis were all entered into logistic regression analysis. The effects of difference in severity were controlled for. The test was essentially two-tailed with level of significance set at $P < 0.05$.

3. Results

Table 1 shows the socio-demographic profile of the participants. Females were the majority (66.3%) and their mean age was 39.9 (±13.3) years. Only 30.5% had up to tertiary education, 59.3% were unemployed, and 58.5% were married. There were no significant socio-demographic differences between patients with PMD and NMD.

As compared with patients with NMD, patients with PMD had significantly higher rates (Table 2) of psychomotor agitation ($P < 0.001$), insomnia ($P < 0.001$), reduced appetite ($P = 0.038$), suicidal ideation ($P = 0.005$), and suicidal attempts ($P = 0.009$). On the other hand, the rates of "other somatic symptoms" and psychomotor retardation were significantly higher in patients with NMD ($P < 0.001$). Similarly patients with PMD had significantly higher overall depression severity rating in comparison to patients with NMD ($P < 0.001$).

The most common psychotic symptoms in patients with PMD were auditory hallucinations (54.26%), persecutory delusions (42.64%), and delusions of reference (33.33%). Others included delusions of guilt, religious delusions, visual hallucinations, somatic delusions, tactile hallucinations, and delusions of jealousy (Table 3).

On regression analysis, psychomotor agitation, suicidal ideation, and insomnia were independently associated with

Table 2: Prevalence of symptoms of depression in patients with PMD versus NMD.

Symptoms	PMD (n = 129) n (%)	NMD (n = 117) n (%)	χ^2	P
Depressed mood	129 (100)	116 (99.1)	1.11*	0.476
Diminished interest	108 (83.7)	95 (81.2)	0.27	0.603
Decreased appetite	70 (54.3)	48 (41.0)	4.31	0.038
Weight loss	41 (31.8)	35 (29.9)	0.10	0.751
Insomnia	127 (98.4)	93 (79.5)	23.34	**<0.001**
Psychomotor agitation	41 (31.8)	10 (8.5)	20.16	**<0.001**
Psychomotor retardation	24 (18.6)	53 (45.3)	20.33	**<0.001**
Fatigue/low energy	98 (76.0)	93 (79.5)	0.44	0.508
Guilt	51 (39.5)	43 (36.8)	0.20	0.654
Worthlessness	63 (48.8)	65 (55.6)	1.11	0.292
Poor concentration	64 (49.6)	56 (47.9)	0.08	0.784
Suicidal ideation	75 (58.1)	47 (40.2)	7.92	**0.005**
Suicidal attempt	23 (17.8)	8 (6.8)	6.73	**0.009**
Other somatic symptoms	38 (29.5)	64 (54.7)	16.11	**<0.001**
HAM-D score	Mean (SD)	Mean (SD)	t	P
HAM-D score	27.64 (3.9)	18.64 (6.1)	13.93	<0.001

*Fisher's correction applied.

Table 3: Profile of psychotic symptoms in patients with psychotic major depression (N = 129).

Symptoms	n (%)
Delusions	
Persecution	55 (42.64)
Reference	43 (33.33)
Guilt	10 (7.75)
Religion	8 (6.20)
Somatic	7 (5.43)
Jealousy	3 (2.32)
Hallucinations	
Auditory	70 (54.26)
Visual	8 (6.20)
Tactile	7 (5.43)

TABLE 4: Logistic regression analysis of depressive symptoms pattern in PMD versus NMD.

Variables	B	SE	Wald	P	OR	95% CI
Psychomotor agitation	.95	.42	5.02	0.025	2.60	1.13–5.96
Psychomotor retardation	−1.29	.34	14.56	<0.001	0.28	0.14–0.54
Insomnia	2.70	.79	11.59	0.001	14.90	3.15–7.57
Decreased appetite	.11	.31	0.13	0.715	1.12	0.61–2.04
Other somatic symptoms	−0.69	.32	4.56	0.033	0.50	0.27–0.94
Suicidal ideation	.86	.33	6.58	0.010	2.36	1.22–4.53
Suicidal attempt	.54	.54	1.00	0.317	1.72	0.59–5.01
Symptom severity	1.66	.81	4.21	0.041	2.54	1.07–4.21

OR: odds ratio.

PMD, while somatic symptoms and psychomotor retardation were predictive of NMD (Table 4).

4. Discussion

This study compared the frequency and severity of depressive symptoms between patients with PMD and NMD in an out-patient psychiatric setting in Nigeria. The prevalence of PMD in the current study sample is higher than those of previous studies in Western populations. Previous authors in Western populations reported that the prevalence of psychotic symptoms in patients with depression is about 19% in community samples and 25% in psychiatric hospital settings [5, 12, 30]. The higher prevalence of PMD in our sample may be attributed to difference in the pattern of service use across settings. Due to low levels of mental health literacy, causal misattribution, and poor access to mental health services in Nigeria, it is plausible that patients are more likely to seek treatment for more severe or psychotic symptoms. In a consecutive sample of out-patient clinic attendees in a similar setting to ours, 61% of depressed patients presenting to services had severe depression [16, 17]. Furthermore, previous studies have documented racial differences in the prevalence and expression of psychotic features in depressed patients [26, 27]. The most common psychotic symptoms in the current sample were auditory hallucinations, persecutory delusions, and delusions of reference. Previous studies have shown that the psychotic symptoms commonly seen in patients with depression are auditory hallucination, paranoid delusions, somatic delusions, delusions of guilt, and tactile hallucinations. The prevalence of tactile hallucination appears lower than that reported among depressed patients in Western population [12, 13].

We found that the symptom profile of patients with psychotic depression differed significantly from that of patients with nonpsychotic depression. This is in keeping with previous research [12, 13, 30, 31]. Our findings of a significantly higher rates of psychomotor agitation, insomnia, and suicidal ideation and attempt in patients with PMD in comparison to NMD are congruent with these reported by Guadiano et al. [12] in a large sample of outpatients with psychotic and nonpsychotic depression in the USA. Other authors have also demonstrated higher prevalence of psychomotor disturbances [13, 15, 32], insomnia [25], and suicidality [13, 22, 33] in patients with PMD.

Patients with PMD had significantly higher rates of reduced appetite than patients with NMD. Previous studies differed regarding this finding. Some authors reported that patients with PMD were more likely to have reduced appetite, [11] while other authors found no significant difference between both groups [12]. In contrast to previous studies, the prevalence of feelings of guilt and worthlessness did not significantly differ between PMD and NMD in the current study. The lack of significant difference in the rates of dysfunctional cognitions between both groups could be attributed to the lower frequency of these symptoms in the current sample, which is not surprising considering the documented rarity of guilt and worthlessness in the phenomenology of depression among Africans [16, 17].

On the other hand, patients with PMD had significantly lower rates of "other somatic symptoms" than those with NMD. Somatic symptoms are commonly expressed by Nigerian patients with depression [20–24]. Ilechukwu [20] found that somatic symptoms were more common in mild and moderate depression than severe depression in a Nigerian clinical population. However, to the best of our knowledge, these somatic symptoms have not been previously shown to be predictive of either PMD or NMD among Africans. Future studies are required to confirm this finding.

The elucidation of patterns of symptoms that are more likely to be associated with PMD, apart from psychotic symptoms which may be underreported, is of clinical significance [10]. Clinician's recognition of these patterns of symptoms could help in overcoming the diagnostic conundrum involved in differentiating PMD from MD. Early identification of PMD is crucial in treatment planning considering its worse clinical course and outcome.

Another important finding is the significantly higher level of symptom severity in PMD than NMD. This reechoes the findings of several authors [12, 31, 33] and reflects the definition of PMD on the basis of severity. However, studies have shown that higher depression scores in PMD are attributable to specific rather than global symptom elevation and greater illness severity is not a specific clinical marker for the presence of psychotic symptoms in patients with depression [11, 34]. Keller et al. [35] noted that the inextricable link between severity and psychosis is a pitfall; they emphasised the need to revise the classification of PMD, which is currently under the severity dimension.

On account of these vital differences in PMD and NMD, which have also been substantiated with neurochemical correlates, it has been argued that PMD is a distinct syndrome from NMD rather than a continuum of NMD manifesting with a greater severity [34–36]. Beyond issues of controversies regarding the classification, of more importance is the clinical/therapeutic significance of these findings. Since PMD responds poorly to conventional antidepressants and is more likely to be associated with resistance to treatment, prompt delineation of PMD from MD will inform better treatment planning [33].

Our study was hospital based and may not be representative of the profile of patients with depression in the general population. We do not know to what extent our cultural inclination or biases affected our clinical interpretation of the symptoms defined as "other somatic symptoms" and how these may apply in other settings. Our findings may also be limited by differences in certain variables such as age of onset of illness, family history, number of episodes of depression, and impact of medications. The latter two factors may be minimal due to the fact that patients were recruited at first contact with psychiatric services and therefore expectedly neuroleptic-naive. However, in the study setting, many patients present late for treatment and the possibility of undisclosed self-medication or unlabelled prescribed medication from other sources cannot be totally ruled out. Though patients with comorbid psychiatric disorders were excluded, due to the cross-sectional nature of the study, it is not known if patients presenting with a depressive episode may eventually evolve to other mood disorder (e.g., bipolar disorder) if followed up longitudinally; this is important considering the evidence that the best predictor of psychosis in the course of mood disorder is bipolar disorder [33]. However, this study has a number of strengths; we provided data from a previously understudied ethnic and cultural setting therefore filling a gap in knowledge. Secondly, participants were also included regardless of their gender and level of education. Thirdly, standardised instruments were used in the assessment of the presence and severity of symptoms. Furthermore, the impact of medications may be minimal because patients were recruited at first contact with services. The availability of collateral information from clinical records and informants is also an improvement on previous studies.

5. Conclusion

In conclusion, the findings of the current study, conducted in a previously understudied ethnic and socio-cultural context, is consistent with previous findings that certain cluster of symptoms may increase the suspicion of occult psychosis in patients with depression. Clinicians should have high index of suspicion of PMD when depression is manifested by psychomotor agitation, insomnia, suicidality, and absence of somatic symptoms. Further studies are required to confirm these findings in our environment. Future studies should consider longitudinal assessments of symptoms in a larger sample.

Conflict of Interests

The authors declare that they have no conflict of interests.

Acknowledgment

The authors would like to thank all the patients who participated in the study and their family members.

References

[1] R. C. Kessler, T. C. Wai, O. Demler, and E. E. Walters, "Prevalence, severity, and comorbidity of 12-month DSM-IV disorders in the national comorbidity survey replication," *Archives of General Psychiatry*, vol. 62, no. 6, pp. 617–627, 2005.

[2] C. Murray and A. Lopez, *The Global Burden of Disease*, Harvard University Press, Cambridge, Mass, USA, 1996.

[3] World Health Organization (WHO), *The International Classification of Mental and Behavioural Disorders*, (ICD-10), WHO, Geneva, Switzerland, 10th edition, 1992.

[4] American Psychiatric Association, *Diagnostic and Statistical Manual of Mental Disorders*, American Psychiatric Association, Washington, DC, USA, 4th edition, 1994.

[5] M. M. Ohayon and A. F. Schatzberg, "Prevalence of depressive episodes with psychotic features in the general population," *The American Journal of Psychiatry*, vol. 159, no. 11, pp. 1855–1861, 2002.

[6] M. Vythilingam, J. Chen, J. D. Bremner, C. M. Mazure, P. K. Maciejewski, and J. C. Nelson, "Psychotic depression and mortality," *The American Journal of Psychiatry*, vol. 160, no. 3, pp. 574–576, 2003.

[7] A. J. Rothschild, "Challenges in the treatment of depression with psychotic features," *Biological Psychiatry*, vol. 53, no. 8, pp. 680–690, 2003.

[8] T. A. Aronson, S. Shukla, K. Gujavarty, A. Hoff, M. DiBuono, and E. Khan, "Relapse in delusional depression: a retrospective study of the course of treatment," *Comprehensive Psychiatry*, vol. 29, no. 1, pp. 12–21, 1988.

[9] B. A. Gaudiano, C. G. Beevers, and I. W. Miller, "Differential response to combined treatment in patients with psychotic versus nonpsychotic major depression," *Journal of Nervous and Mental Disease*, vol. 193, no. 9, pp. 625–628, 2005.

[10] A. J. Rothschild, B. H. Mulsant, B. S. Meyers, and A. J. Flint, "Challenges in differentiating and diagnosing psychotic depression," *Psychiatric Annals*, vol. 36, no. 1, pp. 40–46, 2006.

[11] L. Forty, L. Jones, I. Jones et al., "Is depression severity the sole cause of psychotic symptoms during an episode of unipolar major depression? A study both between and within subjects," *Journal of Affective Disorders*, vol. 114, no. 1–3, pp. 103–109, 2009.

[12] B. A. Gaudiano, D. Young, I. Chelminski, and M. Zimmerman, "Depressive symptom profiles and severity patterns in outpatients with psychotic versus nonpsychotic major depression," *Comprehensive Psychiatry*, vol. 49, no. 5, pp. 421–429, 2008.

[13] M. Thakur, J. Hays, and K. R. R. Krishnan, "Clinical, demographic and social characteristics of psychotic depression," *Psychiatry Research*, vol. 86, no. 2, pp. 99–106, 1999.

[14] A. F. Schatzberg, J. A. Posener, C. DeBattista, B. M. Kalehzan, A. J. Rothschild, and P. K. Shear, "Neuropsychological deficits in psychotic versus nonpsychotic major depression and no mental illness," *The American Journal of Psychiatry*, vol. 157, no. 7, pp. 1095–1100, 2000.

[15] G. Parker, D. Hadzi-Pavlovic, I. Hickie et al., "Distinguishing psychotic and non-psychotic melancholia," *Journal of Affective Disorders*, vol. 22, no. 3, pp. 135–148, 1991.

[16] D. I. Otote and J. U. Ohaeri, "Depressive symptomatology and short-term stability at a Nigerian psychiatric care facility," *Psychopathology*, vol. 33, no. 6, pp. 314–323, 2000.

[17] J. U. Ohaeri and D. I. Otote, "Family history, life events and the factorial structure of depression in a Nigerian sample of inpatients," *Psychopathology*, vol. 35, no. 4, pp. 210–219, 2002.

[18] R. O. A. Makanjuola, "'Ode Ori': A culture-bound disorder with prominent somatic features in Yoruba Nigerian patients," *Acta Psychiatrica Scandinavica*, vol. 75, no. 3, pp. 231–236, 1987.

[19] A. Binitie, "A factor analytical study of depression across cultures (African and European)," *The British Journal of Psychiatry*, vol. 127, no. 12, pp. 559–563, 1975.

[20] S. T. C. Ilechukwu, "Psychiatry in Africa: special problems and unique features," *Transcultural Psychiatric Research Review*, vol. 28, pp. 168–218, 1991.

[21] G. T. Okulate, M. O. Olayinka, and O. B. E. Jones, "Somatic symptoms in depression: evaluation of their diagnostic weight in an African setting," *The British Journal of Psychiatry*, vol. 184, pp. 422–427, 2004.

[22] G. T. Okulate, H. T. Oladapo, and A. Osibogun, "Comparison of three subtypes of depression," *The Nigerian Postgraduate Medical Journal*, vol. 8, no. 1, pp. 41–45, 2001.

[23] G. T. Okulate and O. B. Jones, "Two depression rating instruments in Nigerian patients," *The Nigerian Postgraduate Medical Journal*, vol. 9, no. 2, pp. 74–78, 2002.

[24] P. O. Ebigbo, "Development of a culture specific (Nigeria) screening scale of somatic complaints indicating psychiatric disturbance," *Culture, Medicine and Psychiatry*, vol. 6, no. 1, pp. 29–43, 1982.

[25] K. Ahmed and D. Bhugra, "Depression across ethnic minority cultures: diagnostic issues," World Cultural Psychiatric Review, 2007.

[26] W. A. Vega and R. Lewis-Fernández, "Ethnicity and variability of psychotic symptoms," *Current Psychiatry Reports*, vol. 10, no. 3, pp. 223–228, 2008.

[27] A. L. Whaley and P. A. Geller, "Ethnic/racial differences in psychiatric disorders: a test of four hypotheses," *Ethnicity and Disease*, vol. 13, no. 4, pp. 499–512, 2003.

[28] M. B. First, R. L. Spitzer, J. B. W. Williams, and M. Gibbon, *Structured Clinical Interview for DSM-IV (SCID)*, American Psychiatric Association, Washington, DC, USA, 1997.

[29] M. Hamilton, "Development of a rating scale for primary depressive illness," *The British Journal of Social and Clinical Psychology*, vol. 6, no. 4, pp. 278–296, 1967.

[30] W. Coryell, B. Pfohl, and M. Zimmerman, "The clinical and neuroendocrine features of psychotic depression," *Journal of Nervous and Mental Disease*, vol. 172, no. 9, pp. 521–528, 1984.

[31] E. Lattuada, A. Serretti, C. Cusin, M. Gasperini, and E. Smeraldi, "Symptomatologic analysis of psychotic and non-psychotic depression," *Journal of Affective Disorders*, vol. 54, no. 1-2, pp. 183–187, 1999.

[32] E. Lykouras, D. Malliaras, G. N. Christodoulou et al., "Delusional depression: phenomenology and response to treatment," *Acta Psychiatrica Scandinavica*, vol. 73, no. 3, pp. 324–329, 1986.

[33] D. Souery, L. Zaninotto, R. Calati et al., "Phenomenology of psychotic mood disorders: lifetime and major depressive episode features," *Journal of Affective Disorders*, vol. 135, no. 1–3, pp. 241–250, 2011.

[34] D. V. Jeste, S. C. Heaton, J. S. Paulsen, L. Ercoli, M. J. Harris, and R. K. Heaton, "Clinical and neuropsychological comparison of psychotic depression with nonpsychotic depression and schizophrenia," *The American Journal of Psychiatry*, vol. 153, no. 4, pp. 490–496, 1996.

[35] J. Keller, A. F. Schatzberg, and M. Maj, "Current issues in the classification of psychotic major depression," *Schizophrenia Bulletin*, vol. 33, no. 4, pp. 877–885, 2007.

[36] M. K. Sapru, B. S. S. R. Rao, and S. M. Channabasavanna, "Serum dopamine-β-hydroxylase activity in clinical subtypes of depression," *Acta Psychiatrica Scandinavica*, vol. 80, no. 5, pp. 474–478, 1989.

27

A Low-Cost Point-of-Care Testing System for Psychomotor Symptoms of Depression Affecting Standing Balance

Arindam Dutta,[1] Robins Kumar,[2] Suruchi Malhotra,[2] Sanjay Chugh,[3] Alakananda Banerjee,[2] and Anirban Dutta[4,5]

[1] *The Gnan Systems LLP, Kolkata 700156, India*
[2] *The Dharma Foundation of India, New Delhi 110003, India*
[3] *The Neuro Rehab Services LLP, New Delhi 110048, India*
[4] *The Charité-Universitätsmedizin Berlin, 10117 Berlin, Germany*
[5] *Institut National de Recherche en Informatique et en Automatique (INRIA), 34090 Montpellier, France*

Correspondence should be addressed to Arindam Dutta; arindam.dutta.in@ieee.org

Academic Editor: Charles B. Nemeroff

The World Health Organization estimated that major depression is the fourth most significant cause of disability worldwide for people aged 65 and older, where depressed older adults reported decreased independence, poor health, poor quality of life, functional decline, disability, and increased chronic medical problems. Therefore, the objectives of this study were (1) to develop a low-cost point-of-care testing system for psychomotor symptoms of depression and (2) to evaluate the system in community dwelling elderly in India. The preliminary results from the cross-sectional study showed a significant negative linear correlation between balance and depression. Here, monitoring quantitative electroencephalography along with the center of pressure for cued response time during functional reach tasks may provide insights into the psychomotor symptoms of depression where average slope of the Theta-Alpha power ratio versus average slope of baseline-normalized response time may be a candidate biomarker, which remains to be evaluated in our future clinical studies. Once validated, the biomarker can be used for monitoring the outcome of a comprehensive therapy program in conjunction with pharmacological interventions. Furthermore, the frequency of falls can be monitored with a mobile phone-based application where the propensity of falls during the periods of psychomotor symptoms of depression can be investigated further.

1. Introduction

The World Health Organization (WHO) estimated that major depression is the fourth significant cause of disability for people aged 65 and above [1], where depression is a major contributor to the healthcare costs associated with the elderly population. Depression is a major health issue for elders, yet late-life depression often goes undiagnosed [2]. One in every four among India's elderly (age > 60 years) population is depressed, and around one in 10 experiences a fall that results in fracture [3]. In fact, the elderly population is predicted to increase to 12% of the total population by 2025 [3]. Depressed elderly report decreased independence, poor health, poor quality of life, functional decline, disability, and increased chronic medical problems [1]. Moreover, psychomotor symptoms of depression may contribute to falls among elderly and an associated fear of falling [4]. Here, course of depression, diurnal variation, medication status, gender, and age are associated with psychomotor agitation and retardation [5]. The psychomotor symptoms in depression have unique significance where they have high discriminative validity, may be the only symptoms of depression that distinguish depression subtypes, and are predictive of good response to medicines such as tricyclic antidepressants [5]. Therefore point-of-care testing (POCT) of the psychomotor symptoms of depression is urgently needed in order to screen community dwelling elderly at risk as well as to monitor the course of treatment [2], which takes 2 to 4 weeks to work fully, and a normal course lasts at least 6 months [5].

The costs of such screening of the psychomotor symptoms of depression is important in a low-resource setting, for example, in India, where a low-cost POCT of the psychomotor symptoms of depression was developed and evaluated in this study. In fact, Indian health ministry's working group on noncommunicable disease burden [3] noted that "India will soon become home to the second largest number of elderly in the world. The challenges are unique with this population in India." In accordance, Kumar and colleagues at the Dharma Foundation of India (DFI) conducted a preliminary cross-sectional study on 95 elderly (age > 60 years) subjects from New Delhi and Gurgaon, India [6]. They investigated psychomotor aspects of depression where they found a negative correlation between the Berg Balance Scale (BBS) score [7] and the Geriatric Depression Scale (GDS) score [8]. Also, they found that as age increased, the BBS score decreased and the GDS score increased, leading to poorer balance and depression. Following this alarming insight, DFI conducted a subsampling of 24 community dwelling elderly from their database in India that covered a wide range of BBS and GDS scores, in order to evaluate a low-cost POCT [9] system for the psychomotor symptoms of depression. The first objective of this report is to present the low-cost POCT system for psychomotor symptoms of depression. The second objective is to present the results from the clinical study on 24 community dwelling elderly to evaluate the POCT system. It was hypothesized that the POCT system will be able to capture the psychomotor symptoms of depression in elderly.

2. Methods

2.1. Preliminary Cross-Sectional Study. Kumar and colleagues conducted a cross-sectional study [6] on 104 subjects, who were found through convenient sampling of community dwelling elderly in Delhi and Gurgaon, India. The inclusion criteria of the study were age of elderly 60 years and above, both males and females, and the subjects should have the ability to read and understand either Hindi or English. The exclusion criteria were severe problem with vestibular and visual system, any self-reported history of psychiatric illness excluding depression, cognitive deficits due to any reason, and use of assistive aids for walking, for example, wheel chair, crutch, walker, cane. The evaluation tools used in the study are described below.

(i) Hindi Mental State Examination (HMSE) [10, 11] was developed for the Hindi-speaking semiliterate and illiterate population of rural northern India. The total score possible was 31 where the cut-off score was 19.

(ii) Berg Balance Scale (BBS) [7] consists of 14 common tasks. The 14 items are scored on a 5-point ordinal scale (0 = unable to perform, 4 = independent) based on ability to complete the timed tasks.

(iii) Geriatric Depression Scale (GDS) [8] is a brief questionnaire in which participants are asked to respond to the 30 questions by answering yes or no in reference to how they felt on the day of administration. Scores of 0–9 are considered normal, 10–19 indicate mild depression, and 20–30 indicate severe depression.

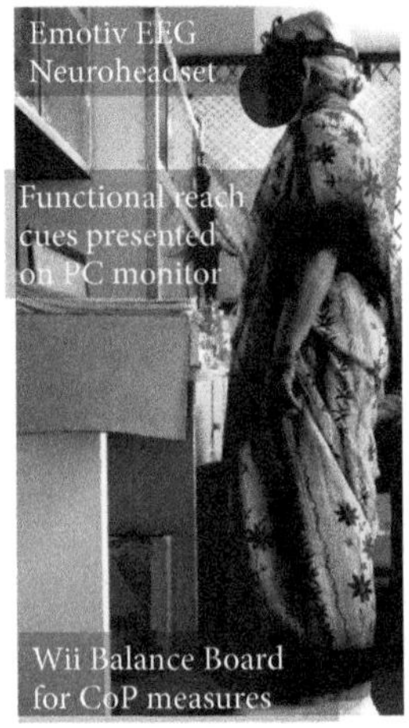

Figure 1: An illustration of the experimental setup.

Only 9 out of 104 subjects were excluded on the basis of the HMSE exclusion criteria, leading to a sample size of 95. The data was then analyzed by statistical software, as described further by Kumar and colleagues [6], where the descriptive statistics were calculated for the age, BBS, GDS, and frequency statistics of Gender. The Pearson correlation and regression analysis were applied to find out the relationship between age, BBS, and GDS. Independent sample t-test was applied to compare the scores of BBS and GDS between males and females.

2.2. Point-of-Care Testing (POCT) of Psychomotor Symptoms of Depression. Following the preliminary cross-sectional study by Kumar and colleagues [6], a convenient subsampling of the community dwelling elderly in India was conducted to select 24 elderly (>60 years) subjects, such that they covered a wide range of BBS and GDS scores. All subjects gave their informed consent for the experiments in compliance with the Helsinki Declaration.

The objective was to evaluate a low-cost POCT system to investigate the psychomotor symptoms of depression affecting standing balance. The experimental setup is shown in Figure 1. The centre of pressure (CoP) was monitored using a Wii Balance Board (Nintendo, USA) [13] and custom software developed using the WiiBrew toolkit [14]. The Wii Balance Board (Wii BB) relayed the 2D ground reaction force information to the PC via Bluetooth [14], while Emotiv EEG Neuroheadset (Emotiv, Australia) relayed EEG data to the PC via their proprietary wireless protocol [12]. The specifications of the EEG Neuroheadset [12] are detailed in the Table 1.

2.2.1. Real-Time Feedback of the Center of Pressure. Wii BB was interfaced with the PC via Bluetooth using the WiiBrew toolkit [14]. The Wii BB has a useable surface of 45 cm × 26.5 cm for standing which was calibrated by placing a variety of known loads at different positions [13]. Wii BB uses four

Table 1: Specifications of the Emotiv EEG Neuroheadset [12].

Number of channels	14 (plus CMS/DRL references)
Channel names (Int. 10–20 locations)	AF3, AF4, F3, F4, F7, F8, FC5, FC6, P3 (CMS), P4 (DRL), P7, P8, T7, T8, O1, O2
Sampling method	Sequential sampling, single ADC
Sampling rate	~128 Hz (2048 Hz internal)
Resolution	16 bits (14 bits effective) 1 LSB = 0.51 μV
Bandwidth	0.2–45 Hz, digital notch filters at 50 Hz and 60 Hz
Dynamic range (input referred)	256 mVpp
Coupling mode	AC coupled
Connectivity	Proprietary wireless, 2.4 GHz band
Battery type	Li-poly
Battery life (typical)	12 hrs
Impedance measurement	Contact quality using patented system

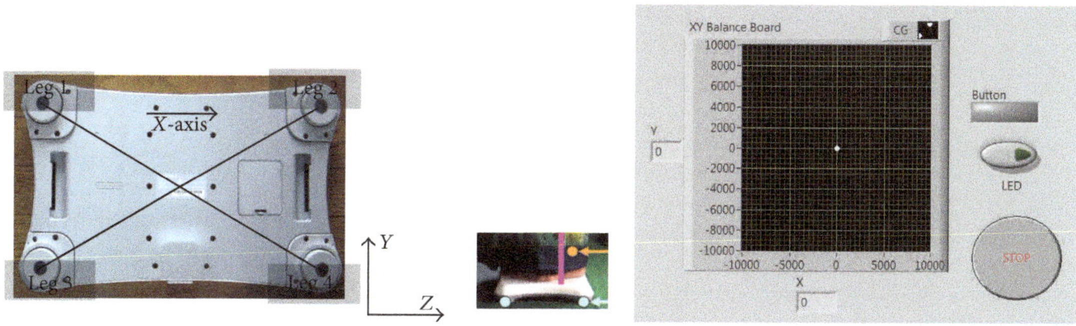

(a) (b)

Figure 2: (a) The load sensors are at the four legs of Wii Balance Board (Wii BB). The origin for Wii BB reference frame was placed on the horizontal standing surface of Wii BB, which was taken at the centre of the four legs as illustrated by the intersection of the diagonals, and the X-direction was assumed from the centre of leg 1 to the centre of leg 2, as shown. The Y-direction was upwards from the horizontal standing surface of Wii BB. (b) Real-time feedback of the center of pressure location.

load sensors at the four legs (shown in Figure 2(a)) to measure the weight. Each sensor at each leg of the Wii BB only measures the vertical component of the force. The CoP can be approximated by interpolating the four vertical forces which was then displayed to the user, as shown at Figure 2(b). The X, Y coordinates of CoP were calculated from the streaming data using the following equation:

$$\text{CoP}(X, Y) = \frac{\sum_{i=1}^{4} \text{Weight}_i(x, y)}{\sum_{i=1}^{4} \text{Weight}_i}, \quad (1)$$

where $\text{Weight}_i(x, y)$ are the coordinates of the ith load sensor in the Wii BB's reference frame, Weight_i is the force recorded by the ith load sensor, and CoP (X, Y) are the coordinates of the CoP in the Wii BB's reference frame. Also, the BBS score was collected to identify those individuals who were classified as "fallers" (BBS below 45) and those individuals who were classified as "nonfallers" (BBS 45 or above).

2.2.2. Offline Analysis of Baseline Resting State EEG. Emotiv EEG Neuroheadset wirelessly relayed EEG data to the PC from 14 channels (International 10–20 system)—AF3, AF4, F3, F4, F7, F8, FC5, FC6, P3 (CMS), P4 (DRL), P7, P8, T7, T8, O1, and O2. Resting state EEG was recorded in eyes-open and eyes-closed conditions during quiet standing for at least 3 minutes. The EEG data were analysed using EEGlab software [15]. The eye-blink artifacts were rejected using EEGlab functions, then the artifact-free continuous EEG was divided into 4.096 seconds epochs using a Hanning time window (epochs were overlapped by 50%), and an estimation of the power spectra was found for the absolute theta (4–7.5 Hz), alpha (7.5–14 Hz), and beta (14–20 Hz) frequency bands for QEEG analysis [16].

Following Grin-Yatsenko and colleagues [16], a three-way analysis of variance ("anovan" in MATLAB R2010a, The MathWorks, Inc., USA) of the absolute EEG power in eyes-closed condition was conducted with the following factors: GDS score (three levels: 0–9, 10–19, 20–30), EEG electrode locations (14 levels), and frequency band (three levels: theta, alpha, and beta). We then performed cluster analysis ("clusterdata" in Matlab R2010a, The MathWorks, Inc., USA) to compute the Euclidean distances between items in the data set and create a hierarchical cluster tree from the data set. Also, Linear Discriminant Classification ("ClassificationDiscriminant.fit" in Matlab R2010a, The MathWorks, Inc., USA) was investigated to evaluate the possibility of classification of depressive patients using eyes-closed EEG power spectra at discriminatory frequency bands and electrode locations, as found using multiple comparison tests ("multcompare" in Matlab R2010a, The MathWorks, Inc., USA).

2.2.3. *Offline Analysis of Psychomotor Symptoms.* A modified functional reach task was used to quantify the subjects' ability to volitionally shift their CoP position as quickly as possible without losing balance while cued with CoP feedback via a graphical user interface (GUI) on PC, as shown in Figures 1 and 2. This modified functional reach task (FRT) resembled the Functional Reach Test, which has been shown to predict risk of falls [17]. During the FRT, the subjects were asked to keep their body rigid and to maintain full feet contact with the Wii BB, while leaning as far as possible from forward, backward, and to right and left sides, as cued by the GUI. The EEG was recorded in eyes-open condition during the consecutive FRT as well as during quiet standing (at least 3 minutes) in-between the FRT. The PT/OT conducting the FRT reported BBS and GDS scores of each elderly subject from a preliminary cross-sectional study (Section 2.1).

The EEG data from 14 channels (International 10–20 system), AF3, AF4, F3, F4, F7, F8, FC5, FC6, P3 (CMS), P4 (DRL), P7, P8, T7, T8, O1, O2, was analysed using EEGlab software [15]. The eye-blink artifacts were rejected using EEGlab functions, then the artifact-free continuous EEG was divided into 4.096 seconds epochs using a Hanning time window (epochs were overlapped by 50%), and the power spectra was estimated for the theta, alpha, and beta frequency bands for QEEG analysis [18]. The evolution of the baseline-normalized EEG power in different frequency bands (normalized by their corresponding baseline eyes-open value) during quiet standing in-between FRT was investigated for different GDS scores, EEG electrode locations, and baseline-normalized cued response time. The cued response time represented latency from visual cue to correct CoP motion out of the 95% confidence boundary of the resting-state CoP cluster in the cued direction—forward, backward, right side, and left side.

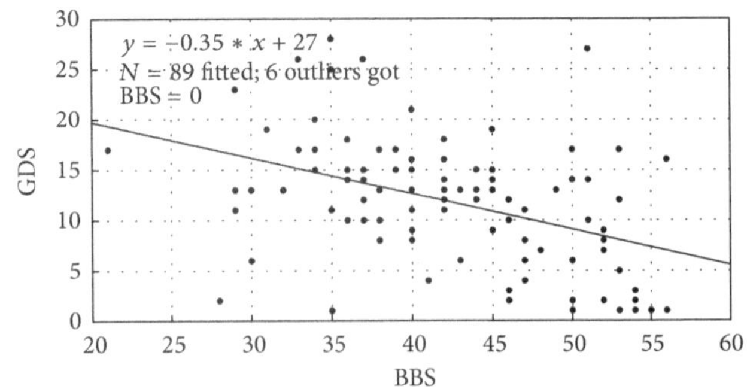

FIGURE 3: Scatter plot between Berg Balance Scale (BBS) and Geriatric Depression Scale (GDS) scores.

TABLE 2: Correlation between age, BBS, and GDS.

		Age	BBS	GDS
Age	Pearson's correlation	1	-0.362^{**}	0.162
	Sig. (2-tailed)		0.000	0.116
BBS	Pearson's correlation	-0.362^{**}	1	-0.423^{**}
	Sig. (2-tailed)	0.000		0.000
GDS	Pearson's correlation	0.162	-0.423^{**}	1
	Sig. (2-tailed)	0.116	0.000	

**Correlation is significant at the $P = 0.01$ level (2-tailed).

TABLE 3: Comparison between male and female with BBS and GDS.

	Gender	$N =$	Mean	Std. deviation	Std. error mean
BBS	Male	51	43.14	8.127	1.138
	Female	44	41.45	7.118	1.073
GDS	Male	51	11.02	6.498	0.910
	Female	44	12.91	6.030	0.909

3. Results

3.1. *Preliminary Cross-Sectional Study.* The descriptive statistics for age were $N = 95$, range = 60–89 years, mean = 70.12 years, std. deviation = 7.27 years. The correlation analysis between age, BBS, and GDS were performed using Pearson's correlation test where Table 2 shows the correlation coefficients. BBS showed a significant negative linear correlation with GDS ($r = -0.423$) and age ($r = -0.362$). GDS had a nonsignificant positive correlation with age ($r = -0.162$) at $P = 0.01$ level. The regression analysis of GDS as the dependent and BBS as the independent variables (predictor) for the analysis of variance showed F-ratio = 20.260, which was higher than the critical value. Therefore the variance attributable to the regression was significant, as shown in Figure 3. Also, the regression analysis of BBS as the dependent variable and age as the independent variable showed F-ratio = 14.030, which was higher than the critical value.

Independent-sample t-test was used to compare the differences in GDS and BBS scores between males and females. Table 3 shows the comparative analysis which includes mean, standard deviation, and standard error of the mean of BBS and GDS scores for the males and females. The t-test failed to reveal a statistically significant difference between the mean of the scores for BBS of male (mean = 43.14, std. deviation = 8.127), and female (mean = 41.45, std deviation = 7.118), $t(93) = 1.065$, $P = 0.289$, $\alpha = 0.05$. As shown in Table 3, the t-test also failed to reveal a statistically significant difference between the mean of the scores for GDS of male (mean = 11.02, std. deviation = 6.498) and female (mean = 12.91, std deviation = 6.030), $t(93) = 1.461$, $P = 0.147$, $\alpha = 0.05$.

3.2. *Point-of-Care Testing (POCT) of Psychomotor Symptoms of Depression.* We avoided using EEG data during eyes-open condition along-with eyes-closed condition (e.g., for alpha attenuation) since substantial eye-blink artifacts appeared for eyes-open condition and not eyes-closed condition, which needed to be filtered with EEGlab. The three-way analysis of variance of absolute EEG power in eyes-closed condition with factors GDS score, EEG electrode location, and frequency bands revealed a significant ($P < 0.01$) main effect of the factors and a significant ($P < 0.01$) interaction effect between GDS score and EEG electrode location, EEG electrode location and frequency band, but nonsignificant ($P = 0.09$) interaction effect between the frequency band and the GDS score. Posthoc analysis revealed an increased spectrum power during eyes-closed condition across all frequency

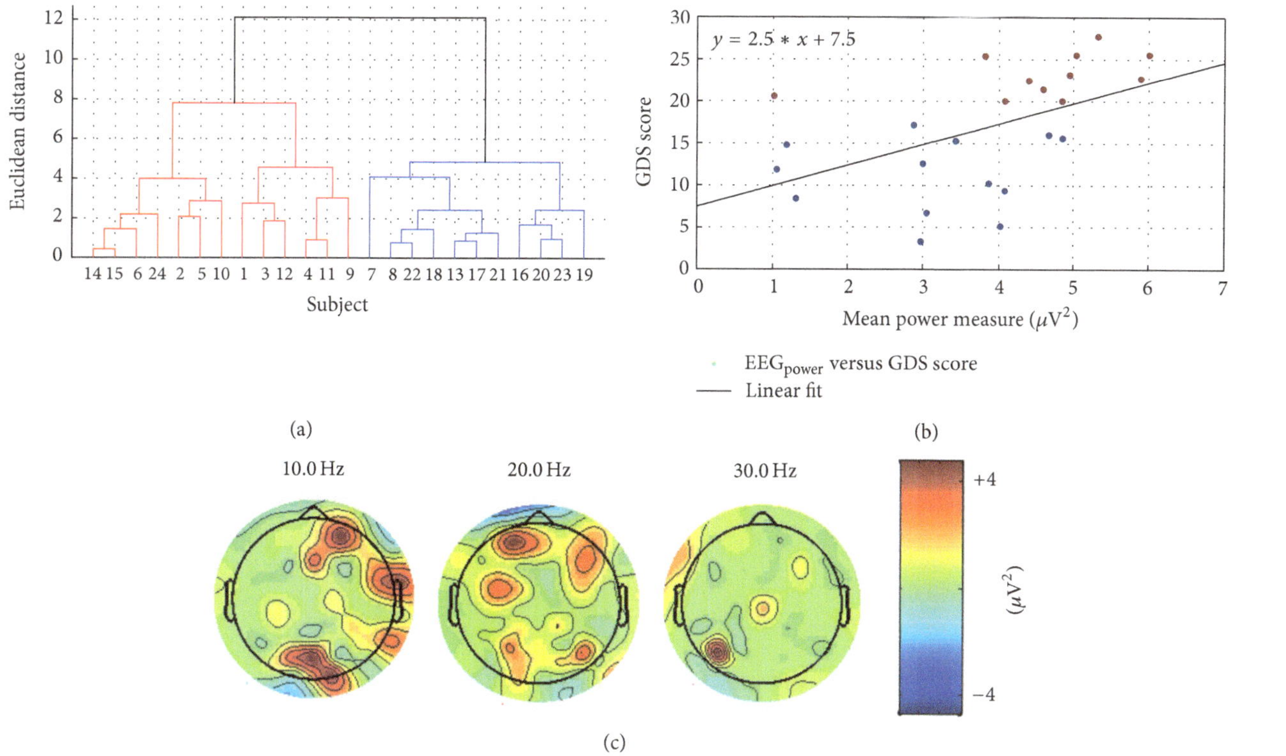

FIGURE 4: (a) Dendrogram plot of the hierarchical cluster tree from the data set—mean power measure at O1, O2, and P8 electrodes averaged over 4–30 Hz versus GDS scores. (b) Scatter plot between GDS scores and mean power measures where marker colors blue for "nondepressed" and brown for "depressed" show the two hierarchical clusters based on the Euclidean distance. (c) Topographic maps of difference EEG spectra at 10 Hz, 20 Hz, and 30 Hz between "depressed" (GDS ≥ 15) and "nondepressed" (GDS < 15) QEEG groups.

bands of the resting state EEG for occipital (O1, O2) and parietal (P8) electrode locations that correlated with worse depression scores. Figure 4(a) shows the dendrogram plot of the hierarchical cluster tree from the data set—mean power measure at O1, O2, and P8 electrodes averaged over 4–30 Hz versus GDS scores. The hierarchical cluster tree reveals primarily two clusters, GDS = 0–15 and GDS = 15–30, that are shown in Figure 4(b) with marker colors blue and brown, respectively, for the scatter plot between GDS scores and mean power measures. In accordance, Linear Discriminant Classification was conducted using mean power measures at O1, O2, and P8 electrodes averaged over 4–30 Hz, where the average percent of classification was found to be >84% for "nondepressed" (GDS = 0–15) QEEG group and >92% for "depressed" (GDS = 15–30) QEEG group.

During the modified functional reach task (FRT), a quicker transition to mental fatigue [18] was found in the "depressed" (GDS ≥ 15) QEEG group as elucidated by a faster increase in the theta band (4–8 Hz) baseline-normalized power in the frontal (F3, F4) electrodes and a faster decrease in the alpha band (8–13 Hz) baseline-normalized power in the parietal (P8) electrodes. Therefore, we defined Theta-Alpha power ratio as a QEEG marker of fatigue, which is the ratio of mean theta band baseline-normalized power in frontal (F3, F4) electrodes to mean alpha band baseline-normalized power in the parietal (P8) electrodes. Figure 5(a) shows the evolution of baseline-normalized response time during FRT and the Theta-Alpha power ratio during quiet standing in-between the FRT in "nondepressed" (GDS < 15) QEEG group while Figure 5(b) shows the same in "depressed" (GDS ≥ 15) QEEG group. In fact, there was a slight initial decrease in the response time in the "nondepressed" (GDS = 0–15) QEEG group before long-term increase due to fatigue, which may be due to initial selective attention to task performance. It was found that the increase in baseline-normalized response time during FRT was quicker in the "depressed" (GDS ≥ 15) QEEG group. Indeed, the baseline-normalized response time correlated with the Theta-Alpha power ratio with Pearson's linear correlation coefficient, $r = 0.2631$ at $P = 0.0096$ level. Also, Pearson's linear correlation coefficient for the "nondepressed" (GDS < 15) QEEG group was $r = 0.2318$ at $P = 0.0631$ level and for the "depressed" (GDS ≥ 15) QEEG group was $r = 0.2160$ at $P = 0.1131$ level, as shown in Figure 6(a). Accordingly, the dendrogram plot of the hierarchical cluster tree from the data set—average slope of the Theta-Alpha power ratio versus average slope of baseline-normalized response time—provided three clusters as shown in Figure 6(b) with blue, red, and green colors, which compared well with the dendrogram plot of the hierarchical cluster tree in Figure 4(a) (compare subject number).

4. Discussion

In this preliminary cross-sectional study, balance (BBS) score had a significant negative linear correlation with depression

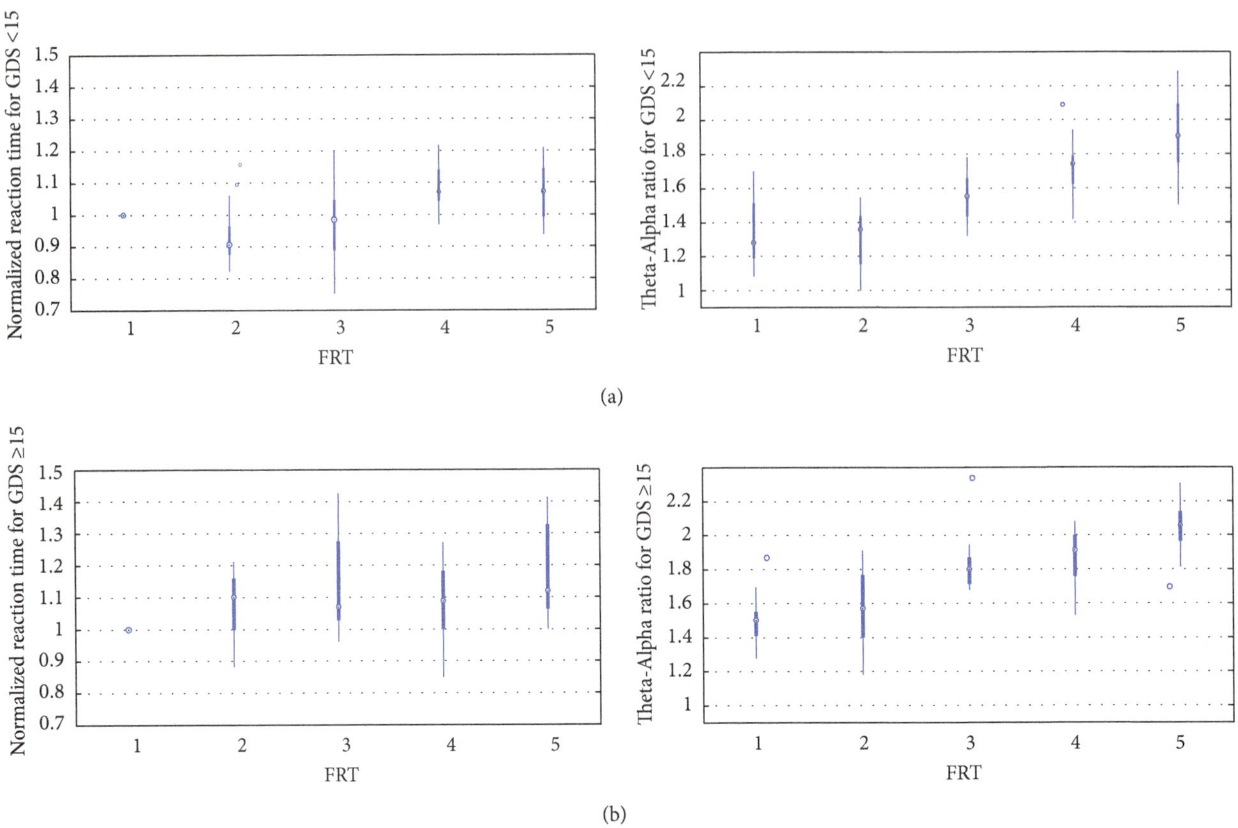

FIGURE 5: Box plot showing the evolution of baseline-normalized cued response time during modified functional reach tasks (FRT) and the Theta-Alpha power ratio during quiet standing in-between FRT for (a) "nondepressed" (GDS < 15) QEEG group and (b) "depressed" (GDS ≥ 15) QEEG group.

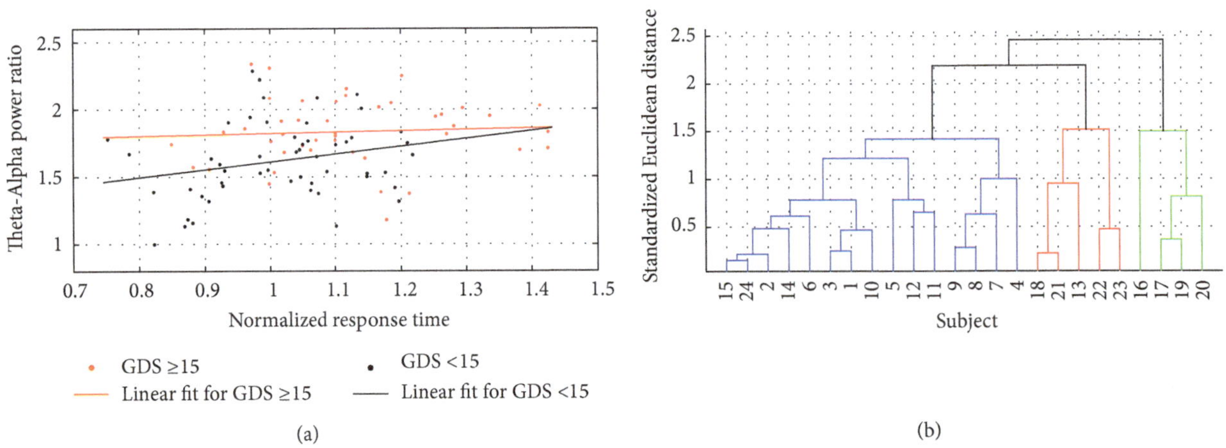

FIGURE 6: (a) Scatter plot between baseline-normalized cued response time and the Theta-Alpha power ratio, and linear regression fit for the "nondepressed" (GDS < 15) and "depressed" (GDS ≥ 15) QEEG groups. (b) Dendrogram plot of the hierarchical cluster tree from the data set—average slope of the Theta-Alpha power ratio versus average slope of baseline-normalized cued response time—providing three clusters shown with blue, red, and green colored linkages.

(GDS) score, which implied that as the depression increased, balance decreased, and vice versa. Since balance (BBS) score also showed a significant negative linear correlation with age, so depression (GDS) score could have been affected by age via balance (BBS) score; however, depression (GDS) score was found to only have a nonsignificant positive correlation with age. Although correlation does not mean causality, but these findings are consistent with those of Kose and colleagues [19], who found that depressive and cognitive symptoms, insufficient mobility, balance impairment and other risk factors are related to each other. In fact, there is a vicious cycle among these parameters. Rochester and colleagues [20] found that cognitive function, depression, physical fatigue, and balance were significantly related to walking speed for functional tasks. These findings are further consistent with those of Suárez and colleagues [21] who found that age-related changes in the neural, sensory, and musculoskeletal systems can lead to balance impairments that affect the ability to move around safely. Newton [22] found through multiple regression analysis that the frequency of performing activities and the comfort in performing activities without the fear of falling significantly contributed to the scores on the balance tests. The probable reason for such a finding may be that balance and depression are both the main risk factors for falls. These findings are consistent with those of Sai and colleagues [23] who had reported many risk factors for falls including a history of falls, lower extremity weakness, balance and gait abnormalities, decreased muscle strength, old age, cognitive impairment, medications, orthostatic hypotension, anemia, female gender, arthritis, and psychological factors including unipolar and bipolar depression and manic depressive disorder. Here, one limitation of our cross-sectional study design was that we did not collect retrospective data on the history of falls. We have now developed an Android application, FallAlert (Gnan Systems LLP, India) [24] to monitor falls using a mobile phone in our future studies.

The QEEG analysis of resting-state EEG showed increased spectrum power across all frequency bands for occipital (O1, O2) and parietal (P8) electrodes that correlated with worse depression (GDS) scores. However, eyes-closed EEG power spectra could reveal only two groups, GDS = 0–15 and GDS = 15–30, where mildly depressed (GDS = 10–19) patients were included either in "nondepressed" (GDS = 0–15) or "depressed" (GDS = 15–30) QEEG groups, making them a mix group. It was possible to classify subjects with only <16% false positive rate and >92% true positive rate using eyes-closed EEG power spectra. Here, monitoring QEEG along with the cued response time during modified functional reach tasks (FRTs) may provide insights into the psychomotor symptoms of depression where a quicker increase in the cued response time and Theta-Alpha power ratio was found in the "depressed" (GDS > 15) QEEG group, which implied a quicker transition to fatigue. In "nondepressed" (GDS ≤ 15) QEEG group there was a slight decrease in the Theta-Alpha power ratio from the baseline resting-state before a long-term increase, which may be attributed to acute effects due to selective attention related to task performance [25]. However in long-term, there was a faster increase in theta band baseline-normalized power in frontal electrodes and a faster decrease in alpha band baseline-normalized power in the parietal electrodes in the "depressed" (GDS > 15) QEEG group. In fact, decreased alpha power activity has been shown to be related to sleepiness, and a decreased high-level information processing is associated with decreased alpha power densities [26]. Therefore, a biomarker of the psychomotor symptoms of depression was investigated using the hierarchical cluster tree from the data set—average slope of the Theta-Alpha power ratio versus average slope of baseline-normalized response time, which provided three clusters that remain to be evaluated in future clinical studies using the motor agitation and retardation scale (MARS) [27]. Nevertheless, we found a good correspondence with the QEEG group where the biomarker of fatigue during FRT was better at discriminating the mild depression and severe depression (compare subject number in Figures 4(a) and 6(b)). Once validated with MARS, the biomarker can be used to plan pharmacological interventions targeting psychomotor symptoms of depression.

The distinctive feature of our study was in monitoring QEEG along with the cued response time during FRT, which provided insights into the psychomotor symptoms of depression. Here, the POCT system may also be used to provide real-time feedback and monitoring of the biomarker, where a comprehensive therapy program can be developed using functional reach training in conjunction with pharmacological interventions. Furthermore, the frequency of falls can be monitored with a freely available mobile phone-based application, FallAlert [24], during such a comprehensive therapy program where the propensity of falls during periods of psychomotor symptoms of depression in elderly can be investigated in an interventional study.

Conflict of Interests

The authors have no conflicts of interest to declare that might raise the question of bias in the work reported or in the conclusions, implications, or opinions stated.

Acknowledgments

Authors acknowledge their gratitude to the reviewers for their insightful comments that helped in improving the paper. R. Kumar is highly indebted to Mrs. Ruby Aikat, ISIC Institute of Rehabilitation Sciences, New Delhi, India, for her invaluable support, inspiring guidance, suggestions, and constant encouragement during this study. R. Kumar would also like to thank Dr. R. K. Sharma (Occupational Therapy Department, Safdarjang Hospital, New Delhi) and Ms. Nidhi Vinaykya for their motivational support. R. Kumar also extends his gratitude to Dharma Foundation of India (Nonprofitable and Charitable Trust) for supporting this cross-sectional study under their "Active Ageing Project." The voluntary help received from all the subjects is gratefully acknowledged. Also, the technical help received from Mr. R. Sehgal is acknowledged who worked on the graphical user interface under funding from the Charpak Scholarship of Excellence Programme, France. The study was supported by Dharma Foundation of India, India; Gnan Systems LLP, India; Neuro Rehab Services LLP, India; IEEE—Engineering Projects in Community Service, India; Charpak Scholarship of Excellence Programme, France.

References

[1] B. G. Pollock and C. F. Reynolds III, "Depression late in life," *The Harvard Mental Health Letter*, vol. 17, no. 3, pp. 3–5, 2000.

[2] B. D. Lebowitz, J. L. Pearson, L. S. Schneider et al., "Diagnosis and treatment of depression in late life: consensus statement

update," *Journal of the American Medical Association*, vol. 278, no. 14, pp. 1186–1190, 1997.

[3] Union health ministry's working group on non-communicable disease burden in India, 2013, http://planningcommission.nic.in/aboutus/committee/wrkgrp12/health/WG_3_2non_communicable.pdf.

[4] G. A. R. Zijlstra, J. C. M. van Haastregt, J. T. M. van Eijk, E. van Rossum, P. A. Stalenhoef, and G. I. J. M. Kempen, "Prevalence and correlates of fear of falling, and associated avoidance of activity in the general population of community-living older people," *Age and Ageing*, vol. 36, no. 3, pp. 304–309, 2007.

[5] C. Sobin and H. A. Sackeim, "Psychomotor symptoms of depression," *American Journal of Psychiatry*, vol. 154, no. 1, pp. 4–17, 1997.

[6] R. Kumar, R. Aikat, and A. Banerjee, "Relationship between balance and depression in elderly," in *Proceedings of the the 2nd IASTED International Conference on Assistive Technologies*, 2012.

[7] K. Berg, "Measuring balance in the elderly: preliminary development of an instrument," *Physiotherapy Canada*, vol. 41, no. 6, pp. 304–311, 1989.

[8] J. A. Yesavage, T. L. Brink, and T. L. Rose, "Development and validation of a geriatric depression screening scale: a preliminary report," *Journal of Psychiatric Research*, vol. 17, no. 1, pp. 37–49, 1982.

[9] A. Dutta, A. Banerjee, and A. Dutta, "Low-cost visual postural feedback with Wii balance board and Microsoft Kinect—a feasibility study," in *Proceedings of the IEEE Point-of-Care Healthcare Technologies (PHT '13)*, pp. 291–294, 2013.

[10] M. Ganguli and S. Dube, "Depressive symptoms, cognitive impairment and functional impairment in a rural elderly population in India," *International Journal of Geriatric Psychiatry*, vol. 14, no. 10, pp. 807–820, 1999.

[11] M. Ganguli, G. Ratcliff, V. Chandra et al., "A Hindi version of the MMSE: the development of a cognitive screening instrument for a largely illiterate rural elderly population in India," *International Journal of Geriatric Psychiatry*, vol. 10, no. 5, pp. 367–377, 1995.

[12] The Emotiv EEG Neuroheadset specifications, 2013, http://emotiv.wikia.com/wiki/Emotiv_EPOC.

[13] F. Koslucher, M. G. Wade, B. Nelson, K. Lim, F. C. Chen, and T. A. Stoffregen, "Nintendo Wii Balance Board is sensitive to effects of visual tasks on standing sway in healthy elderly adults," *Gait Posture*, vol. 36, no. 3, pp. 605–608, 2012.

[14] The WiiBrew website, 2013, http://wiibrew.org/wiki/Wii_Balance_Board.

[15] A. Delorme and S. Makeig, "EEGLAB: an open source toolbox for analysis of single-trial EEG dynamics including independent component analysis," *Journal of Neuroscience Methods*, vol. 134, no. 1, pp. 9–21, 2004.

[16] V. A. Grin-Yatsenko, I. Baas, V. A. Ponomarev, and J. D. Kropotov, "EEG power spectra at early stages of depressive disorders," *Journal of Clinical Neurophysiology*, vol. 26, no. 6, pp. 401–406, 2009.

[17] P. W. Duncan, S. Studenski, J. Chandler, and B. Prescott, "Functional reach: predictive validity in a sample of elderly male veterans," *Journals of Gerontology*, vol. 47, no. 3, pp. M93–M98, 1992.

[18] T. C. Hankins and G. F. Wilson, "A comparison of heart rate, eye activity, EEC and subjective measures of pilot mental workload during flight," *Aviation Space and Environmental Medicine*, vol. 69, no. 4, pp. 360–367, 1998.

[19] N. Kose, S. Cuvalci, G. Ekici, A. S. Otman, and M. G. Karakaya, "The risk factors of fall and their correlation with balance, depression, cognitive impairment and mobility skills in elderly nursing home residents," *Saudi Medical Journal*, vol. 26, no. 6, pp. 978–981, 2005.

[20] L. Rochester, V. Hetherington, D. Jones et al., "Attending to the task: interference effects of functional tasks on walking in Parkinson's disease and the roles of cognition, depression, fatigue, and balance," *Archives of Physical Medicine and Rehabilitation*, vol. 85, no. 10, pp. 1578–1585, 2004.

[21] H. Suárez, A. Suárez, and L. Lavinsky, "Postural adaptation in elderly patients with instability and risk of falling after balance training using a virtual-reality system," *International Tinnitus Journal*, vol. 12, no. 1, pp. 41–44, 2006.

[22] R. A. Newton, "Balance screening of an inner city older adult population," *Archives of Physical Medicine and Rehabilitation*, vol. 78, no. 6, pp. 587–591, 1997.

[23] A. J. Sai, J. C. Gallagher, L. M. Smith, and S. Logsdon, "Fall predictors in the community dwelling elderly: a cross sectional and prospective cohort study," *Journal of Musculoskeletal Neuronal Interactions*, vol. 10, no. 2, pp. 142–150, 2010.

[24] The FallAlert Android App, 2013, https://play.google.com/store/apps/details?id=com.gnansys.fallalert.

[25] M. A. S. Boksem, T. F. Meijman, and M. M. Lorist, "Effects of mental fatigue on attention: an ERP study," *Cognitive Brain Research*, vol. 25, no. 1, pp. 107–116, 2005.

[26] C. Stampi, P. Stone, and A. Michimori, "A new quantitative method for assessing sleepiness: the alpha attenuation test," *Work and Stress*, vol. 9, no. 2-3, pp. 368–376, 1995.

[27] C. Sobin, L. Mayer, and J. Endicott, "The motor agitation and retardation scale: a scale for the assessment of motor abnormalities in depressed patients," *Journal of Neuropsychiatry and Clinical Neurosciences*, vol. 10, no. 1, pp. 85–92, 1998.

Permissions

All chapters in this book were first published in DRT, by Hindawi Publishing Corporation; hereby published with permission under the Creative Commons Attribution License or equivalent. Every chapter published in this book has been scrutinized by our experts. Their significance has been extensively debated. The topics covered herein carry significant findings which will fuel the growth of the discipline. They may even be implemented as practical applications or may be referred to as a beginning point for another development.

The contributors of this book come from diverse backgrounds, making this book a truly international effort. This book will bring forth new frontiers with its revolutionizing research information and detailed analysis of the nascent developments around the world.

We would like to thank all the contributing authors for lending their expertise to make the book truly unique. They have played a crucial role in the development of this book. Without their invaluable contributions this book wouldn't have been possible. They have made vital efforts to compile up to date information on the varied aspects of this subject to make this book a valuable addition to the collection of many professionals and students.

This book was conceptualized with the vision of imparting up-to-date information and advanced data in this field. To ensure the same, a matchless editorial board was set up. Every individual on the board went through rigorous rounds of assessment to prove their worth. After which they invested a large part of their time researching and compiling the most relevant data for our readers.

The editorial board has been involved in producing this book since its inception. They have spent rigorous hours researching and exploring the diverse topics which have resulted in the successful publishing of this book. They have passed on their knowledge of decades through this book. To expedite this challenging task, the publisher supported the team at every step. A small team of assistant editors was also appointed to further simplify the editing procedure and attain best results for the readers.

Apart from the editorial board, the designing team has also invested a significant amount of their time in understanding the subject and creating the most relevant covers. They scrutinized every image to scout for the most suitable representation of the subject and create an appropriate cover for the book.

The publishing team has been an ardent support to the editorial, designing and production team. Their endless efforts to recruit the best for this project, has resulted in the accomplishment of this book. They are a veteran in the field of academics and their pool of knowledge is as vast as their experience in printing. Their expertise and guidance has proved useful at every step. Their uncompromising quality standards have made this book an exceptional effort. Their encouragement from time to time has been an inspiration for everyone.

The publisher and the editorial board hope that this book will prove to be a valuable piece of knowledge for researchers, students, practitioners and scholars across the globe.

List of Contributors

Sareh Zarshenas, Parsa Houshvar and Ali Tahmasebi
Department of OccupationalTherapy, School of Rehabilitation Sciences, Isfahan University of Medical Sciences, Isfahan, Iran

Gloria Angeletti, Chiara Santucci and Valeria Savoja
Department of Neurosciences, Mental Health and Sensory Functions and Department of Psychiatry, Sant'Andrea Hospital, Sapienza University of Rome, 00189 Rome, Italy

Maurizio Pompili and Marco Innamorati
Department of Neurosciences, Mental Health and Sensory Functions and Department of Psychiatry, Suicide Prevention Center, Sant'Andrea Hospital, Sapienza University of Rome, 1035 Via di Grottarossa, 00189 Rome, Italy

Mark Goldblatt
McLean Hospital, Belmont, MA, USA
Department of Psychiatry, Harvard Medical School, Cambridge, MA 02138, USA

Paolo Girardi
Department of Neurosciences, Mental Health and Sensory Functions and Department of Psychiatry, Sant'Andrea Hospital, Sapienza University of Rome, 00189 Rome, Italy
Department of Neurosciences, Mental Health and Sensory Functions and Department of Psychiatry, Suicide Prevention Center, Sant'Andrea Hospital, Sapienza University of Rome, 1035 Via di Grottarossa, 00189 Rome, Italy
Villa Rosa Medical Research Centre, Viterbo, Italy

Loren L. Toussaint and Justin C.Marschall
Department of Psychology, Luther College, 700 College Dr., Decorah, IA 52101, USA

David R.Williams
Department of Society, Human Development, and Health, Harvard University, Boston, MA 02115, USA
Department of African and African American Studies, Harvard University, Cambridge, MA 02138, USA
Department of Sociology, Harvard University, Cambridge, MA 02138, USA

JawaherMasmoudi, Rahma Damak, Uta Ouali and Abdelaziz Jaoua
Department of Psychiatry A, University Medical Center H´edi Chaker, 3000 Sfax, Tunisia

Hela Zouari and Nouri Zouari
Department of Functional Exploration and Metabolic Diseases, University Medical Center Habib Bourguiba, 3000 Sfax, Tunisia

Anouar Mechri
Department of Psychiatry, University Medical Center Fattouma Bourguiba, 5000 Monastir, Tunisia

Diana Sarokhani
Student Research Committee, Ilam University of Medical Science, P.O. Box 69311-57793, Ilam, Iran
Department of Computer, Faculty of Engineering, Malayer University, P.O. Box 95863-65719, Hamadan, Iran

Yousef Veisani
Student Research Committee, Ilam University of Medical Science, P.O. Box 69311-57793, Ilam, Iran
Psychosocial Injuries Research Center, Ilam University of Medical Science, P.O. Box 69315-138, Ilam, Iran

Mohamad Taher Sarokhani
Student Research Committee, Ilam University of Medical Science, P.O. Box 69311-57793, Ilam, Iran
Science and Research Branch, Islamic Azad University, Kermanshah, Iran

Ali Delpisheh
Department of Clinical Epidemiology, Ilam University of Medical Sciences, P.O. Box 69315-138, Ilam, Iran
Psychosocial Injuries Research Center, Ilam University of Medical Science, P.O. Box 69315-138, Ilam, Iran

Rohollah Esmaeli Manesh
Eslamabad Payame Noor University, Kermanshah, Iran

Kourosh Sayehmiri
Social Medicine Department, Medicine Faculty, Ilam University of Medical Sciences, P.O. Box 69315-138, Ilam, Iran

JoukoMiettunen, Matti Isohanni and Juha Veijola
Department of Psychiatry, Institute of Clinical Medicine, University of Oulu, P.O. Box 5000, 90014 Oulu, Finland
Clinic of Psychiatry, Oulu University Hospital, Oulu, Finland

Tiina Paunio
Department of Chronic Disease Prevention, National Institute for Health and Welfare, Haartmaninkatu 8, 00251 Helsinki, Finland

Nelson Freimer
UCLA Center for Neurobehavioral Genetics, Semel Institute for Neuroscience and Human Behavior, Gonda Building, Room 3506, 695 Charles E. Young Drive South, Los Angeles, CA 90095, USA

Anja Taanila
Institute of Health Sciences, University of Oulu, P.O. Box 5000, 90014 Oulu, Finland
Unit of General Practice, Oulu University Hospital, 90029 Oulu, Finland

Jesper Ekelund
Department of Mental Health and Substance Use Services, National Institute for Health and Welfare, P.O. Box 30, 00271 Helsinki, Finland

Marjo-Riitta Järvelin
Institute of Health Sciences, University of Oulu, P.O. Box 5000, 90014 Oulu, Finland
Department of Epidemiology and Biostatistics, Imperial College London, London SW7 2AZ, UK

Matti Joukamaa
Social Psychiatry Unit, School of Health Sciences, University of Tampere, 33014 Tampere, Finland
Department of Psychiatry, Tampere University Hospital, Tampere, Finland

Dirk Lichtermann
Methadone Maintenance Clinic "Caf´e Ersatz", Münsterstraße 18, 53111 Bonn, Germany

Heli Koivumaa-Honkanen
Department of Psychiatry, University of Eastern Finland and Kuopio University Hospital, P.O. Box 1777, 70211 Kuopio, Finland
Department of Psychiatry, South-Savonia Hospital District, Mikkeli, Finland
Department of Psychiatry, North Karelia Central Hospital, Joensuu, Finland
Department of Psychiatry, SOSTERI, Savonlinna, Finland
Department of Psychiatry, SOTE, Iisalmi, Finland
Department of Psychiatry, Lapland Hospital District, Rovaniemi, Finland

Harold G. Koenig
Departments of Psychiatry and Medicine, Duke University Medical Center, Box 3400 Medical Center, Durham, NC 27705, USA
Department of Medicine, King Abdulaziz University, Jeddah 21413, Saudi Arabia

Barbara P. Yawn, Susan Bertram and PeterWollan
Department of Research, Olmsted Medical Center, Rochester, MN 55904, USA

Ardis L. Olson
Departments of Pediatrics and Community and Family Medicine, Dartmouth Medical School, Dartmouth Medical School, Hanover, NH 03755, USA

Wilson Pace
National Research Network, American Academy of Family Physicians, Leawood, KS 66211, USA

Allen J. Dietrich
Department of Community and Family Medicine, Dartmouth Medical School, Hanover, NH 03735, USA

Gopal K. Singh,Mary Kay Kenney, Reem M. Ghandour, Michael D. Kogan and Michael C. Lu
US Department of Health and Human Services, Health Resources and Services Administration, Maternal and Child Health Bureau, 5600 Fishers Lane, Room 18-41, Rockville, MD 20857, USA

Yousef Veisani
Student Research Committee, Ilam University of Medical Sciences, P.O. Box 69311-57793, Ilam, Iran
Department of Clinical Epidemiology, Faculty of Medicine, Ilam University of Medical Sciences, P.O. Box 69315-138, Ilam, Iran

Ali Delpisheh and Kourosh Sayehmiri
Department of Clinical Epidemiology, Faculty of Medicine, Ilam University of Medical Sciences, P.O. Box 69315-138, Ilam, Iran
Prevention of Psychosocial Injuries Research Centre, P.O. Box 69311-57793, Ilam, Iran

Shahab Rezaeian
Department of Epidemiology, School of Health & Nutrition, Shiraz University of Medical Sciences, P.O. Box 71348-14366, Shiraz, Iran

Megumi Haruna
Division of Health Sciences & Nursing, Department of Midwifery andWomen's Health, Graduate School of Medicine, University of Tokyo, 7-3-1 Hongo, Bunkyo, Tokyo 113-0033, Japan

Mariko Minatani and Sachiko Kita
Division of Health Sciences & Nursing, Department of Midwifery andWomen's Health, Graduate School of Medicine, University of Tokyo, 7-3-1 Hongo, Bunkyo, Tokyo 113-0033, Japan
Kitamura Institute of Mental Health Tokyo, 101 Akasaka 8-5-13,Minato, Tokyo 107-0052, Japan

Yukiko Ohashi
Kitamura Institute of Mental Health Tokyo, 101 Akasaka 8-5-13,Minato, Tokyo 107-0052, Japan

Toshinori Kitamura
Kitamura Institute of Mental Health Tokyo, 101 Akasaka 8-5-13,Minato, Tokyo 107-0052, Japan
Nagoya University, 65 Tsurumai-cho, Showa, Nagoya, Aichi 466-8550, Japan

Kyoko Sakanashi
Department ofWomen's Health and Mother-Child Nursing, Faculty of Life Sciences, Kumamoto University, 4-24-1 Kuhonji, Chuo, Kumamoto 862-0976, Japan

Tomoko Tanaka
Aso Health Center, 1204 Uchimaki, Aso, Kumamoto 869-2301, Japan

Hans Christian B. Vangberg, Kjersti R. Lillevoll, Knut Waterloo and Martin Eisemann
Department of Psychology, University of Tromsø, 9037 Tromsø, Norway

James A. Cartreine
Department of Psychiatry, Brigham and Women's Hospital, Harvard Medical School, 1249 Boylston Avenue 3rd floor, Boston, MA 02215, USA
Harvard Medical School, Boston, MA 02215, USA

Trina E. Chang
Harvard Medical School, Boston, MA 02215, USA
Department of Psychiatry, Massachusetts General Hospital, Harvard Medical School, Boston, MA 02114, USA

Janette L. Seville
Department of Psychiatry, Dartmouth-Hitchcock Medical Center, Dartmouth Medical School, Lebanon, NH 03756, USA

Luis Sandoval and Mark T. Hegel
Department of Educational Psychology, University of Texas at Austin, Austin, TX 72705, USA

John B. Moore and Shuai Xu
Harvard Medical School, Boston, MA 02215, USA

James A. Cartreine
Department of Psychiatry, Brigham and Women's Hospital, Harvard Medical School, 1249 Boylston Avenue 3rd floor, Boston, MA 02215, USA
Harvard Medical School, Boston, MA 02215, USA

Trina E. Chang
Harvard Medical School, Boston, MA 02215, USA
Department of Psychiatry, Massachusetts General Hospital, Harvard Medical School, Boston, MA 02114, USA

John B. Moore and Shuai Xu
Harvard Medical School, Boston, MA 02215, USA

Janette L. Seville and Mark T. Hegel
Department of Psychiatry, Dartmouth-Hitchcock Medical Center, Dartmouth Medical School, Lebanon, NH 03756, USA

Luis Sandoval
Department of Educational Psychology, University of Texas at Austin, Austin, TX 72705, USA

Claudio Imperatori
Universitá Europea di Roma, 00163 Rome, Italy

Marco Innamorati
Universitá Europea di Roma, 00163 Rome, Italy
Istituto Skinner, 00184 Rome, Italy
DISPUTer, Dipartimento di Scienze Psicologiche, Umanistiche e del Territorio, "G. d'Annunzio" University, 66100 Chieti, Italy

Stella Tamburello, Anna Contardi and Antonino Tamburello
Universitá Europea di Roma, 00163 Rome, Italy
Istituto Skinner, 00184 Rome, Italy

Aristide Saggino and Michela Balsamo
DISPUTer, Dipartimento di Scienze Psicologiche, Umanistiche e del Territorio, "G. d'Annunzio" University, 66100 Chieti, Italy

Michela Balsamo, Maria Rita Sergi and Aristide Saggino
DISPUTer, Dipartimento di Scienze Psicologiche, Umanistiche e del Territorio, "G. d'Annunzio" University, 66100 Chieti, Italy

Marco Innamorati
DISPUTer, Dipartimento di Scienze Psicologiche, Umanistiche e del Territorio, "G. d'Annunzio" University, 66100 Chieti, Italy
Universit`a Europea di Roma, 00163 Rome, Italy
Istituto Skinner, 00184 Rome, Italy

Claudio Imperatori
Universitá Europea di Roma, 00163 Rome, Italy

Martino Belvederi Murri
Division of Psychiatry, Department of Neurosciences, University of Parma, 43100 Parma, Italy

Massimo Continisio and Antonino Tamburello
Universitá Europea di Roma, 00163 Rome, Italy
Istituto Skinner, 00184 Rome, Italy

Richard R. Dopp and Ann J.Mooney
Child and Adolescent Psychiatry Section, Department of Psychiatry, University of Michigan, 4250 Plymouth Road, Ann Arbor, MI 48109-2700, USA

Cheryl King
Departments of Psychiatry and Psychology, University of Michigan, 4250 Plymouth Road, Ann Arbor, MI 48109-2700, USA

Roseanne Armitage
Departments of Psychiatry and Psychology, University of Michigan, 4250 Plymouth Road, Ann Arbor, MI 48109-2700, USA
Sleep and Chronophysiology Laboratory, University of Michigan, 4250 Plymouth Road, Ann Arbor, MI 48109-2700, USA

Justin K. Benzer, James F. Burgess, Jennifer L. Sullivan, David C.Mohr, MarkMeterko and Irene E. Cramer
Center for Organization, Leadership, and Management Research, VA Boston Healthcare System, Boston, MA 02130, USA
Boston University School of Public Health, Boston, MA, USA

Sarah Beehler and ChristopherMiller
Center for Organization, Leadership, and Management Research, VA Boston Healthcare System, Boston, MA 02130, USA

Andualem Mossie
Department of Biomedical Sciences, College of Health Sciences, Jimma University, Ethiopia

Dagmawi Kindu
College of Health Sciences, Debre Tabor University, Ethiopia

Alemayehu Negash
Department of Psychiatry, College of Health Sciences, Jimma University, Ethiopia

ArjanW. Braam
Longitudinal Aging Study Amsterdam, Department of Epidemiology and Biostatistics, EMGO Institute for Health and Care Research, VU University Medical Center Amsterdam, Van der Boechorststraat 7, 1081 BT Amsterdam, The Netherlands
Department of Emergency Psychiatry & Department of Specialist Training, Altrecht Geestelijke Gezondheidszorg, Utrecht, The Netherlands

Marianne Klinkenberg
Integraal Kankercentrum Nederland, Amsterdam, The Netherlands

Henrike Galenkamp and Dorly J. H. Deeg
Longitudinal Aging Study Amsterdam, Department of Epidemiology and Biostatistics, EMGO Institute for Health and Care Research, VU University Medical Center Amsterdam, Van der Boechorststraat 7, 1081 BT Amsterdam, The Netherlands

A. C.McFarlane
Department of Psychiatry, Centre for Traumatic Stress Studies, The University of Adelaide, Adelaide SA 5000, Australia

RichardWilliams
Mental Health Strategy, Welsh Institute for Health and Social Care, University of Glamorgan and Ty Bryn, St Cadoc's Hospital, Aneurin Bevan Health Board, NHS Wales, Lodge Road, Caerleon, Gwent NP 18 3XQ, UK

Amanda J. Nguyen, Emily E. Haroz, TamarMendelson and Judith Bass
Department of Mental Health, Johns Hopkins School of Public Health, 624 North Broadway, 8th Floor, Baltimore, MD 21205, USA

Patricia A. Findley
School of Social Work, Rutgers University, New Brunswick, NJ 08901, USA

Chan Shen
Department of Biostatistics, MD Anderson Cancer Center, The University of Texas, Houston, TX 77030, USA

Usha Sambamoorthi
Department of Pharmaceutical Systems and Policy, School of Pharmacy, West Virginia University, Morgantown, WV 26506, USA
Department of Community Health and Preventive Medicine, Morehouse School of Medicine, Atlanta, GA 30310, USA

Carley J. Pope and Dwight Mazmanian
Department of Psychology, Lakehead University, 955 Oliver Road,Thunder Bay, ON, Canada P7B 5E1

Luigi Grillo
Via Ragazzi del 99,No. 45, 20010 San Giorgio su Legnano, Italy

Laurel L. Hourani, JasonWilliams, Valerie Forman-Hoffman,Marian E. Lane,
BelindaWeimer and RobertM. Bray
Behavioral Health and Criminal Justice Division, RTI International, 3040 Cornwallis Road, P.O. Box 12194, Research Triangle Park, NC 27709, USA

Increase Ibukun Adeosun and Oyetayo Jeje
Federal Neuropsychiatric Hospital, Yaba, 8 Harvey Road, PMB 2008, Lagos, Nigeria

Arindam Dutta
The Gnan Systems LLP, Kolkata 700156, India

Robins Kumar, SuruchiMalhotra and Alakananda Banerjee
The Dharma Foundation of India, New Delhi 110003, India

Sanjay Chugh
The Neuro Rehab Services LLP, New Delhi 110048, India

and Anirban Dutta
The Charité-Universit¨atsmedizin Berlin, 10117 Berlin, Germany
Institut National de Recherche en Informatique et en Automatique (INRIA), 34090 Montpellier, France

Index

O

P

Q

R

S

T

V

W